PRINCIPLES OF NUTRITION AND DIET THERAPY

Barbara Luke, R.N., R.D., M.A., M.P.H.

Instructor, Home Economics and Nutrition, New York University;
Professional Associate in Obstetrics/Gynecology, New York Hospital, New York;
Staff Associate in Obstetrics/Gynecology (Nutrition), Cornell University Medical College,
Ithaca, New York

PRINCIPLES OF NUTRITION AND DIET THERAPY

LITTLE, BROWN
AND COMPANY
BOSTON/TORONTO

CONTENTS

Preface *ix*

PREFACE

This book is written for life science undergraduates, particularly those considering entering training in one of the health-related fields. Little or no knowledge of chemistry or biology is assumed, although what is learned in this textbook will certainly help in other life science courses. Every effort has been made to include current references from a variety of disciplines, including nursing, pharmacy, and medicine, with the main emphasis naturally being on nutrition. Nearly one-half of this textbook is devoted to presenting a solid foundation of the basic principles of nutrition; the second half of the book utilizes these principles in their clinical application. In keeping with newer thinking in the health field, over one-fourth of the book is devoted to the attainment and maintenance of health.

The four parts of this text are as follows: Part 1, Introduction; Part 2, Foods: Understanding Their Composition and Nutritive Value; Part 3, Nutrition in Health; and Part 4, Therapeutic Application of Nutrition. In addition to the nine chapters devoted to the food elements and gastrointestinal function, Part 2 includes nine chapters on the nature of foods, additives, toxicology, and labeling in order to reflect a personal philosophy that the study of nutrition should begin with a solid understanding of foods, analogous to learning the alphabet before speaking a new language. Part 3 is divided into an overview and a discussion of the life cycle and life-style considerations. The main emphasis of these 13 chapters is health and how to assess and maintain that state through a range of personal habits and stages in life. Part 4 is divided into principles and specific diet therapy regimens. These 12 chapters are built on the knowledge gained throughout the book and describe the most dramatic role of nutrition: the prevention, treatment, or cure of disease. A glossary is included for those unfamiliar with new terms. Case studies, with questions and answers, are used in some chapters of Part 4 to help the student utilize and understand the principles presented. The answers to these case studies are given after the final chapter. References and Suggested Readings appear at the end of each chapter for those who wish to pursue a topic further.

Writing a book of this size naturally involved the support and help of many people. I am grateful to the staffs at the Columbia University Health Sciences Library, Ohio State University Health Sciences Library, and the University of Cincinnati Health Sciences Library for their assistance on numerous occasions. I am indebted to Mary Ann Jonaitis, R.N., M.S., for her help in obtaining articles and for her support and encouragement. I also wish to thank professional associates and personal friends for their interest and best wishes, especially Dr. Allan R. Shade and Betsey and Neil Mason. The staff at Little, Brown and Company, particularly Susan F. Pioli, Book Editor, have been wonderful to work with. Special thanks goes to Ann F. West, Nursing Developmental Editor, whose humor, patience, good judgment, and "purple crayon" have made her a joy to work with. To Mrs. Venonne Waldron, I owe many thanks for her expert and efficient typing and emotional support as I became a new mother midway through the writing of this manuscript. My thanks also go to Kimble Pendleton Mead for his imaginative, wonderful drawings that brought humor to this textbook. The most thanks of all go to my husband, Paul Wissel, who helped me through the four years it took to complete this book with humor, strength, advice, and encouragement, all wrapped in a very special kind of love.

B. L.

Part 1

INTRODUCTION

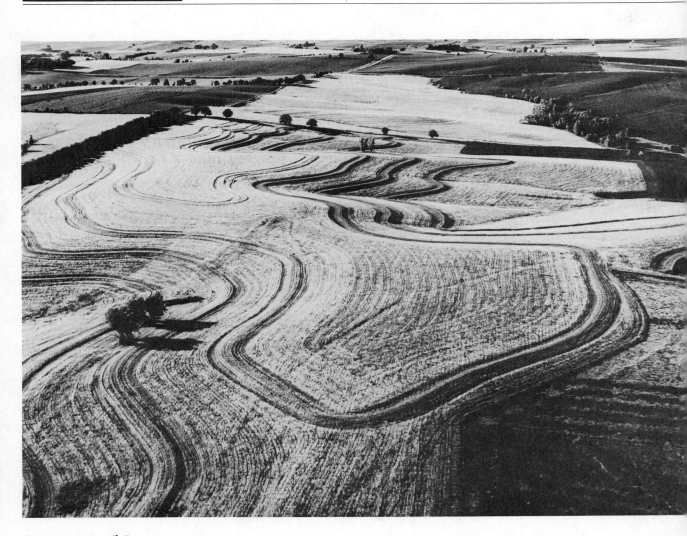

(Courtesy U.S. Soil Conservation Service, issued by F.A.O.)

THE STUDY OF NUTRITION

Early humans probably used trial and error to discover which of the flora and fauna in the environment was edible. With experience, certain substances became valued for their medicinal or healing qualities, and specific diets were prescribed for various maladies. Through such experimentation, the art of nutrition was born, thousands of years before the biochemical discoveries of the nineteenth and twentieth centuries also made it a practice.

"Necessity is the mother of invention" also applies to many historical developments in nutrition. Some of the most far-reaching inventions stemmed from the need to feed armies during wartime. Others came about through private enterprise or imaginative inventors. Today, nutrition is still both an art and a science, and as such is practiced by many members of the health care team. Although the nutritionist or dietitian assumes major responsibility for the nutritional care of the patient, almost every other discipline becomes involved, whether in reinforcing the principles taught, providing laboratory or anthropometric data, or advising about the interactions with medications or other therapeutic regimens.

Chapter 1

THE ART AND SCIENCE OF NUTRITION

The science of nutrition may have been born with modern biochemistry in this century, but the art of nutrition dates back far before the written word. Herbs, roots, various tree barks, and even unconventional parts of animals have been medicinal and dietary prescriptions for the treatment of a wide variety of ailments for thousands of years. Many of these treatments have survived the test of time and may be found in the modern-day pharmacopoeia. Much of what worked empirically centuries ago has been scientifically demonstrated to be effective today. (Our medical and dietary debt to the distant past is explored in more detail in Chap. 37.)

Immemorially, humankind has been faced with the perpetual challenge of change. Our response to this change not only has permitted our survival, but has spurred on our growth and evolution to the present level of advanced technology. Food is one of the basic necessities for survival, and much of human reasoning and creativity over the centuries has been directed at its acquisition, preservation, improvement, and distribution. As long ago as 2000 B.C. such preservation techniques as sun drying, salting, cooling, pickling, and fermenting were in wide practice, although the principles underlying these methods were unknown or were based on religion, taboos, myths, or the alchemist's imagination [1]. Most of these methods of preservation were developed by accident or as the result of a real need, such as the need to preserve food for times of famine or for special religious events.

Perhaps the first major event in the development of agriculture was the use of a *digging stick* to lay seed in the ground in separate holes. This first step probably occurred about 4000 B.C. in the fertile river basin of the Nile region in Egypt. The concept that the year was divided into cycles soon followed, leading to the development of the 360-day calendar and a system of irrigation to control water. The next major invention occurred about 3000 B.C., a plow with a *forward-curving blade* (Fig. 1-1). This innovation permitted greater amounts of land to be tilled, increased food production, and led to the ability of a society to support more members who were not food producers. From these beginnings, Egyptian civilization evolved. The most powerful members of Egyptian society were those who were knowledgeable about the seasons from astronomy and who had control of the water supply. Because of increasing population and the threat of droughts, the Egyptians were the first people to store grain, first in pottery and later in separate granaries. Central milling was established to grind the grain. During this time also the art and science of wine making was developed.

Because of the surplus of grain and other foodstuffs, specialized services and industries could develop, such as pottery making, baking, weaving, and brewing. As the society became more complex, the need for mathematics and tools

Adapted from T. P. Labuza and A. E. Sloan, Force of change: From Osiris to open dating. *Food Technology* 35:34, 1981. Courtesy of Institute of Food Technologists, Chicago.

developed. The solutions to the real and perceived needs of the time, influenced by climate, nature, and pure accident, resulted in making Egypt the most powerful empire of its time.

The next major development in agriculture was the *waterwheel*, which was brought from China to Egypt about 100 B.C. In Egypt it was used to supplement slave and oxen power in the mills for grinding grain and irrigating the fields.

The daily diet for the average Egyptian depended largely on his position in society. The diet probably included baked bread or crackers; wine or beer made from barley; salted, dried, or raw fish; and raw or salted wild game. During harvest time such vegetables as lettuce, lentils, and cucumber were also available. During droughts, the diet generally consisted of beer and bread.

After the fall of the Roman Empire, the diet of the general populace deteriorated. Fresh fruits were available only during the harvest, and fresh meat was scarce. Cereals became the mainstay of the daily diet, supplemented with salted fish for those living near the coasts.

All that was then known about astronomy was compiled by Claudius Ptolemy of Alexandria, Egypt, around A.D. 127–151. His works, the *Mathematibe Syntaxis*, were used until the fall of the Roman Empire in A.D. 500. They were rediscovered some 800 years later, when Alfonso the Wise of Spain established a school to translate the texts and star tables. Together with the development of the *lateen sail* and *sternpost rudder*, these books helped open trade routes from Europe to the Orient, Africa, and the New World. These explorations brought

FIG. 1-1. A plow with a forward-curving blade similar to the plow first used in Egypt around 3000 B.C. (WHO photo by Bob Miller.)

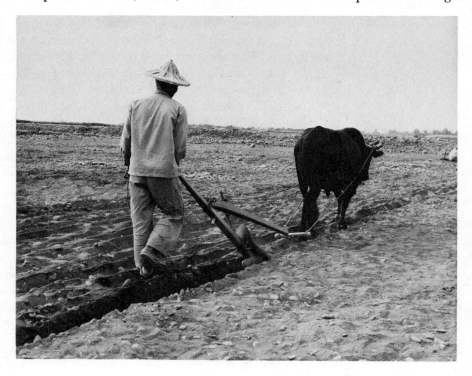

back such new foods as potatoes, maize, coffee, tea, sugar cane, and a wider variety of spices for preservation.

A series of technologic improvements in agriculture occurred in Europe at this same time. The *moldboard plow* was introduced from the Slavic countries in the sixth century; its deep blade permitted planting in well-forested areas. In addition, introduction of the *horse harness* permitted the replacement of the ox by the horse as a plow animal, doubling the amount of acreage tilled daily. The development of the *horseshoe* allowed the horse to work under all kinds of weather conditions, thereby increasing production. Rotation of crops and the use of legumes to fertilize the soil also increased output.

Between A.D. 1000 and 1600, several other major innovations helped pave the way for the Industrial Revolution. Greater use of the *geared waterwheel* enabled the European peasants to mill their own grain. The *cammed waterwheel* was utilized to crush malt for beer and to power bellows for blast furnaces to make metals. During the 1200s a clock was first used for controlling working hours and later in navigation. The *loom* and *spinning wheel* were invented in the 1300s for making cloth. In the 1400s the printing press and cheap rag paper were first introduced for communication.

Despite these major inventions and developments in agriculture and industry, methods of food preservation remained essentially the same as during the Egyptian period. The Pilgrims who came to America in the early 1600s lived on crackers, oatmeal, biscuits, bacon, dried or salted codfish, smoked herring, black-eyed peas, and a few vegetables. The Indians of the New World introduced them to sweet potatoes, corn, cranberries, and peanuts. Because of limited methods of preservation, the period of late winter and early spring became known as the "six-week want" [2].

The beginnings of the Industrial Revolution in Europe led to an exodus of laborers to the New World in an effort to preserve job security. The development of mass production techniques, including production lines and interchangeable parts, permitted the utilization of unskilled labor and decreased the dependency on skilled labor.

After the French Revolution, Emperor Napoleon was plagued by the constant problem of supplying his troops with adequate food. As a result, he established the Society for the Encouragement of Industry, which was to produce a number of important discoveries. In 1816 Magendie, through this Society, did some of the original groundwork on the study of proteins. Through the experimental feeding of dogs, he showed that nitrogen-containing foods were essential to life. This initial work led to the concept of biologic value, developed by Karl Thomas in 1909, to describe the quality of proteins; the discovery of the amino acids (the last indispensable one, threonine, was discovered by W. C. Rose and associates in 1935); and, finally, the concept of essential amino acids, advanced by Rose in 1938.

The need for new and better methods of food preservation was met by Nicolas Appert, also through this Society. This Frenchman developed the following effec-

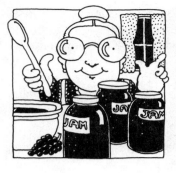

tive technique: He placed foods in bottles, heated them in boiling water, then corked and wired the bottles shut and heated them again. Food treated in this manner could be preserved for many years. He published his method in 1810, under the title *The Book of All Households, or the Art of Preserving, for Many Years, All Animal and Vegetable Substances.* Although the process of heat preservation had been perfected, the scientific principles underlying its success were still unknown.

Appert's technique was modified for use with canned foods by the Englishmen Gamble, Donkin, and Hall in 1811. These canned foods were taken on the first expedition to the Arctic in 1815, and by 1818 they were supplying the Royal Navy. In the 1820s William Underwood established a seafood cannery in Boston. Because the cans were made by hand, the process was both expensive and time-consuming. The canning process itself was long, about 6 hours for canned beef, and the original cans could be opened only with a hammer and chisel. Improvements continued to be made, including a more easily opened can that had been soldered shut with lead, and decreased processing time. The success of the canning business was bolstered by the increased needs of the American Civil War.

Although Roger Bacon had invented the inverted magnifying glass in the 1200s and Anton van Leeuwenhoek the microscope in the 1600s, the connection between microorganisms and food spoilage was not made until Louis Pasteur's work in 1864. The beer industry of France had hired Pasteur to investigate why a batch would sometimes fail. He discovered that the killing of microorganisms by heat was the scientific principle behind preservation. In 1896 the first scientific papers connecting Pasteur's concepts and Appert's techniques were presented. In 1908, Harvey Wiley of the U.S. Department of Agriculture's Bureau of Chemistry established standards on canning for the enforcement of the Pure Foods and Drug Act.

The process of canning continued to change and improve through the development of better steel and the enameling of cans to prevent erosion. Because of Napoleon's need to feed his army, the eating habits of America (and much of the world) began to change dramatically.

Refrigeration, another method of food preservation, was also developed in the early 1800s. Natural ice had been used, however, since ancient times to cool and store foods. In North America, the cutting of ice from lakes in the North and selling it in the South was a common practice in the 1700s. An early attempt at mechanical refrigeration was made by John Gorrie in Florida in 1838. He ran a hospital for malaria patients and felt that by lowering their temperatures he could help cure the disease. He was granted a U.S. patent in 1851 for a refrigeration device based on air compression. That same year an Australian, Harrison, patented a similar machine with the intent of using it for meat shipment and preservation. Gorrie's invention was rejected at the time, but his ideas were carried back to France where a refrigeration device, based on an ammonia absorption system, was patented.

Because of rapid population growth during the 1860s, England was experiencing a food shortage. Investors from Australia and Argentina made several attempts, successful and unsuccessful, at using refrigeration to preserve meat during trans-Atlantic shipping.

The Germans were interested in perfecting the technique of refrigeration because their process of making lager beer included cooling during fermentation and storage. The first practical refrigeration system, based on Gorrie's principles, the new thermodynamics, and the current ideas on the ammonia compressor systems, was developed by Carl von Linde in 1853 for a Munich brewery. During the next 75 to 80 years, however, most refrigeration units were too large or too expensive for home use and were mainly used in industry. By the 1930s and early 1940s inexpensive home-scale units were developed by Westinghouse, General Electric, and others to meet the needs of the individual consumer.

Interest in freezing as a method of food preservation was limited to shipping meat overseas during the 1800s. The first commercial ice cream plant opened in Baltimore in 1851 and sold directly to the consumer. Fish were frozen for export from the United States by 1880. It was not until 1923, when Clarence Birdseye of Gloucester, Massachusetts, opened his own frozen food business did commercial consumer-pack frozen food become available. Birdseye was bought out by the Postum Company (later to become the General Foods Corporation) in 1929 for $22 million. Improvements in processing, including blanching of fruits and vegetables before freezing to destroy enzymes, led to better frozen food products. In addition, the demands for dried and canned foods by the American troops during World War II boosted the use of frozen foods at home.

The food industry in America really began during the late nineteenth and early twentieth centuries, when the country began to shift from rural communities to urban centers. Through research and development, the food industry applied the newest scientific knowledge while attempting to meet the needs of changing lifestyles. Many billion-dollar businesses of today were begun as one-man operations by a man with an idea. Henry J. Heinz started by selling bottled horseradish in Pennsylvania at the age of 25. J. H. Kraft, a pioneer in canning cheese, began by selling cheese wrapped in foil or in glass jars from a wagon in the streets of Chicago [3].

In the 184 years since 1800, three major innovations in food preservation (canning, refrigeration, and freezing) have made a wide variety of foods available all year. Developments since 1950 are mostly based on the incorporation of the principles of science to replace art, or methods to reduce energy consumption [1]. Some of these newer innovations include freeze-drying, irradiation, microwave cooking, synthetic foods, and genetic manipulation. New challenges to food technology include meal preparation and cleanup in the null-gravity environment of space travel. Foods chosen for recent space travel were rehydratable, irradiated, and of intermediate moisture content [4].

From 3000 B.C. to A.D. 1800, the only major change in the food system was in the way food was produced on the farm. From 1800 to the present, scientific breakthroughs brought about new food preservation techniques. In the future, changes will probably be related to nutrition, health, and toxicology. As an art nutrition is ancient, but as a science it has just begun.

References

1. Labuza, T. P., and Sloan, A. E.   Force of change: From Osiris to open dating. *Food Tech.* 35:34, 1981.
2. Institute of Food Technologists.   *Food of Our Fathers.* Chicago: Institute of Food Technologists, 1976.
3. Schaefer, A. E.   Immigrants: Diets and dietary problems. *School Foodservice J.* 30:61, 1976.
4. Stadler, C. R., et al.   Food system for Space Shuttle Columbia. *J. Am. Diet. Assoc.* 80:108, 1982.

Suggested Readings

Bitting, A. W.   *Appertizing on the Art of Canning: Its History and Development.* San Francisco: Trade Pressroom, 1937.
Brown, G. E., Jr.   Agriculture: A key to adequate food and nutrition for the people of the world. *Nutr. Rev.* 16:18, 1981.
Drummond, J. C., and Wilbraham, A.   *The Englishman's Food: A History of Five Centuries of English Diet.* London: Jonathan Cape, 1957.
Grivetti, L., Ghalioungui, P., and Darby, W. J.   *Food: The Gift of Osiris.* London: Academic, 1976.
Pearcy, G. E.   *World Food Scene.* Redondo Beach, Calif.: Plycon Press, 1980.
Storck, J., and Teague, W. D.   *Flour for Man's Bread.* Minneapolis: University of Minnesota Press, 1952.
Verrill, A. H.   *Foods America Gave the World.* Boston: L. C. Page, 1937.
Wilson, C. A.   *Food and Drink in Britain from Stone Age to Recent Times.* London: Constable, 1973.

Chapter 2

NUTRITION AND THE HEALTH CARE TEAM

Health care in the United States has changed dramatically in the past 50 years. New disciplines, such as perinatology and thanatology, have been developed, while the roles of traditional professions have broadened to keep pace with changing health care needs. Nutrition is a field whose growth this century has been unprecedented. A wide variety of other disciplines, including medicine, pharmacology, biochemistry, microbiology, food science, agriculture, and home economics, have contributed to its advances and discoveries. Clinical dietetics has changed its focus from curing deficiency diseases to searching for the role of diet in the cause of chronic degenerative diseases and examining the importance of diet in maintaining health.

Today, health care is an interdisciplinary effort, with each member of the professional team reinforcing the therapeutic regimens of the other members. Underlying all therapies, whether they are medical, surgical, or pharmacologic, is the need to maintain optimal nutritional status for the maximal patient response to all regimens. For this reason, the principles of nutrition are taught as part of the basic education in nearly every health discipline, often with emphasis on the clinical application of the newer theories.

The Nutritionist

The *nutritionist*, or *dietitian*, is the health professional whose primary responsibility is the nutritional care of the patient. A *registered dietitian* is a person who has completed an undergraduate program approved by the American Dietetic Association (ADA) as well as a dietetic internship or sponsored work period, and has passed the registration examination given by the ADA. Once licensed, the registered dietitian must maintain registration by obtaining at least 90 hours of continuing education credit every 5 years. This can be done through publishing, lectures, formal classes, in-service instruction, or a number of other methods. In this way, registered dietitians keep up with the latest in their field, assuring that the care they provide patients is of the best quality. As part of their work in hospitals, they monitor dietary intake and, in collaboration with the physician, adjust the daily diet to meet changes in laboratory values, clinical state, and new information obtained from diagnostic tests.

The Physician

Responsible for the medical (or surgical) care of the patient, the *physician* orders and interprets diagnostic tests, plans the therapeutic regimen, requests consultations from professionals in other disciplines, and writes orders for interdisciplinary care.

The Nurse

The *nurse* carries out the nursing component of care, reevaluating and changing it in concert with recommendations of team conferences and the changing clinical state of the patient. As the person responsible for administering the therapeutic regimen and often the person explaining its importance to the patient, the nurse plays a vital role in the management of nutritional therapy, patient compliance, and ultimately, the effectiveness of treatment. Often the nurse will work closely with a dietitian to carry out the optimal plan of care. Ideally, the nurse should educate the patient about the importance of diet to overall health, not just as a relief to a particular physiologic disorder. Patients should be informed about the elements of a well-balanced diet and encouraged to take responsibility for their own and their family's eating patterns.

THE NURSING PROCESS IN NUTRITION

The goals for nutritional care of the patient include maintaining optimal nutritional status, correcting nutritional deficiencies, and preparing the patient for discharge [1]. Integrating nutritional care with other aspects of patient care, the nurse will often apply the *nursing process* to care situations. Following is a brief overview of the application of the steps of the nursing process—assessment, planning, implementation, and evaluation—to nutrition [2].

Assessment of nutritional status is a key to the understanding of nutritional imbalance. It consists of the diet history, physical examination (including anthropometric measurement), and laboratory testing. The assessment of nutritional status is discussed in detail in Chapter 22. Once data have been collected, the nurse will analyze it in order to come to some conclusion(s) about a nutritionally related problem, culminating with a *nursing diagnosis*, a clear statement of the patient's health status and concerns that can be affected by nursing intervention [3]. Examples of nursing diagnoses related to nutrition include poor nutritional intake due to the following:

1. Lack of knowledge about the four food groups.
2. Problems of metabolism
3. Problems of eating (such as arthritis, which may limit ability to use utensils)
4. Anorexia (loss of appetite) related to effects of medication (such as antibiotics)
5. Lack of desire to eat caused by (for instance) depression

Often, as in the case of a metabolism problem, a physician or dietitian will be called in for more extensive assessment and later, planning.

In the *planning* phase of the nursing process, the nurse will first have to decide who will be responsible for carrying out the nutritional care plan—the patient, the nurse or other health professional, or the patient supported by family and/or friends. It will be important to set goals with full participation by the patient, otherwise compliance will not be guaranteed (see Fig. 2-1). Both long- and short-term goals should be set and the nurse should explain to the patient how progress will be measured.

Motivation is essential to patient compliance, and it is often necessary for the nurse to back up a proposed diet with explanations of the scientific principles

FIG. 2-1. It is important to include the patient in all aspects of nutrition care planning. (From B. Kemp and A. Pillitteri, *Framework for Nursing Practice*. Boston: Little, Brown, 1984.)

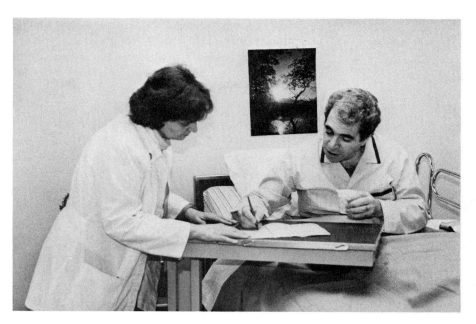

related to it. Even more important may be the ability of the nurse to recognize that many external elements will affect the patient's willingness and/or ability to comply with a given diet. The symbolism of food to that person (keeping in mind that hospitalization often distorts the meaning of food to a patient, making it play either an overimportant or underimportant role [1]), food preferences, age group, religious and cultural values, availability of certain foods, cooperation of the food preparer, cost of the new diet plan, and physical limitations are only some of the elements that will affect the ultimate success of a proposed nutritional plan [4]. The *implementation* of a nutritional care plan (which may consist of a diet or a better eating pattern) includes education and supervision of dietary intake through observation or actual provision of nutritional substances (such as intravenous feeding). (Education will be discussed in more detail in Chapter 31; age group considerations are covered in Chapters 23 through 29; and intravenous and parenteral nutrition are discussed in Chapter 35. Specific diet plans are discussed in relation to specific disorders in Section IX, Nutritional Therapy in Disease.)

Implementation may also mean, in the case of hospitalized patients, helping people to enjoy their meals more. This may include protecting temperature and taste of food when it is served; scheduling other events (visits or tests) so that they don't interfere with meals; promoting patient comfort at mealtime; and providing a pleasant eating environment [4].

Evaluation of the nutritional plan requires many of the same measures used for the initial nutritional assessment. It is important also to evaluate the patient's response to a diet to determine whether any changes should be made for better compliance. Daily follow-up may be necessary at first to help patients develop confidence in their ability to successfully manage their own diet patterns [1]. Evaluation is a continuous process; as health status changes, plans will also change, requiring constant evaluation and reevaluation.

Other Disciplines

Persons in several other disciplines may or may not become involved in the care of a particular patient, depending on the diagnosis and planned therapeutic regimens. The *pharmacist* prepares all drug therapy ordered by the physician and serves as a resource person for the health care team on drug interactions and incompatibilities. The *physical therapist* may be called in to help plan and implement the physical rehabilitation of a patient, particularly after surgery or major trauma. *Respiratory therapists* implement any treatment involving administration of medications or fluids via the respiratory system, as well as therapeutic regimens to rehabilitate compromised lung capacity.

Members of all of these professions, in carrying out their individual programs of care, must know how their therapy complements the actions of other therapies of the health care team. The pharmacist must know how each drug administered will affect the patient's nutritional status. The nutritionist must know how the exercises prescribed by the physical therapist will influence the patient's protein and calcium requirements. The nurse must know the practical aspects of a special diet when questioned by a patient's spouse during visiting hours. In this way, the overall therapeutic regimen will be beneficial and the health team effective in achieving its goals.

References

1. Moran, J. Nutritional Care of Hospitalized Patients. In E. A. Hincker and L. Malasanos (eds.), *The Little, Brown Manual of Medical-Surgical Nursing*. Boston: Little, Brown, 1983.
2. Marriner, A. *The Nursing Process: A Scientific Approach to Nursing Care* (3rd ed.). St. Louis: Mosby, 1983.
3. Griffith, J. W., and Christensen, P. J. *Nursing Process: Application of Theories, Frameworks, and Models*. St. Louis: Mosby, 1982. P. 111.
4. Kemp, B., and Pillitteri, A. Nutrition in Health. In B. Kemp and A. Pillitteri, *Fundamentals of Nursing: A Framework for Practice*. Boston: Little, Brown, 1984.

Suggested Reading

Bodinski, L. *The Nurse's Guide to Diet Therapy*. New York: Wiley, 1982.

Part 2

FOODS: UNDERSTANDING THEIR COMPOSITION AND NUTRITIVE VALUE

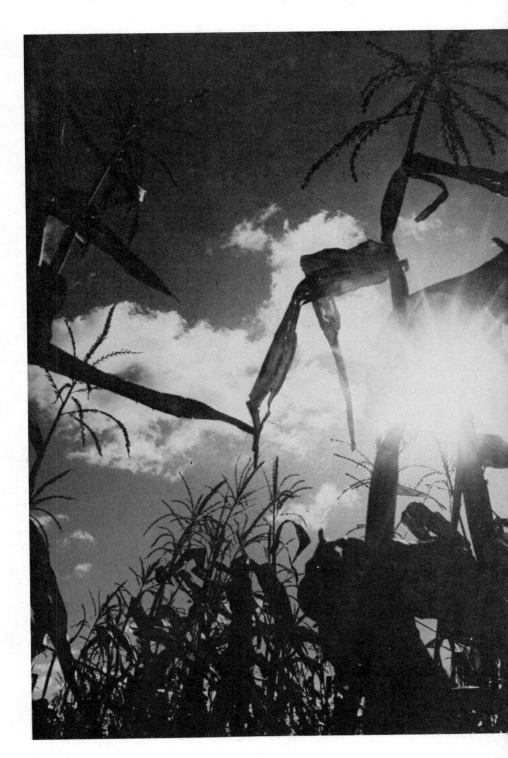

COMPOSITION AND UTILIZATION OF FOODS

In the following nine chapters the components of foods are translated into their roles in metabolism. The uniqueness of each micronutrient (those eaten in small quantities) and macronutrient (those eaten in large quantities) is defined during health, as well as alterations in requirements during special periods, such as growth or illness.

Since food is actually the alphabet of the language of nutrition, the effects of cooking, storage, and processing on nutrient composition and availability is also presented in each chapter. In studying nutrition, it is important to be able to mentally move easily from the kitchen to the biochemical laboratory, with a thorough understanding of the principles involved at each step. The transition from cook to chemist is stressed in this unit.

Chapter 3

PROTEINS AND AMINO ACIDS

Proteins hold a central position in the architecture and functioning of all living matter. They are the major components of bones, skin, hair, and muscle, and they play a variety of vital roles in other living processes. As catalysts, protein enzymes speed the reactions of metabolism; as hemoglobin and myoglobin, proteins facilitate oxygen transport; and as hormones, proteins act as regulators of metabolism. Proteins also serve as storehouses for the genetic information characteristic of a species. A classification of proteins by their biologic function is given in Table 3-1.

The modern-day knowledge of proteins has its beginnings in the development of organic chemistry and the advances in agriculture during the nineteenth century. Proteins were at first called albuminous substances since they were found in abundance in egg white, which is *albumen* in Latin. In 1838 the Dutch chemist Gerard Johann Mulder (1802–1880) emphasized the importance of the albuminous substances by coining the term *protein,* from the Greek work *proteios* meaning "of prime importance." The French chemist Jean Baptiste Boussingault (1802–1887), in studying the nitrogen requirements of plants, found that plants could store nitrogen without an apparent source. It is now known that certain bacteria in the root nodules convert nitrogen into protein. He also demonstrated the relation between the nitrogen content of foods and growth rates, concluding that some proteins were more useful to the body than others. The German chemist Justus von Liebig (1805–1873) continued Boussingault's work and looked to the soil and agriculture for answers to the nitrogen mystery. He realized that plants obtain nitrogen from nitrates, soluble nitrogenous compounds in the soil, and that animal fertilizers contribute this vital nitrogen.

By 1900 a dozen different amino acids had been identified, including tryptophan, which was isolated by the English biochemist Frederick Gowland Hopkins (1861–1947). By combining tryptophan with the incomplete protein zein from corn, Hopkins was able, experimentally, to support life, and to demonstrate the "essentiality" of certain amino acids. Hopkins was also the first to suggest that one or more "accessory factors" (later termed *vitamins*) present in certain foods were vital to life (see Chaps. 8 and 9).

Emil Fischer (1852–1919), the German chemist, probably did more for the study of biochemistry and, in particular, proteins than any other scientist. He determined the manner in which amino acids are combined within the protein molecule, identified the actions of enzymes and their "lock and key" relationships with substrates, and described the synthesis of protein from amino acid molecules.

As the sciences grew and more sophisticated tools were developed, the mystery of proteins began to unfold. Although much is still unknown, some of the greatest scientific discoveries of the twentieth century have been in the study of proteins. Among these breakthroughs were the determination of the amino acid sequences of insulin by the English biochemist Frederick Sanger (b. 1918) and of

TABLE 3-1. Classification of proteins by biologic function

Type	Examples	Occurrence or function
Enzymes	Hexokinase	Phosphorylates glucose
	Lactate dehydrogenase	Dehydrogenates lactate
	Cytochrome c	Transfers electrons
	DNA polymerase	Replicates and repairs DNA
Storage proteins	Ovalbumin	Egg white protein
	Casein	A milk protein
	Ferritin	Iron storage in spleen
	Gliadin	Seed protein of wheat
	Zein	Seed protein of corn
Transport proteins	Hemoglobin	Transports O_2 in blood of vertebrates
	Hemocyanin	Transports O_2 in blood of some invertebrates
	Myoglobin	Transports O_2 in muscle cells
	Serum albumin	Transports fatty acids in blood
	β_1-Lipoprotein	Transports lipids in blood
	Iron-binding globulin	Transports iron in blood
	Ceruloplasmin	Transports copper in blood
Contractile proteins	Myosin	Thick filaments in myofibril
	Actin	Thin filaments in myofibril
	Dynein	Cilia and flagella
Protective proteins in vertebrate blood	Antibodies	Form complexes with foreign substances
	Complement	Forms complexes with some antigen-antibody systems
	Fibrinogen	Precursor of fibrin in blood clotting
	Thrombin	Component of clotting mechanism
Toxins	*Clostridium botulinum* toxin	Causes bacterial food poisoning
	Diphtheria toxin	Bacterial toxin
	Snake venoms	Enzymes that hydrolyze phosphoglycerides
	Ricin	Toxic protein of castor bean
	Gossypol	Toxic protein of cottonseed
Hormones	Insulin	Regulates glucose metabolism
	Adrenocorticotropic hormone	Regulates corticosteroid synthesis
	Growth hormone	Stimulates growth of bones
Structural proteins	Viral coat proteins	Sheath around nucleic acid
	Glycoproteins	Cell coats and walls
	α-Keratin	Skin, feathers, nails, hooves
	Sclerotin	Exoskeletons of insects
	Fibroin	Silk of cocoons, spider webs
	Collagen	Fibrous connective tissue (tendons, cartilage)
	Elastin	Elastic connective tissue (ligaments)
	Mucoproteins	Mucous secretions, synovial fluid

Source: A. L. Lehninger, *Biochemistry: The Molecular Basis of Cell Structure and Function* (2nd ed.). New York: Worth, 1975. P. 64.

hemoglobin by the English biochemist Max Perutz (b. 1914). The helical structure of DNA and the model for protein synthesis were discovered by the American biochemist J. D. Watson (b. 1928) and the English biochemist F. H. C. Crick (b. 1916). For their outstanding contributions to science, each of these men was honored with the Nobel prize.

Amino Acids

Unlike carbohydrates and lipids, proteins are not multiples of a single subunit but are composed of 20 amino acids present in characteristic proportions and linked in a specific sequence in each protein. The three-dimensional structure and many of the biologic properties of proteins are determined largely by the kinds of amino acids present, the order in which they are linked, and the spatial relation of one amino acid to another.

Each amino acid is composed of an amino group (NH_2) at one end and a carboxyl group (COOH) at the other, each linked to a common carbon atom (called the alpha carbon) in the middle. The identity of an individual amino acid is determined by a third group, the *residue* (R), or side chain, also linked to the alpha carbon (Fig. 3-1). The residues differ in size, shape, and chemical reactivity, giving each amino acid unique properties. The 20 common amino acids are shown in Table 3-2.

ESSENTIAL AND NONESSENTIAL AMINO ACIDS

Through the course of evolution, humans have lost the ability to synthesize the carbon chains of certain amino acids normally present in most proteins. Those amino acids that cannot be made by the human body at a rate adequate to meet metabolic requirements have been termed *essential amino acids.* They must be obtained in a ready-made form from the daily diet. The remaining amino acids, termed *nonessential,* are no less important, but their structures can be synthesized in the body from dietary components.

The list of essential amino acids is different for each animal species. The physiologic state of the organism also determines which amino acids are essential: For instance, histidine is essential in the human diet to maintain normal growth only during childhood. One essential amino acid, arginine, is synthesized in the body, but too slowly to meet metabolic demands. It is known that eight other amino acids are essential in the human and must be supplied by dietary sources: lysine, tryptophan, threonine, methionine, phenylalanine, leucine, valine, and isoleucine.

FIG. 3-1. An alpha amino acid. (R = residue or side chain; α shows alpha carbon.)

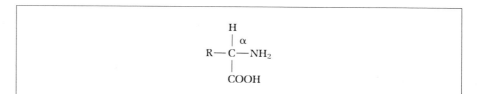

TABLE 3-2. The twenty common amino acids

Structural formula	Common name	Three-letter abbreviation
A. Amino acids with nonpolar side chains		
$H-CHCO_2^-$ $\quad\quad\mid$ $\quad +NH_3$	Glycine	Gly
$CH_3-CHCO_2^-$ $\quad\quad\quad\mid$ $\quad\quad +NH_3$	Alanine	Ala
$(CH_3)_2CH-CHCO_2^-$ $\quad\quad\quad\quad\mid$ $\quad\quad\quad +NH_3$	Valine*	Val
$(CH_3)_2CHCH_2-CHCO_2^-$ $\quad\quad\quad\quad\quad\mid$ $\quad\quad\quad\quad +NH_3$	Leucine*	Leu
CH_3 $\mid$ $CH_3CH_2CH-CHCO_2^-$ $\quad\quad\quad\quad\mid$ $\quad\quad\quad +NH_3$	Isoleucine*	Ile
phenyl$-CH_2-CHCO_2^-$ $\quad\quad\quad\quad\mid$ $\quad\quad\quad +NH_3$	Phenylalanine*	Phe
CH_2 $\diagup \quad \diagdown CHCO_2^-$ $CH_2 \quad\quad \mid$ $\quad \diagdown \quad NH_2^+$ CH_2	Proline	Pro
B. Amino acids with polar but neutral side chains		
indole$-CH_2-CHCO_2^-$ $\quad\quad\quad\quad\mid$ $\quad\quad\quad +NH_3$	Tryptophan*	Trp
$HOCH_2-CHCO_2^-$ $\quad\quad\quad\mid$ $\quad\quad +NH_3$	Serine	Ser
CH_3 $\mid$ $HOCH-CHCO_2^-$ $\quad\quad\quad\mid$ $\quad\quad +NH_3$	Threonine*	Thr
$HO-$phenyl$-CH_2-CHCO_2^-$ $\quad\quad\quad\quad\quad\mid$ $\quad\quad\quad\quad +NH_3$	Tyrosine	Tyr

TABLE 3-2 (CONTINUED)

Structural formula	Common name	Three-letter abbreviation
$HSCH_2—CHCO_2^-$ $\quad\quad\quad\;\; |$ $\quad\quad\quad +NH_3$	Cysteine	Cys
$CH_3SCH_2CH_2—CHCO_2^-$ $\quad\quad\quad\quad\quad\quad |$ $\quad\quad\quad\quad\quad +NH_3$	Methionine*	Met
$\quad O$ $\quad\quad\diagdown\!\!\!\!\diagup$ $\quad\quad\quad CCH_2—CHCO_2^-$ $\diagup\quad\quad\quad\quad |$ $NH_2\quad\quad +NH_3$	Asparagine	Asn
$\quad O$ $\quad\quad\diagdown\!\!\!\!\diagup$ $\quad\quad\quad CCH_2CH_2—CHCO_2^-$ $\diagup\quad\quad\quad\quad\quad |$ $NH_2\quad\quad\quad +NH_3$	Glutamine	Gln
C. Amino acids with acidic side chains		
$HO_2CCH_2—CHCO_2^-$ $\quad\quad\quad\quad |$ $\quad\quad\quad +NH_3$	Aspartic acid	Asp
$HO_2CCH_2CH_2—CHCO_2^-$ $\quad\quad\quad\quad\quad\quad |$ $\quad\quad\quad\quad\quad +NH_3$	Glutamic acid	Glu
D. Amino acids with basic side chains		
$NH_2CH_2CH_2CH_2CH_2—CHCO_2^-$ $\quad\quad\quad\quad\quad\quad\quad\quad |$ $\quad\quad\quad\quad\quad\quad\quad +NH_3$	Lysine*	Lys
$\quad\quad NH$ $\quad\quad ||$ $NH_2CNHCH_2CH_2CH_2—CHCO_2^-$ $\quad\quad\quad\quad\quad\quad\quad\quad |$ $\quad\quad\quad\quad\quad\quad\quad +NH_3$	Arginine*	Arg
$\quad\; H$ $\quad\; |$ $\quad\; N$ $\diagup\;\diagdown$ $HC\quad\; C—CH_2—CHCO_2^-$ $||\quad\; ||\quad\quad\quad\; |$ $N—CH\quad\quad +NH_3$	Histidine*	His

*These amino acids cannot be made by the body but must be obtained from the food we eat.
Source: G. H. Schmid, *The Chemical Basis of Life: General, Organic, and Biological Chemistry for the Health Sciences.* Boston: Little, Brown, 1982.

TABLE 3-3. Amino acids essential for nitrogen balance in humans

Amino acid	Minimum daily requirements (gm)	Recommended daily requirement (gm)
L-Tryptophan	0.25	0.5
L-Phenylalanine	1.10	2.2
L-Lysine	0.80	1.6
L-Threonine	0.50	1.0
L-Valine	0.80	1.6
L-Methionine	1.10	2.2
L-Leucine	1.10	2.2
L-Isoleucine	0.70	1.4

Source: W. C. Rose, *Federation Proceedings* 8:546, 1949.

The classic experiments by Rose with normal adult human subjects established the amounts of these essential amino acids required for *nitrogen balance,* the metabolic state of an organism when the nitrogen intake (from foods) equals the nitrogen output in urine, feces, and perspiration [1]. The minimum and recommended intakes of essential amino acids needed to maintain nitrogen balance in normal adult humans are given in Table 3-3.

Several essential amino acids such as methionine and phenylalanine directly supply the materials for other, nonessential, amino acids; consequently the basic dietary requirements for them are high. Both cystine and cysteine derive their sulfur uniquely from methionine. Tyrosine is formed in one step from the essential amino acid phenylalanine; therefore the required amount of phenylalanine allows for both tyrosine and phenylalanine requirements.

Of the nonessential amino acids, alanine, aspartic acid, and glutamic acid can be made via the transfer of an amino group from one compound to another from alpha-keto acids, which arise in the citric acid cycle during metabolism. Proline is made from glutamic acid. Serine is made as a by-product during glycolysis, and glycine is synthesized from serine.

INDIVIDUAL AMINO ACIDS

The following is a brief description of some of the amino acids, highlighting their structure and principal functions:

GLYCINE

The demand for this nonessential amino acid is enormous during periods of rapid growth. Glycine, the simplest amino acid, is important in the production of porphyrins (compounds essential to the formation of hemoglobin), creatine, the conjugated bile salts, and two of the four bases of deoxyribonucleic acid (DNA): the purines adenine and guanine. Glycine also aids in the elimination of toxic phenols from the liver and is essential to the production of connective tissue.

GLUTAMIC ACID

This amino acid readily gives up its amino group, giving rise to the formation of nonessential amino acids in the body. Glutamic acid is the predominant amino acid in wheat protein (gliadin). In its purified form, as monosodium glutamate, it is used as a flavor enhancer in cooking, particularly in Chinese food, and in many manufactured or "processed" foods. Glutamic acid is important in the metabolism of ammonia and in the synthesis of gamma-aminobutyric acid (GABA), considered the primary inhibitory neurotransmitter in the brain (that is, GABA works to prevent a nerve cell from discharging a nerve impulse).

PHENYLALANINE AND TYROSINE

These two amino acids and tryptophan are unique because they contain a benzene ring in their structures. The ring is used in the body's production of the hormones epinephrine (adrenaline) and thyroxine and the pigment melanin, which occurs in the hair, the skin, and the choroid lining of the eye. In Addison's disease, the failure of the adrenal glands to make epinephrine leads to the diversion of phenylalanine and tyrosine to melanin production, resulting in a deepening of skin pigmentation. The body can convert phenylalanine to tyrosine but not vice versa, making the former a dietary essential.

TRYPTOPHAN

One important role of tryptophan is as a precursor of nicotinic acid (niacin), one of the B-complex vitamins. As nicotinamide, tryptophan is a constituent of the coenzymes nicotinamide-adenine dinucleotide (NAD) and nicotinamide-adenine dinucleotide phosphate (NADP), which act as hydrogen and electron acceptors and function in the metabolism of proteins, fats, and carbohydrates and in cellular respiration. Tryptophan is also the precursor of serotonin (5-hydroxytryptamine), a substance that causes constriction of blood vessels in many tissues and acts as a neurotransmitter in the central nervous system.

HISTIDINE

As mentioned earlier, the body is unable to synthesize sufficient amounts of the basic ring structure of the histidine molecule during childhood, so histidine is an essential amino acid at that time. Once the ring is provided, an amino group can be added without difficulty. Histidine is converted to histamine by the removal of its carboxyl group. Histamine, which is normally found in the intestine and many other tissues, stimulates the secretion of hydrochloric acid by the stomach.

PROLINE

The structure of proline consists primarily of a pyrrole ring. The ring structure is part of the porphyrins, which form hemoglobin and the cytochromes. Both porphyrin and vitamin B_{12} (cyanocobalamin) contain four pyrrole rings.

ARGININE

This amino acid is necessary for the formation of urea by the liver.

LYSINE

This essential amino acid is important because it is lacking in most vegetable seed proteins, with the exception of peas and beans. For this reason, lysine is the amino acid most likely to be deficient in the vegetarian diet.

CYSTEINE, CYSTINE, AND METHIONINE

These amino acids are the primary sources of sulfur in the diet. Both cystine and cysteine can be made from methionine, but not vice versa; therefore methionine is a dietary essential. Sulfur is an important component in one type of protein bonding (see Proteins below) and is partly responsible for the three-dimensional structures of insulin and of keratin in hair.

Proteins

As the foregoing description demonstrates, the individual amino acids are unique and can profoundly influence the body's metabolism. These separate building blocks take on even greater significance when linked in a specific sequence as polypeptide chains, and when arranged in precise and specific spatial organization as proteins.

STRUCTURE AND BONDING

Each amino acid can be thought of as a simple structural unit, a monomer, which, when bonded to other amino acids, forms a larger whole, a polymer. The amino acids always link up so that the amino group of one joins to the carboxyl group of the adjacent amino acid, forming a *peptide bond*. In forming the peptide bond, the amino group gives up one hydrogen atom and the carboxyl group gives up one hydrogen and one oxygen atom, thus removing one molecule of water (H_2O) (Fig. 3-2). The linking of these monomers, the amino acids, forms the repeating peptide units in a polypeptide chain. *Hydrolysis* is the rupture of these bonds, with the addition of water, to yield smaller peptide chains and individual amino acids. A protein molecule consists of one or more polypeptide chains, each chain containing from approximately twenty to several hundred

FIG. 3-2. Amino acids united by a peptide bond.

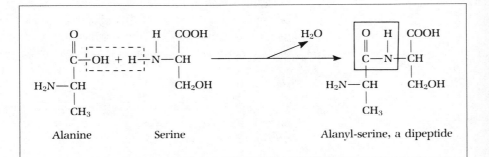

amino acid residues. The specific sequence of amino acids linked by peptide bonds and the sequence of the polypeptide chains constitute the *primary structure* of the protein.

The long polypeptide chain of each protein is folded in a unique configuration, its *secondary structure,* which is intrinsically related to its biologic activity. In 1937, Mirsky and Pauling suggested that *hydrogen bonding* was a major factor in maintaining the folded structure of the peptide chain. The hydrogen bond is formed because of the tendency of the hydrogen atom to share the electrons of an oxygen atom (Fig. 3-3). In many proteins, the hydrogen bonding produces a regular coiled arrangement of the polypeptide chain, called the *alpha helix* (Fig. 3-4). This structure is maintained by the hydrogen bonds between the C=O and N—H groups of a single peptide chain. Individual hydrogen bonds are comparatively weak, but the reinforcing action of a large number of such bonds in the protein molecule produces a relatively stable structure. These bonds can be broken in the unfolding process that occurs during *denaturation,* which is the disorganization of the component amino acids that occurs with exposure to moderate heat, agitation, ultraviolet light, alcohol, mild acids or alkali, salt, sugar, or the process of freezing.

Another type of bonding involved in maintaining the specific folding of the polypeptide chain is *disulfide linkage.* In polypeptide chains containing cysteine, cystine, or methionine, the disulfide bond is the union of two parallel peptide chains by a sulfur–sulfur (S—S) linkage (Fig. 3-5). This is a stable bond not readily broken under the usual conditions of denaturation.

The *tertiary structure* of a protein is its spatial conformation in three dimensions. This arrangement and interrelationship of the twisted chains of protein into specific layers of fibers is preserved by hydrogen bonds, disulfide bonds, hydrophobic bonds, and ionic bonds. Like disulfide linkages, *hydrophobic bonds* result from the nature and sequence of the individual amino acids in the polypeptide chain. The residues, or side chains, of alanine, valine, leucine, isoleucine, phenylalanine, tyrosine, methionine, and tryptophan are essentially hydrophobic ("water fearing"), meaning that they have little or no attraction for

FIG. 3-3. Hydrogen bonds.

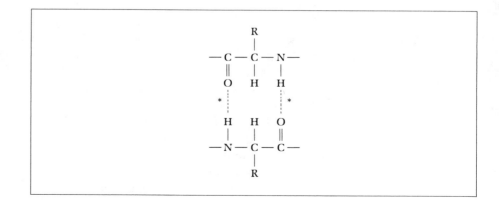

FIG. 3-4. Alpha-helical structure of a polypeptide segment
showing the sites of intrachain
hydrogen bonds. (From I.
Danishefsky, *Biochemistry for
Medical Sciences.* Boston: Little, Brown, 1981.)

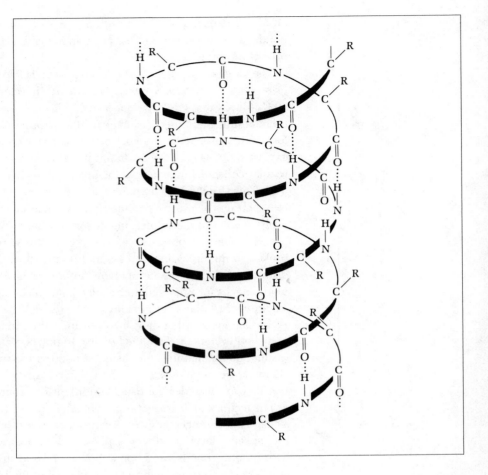

water molecules. Such residues can closely approach each other to form links with different parts of the peptide chain or to bind separate chains together. When large regions of peptide chains involve only hydrophobic residues, the exclusion of water results in a very tightly bonded structure. Hydrophobic bonding also serves to bring together groups that can form hydrogen bonds or ionic bonds in the absence of water, thereby aiding in the stability of the overall structure of the protein molecule. Also involved in protein-protein interactions, hydrogen bonding plays an important role in the formation of enzyme-substrate complexes and antigen-antibody interactions. *Ionic bonds* result from the attraction of negatively and positively charged residues that have come into juxtaposition. Because ions are strongly attracted to water (strongly hydrated), ionic bonds are stable only in the hydrophobic portions of the protein molecule, where they contribute to the overall stabilization of the protein structure.

In proteins that contain more than a single peptide chain, the *quaternary structure* is the spatial relationship among the separate chains or subunits, each

FIG. 3-5. Two peptide chains united by a disulfide linkage.

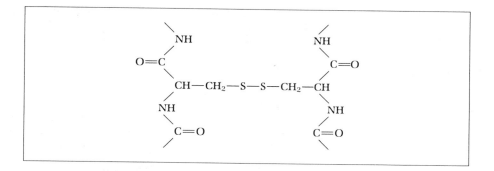

with its own primary, secondary, and tertiary structure. This higher level of organization may be essential to the biologic activity of the protein, as in hemoglobin, insulin, and enzyme proteins (Fig. 3-6).

The amino acid sequence and character of the primary polypeptide chain determines the secondary, tertiary, and quaternary structures of an individual protein. Once the chain is formed, the residues or side chains give each protein its own distinctive nature by directing the specific convolution and aggregation of the coiled chains. In addition to providing structural stability, the side chains contribute to the precise interactions of proteins and serve as reactive sites of attachment for groups other than amino acids.

CLASSIFICATION

Proteins may be classified according to their overall shape (such as fibrous or globular), their composition (*simple*, such as egg albumin, or *conjugated*, such

FIG. 3-6. The quaternary structure of hemoglobin. The hemoglobin molecule is made up of four polypeptide chains: two identical alpha chains and two identical beta chains. Each chain encloses a heme molecule. (From G. H. Schmid, *The Chemical Basis of Life: General, Organic, and Biological Chemistry for the Health Sciences.* Boston: Little, Brown, 1982.)

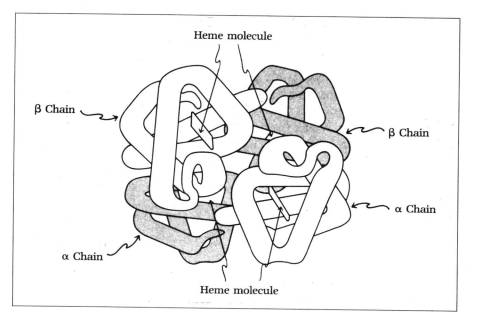

as hemoglobin), or their function. A variety of different types of proteins and their functions are discussed below.

FIBROUS PROTEINS

Fibrous proteins, as their name implies, are shaped like threads or rope and are structurally very strong. Their coiled polypeptide chains are usually arranged along a single dimension, tightly linked, and are often in parallel bundles. They are insoluble and very resistant to digestion by proteolytic enzymes. Examples of fibrous proteins include *keratin* (silk, wool, skin, hair, horns, nails, hooves, and quills) and *collagen* and *elastin* (connective tissue and bone).

Keratins

Keratins include the structural protein elements of skin as well as the biologic derivatives of ectoderm, such as hair, wool, scales, feathers, quills, nails, hooves, and silk. Keratin is the only protein not dissolved by the hydrolytic enzymes of the human digestive tract and are divided into two classes: alpha keratin and beta keratin. The condensed form, alpha keratin, can be changed to beta keratin by unfolding. The *alpha keratins* contain a high percentage of cystine residues and thus have many disulfide cross linkages; they also contain most of the common amino acids. The hard, brittle proteins of horns and nails are alpha keratins that have a high cystine content (up to 22%). The softer, more flexible alpha keratins of skin, hair, and wool contain only about 10 to 14% cystine. In contrast, the *beta keratins* do not contain any cystine or cysteine but are composed of amino acids with small side chains, such as glycine, alanine, and serine. The beta keratins are found in the scales, claws, and beaks of reptiles and birds and in the fibers spun by spiders and silkworms. Another important difference between the alpha and beta keratins is their reaction to heating: The beta keratins stretch to almost double their original length when exposed to moist heat and contract to normal length on cooling. The alpha keratins do not stretch at all under these conditions.

Collagen

Collagen is the most abundant of all proteins in higher animals, accounting for one-third or more of the total body protein. The arrangement of collagen fibers depends on the particular biologic function of the collagen. For example, the collagen fibers in cowhide form an interlocking network laid down in sheets; myosin, the major protein in muscle, undergoes a change in its structure during muscle contraction and relaxation. Although insoluble in water and resistant to digestive enzymes, collagen is converted into easily digestible, soluble *gelatins* by boiling in water, dilute acids, or alkalis. This conversion into a mixture of polypeptides is nonreversible. Collagens contain over 20% proline and hydroxy-proline, amino acids rarely found in other proteins. Most collagen lacks cystine and cysteine and contains about 35% glycine and 11% alanine, thus resembling the beta keratins in composition. The secondary structure of collagen is a triple

FIG. 3-7. The structure of two different proteins: collagen, a fibrous protein, and a globular protein.
A. The helical structure of tropocollagen.
B. The triple helix formed by three tropocollagen helices winding about each other.
C. A globular protein made up of a single alpha-helical coil. (From G. H. Schmid, *The Chemical Basis of Life: General, Organic, and Biological Chemistry for the Health Sciences.* Boston: Little, Brown, 1982.)

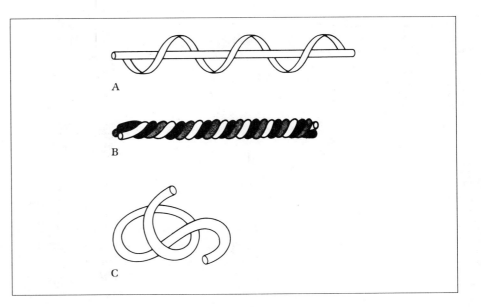

helix made up of units of tropocollagen. No other protein contains a similar triple helix structure (Fig. 3-7A, B).

Elastin, another fibrous protein, is the elastic connective tissue present in ligaments, tendons, arteries, and other resilient tissues. It is unique because its polypeptide chains are connected to form a stretchy, two-dimensional sheet, like a trampoline net. The fibers in tendons are arranged in parallel bundles to give maximum strength. Elastin is similar to collagen, but cannot be converted to gelatin.

GLOBULAR PROTEINS

Globular proteins are more complex than fibrous proteins. They are characterized by the presence of peptide chains that are folded or coiled into compact three-dimensional structures. Each type of globular protein has a distinctive folding pattern, or tertiary structure (Fig. 3-7C). On heating, globular proteins undergo denaturation, yielding unfolded, random conformations of their polypeptide chains and losing their biologic activity (Fig. 3-8). Globular proteins, which are involved in a diversity of specialized biologic activities, include enzymes, oxygen-carrying proteins (e.g., hemoglobin and myoglobin), and protein hormones (e.g., insulin).

Most of the globular proteins whose structures are known are enzymes, proteins capable of catalyzing certain chemical reactions in the cell. These organic catalysts, produced by living organisms, are of vital importance in digestion, metabolism, synthesis, blood clotting, and respiration. Many enzymes are named by adding the suffix *-ase* to the substrate, or the molecule on which the

FIG. 3-8. The denaturation and renaturation of protein. (From G. H. Schmid, *The Chemical Basis of Life: General, Organic, and Biological Chemistry for the Health Sciences.* Boston: Little, Brown, 1982.)

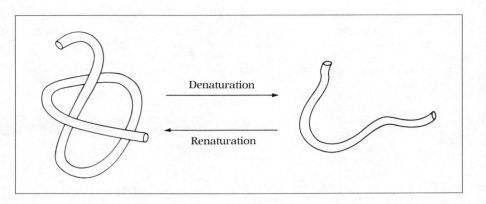

enzyme exerts catalytic action. For instance, the enzyme lactase is so named because it catalyzes lact*ose*. In the tertiary structure, the functional groups of certain specific amino acids are held in proximity to one another. This region of the protein molecule is capable of binding a particular substrate molecule and catalyzing a chemical change. The region at which the catalytic activity occurs is named the *active site*. Some enzymes depend only on their structure as proteins for activity, while others require one or more nonprotein components, *cofactors,* for potency. The enzyme may require a coenzyme, an organic molecule, or a *metal ion*, or both. If the coenzyme cannot be synthesized in the living system but is required in the diet, it is referred to as a *vitamin*. The metal ion may bridge the substrate and enzyme, stabilize the enzyme in a catalytically active form, or act as the primary catalytic center. Enzymes can be inactivated by heat. This inactivation is brought about by a drastic change in the structure of the protein, denaturation. Enzymes are also inactivated by acids, concentrated sugar solutions, sulfur dioxide, and hydrogen sulfide. Vitamins are discussed in more detail in Chaps. 8 and 9.

Glutelins and Prolamines

These are the chief proteins of plants. Glutelins, present in cereals, include glutenin in wheat, and oryzenin in rice. Wheat is unique among cereals because its gluten is capable of forming a dough that will retain the gas that is produced during fermentation and, on baking, will yield a light, well-aerated bread. Rye has a small amount of gluten and is therefore much more difficult to bake with. Barley, maize, millet, oats, and rice cannot be made into bread, but their grains may be eaten after boiling or made into flour for porridge or meal (see Chap. 12 for more details).

Protamines and Histones

These are basic proteins of low molecular weight, usually combined with nucleic acids. Large amounts of protamine are found in cellular nucleoproteins. Protamines are used commercially in the production of delayed-action insulins such as neutral protamine Hagedorn (NPH) insulin and protamine zinc insulin (PZI).

Most of the proteins discussed thus far, with the exception of certain types of enzymes, have contained only amino acids or derivatives of amino acids. As shown in Table 3-4, this type of protein is termed a *simple protein.* A protein that contains some nonprotein substance, a prosthetic group, is called *conjugated protein.* Examples of this latter type include nucleoproteins (with nucleic acids), glycoproteins (with carbohydrate), lipoproteins (with lipids), and metalloproteins (with a metal). A summary of simple and conjugated proteins and their characteristics is given in Table 3-4.

Digestion and Metabolism
ALTERATION OF FOOD PROTEINS BY COOKING

With the exception of the insoluble fibrous protein keratin, which is not hydrolyzed by digestive enzymes, food proteins are generally readily digested under normal conditions. Most food proteins (e.g., egg white), when subjected to temperatures of 100°C (212°F) or above during the normal process of cooking, *coagulate* (change from a liquid to a solid state). Heating to coagulation temperatures causes *polymerization,* the formation of a complex molecule from the union of a number of simpler ones. Superheated steam, in the absence of air, as in pressure cooking, causes hydrolysis of proteins. This process breaks down the proteins collagen and elastin in connective tissue, the proteins responsible in part for the toughness of meat. Dry heat may cause *oxidation,* the chemical addition of oxygen. Once a protein has undergone any of these changes, its specific properties, e.g., enzymatic, hormonal, or immunologic, are permanently destroyed. Proper cooking actually facilitates digestion and utilization by partially breaking down the protein structure, e.g., cooked egg albumin is more readily digested than raw. Excessive or prolonged heating may actually produce additional linkages, decreasing the digestability of the protein. An example is the decreased physiologic availability of lysine, tryptophan, and other amino acids in toasted cereal products [2, 3, 4]. Lysine, for example, links with carbohydrate, forming a resistant bond, as a result of high heat. For this reason, the brown crust of bread and toasted cereals contain less available lysine.

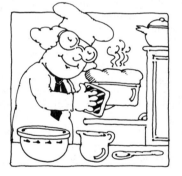

Proteins may undergo a lesser change when their secondary, tertiary, and quaternary structures are altered during *denaturation.* The denaturation process involves some disorganization of the specific arrangement of the component amino acids, often reversible once normal conditions are restored (Fig. 3-8). Most enzymes lose their specific properties once denatured. Proteins are most easily denatured at their *isoelectric point,* that pH at which the electric charges on their amino (NH_2—) and carboxyl (COOH—) groups balance exactly. Many techniques in cooking involve denaturation in preparation for the final coagulation. Examples include beating eggs before frying them in making scrambled eggs and pounding meat to tenderize it before roasting.

DIGESTION OF PROTEIN

Free amino acids are found only in small quantities in natural foodstuffs. Because most dietary proteins are polypeptide chains ranging in molecular weight from about five thousand to many millions, they are too large to pass through

TABLE 3-4. Classification of proteins by composition

Protein	Occurrence	Characteristics
Simple proteins		
Albumins	Blood (serum albumin); milk (lactalbumin); egg white (ovalbumin); lentils (legumelin); kidney beans (phaseolin); wheat (leucosin)	Globular protein; soluble in water and dilute salt solutions; precipitated by saturated solution and coagulated by heat; found in both plant and animal tissues
Globulins	Blood (serum globulin); muscle (myosin); potato (tuberin); Brazil nuts (excelsin); hemp (edestin); lentils (legumin)	Globular protein; sparingly soluble in water; soluble in dilute neutral solutions; precipitated by dilute ammonium sulfate and coagulated by heat; distributed in both plant and animal tissues
Glutelins	Wheat (glutenin); rice (oryzenin)	Insoluble in water and dilute salt solutions; soluble in dilute acids; found in grains and cereals
Prolamines	Wheat and rye (gliadin); corn (zein); rye (secalin); barley (hordein)	Insoluble in water and absolute alcohol; soluble in 70% alcohol; high in amide nitrogen and proline; occur in grain seeds
Protamines	Sturgeon (sturine); mackerel (scombrine); salmon (salmine); herring (clupeine)	Soluble in water; not coagulated by heat; strongly basic; high in arginine; associated with DNA; occur in sperm cells
Histones	Thymus gland, pancreas; nucleoproteins (nucleohistone)	Soluble in water, salt solutions, and dilute acids; insoluble in ammonium hydroxide; yield large amounts of lysine and arginine; combined with nucleic acids within cells
Scleroproteins or albuminoids	Connective tissue and hard tissues	Fibrous protein; insoluble in all solvents and resistant to digestion
Collagen	Connective tissues, bones, cartilage, and gelatin	Resistant to digestive enzymes but altered to digestible gelatin by boiling water, acid, or alkali; high in hydroxyproline
Elastin	Ligaments, tendons, and arteries	Similar to collagen but cannot be converted to gelatin
Keratin	Hair, nails, hooves, feathers, and horn	Partially resistant to digestive enzymes; contains large amounts of sulfur, as cystine
Conjugated proteins		
Nucleoproteins	Cytoplasm of cells (ribonucleoprotein); nucleus of chromosomes (deoxyribonucleoprotein); viruses and bacteriophages	Contain nucleic acid, nitrogen, and phosphorus; present in chromosomes and in all living forms as a combination of protein with either DNA or RNA
Mucoproteins	Saliva (mucin); egg white (ovomucoid)	Proteins combined with amino sugars, sugar acids, and sulfates; contain more than 4% hexosamine
Glycoproteins	Bone (osseomucoid); tendons (tendomucoid); cartilage (chondromucoid)	Same as mucoproteins except contain less than 4% hexosamine
Phosphoproteins	Milk (casein); egg yolk (ovovitellin)	Phosphoric acid joined in ester linkage to protein
Chromoproteins	Hemoglobin; myoglobin; flavoproteins; respiratory pigments; cytochromes	Protein compounds with nonprotein pigment such as heme; colored proteins
Lipoproteins	Serum lipoprotein; brain, nerve tissues; milk; eggs	Water-soluble proteins conjugated with lipids; found dispersed widely in all cells and all living forms

TABLE 3-4 (CONTINUED)

Protein	Occurrence	Characteristics
Metalloproteins	Ferritin; carbonic anhydrase; ceruloplasmin	Proteins combined with metallic atoms that are not part of a nonprotein prosthetic group
Derived proteins		
Proteans	Edestan (from edestin) and myosan (from myosin)	Result from short action of acids or enzymes; insoluble in water
Proteoses	Intermediate products of protein digestion	Soluble in water, uncoagulated by heat, and precipitated by saturated ammonium sulfate; result from partial digestion of protein by pepsin or trypsin
Peptones	Intermediate products of protein digestion	Same properties as proteoses except that they cannot be salted out; of smaller molecular weight than proteoses
Peptides	Intermediate products of protein digestion	Two or more amino acids joined by a peptide linkage; hydrolyzed to individual amino acids

Source: R. T. Lagua, V. S. Claudio, and V. F. Thiele, *Nutrition and Diet Therapy* (2nd ed.). St. Louis: Mosby, 1974. Pp. 264–265.

membranes and therefore cannot be absorbed directly by the gastric and intestinal mucosa. Dietary proteins must be hydrolyzed into their amino acid components to enter the circulation and be utilized for protein synthesis. This hydrolytic digestion occurs in the protected environment of the lumen of the gastrointestinal tract, where the hydrolytic enzymes do not have access to the organism's own cell contents. To protect the tissue in which they are produced, enzymes are synthesized in an inactive form, termed *proenzymes* or *zymogens*, which are activated in the lumen of the gastrointestinal tract. Lysis, or breaking off, of additional lengths of peptide chain under the conditions necessary for activation results in the formation of an active enzyme. Hydrolysis of the peptide bonds of proteins is carried out by the class of enzymes termed *proteases*. The *proteolytic*, or protein-splitting, enzymes, found in gastric juice, pancreatic juice, and the brush border of the intestinal epithelial cells, hydrolyze specific types of peptide linkages. A special enzyme is required for each specific linkage. This explains the diversity of proteolytic enzymes and why no single enzyme can usually digest protein to its constituent amino acids.

GASTRIC DIGESTION

Pepsin is the major proteolytic enzyme in the stomach. The zymogen precursor of pepsin, pepsinogen, is formed and secreted by cells in the gastric mucosa. It is converted to pepsin both by the acidity of the gastric juice and by pepsin itself (that is, it is *autocatalytic*). A small amount of pepsin can cause the activation of the remaining pepsinogen. The native proteins of the diet or proteins denatured by cooking are the substrates for peptic activity in the stomach. Although pepsin does liberate free amino acids from proteins, it does so very slowly. Since food remains in the stomach for a limited time, pepsin hydrolyzes dietary proteins mainly into a mixture of polypeptides.

Pepsin is unique in its ability to digest all the different types of dietary proteins, including collagen, a protein that is affected little by other digestive enzymes. Because collagen is a major constituent of intercellular connective tissue, its breakdown is vital if other digestive enzymes are to penetrate and digest the cellular protein contents of meats. If hydrochloric acid production is insufficient to maintain the gastric contents at the pH necessary for peptic action (about 1.8 to 2.0), protein (and therefore, collagen) digestion in the stomach may be very limited, as seen in *pernicious anemia*. In *achylia* the absence of pepsin and hydrochloric acid from the gastric contents hinders protein digestion in the stomach. Any condition that leads to impaired peptic activity in the stomach will result in poor digestion of meats.

Pepsin only begins the process of protein digestion, splitting proteins into large polypeptides. Pepsin also initiates clotting, the first step in the digestion of milk. The first time a baby "spits up," the appearance of the milk may surprise a mother: it has already been processed into clumps and liquids.

INTESTINAL DIGESTION

The stomach contents, or *chyme*, pass through the pyloric valve into the duodenum, the first part of the small intestine. The pancreatic and biliary ducts open into the duodenum at a point very close to the pylorus (see Chap. 11). The alkaline pancreatic and biliary secretions neutralize the acid of the chyme and inactivate the gastric enzymes. The pH is changed to alkaline, which is necessary for the action of the enzymes contained in the pancreatic and intestinal juices and for the final hydrolysis of proteins.

The pancreas secretes a slightly alkaline fluid containing inactive zymogen precursors of several proteases: *trypsinogen, proelastase,* and several *chymotrypsinogens* (all endopeptidases), and *procarboxypeptidases A* and *B* (both exopeptidases). An intestinal enzyme, *enterokinase,* specifically and rapidly converts trypsinogen to *trypsin* by proteolytic cleavage. Trypsin is responsible for the conversion of all other inactive zymogens, including trypsinogen, to their active forms. The chymotrypsinogens are converted to *chymotrypsins;* the procarboxypeptidases to *carboxypeptidases.*

The alkaline pancreatic juices provide the optimal pH for the hydrolytic action of the pancreatic enzymes, each of which has a specific action. Trypsin acts on peptide linkages involving the carboxyl groups of the amino acids arginine and lysine. The chymotrypsins are most active on the peptide bonds involving the carboxyl groups of phenylalanine, tyrosine, methionine, and tryptophan. The action of all the enzymes is additive, resulting in the progressive hydrolysis of large polypeptides to small peptides and amino acids.

Enzymes that hydrolyze peptide bonds are also contained within the mucosa of the small intestine. These *aminopeptidases* and *dipeptidases*, enzymes that break down peptides into free amino acids, may be secreted into the intestinal juice to act within the lumen of the intestine, although mostly they function within the cells of the mucosa itself.

The successive action of the proteolytic enzymes in the stomach and small intestine results in the complete hydrolysis of most of the dietary protein into amino acids. Although trypsin and chymotrypsin act more rapidly and completely if preceded by the action of pepsin, these two pancreatic enzymes alone can release amino acids from proteins. Thus surgical removal of part of the stomach does not seriously impair the utilization of dietary protein. However, if there is extensive destruction of pancreatic tissue or obstruction of the pancreatic ducts, limiting the quantity of enzymes reaching the duodenum, major amounts of undigested dietary protein will pass through the gastrointestinal tract unabsorbed. The gastric and intestinal enzymes and their actions are summarized in Table 3-5.

AMINO ACID ABSORPTION

The emptying of the stomach, movement of chyme through the intestines, proteolytic breakdown, and subsequent absorption of amino acids are so coordinated that free amino acids do not accumulate in the intestinal lumen, but rather are absorbed at about the same rate that they are liberated from the dietary proteins. Within 15 minutes after ingestion, amino acids are absorbed by the intestine, enter the portal circulation, and can be detected in the blood. Maximal concentrations are attained 30 to 50 minutes after eating. Absorption occurs chiefly in the small intestine but may be impaired by anoxia (lack of oxygen) or in the presence of metabolic poisons or inhibitors.

A mixture of amino acids and small peptides (not greater than 8 amino acid residues) is presented for absorption by the cells of the intestinal mucosa. Some of these small peptides, as well as an occasional undigested protein, may penetrate the intestinal mucosa and appear in the blood. This phenomenon is of importance in mammalian life since, in the very young of most species, the permeability of the mucosa is greater than in the adult, which permits passage of antibodies from the *colostrum*. Colostrum is secreted by the mammary glands during the first few days after delivery; chief among its protein components are immunoglobulins responsible for the immunity of the newborn. To ensure the availability of the antibodies, colostrum contains a protein that is a potent trypsin inhibitor. Together with a low concentration of proteolytic enzymes in the digestive fluids, these factors may lead to the absorption of sufficient undigested proteins to cause immunologic sensitization (the production of antibodies against a foreign protein). This may be the basis for allergic reactions toward some food proteins, e.g., milk and eggs, and the transmission of such sensitivities from mother to child through the breast milk.

The concentrations of amino acids absorbed in the portal blood do not correspond completely to the distribution found in the protein food. This discrepancy is due to two factors: First, certain amino acids are transformed into other forms during absorption. Most commonly, aspartate and glutamate are converted to alanine [5]. Normally, aspartate and glutamate are found in very low concentra-

TABLE 3-5. Gastric and intestinal enzymes and their actions

Site	Stomach	Small intestine						
		Endopeptidases (proteinases)			Exopeptidases (peptidases)			
Optimum pH	1.8–2.0	8.0–9.0			7.0–7.5			
Proenzyme (zymogen)	Pepsinogen	Trypsinogen	Chymotrypsinogen	Proelastase	Procarboxypeptidase A	Procarboxypeptidase B		
Enzyme	Pepsin	Trypsin	Chymotrypsin	Elastase	Carboxypeptidase A	Carboxypeptidase B	Dipeptidase	Aminopeptidase
Substrate (specific peptide linkages)	Carboxyl group of phenylalanine, tryptophan, and tyrosine	Carboxyl group of arginine, lysine	Carboxyl group of phenylalanine, tryptophan, tyrosine, and methionine	Carboxyl group of nonpolar amino acids	Carboxyl terminal of amino acids (aromatic or aliphatic)	Carboxyl terminal of basic amino acids: arginine, lysine, and histidine	Carboxyl terminal of dipeptides	Amino terminal of dipeptides
Product	Polypeptides	Small peptides and amino acids			Amino acids			

tions in the blood. High levels, as in parenteral feedings, have been found to be harmful [6]. This may be due to the chelating, or binding, effect of these two amino acids, limiting the availability of essential ions of such elements as calcium and magnesium. The Chinese Restaurant Syndrome of headache and malaise after eating Chinese food has been attributed to the liberal use of monosodium glutamate in Chinese cooking. It may be that the intestine's ability to convert glutamate to alanine is exceeded by the quantity of glutamate in the food, so that a large quantity of glutamate is absorbed before it can be converted. The second factor influencing blood levels of amino acids is that the absorption of certain amino acids may be specifically inhibited by the presence of other amino acids. Animal studies suggest that there is competition among amino acids for the selective, specific processes responsible for intestinal absorption, and that the absorption of amino acids is an active function of the intestinal mucosa, although the exact mechanisms are not fully understood [6]. Similarly, it has long been known that in diseases in which the functional integrity of the intestinal wall has been compromised, e.g., in *sprue* or *ulcerative colitis*, intestinal absorption of amino acids is impaired. Immediately after surgical removal of a portion of the small intestine (as in intestinal bypass surgery for morbid obesity), there is a profound disturbance in the ability to absorb amino acids. After 5 or 6 months, however, the remaining small intestine usually hypertrophies (enlarges) to the extent that it almost completely restores the total capacity for amino acid absorption. This hypertrophy, or new growth, is a functional adaptation of the remaining intestine to the increased physiologic demands.

When the carefully regulated release of amino acids into the small intestine for absorption is disturbed after such surgical procedures as a *total gastrectomy*, impaired protein utilization and loss of fecal nitrogen result. This inefficiency is most probably due to the loss of regulated gastric emptying and its influence on the timed release of amino acids. Undigested proteins, peptides, and unabsorbed amino acids pass on to the lower intestinal tract, where they are exposed to the action of the intestinal bacteria. The intestinal microorganisms may *decarboxylate* (removal of a carboxyl group from) certain amino acids, converting them to toxic, pharmacologically active compounds, such as histamine from histidine, tyramine from tyrosine, and tryptamine from tryptophan. The *deamination* of (removal of an amino group from) certain amino acids and subsequent intestinal absorption of ammonia leads to the toxic rise in blood ammonia levels seen in hepatic diseases. Destruction of methionine and cystine by microbial action in the intestines leads to the abnormal accumulation of sulfur-containing compounds in the blood.

HEPATIC AMINO ACID METABOLISM

The absorbed amino acids are carried in the portal blood to the liver, the principal site of their metabolism. From these amino acids, the liver synthesizes proteins for its own requirements. It also synthesizes several protein components of plasma and nitrogen-containing compounds, such as purines, pyrimidines, uric acid, nicotinic acid, and creatine. In addition, the liver produces a balanced mixture of amino acids for other organs, which it delivers via the blood. Finally, the liver synthesizes nonessential amino acids and provides for the disposal of surplus amounts of both nitrogen and the carbon chains of amino acids.

Nitrogen Balance and Protein Dynamics
THE AMINO ACID POOL

By entering the hepatic metabolic system, dietary proteins join the body's "amino acid pool" and the state of *dynamic equilibrium* between tissue proteins (endogenous source) and dietary proteins (exogenous source). The uptake of amino acids by tissues is in direct proportion to growth needs, e.g., fetal tissue, tumors, and rejuvenating organs incorporate amino acids at a much faster rate than do normal adult tissues. Organs with a rapid turnover of cells, such as intestinal mucosa, which renews itself every 1 to 3 days, extract required amino acids from the metabolic pool at a faster rate than do red blood cells, which have a life span of 120 days. Amino acids and the products of amino acid metabolism are also constantly being added to the circulation by the breakdown of old proteins. Thus, the sources of the body's amino acid pool are indistinguishable, and at any given moment include both exogenous components (from dietary intake) and endogenous components (from tissue breakdown). For example, arginine is arginine whether it was from the breakdown of a red blood cell or a recently digested steak. Although protein is not stored in the body in the same sense that fat or certain vitamins are, almost one-fourth of the body tissues can be mobilized without compromising vital functions. For this reason, the body can adjust to total starvation for as long as 30 to 50 days, and partial starvation for even longer periods, without detriment, if tissues are eventually restored to their normal protein composition (see Chap. 34).

NITROGEN BALANCE

On the average, protein is composed of 16% nitrogen, with 1 gm of nitrogen being equal to 6.25 gm of protein. One gram of protein can provide 4 calories. Under normal conditions the human body is in a state of *nitrogen balance*, that is, the nitrogen intake from dietary sources is equal to the nitrogen excretion in the feces, urine, and skin. Fecal losses include undigested dietary proteins and, from endogenous sources, the sloughed off cells of the intestinal mucosa, enzymes from digestive juices, and bacterial cells. These fecal losses are also influenced by the amount of food consumed, its digestibility, and its fiber content. Urinary losses include deaminated amino acids, excreted mainly as urea and ammonia, and the nonprotein nitrogenous end products of creatine, uric acid, and others. When the dietary protein intake exceeds the tissue maintenance requirements, the surplus is excreted and not stored, thus increasing the amount of urinary nitrogen. Loss of nitrogen through skin, hair, nails, and perspiration is extremely difficult to measure and varies widely with climatic conditions.

The daily losses of nitrogen in the normal adult male average about 2.5 gm; with profuse sweating, losses from the skin can be as high as an additional 3.75 gm of nitrogen (equal to 23.4 gm of protein) in 24 hours. During all phases of the life cycle, there is a continuous loss and entry of nitrogenous compounds in the body. Hormonal influences, metabolic needs, state of health or illness, and environmental factors all determine the daily nitrogen requirements and balance.

When the intake of nitrogen exceeds the output, the body is in a state of "positive" nitrogen balance, also termed *anabolism*. This occurs during periods of growth (infancy, childhood, pregnancy), convalescence from a debilitating disease or malnutrition, and during physical training when new muscle tissue is being formed. Growth or repair may occur despite an overall "negative" balance, when other organs provide the required amino acids for a growing tissue. An inadequate protein intake during pregnancy and lactation mobilizes maternal tissue to provide amino acids for the growing fetus or the synthesis of milk. In rapidly growing tumors, the breakdown of normal tissue provides the amino acids needed for protein synthesis.

When the nitrogen output exceeds the intake, a state of "negative" nitrogen balance, or *catabolism*, results. For the synthesis of protein to occur, all essential amino acids must be present in sufficient amounts. If one is present to a limited extent, protein synthesis will continue for only as long as the supply lasts; this amino acid is the *limiting amino acid*. If one or more essential amino acids are missing (that is, *incomplete protein*), the remaining amino acids will not be stored for later synthesis, but will be deaminated and used for energy. If the caloric intake is insufficient to spare protein for tissue synthesis, dietary and tissue proteins will be catabolized for energy. Following trauma and burns and during illness, fever, and periods of fear, stress, and anxiety, protein catabolism is greatly increased (see Chap. 36).

HORMONAL INFLUENCE

Much of the variation in balance and mobilization of tissue nitrogen is mediated through the action of hormones. Growth hormone, from the anterior pituitary, has an anabolic effect on nitrogen balance during infancy and childhood. During adolescence and puberty the sex hormones, estrogens and androgens, facilitate positive nitrogen balance. In normal amounts, thyroid hormone also stimulates growth. Insulin promotes the entry of amino acids into the cells, indirectly aiding anabolism. The hormones that increase catabolism are the adrenocortical hormones, epinephrine and norepinephrine, released during periods of stress or injury. These hormones stimulate the breakdown of tissue proteins to yield glucose.

QUALITY OF PROTEIN

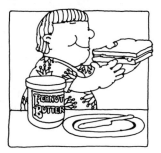

The prime consideration in evaluating the nutritional value of a protein is the relation of its amino acid composition to that required for tissue growth, repair, and maintenance. A protein that contains all amino acids in the proportions needed will be more completely utilized than one with a limited quantity of one or more of the essential amino acids (the limiting amino acid), which would result in the others being wasted. The nitrogen from the remaining amino acids cannot be stored, and nitrogen equilibrium cannot be sustained, regardless of how complete the diet is in other respects (Fig. 3-9). If, however, another protein containing the missing amino acid in adequate amounts is added at the same meal and in the presence of sufficient calories, protein synthesis can continue

FIG. 3-9. Incomplete protein. Many countries suffer severely from malnutrition—even while there are surpluses of food on the market. In this case, even these large quantities of corn cannot make up for the lack of other necessary amino acids. (WHO photo by P. Almasy.)

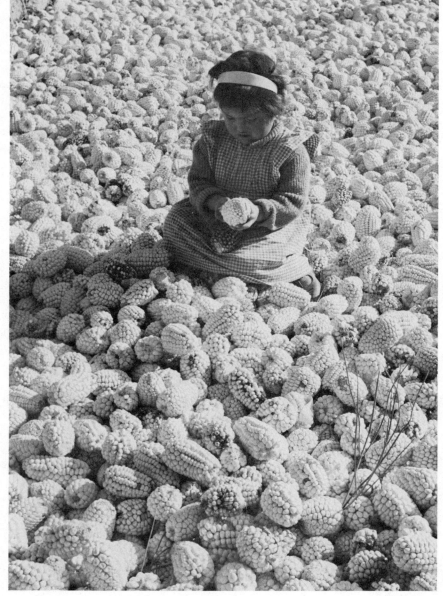

and nitrogen equilibrium can be maintained. The ability of proteins to complement each other's amino acid deficiencies is termed *supplementary value.* In order for complementary protein foods to match amino acid requirements, both foods must be ingested within the same recipe or meal. If eaten several hours apart, the effect is as if they were consumed separately, and neither incomplete protein can be utilized for protein synthesis.

The efficiency of a protein source can be evaluated experimentally by its capacity to maintain the nitrogen balance or promote growth. This is done by measuring the amounts of nitrogen retained by the body: The higher the amount of nitrogen retained, the higher the quality of the protein. The Food and Agriculture Organization (FAO) of the United Nations determines the *biologic value* (BV) of proteins, based on this method, and sets world standards. The biologic value of the protein, the percentage of true digestible protein utilized by the body, is expressed as

$$BV = \frac{\text{Dietary nitrogen} - \text{urinary nitrogen} - \text{fecal nitrogen}}{\text{Dietary nitrogen} - \text{fecal nitrogen}}$$

The biologic value estimation does not account for losses of nitrogen in digestion. Another measure of protein quality, which does include this factor, is the *net protein utilization* (NPU), expressed as

$$NPU = \frac{\text{Retained nitrogen}}{\text{Intake of nitrogen}}$$

By measuring growth on a fixed amount of dietary protein, the efficiency of a protein can also be determined. This index, the *protein efficiency ratio* (PER), is used in determining daily protein requirements, and is expressed as

$$PER = \frac{\text{Weight gained}}{\text{Nitrogen intake}}$$

In a diet with a PER or NPU of 70 or greater, the U.S. Recommended Dietary Allowance (RDA) is about 45 gm. In diets with the PER less than 70, more protein is needed, and the recommendation is increased to 65 gm.

Generally, animal proteins are of a higher biologic value than are vegetable proteins, since their amino acid distribution more closely approximates that of body tissue. Careful planning, however, can assure a healthy and nutritious diet from nonanimal protein sources. Table 3-6 summarizes the amino acid strengths, deficiencies, and NPU values of various foods. Since protein foods within the same group generally have a similar amino acid composition and therefore the same known strengths and weaknesses, proteins from different groups can be mixed within a recipe or meal to ensure an intake of all essential amino acids, or *complete protein.* In 1971, Frances Moore Lappé published a revolutionary book based on this idea, and her guide to combining protein sources is given in Fig. 3-10. Her book provides an excellent and sound guide to wholesome vegetarian eating as well as to the relative costs, advantages, and disadvantages of animal and vegetable proteins (see Suggested Readings).

QUANTITY OF PROTEIN AND RECOMMENDED INTAKES

By feeding experimental diets in which a mixture of amino acids is the sole source of nitrogen, the manipulation of each essential amino acid can determine the requirements for nitrogen balance and growth. The estimated amino acid

TABLE 3-6. Amino acid strengths, deficiencies, and net protein utilization (NPU) values in selected foods

Food	NPU	Amino acid composition	
		Deficiency	Strength
Dairy*		None	Lysine
Egg	94		
Milk	82		
Seafood*		None	Lysine
Haddock	80		
Tuna	80		
Meats and poultry*		None	Lysine
Beef	67		
Pork	67		
Chicken	65		
Lamb	65		
Grains and cereals		Isoleucine and lysine	None
Oatmeal	66		
Wheat	60		
Barley	60		
Rice	57		
Most flours	40–60		
Nuts and seeds		Isoleucine and lysine	Tryptophan
Cashews	58		
Walnuts	50		
Peanuts	43		
Legumes		Tryptophan, methionine, and cysteine	Lysine
Peas	47		
Beans	38		
Lentils	30		

*Complete proteins containing all essential amino acids.
Source: Compiled from data in F. M. Lappé, *Diet for a Small Planet*. New York: Ballantine Books, 1971. Pp. 68–99.

requirements are summarized in Table 3-7. As shown in the last two columns, the infant's requirements of the individual amino acids range from 4 to 12 times the amounts needed by the adult per unit of weight. This is because the amount needed for growth is much greater than that for maintenance. As the growth rate slows, the need for protein is reduced, but until after puberty, it remains greater than adult requirements. The U.S. RDAs reflect this: 2.2 gm per kilogram body weight for infants under 6 months; 2.0 gm per kilogram for infants 6 months to 1 year; 1.8 gm per kilogram for children ages 1 to 3 years; 1.1 gm per kilogram, ages 4 to 10; 1.0 gm per kilogram, ages 11 to 14; 0.9 gm per kilogram, ages 15 to 18; and 0.8 gm per kilogram, ages 19 and over. During pregnancy the RDA increases by 30 gm; during lactation, 20 gm. As might be suspected, a deficiency of protein most severely affects growing children (see Chap. 34).

The first authoritative body to attempt to establish a standard of protein intake

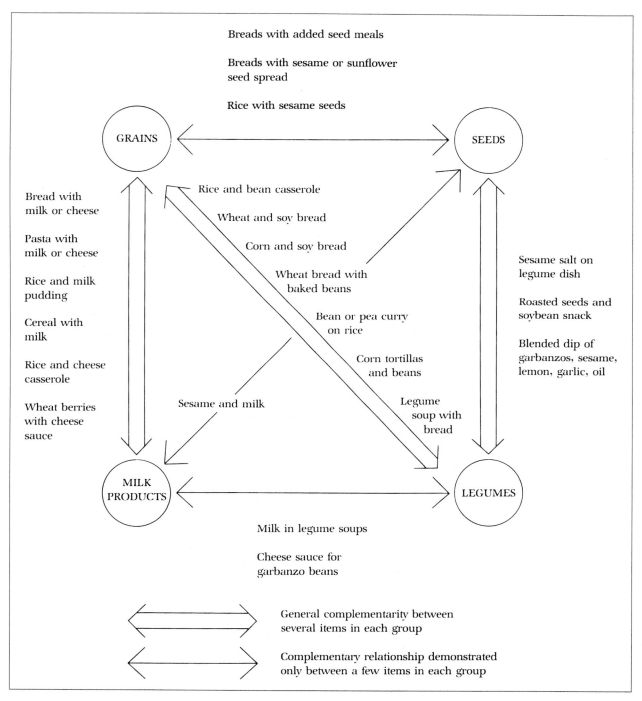

FIG. 3-10. Summary of complementary protein relationships. (From F. M. Lappé, *Diet for a Small Planet.* New York: Ballantine Books, 1971.)

45

TABLE 3-7. Amino acids required to maintain nitrogen balance in adults and growth in infants under 6 months

Amino acid	Man (mg/day)	Woman (mg/day)	Combined adult values (mg/kg body weight/day)	Infant (mg/kg body weight/day)
Histidine	0	0	0	28
Isoleucine	700	550	10	70
Leucine	1100	730	14	161
Lysine	800	545	12	103
Methionine and cystine	1100	700	13	58
Phenylalanine and tyrosine	1100	700	14	125
Threonine	500	375	7	87
Tryptophan	250	168	4	17
Valine	800	622	10	93

Source: Food and Agriculture Organization of the United Nations, Joint FAO/WHO ad hoc Expert Committee. *WHO Tech. Rep. Ser.* 522, 1973.

was the League of Nations in 1936. Their empirical recommendation of 1 gm/kg body weight/day was widely accepted and is still used as a guide. In 1957, 1965, and 1973 the FAO of the United Nations attempted to define their own standards, based on physiologic needs and the biologic tests discussed previously. Based on mixed dietary protein with an NPU of 70, they suggest, for a normal man, about 53 gm per day, or 0.57 gm/kg/day, or about 7.0 percent of the daily total caloric intake.

References

1. Rose, W. C.   Amino acid requirements of man. *Fed. Proc.* 8:546, 1949.
2. Morgan, A. F.   The effect of heat upon the biological value of cereal proteins and casein. *J. Biol. Chem.* 90:771, 1931.
3. Rice, E. E., and Beuk, J. F.   The effect of heat upon the nutritive value of protein. *Adv. Food Res.* 4:233, 1953.
4. Frazier, E., Cannon, P. R., and Hughes, R. H.   The problem of heat injury to dietary protein. *Food Res.* 18:91, 1953.
5. Neame, K. D., and Wiseman, G.   The transamination of glutamic and aspartic acids during absorption by the small intestine of the dog in vivo. *J. Physiol. (Lond.)* 135:442, 1957.
6. Pinsky, J., and Geiger, E.   Intestinal absorption of histidine as influenced by tryptophan in the rat. *Proc. Soc. Exp. Biol. Med.* 81:55, 1952.

Suggested Readings

Berry, R. E.   Tropical fruits and vegetables as potential protein sources. *Food Technol.* 35:45, 1981.
Cooper, M. D., and Lawton, A. R.   The development of the immune system. *Sci. Am.* 231:58, 1974.
Delwiche, C. C.   The nitrogen cycle. *Sci. Am.* 223:136, 1970.

Dickerson, R. E.   The structure and history of an ancient protein. *Sci. Am.* 226:58, 1972.

Doty, P.   Proteins. *Sci. Am.* 197:173, 1957.

Edelman, G. M.   The structure and function of antibodies. *Sci. Am.* 223:34, 1970.

Ewald, E. B.   *Recipes for a Small Planet.* New York: Ballantine, 1973.

Food and Agriculture Organization of the United Nations. Eight Reports of Joint FAO/WHO Expert Committee on Nutrition (FAO Nutrition Meetings Report Series No. 49). *WHO Tech. Rep. Ser.* 477, 1971.

Food and Agriculture Organization of the United Nations. Handbook on nutritional requirements (FAO Nutritional Studies No. 28). *WHO Mon. Ser.* 61, 1974.

Friedman, M. (ed.)   *Protein Crosslinking: Nutritional and Medical Consequences.* New York: Plenum, 1977. Pp. 740.

Lappé, F. M.   *Diet for a Small Planet.* New York: Ballantine, 1971.

Light, A.   *Proteins: Structure and Function.* Englewood Cliffs, N.J.: Prentice-Hall, 1974.

Mayer, M. M.   The complement system. *Sci. Am.* 229:54, 1973.

Perutz, M. F.   The hemoglobin molecule. *Sci. Am.* 211:64, 1964.

Perutz, M. F.   Hemoglobin structure and respiratory transport. *Sci. Am.* 239:92, 1978.

Sanger, F.   The Chemistry of Insulin. In *Nobel Lectures: Chemistry, 1942–1962.* Amsterdam: Elsevier, 1964. Pp. 544–556.

Schwabe, C. W.   *Unmentionable Cuisine.* Charlottesville: University Press of Virginia, 1980. Pp. 476.

Scrimshaw, M. S.   World need for protein. *J. Am. Oil Chem. Soc.* 58:389, 1981.

Sharon, N.   Glycoproteins. *Sci. Am.* 230:78, 1974.

World soya conference. *Food Eng.* 53:83, 1981.

Yung-Shung, C.   Soybean protein food in China. *J. Am. Oil Chem. Soc.* 58:96A, 1981.

Zuckerkandl, E.   The evolution of hemoglobin. *Sci. Am.* 212:110, 1965.

Chapter 4

CARBOHYDRATES

Carbohydrates are the main and preferred fuel of the human body; a constant supply is vital to the functioning of most systems, the nervous system in particular. Carbohydrates constitute the largest portion of the food consumed in the world by humans and other animals. They represent over 45 percent of the diet in America, and as much as 90 percent of the diet in such countries as China and Japan, where rice is the staple food. Synthesized by green plants from carbon dioxide and water in the presence of sunlight, carbohydrates are produced during photosynthesis. During this process, light energy is converted to chemical energy, which is stored in the plant structure and released on metabolism. The carbohydrates of the plant kingdom provide the major energy fuel on which the animal kingdom depends.

Carbohydrates are also components in the biosynthesis of other vital compounds, such as amino acids and fatty acids, and structural components of biologically important compounds, such as glycolipids, glycoproteins, heparin, nucleic acids, and cartilage.

Photosynthesis

Solar energy is the ultimate source of energy for nearly all organisms, through the operation of food chains. The energy captured during the process of photosynthesis provides over 90 percent of all energy used by humankind for heat, light, power, and food. The light absorbed by chlorophyll-containing plant cells provides this prime source of energy in the biosphere. *Photosynthesis*, the process whereby light (electromagnetic) energy is converted into chemical energy, occurs in organized subcellular bodies called *chloroplasts*. The energy from light is utilized to change, or *fix*, carbon dioxide (CO_2) into carbohydrate, in a process which is the reverse of the oxidation of glucose.

Photosynthesis occurs in two major phases. In the first phase (termed *light reactions*, or the light phase), light energy is captured by light-absorbing pigments and is converted into the chemical energy of *ATP* (adenosine triphosphate) and certain reducing agents, particularly *NADPH* (the reduced form of nicotinamide-adenine dinucleotide phosphate). Hydrogen atoms are removed from water molecules and are used to reduce (add electrons to) $NADP^+$, resulting in the by-product of molecular oxygen. At the same time, ADP (adenosine diphosphate) is *phosphorylated* (an energy-rich phosphate bond is formed). Water serves as an electron donor, and NADPH and ATP are the results of the conversion of light energy into chemical energy. The light phase can be summarized as

$$H_2O + NADP^+ + \underset{\substack{\text{(inorganic}\\ \text{phosphate)}}}{P_i} + ADP \xrightarrow{\text{light}} \underset{\text{(oxygen)}}{O_2} + NADPH + H^+ + ATP$$

During the second phase (*dark reactions*, or the dark phase), the energy-rich products of the first phase, NADPH and ATP, are used to reduce carbon dioxide, yielding glucose. The free energy required for biosynthesis is provided by the phosphate bond energy of ATP and by the reducing ability of NADPH and other coenzymes. Simultaneously, NADPH is reoxidized to $NADP^+$ and ATP is broken down again to ADP and phosphate. The second phase, which is brought about by enzyme-catalyzed reactions and does not require light, can be summarized as

$$CO_2 + NADPH + H^+ + ATP \longrightarrow C_6H_{12}O_6 + NADP^+ + ADP + P_i$$
$$\text{(glucose)}$$

By combining the two phases, the balanced overall scheme for photosynthesis can be shown as

$$6\ CO_2 + 6\ H_2O \xrightarrow{\text{light}} C_6H_{12}O_6 + 6\ O_2$$
(carbon   (water)   (glucose)   (oxygen)
dioxide)

This deceptively simple conversion, which has never been duplicated by humans, captures only about one-tenth of one percent of the energy received from the sun. Yet this seemingly small percentage is equivalent to 150 to 200 billion tons of dry organic matter, namely the earth's major ecosystems: the forests, grasslands, marshes, estuaries, oceans, rivers, tundras, and deserts [1]. Green plants are considered the primary producers of the biosphere, and although forests cover only about a tenth of the earth's surface, they "fix" almost half of the total energy of the biosphere.

Classification, Structure, and Bonding

Carbohydrates are composed of carbon, hydrogen, and water and may be classified according to their molecular structure, components, and types of bonding. The simplest division is by the length of the basic carbon chain.

MONOSACCHARIDES

Also termed *simple sugars* are carbohydrates that cannot be broken down or *hydrolyzed* into a simpler form. Monosaccharides contain three to seven carbon atoms and are often subdivided by the number of carbon atoms present: *Trioses* (three carbon atoms) are formed in the metabolic breakdown of *hexoses* (six carbon atoms); *tetroses* (four carbon atoms) and *pentoses* (five carbon atoms) are important as constituents of nucleic acids and as coenzymes. Only hexoses are of major dietary importance—glucose, galactose, fructose, and mannose are hexoses. All hexoses have the same empirical formula, $C_6H_{12}O_6$, but differ in the spatial arrangement around the carbon atoms. Glucose, galactose, and mannose have an aldehyde group (—CHO) and are considered aldohexoses; fructose contains a ketone group (C=O) and is therefore a ketohexose. The D- (dextro-) or L- (levo-) designation is determined by the spatial relationship of the —H and

FIG. 4-1. The L- and D- config-uration of glucose. (From H. A. Harper, *Review of Physiologi-cal Chemistry* [17th ed.]. Los Altos, Calif.: Lange Medical, 1979.)

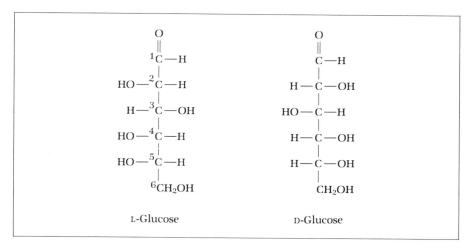

L-Glucose   D-Glucose

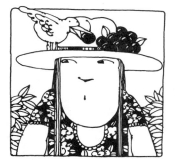

—OH groups around the carbon atom adjacent to the terminal primary alcohol carbon (C-5, in glucose) (Fig. 4-1). When the —OH is on the left, the sugar is a member of the L- series; when it is on the right, it is a member of the D- series. Most monosaccharides occurring in human metabolism are of the D- configura-tion (Fig. 4-1).

Glucose, the chief end product of carbohydrate digestion, is the principal sugar in the blood and serves as the body's major metabolic fuel. Its structure, which may be written as a straight chain formula, is a six-member ring containing one oxygen atom. Its chemical properties come from its ring structure, which x-ray diffraction analysis shows more accurately to be bent, or in the form of a chair (Fig. 4-2). Also known as dextrose, grape sugar, or corn sugar, glucose is water soluble and is found in such sweet fruits as grapes, berries, and oranges, and in some vegetables, including sweet corn and carrots.

Fructose, also termed *levulose* or fruit sugar, is a highly soluble sugar that does not readily crystallize (Fig. 4-3A). Fructose is a product of the hydrolysis of sucrose (cane sugar) and is sweeter than sucrose. Fructose is most prevalent in honey and ripe fruits and vegetables.

Galactose is not found free in nature; it is found only as a by-product of the hydrolysis (breakdown) of lactose. It is also a constituent of cerebrosides (gly-colipids found in the brain) and certain polysaccharides (Fig. 4-3B).

Mannose also is not found free in nature; it is found in legumes in the form of mannosan, a partially digestible polysaccharide. It is also a constituent of poly-saccharides of albumins, globulins, and mucoids (Fig. 4-3C).

Deoxysugars are pentoses (five carbons) in which a hydroxyl group (—OH) attached to the ring has been replaced by a hydrogen atom. They include ribose, a constituent of riboflavin (a B-complex vitamin), ribonucleic acid (RNA), and deoxyribonucleic acid (DNA). RNA and DNA molecules are composed of inter-twining sugar-phosphate chains of ribose or deoxyribose and four paired nitrog-enous bases attached to the chain by hydrogen bonding. Together, they contain

FIG. 4-2. α-D-glucose.

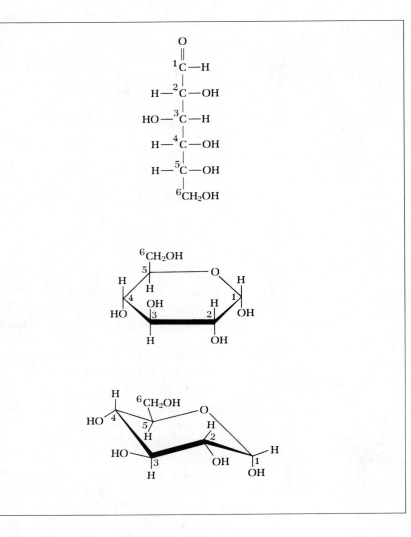

and transmit the genetic code distinctive to the cell and characteristic of the particular species.

DISACCHARIDES

These double sugars are composed of two monosaccharide residues joined by a *glycosidic linkage* with the loss of one molecule of water (*condensation*). Water-soluble, diffusible, and crystallizable, they vary in sweetness (Table 4-1) and can be split into simple sugars (monosaccharides) by acid hydrolysis or by digestive enzymes.

Sucrose, also known as cane, beet, or table sugar, contains a molecule each of glucose and fructose joined in a β, 1-2 glycosidic linkage (Fig. 4-4A). It is found in sugar cane, sugar beets, brown sugar, sorghum, molasses, and maple syrup. Some fruits and vegetables may also contain small amounts of sucrose.

FIG. 4-3.
A. D-Fructose.
B. D-Galactose.
C. D-Mannose.

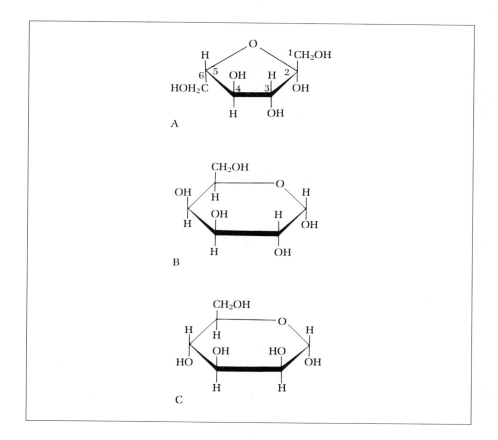

Lactose, also called milk sugar, contains a molecule each of glucose and galactose in a β, 1-4 glycosidic linkage (Fig. 4-4B). This sugar is produced by mammals and is the only carbohydrate of animal origin of significance in the diet. It is about one-sixth as sweet as sucrose, and its concentration in milk ranges from 2 to 8 percent, depending on the animal species. Human milk contains about twice as much lactose as does cow's milk.

Maltose, also called malt sugar, is composed of two molecules of glucose joined in an α, 1-4 glycosidic linkage (Fig. 4-4C). Formed mostly as an intermediate product in the hydrolysis of starch, maltose does not occur in appreciable quantities in food. It is present during the fermenting of grains in beer and in malted breakfast cereals. It is also used with dextrins as the carbohydrate source in infant formulas.

POLYSACCHARIDES

Polysaccharides are complex compounds that result from the condensation of many monosaccharides and are of relatively high molecular weight. Polysaccharides contain more than 10 sugar units, are amorphous rather than crystalline, are neither sweet nor soluble in water, and vary in degree of digestibility.

TABLE 4-1. Relative sweetness of selected sugars and sweeteners

Sugar or sweetener	Sweetness (%)
Nutritive sugars	
Sucrose (reference sugar)	100
Fructose	173
Glucose	74
Glycine	70
Glycerol	60
Sorbitol	60
Maltose	33
Lactose	16
Nonnutritive sweeteners	
Saccharin	550
Dulcin	250
Cyclamates	30

Source: R. T. Lagua, V. S. Claudio, and V. F. Thiele, *Nutrition and Diet Therapy* (2nd ed.). St. Louis: Mosby, 1974. P. 220.

These sugars are composed of glucose plus molecules joined together by two types of linkages: 1-4 and 1-6. The 1-4 linkage (bonded at the first and fourth carbons in the ring) forms straight chains; the 1-6 linkage (first and sixth carbons) joins at the point where one straight chain branches from another. By utilizing both types of linkages highly branched structures are formed.

Starch is the storage form of carbohydrate in plants. It consists of two types of compounds, amylose and amylopectin. *Amylose,* composed of long straight chains of glucose (up to several hundred glucose units) is joined by α, 1-4 glycosidic linkages and makes up 15 to 20 percent of the total starch granule. *Amylopectin* is composed of shorter, branched chains of glucose with both alpha, 1-4 and alpha, 1-6 linkages. The starch granules are encased in a celluloselike wall, distinctive in size and shape for each plant species. Starch is broken down by the splitting off of maltose units, which in turn are hydrolyzed into glucose. Starch is considered a *glucosan* because it yields only glucose on hydrolysis. *Dextrins* are the large, partially degraded glucose polymer units formed as intermediates during hydrolysis. These partially degraded polysaccharides undergo progressive attrition by hydrolysis, with the end product being glucose. Dextrins are also produced when flour is browned and when bread is toasted. The structure of starch is shown in Fig. 4-5.

Inulin is a starch found in tubers and the roots of artichokes, dandelions, and dahlias. It is considered a *fructosan* because on hydrolysis it yields only fructose. Clinically, it is used in testing kidney function and the glomerular filtration rate, since it is completely filtered by the glomeruli and is neither reabsorbed nor excreted by the kidney tubules.

Glycogen, also called animal starch, is similar in structure to the amylopectin of starch, but has a higher percentage of 1-6 linkages and therefore more branched chains of glucose. It is rapidly synthesized from glucose in the liver and

FIG. 4-4. Disaccharides.
A. Sucrose.
B. Lactose.
C. Maltose.

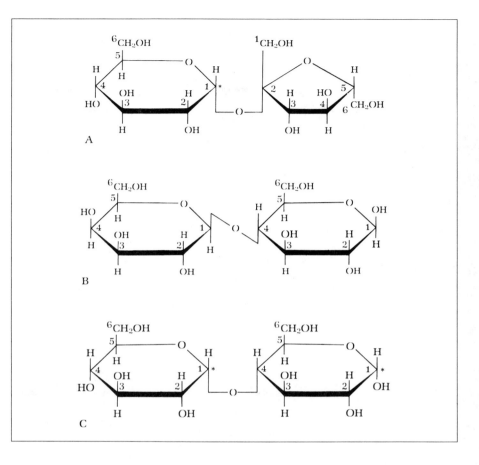

muscle and accounts for about 2 to 8 percent and 1 percent of their weights, respectively. Its structure is shown in Fig. 4-6.

Insoluble polysaccharides include cellulose, pectins, agar, carrageenan, and alginates. *Cellulose* is the most abundant organic compound in the world, comprising about half of the carbon in vegetation. It serves as the structural component of plant tissues and is found in the skins of fruits, the coverings of seeds, and the structural parts of plants. There is no enzyme in the human gastrointestinal tract capable of digesting this polysaccharide, so it passes through undigested, providing roughage and bulk for optimal functioning of the lower bowel and for maintaining muscle tone of the colon. *Ruminants* (animals having stomachs with four cavities) such as cows can utilize cellulose because of specific enzymes in the *rumen*, the first compartment of the stomach. Thus they can derive nutrients from what is considered an indigestible dietary constituent for humans. Because cows can break down cellulose, they are able to obtain a large portion of their energy from it. *Pectins* are found in ripe fruits and, because of their ability to absorb water and form gels, are used in making jellies. *Agar* is a polysac-

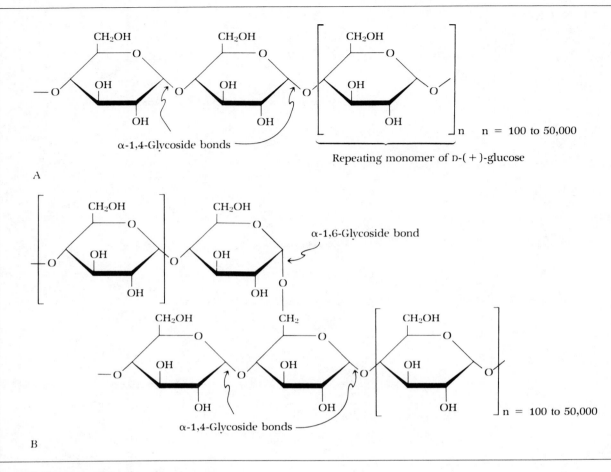

FIG. 4-5. Structure of starch.
A. Amylose.
B. Amylopectin. (From G. H. Schmid, *The Chemical Basis of Life: General, Organic, and Biological Chemistry for the Health Sciences*. Boston: Little, Brown, 1982.)

charide obtained from seaweed and is useful for its gelling properties and as a culture medium for bacteria in the laboratory. *Carrageenan* (Irish moss) and *alginates*, from seaweed, are used to enhance the smoothness of food such as ice cream and evaporated milk.

CARBOHYDRATE DERIVATIVES

Sugars that have reacted chemically to form various other compounds are called *carbohydrate derivatives*. Such derivatives include glycosides, amino sugars, sorbitol, and ascorbic acid. *Glycosides* are compounds formed from the condensation of a sugar and a hydroxyl group of a second compound, which may or may not be another sugar. If the first sugar is glucose, the resulting glycoside is glucoside; if galactose, galactoside; and so on. These compounds are found in drugs and spices, and as constituents of animal tissues. The *cardiac glycosides* are among the best-known drugs and contain steroids as the second compound; they include derivatives of digitalis and strophanthin (ouabain) and antibiotics

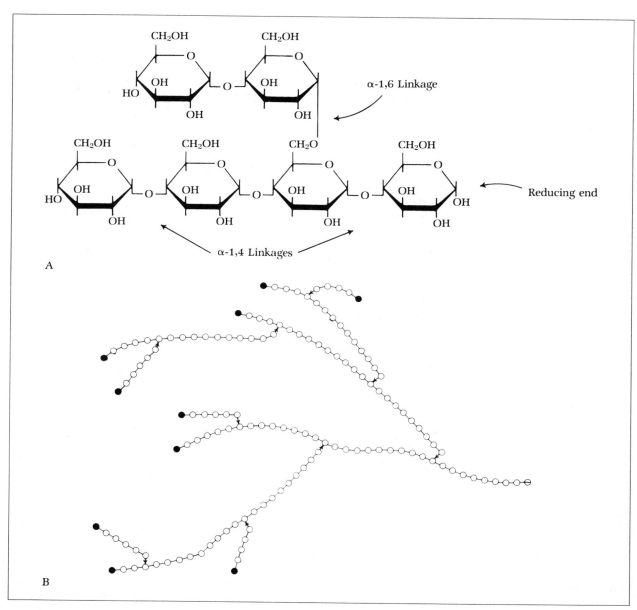

FIG. 4-6.
A. Types of linkages in glycogen.
B. General structure of glycogen. ⊖, reducing end; ●,
   nonreducing ends; ○—○,
   α, 1-4 linkage; ○←○, α,
   1-6 linkage (branch point).
   Each chain is extended and
   branched further, producing
   a polysaccharide of high
   molecular weight. (From I.
   Danishefsky, *Biochemistry
   for Medical Sciences.* Boston:
   Little, Brown, 1981.)

such as streptomycin. Glycosides are also components of steroid and adrenal hormones. *Amino sugars,* sugars containing an amino group ($—NH_2$), include such compounds as D-glucosamine (part of *hyaluronic acid,* which binds water in the interstitial spaces and acts as a shock absorber in the joints), D-galactosamine (part of *chondroitin,* a constituent of cartilage), and D-mannosamine (a mucoprotein). The antibiotics erythromycin and carbomycin are also amino sugars. *Sorbitol,* a sugar alcohol, is sweet and water soluble. Because almost 70 percent of it can be metabolized without appearing in the blood as glucose, it is often recommended as a substitute for table sugar in diets for diabetics. *Ascorbic acid,* also called vitamin C, is a water-soluble hexose derivative. It is synthesized by plants and by some animals but not by humans.

Other carbohydrates in body compounds include *heparin,* a mucopolysaccharide that prevents the clotting of blood; *galactolipins,* constituents of nervous tissue; *glucuronic acid,* a mucopolysaccharide that acts as a detoxifying agent in the liver by combining with toxic chemical and bacterial by-products; and *chitin,* a constituent of the hard outer shell of insects and crustaceans.

Carbohydrates in Foods

Sugars are the simplest of organic foods. Besides adding flavor to foods, they also alter the degree of hydration, increase the moisture-retaining abilities, alter the color and texture of fruit products, and influence the viscosity of starch paste and the firmness of gelatin and pectin gels. Since the complex carbohydrates (starches) will be discussed at length in several chapters in Section III, only the sugars will be covered here. The composition of selected sugars is given in Table 4-2; that of selected carbohydrate-rich foods is given in Table 4-3.

Sucrose, the most common sugar used in the United States, is generally manu-

TABLE 4-2. Composition of selected sugars, per tablespoon

Sugar	Calories	Carbohydrates (gm)	Iron (mg)	Thiamine (μg)	Riboflavin (μg)	Niacin (mg)	Ascorbic acid (mg)	Vitamin A (IU)	Vitamin D (IU)
Corn syrup	57	14.8	0.8	0	2	tr	0.1	0	0
Honey	64	16.4	0.2	2	14	tr	1.0	0	0
Maple syrup	50	12.8	0.2	—	—	—	—	—	—
Molasses									
1st extraction	50	13.0	0.9	14	12	tr	—	—	—
2nd extraction	46	12.0	1.2	—	—	—	—	—	—
3rd extraction	43	11.0	2.3	56	50	0.4	—	—	—
Chocolate syrup	49	11.7	0.4	7	28	0.05	—	—	—
Sorghum	52	13.4	2.4	—	—	—	—	—	—
Brown, dark	52	13.4	0.4	—	—	—	—	—	—
White, granulated	46	11.9	—	—	—	—	—	—	—
Treacle, black	53	13.4	1.8	—	—	—	—	—	—

tr = trace.

Source: C. F. Church and H. N. Church, *Food Values of Portions Commonly Used* (12th ed.). Philadelphia: Lippincott, 1975. Pp. 72–73.

TABLE 4-3. Composition of selected carbohydrate-rich foods

Food	Amount	Calories	Protein (gm)	Carbohydrate (gm)	Fiber (gm)	Fat (gm)	Iron (mg)	Thiamine (μg)	Riboflavin (μg)	Niacin (mg)	Ascorbic acid (mg)	Vitamin A (IU)	Vitamin D (IU)
Breads													
Cracked wheat	1 slice	60	2.0	12.0	0.1	0.1	0.3	30	20	0.3	tr	tr	—
White, enriched	1 slice	62	2.0	11.6	tr	0.7	0.6	60	50	0.6	tr	tr	—
Whole wheat	1 slice	56	2.4	11.0	0.4	0.7	0.5	60	20	0.6	tr	tr	—
Iced coffee cake	1 small	196	3.9	31.6	tr	6.1	0.8	100	110	0.7	—	214	—
Danish pastry	1 small	148	2.6	16.0	0.1	8.2	0.3	20	50	0.3	tr	108	—
Sugar doughnut	1 average	151	2.1	21.7	tr	6.5	0.6	70	60	0.5	tr	41	—
Grains and pasta													
Oatmeal, cooked	1 cup	148	5.4	26.0	0.5	2.8	1.7	220	50	0.4	—	—	—
White rice, cooked	¾ cup	103	2.1	22.5	0.1	0.1	0.2	20	8	0.5	—	—	—
Corn grits, cooked	1 cup	123	2.9	26.8	0.2	0.2	0.7	90	70	1.0	—	145	—
Spaghetti, cooked	1 cup	216	7.3	44.0	0.1	0.7	1.6	260	150	2.0	—	—	—
Wheat germ	3 tbsp	102	7.4	13.1	0.7	3.1	2.6	560	190	1.2	—	—	—
Fruits (all raw, fresh)													
Apple	1 medium	87	0.3	21.7	1.5	0.9	0.5	40	30	0.2	6	140	—
Avocado	½, pitted	167	2.1	6.3	1.6	16.4	0.6	110	200	1.6	14	290	—
Banana	1 small	85	1.1	22.2	0.5	0.2	0.7	50	60	0.7	10	190	—
Cantaloupe	¼ melon	30	0.7	7.5	0.3	0.1	0.4	40	30	0.6	33	3400	—
Figs	2 large	80	1.2	20.3	1.2	0.3	0.6	60	50	0.4	2	80	—
Orange	1 medium	73	1.5	18.3	0.8	0.3	0.6	150	60	0.6	80	300	—
Peach	1 medium	38	0.6	9.7	0.6	0.1	0.5	20	50	1.0	7	1330	—
Pear	½ medium	61	0.7	15.3	1.4	0.4	0.3	20	40	0.1	4	20	—
Tomato	1 small	22	1.1	4.7	0.5	0.2	0.5	60	40	0.7	23	900	—
Vegetables (cooked)													
Beans, kidney	⅖ cup	118	7.8	21.4	1.5	0.5	2.4	110	60	0.7	—	tr	—
Broccoli	1 large stalk	26	3.1	4.5	1.5	0.3	0.8	90	200	0.8	90	2500	—
Corn, sweet	1 medium ear	96	3.5	22.1	0.7	1.0	0.7	150	120	1.7	12	400	—
Lentils	⅔ cup	106	7.8	19.3	1.2	tr	2.1	70	60	0.6	—	20	—
Peas	½ cup	102	7.2	18.0	1.5	0.4	1.5	220	90	0.9	—	36	—
Potato, baked	1 medium	139	3.9	31.7	0.9	0.2	1.0	150	60	2.6	30	tr	—
Squash, winter	½ cup	63	1.8	15.4	1.8	0.4	0.8	50	130	0.7	13	4200	—

tr = trace

Source: C. F. Church and H. N. Church, *Food Values of Portions Commonly Used* (12th ed.). Philadelphia: Lippincott, 1975.

factured from sugar cane or sugar beets (Fig. 4-7). Although these two sources differ in the types of impurities in the unrefined state, marketed white sugar is 99.9 percent pure sucrose, regardless of the source. *White sugar* is produced by concentrating sugar cane or sugar beet juice, centrifuging the crystals, and then purifying them. *Raw sugar* is an intermediate product of sucrose crystals still covered with a film of nonsucrose impurities. *Brown sugar* is sucrose crystals with a film of dark-colored syrup, which gives the sugar its characteristic color and flavor. The color varies with the amount of refinement. The sucrose and

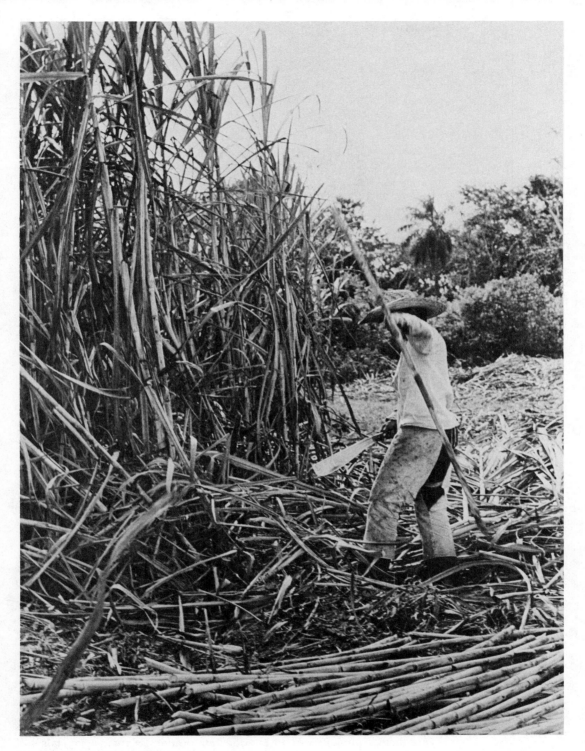

FIG. 4-7. Harvesting sugar cane
in Bolivia. (FAO photo by T.
Kamphuis.)

moisture content vary from 91 percent and 2 percent, respectively, for dark brown sugar to 90 percent and 4 percent for yellow [2]. *Molasses* is the syrup separated from the crystals in the manufacture of sucrose. It usually is produced through three extractions, the final being *blackstrap,* the highest in nutrients. *Invert sugar* is manufactured by heating sucrose in dilute acid. It is more soluble than sucrose and because of its fructose content has better moisture-retaining properties.

Corn syrup is manufactured by the hydrolysis of corn starch to produce a mixture of glucose, maltose, dextrins, and higher polymers of glucose. It can also be produced from other starches, including potato, rice, and barley.

Honey is a natural syrup, varying in composition and flavor with the plant source of the nectar, processing, and storage. Its principal carbohydrates are glucose and fructose. Its sweetness varies with concentration and degree of crystallization, although generally it is considered to be about 70 to 75 percent as sweet as sucrose.

Maple syrup is made from the sap of the sugar maple. The sap contains about 2 percent solids, mostly sucrose, which are concentrated by boiling. The evaporation at atmospheric pressure causes the pH to become alkaline enough to induce polymerization of the hexose, with resultant browning.

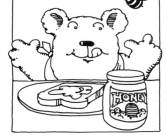

Digestion and Metabolism

Although carbohydrates are involved in many compounds and activities, their primary function is to provide energy to the organism. On oxidation by the body, each gram of carbohydrate yields four calories. There is no "essential" dietary carbohydrate, since glucose and other carbohydrate structures can all be synthesized from noncarbohydrate sources, but it does command a central role in sparing other nutrients from providing energy for metabolism, and it aids in the digestion, absorption, and utilization of other components of the diet.

ALTERATIONS IN CARBOHYDRATES BY COOKING AND OTHER PROCESSES

THICKENING AGENTS

Heating a polysaccharide (e.g., starch) in an aqueous environment results in increased digestibility. The swelling and rupture of the polysaccharide molecules permit greater enzymatic action during digestion. Although insoluble in cold water, starch, when mixed with liquid and heated, swells. The mixture increases in viscosity and forms a paste—thus the thickening ability of cornstarch and flour in gravies and puddings. Mixtures of starch and acid ingredients (lemon pudding, salad dressing) may become thin because of hydrolysis of the starch molecule.

HYDROLYSIS

Because neither glucose nor fructose crystallizes readily, each aids in maintaining other sugars in solution, as in the preparation of cane syrup from sucrose and in preventing the crystallization, and consequent gritty texture, of sucrose in candy or jelly.

FERMENTATION

Simple sugars and disaccharides may be easily fermented by bacteria and yeast. The manufacture of alcoholic beverages is through the fermentation of glucose by yeast. Fermenting barley produces malt syrups. Lactose is fermented by lactic acid–producing microorganisms.

PRESERVATION

Sugar acts as a preservative by lowering the water activity of the food in which it is used and thereby inhibiting microbial growth [3]. The water activity is measured by determining the water vapor of the food and dividing it by the vapor pressure of pure water at the same temperature. The growth of bacteria is inhibited at water activities less than 0.90; the growth of yeasts, at activities lower than 0.75; and the growth of molds, at activities lower than 0.65. For more detailed discussion, see Chap. 19.

BROWNING

In carbohydrate-containing foods, browning is the result of three possible reactions. The first is the *Maillard reaction* (nonenzymatic browning) [4], which is a reaction between proteins and sugars not requiring oxygen. Many foods (products) depend on this reaction for the development of their characteristic flavor: maple syrup and coffee. *Enzymatic browning* occurs in the presence of oxygen, as when cut fruits or vegetables are exposed to air. *Carmelization*, which does not require oxygen, occurs in foods with sugar when heated to high temperatures.

DIGESTION

Most carbohydrates in foods are in the form of polysaccharides and disaccharides and must be hydrolyzed into simple hexose sugars before being absorbed. Disaccharides and polysaccharides are converted to monosaccharides by the enzymes present in saliva (ptyalin), pancreatic secretions (pancreatic amylase), and the mucosa of the small intestine (disaccharidases). Digestion is initiated in the mouth by the starch-splitting action of the salivary enzyme *ptyalin;* its digestive action continues to some degree in the stomach. Ptyalin, a kind of amylase, hydrolyzes starch into dextrins and maltose and depends on a neutral or alkaline pH; its enzymatic activity is inhibited by an acid environment. In the intestinal tract, *pancreatic amylase* hydrolyzes the remaining starch to dextrins and maltose. The amylases, in saliva and pancreatic juice, can only attack 1-4 linkages. The intestinal *disaccharidases* split disaccharides such as maltose, lactose, and sucrose into their monosaccharide components, liberating glucose, galactose, and fructose. The majority of dietary carbohydrate is presented to the intestinal mucosa as disaccharides to be split by glycosidases or disaccharidases present in the *brush border* of the mucosal cells. These disaccharides are broken down to the monosaccharides glucose, fructose, and galactose; other monosaccharides include mannose from glycoproteins and pentoses derived from the digestion of nucleic acids. Hydrolysis takes place within the mucosal cells of the thrush border, and the monosaccharide products are then secreted into the portal circulation.

PHYSIOLOGIC ABSORPTION   Each disaccharide is absorbed at a different site along the small intestine, which results in the most efficient assimilation. Lactose is absorbed at the duodenum and proximal jejunum; maltose, at the jejunum and proximal ileum; and sucrose, at the distal jejunum and ileum. Logically, the concentration of specific disaccharidase is greatest at the site where it is absorbed, although all may be found, but in lower concentrations, along the entire small intestine.

Absorption of monosaccharides in the small intestine involves two distinct processes. *Nonspecific, passive,* or *simple diffusion* is governed by the sugar concentration gradient between the intestinal lumen and the mucosal cells, and between the mucosal cells and the blood plasma. *Active transport* is independent of concentration gradients and requires energy, which is provided by glucose within the intestinal tissue. Also called the *sodium pump* and *mobile carrier system,* active transport works by pumping sodium out of the mucosal cell and sugar in. Its energy is provided by glucose within the epithelial cell. Active transport involves phosphorylation of the sugar in the cells of the intestinal mucosa and hydrolysis of the disaccharide. Glucose, galactose, and fructose are subject to both types of absorption, unlike other five-carbon and six-carbon sugars [5]. They are therefore pulled into the bloodstream more rapidly than other sugars. Their specific absorption rates are independent of their concentration in the intestinal lumen. Glucose and galactose are absorbed at about equal rates; fructose is absorbed about half as rapidly, but faster than other sugars.

The absorption of glucose is influenced by the general condition of the organism. Malabsorption occurs with infections, intoxication, prolonged undernutrition, and vitamin deficiencies (especially of thiamin, pantothenic acid, and pyridoxine). The period of contact of the sugar with the absorptive surface is also important: Absorption is decreased with increased intestinal motility, as in diarrheal conditions. Structural or functional abnormalities of the mucous membrane can alter glucose absorption: It is decreased in inflammation (enteritis), edema (congestive heart failure), celiac disease, and hypothyroidism and increased in hyperthyroidism.

Disaccharidase deficiency, of which lactose intolerance is the most common, also produces malabsorption of carbohydrate. Three types of lactose intolerance, or lactase deficiency, are generally recognized: the rare, *congenital* form, considered an inborn error of metabolism; the temporary *acquired lactose intolerance,* due to inflammation of or damage to the epithelial mucosa; and the most common, *primary adult low lactase activity,* also known as isolated or racial lactose intolerance. This last type afflicts major portions of the world's population [6]. The symptoms of lactose intolerance—bloating, flatulence, pain, and diarrhea—are secondary to the osmotic effect of unhydrolyzed lactose and its fermentation by intestinal bacteria to produce lactic acid and short-chain fatty acids, with resultant bowel irritation. It is diagnosed by an intestinal biopsy and lactose determination or, less accurately, by the oral lactose tolerance test.

HEPATIC METABOLISM OF CARBOHYDRATES

After absorption into the portal blood, the monosaccharides are processed through the liver before entering the systemic circulation. In the liver, galactose and fructose are converted to glucose. The liver serves as the clearinghouse for the metabolism, conversion, and distribution of glucose to all body systems. Thus the liver's functional state has a profound influence on the carbohydrate metabolism of the entire organism. The amount of glucose in the systemic circulation is the result of the functioning of two groups of opposing hepatic processes. The first includes the *extraction and degradation of glucose* from the blood. The glucose is utilized for energy production, storage, and synthesis of other compounds. The second includes the *synthesis and release of glucose* to the blood, by the formation of blood sugar from nonglucose hexoses, conversion of glycogen to blood glucose, and the renal and hepatic synthesis of blood glucose from noncarbohydrate sources.

EXTRACTION AND DEGRADATION OF GLUCOSE
Oxidation for Energy
The normal fasting blood sugar ranges from 70 to 90 mg per 100 ml; the blood sugar level rises after a carbohydrate-rich meal, when hexose sugars are actively absorbed from the digested food in the intestinal lumen, to 140 to 150 mg per 100 ml. This rise is counteracted by hepatic energy metabolism and storage against future need, with the resultant return to normal blood sugar levels of 80 to 100 mg per 100 ml soon after eating. If the blood sugar level reaches 160 to 180 mg per 100 ml, some glucose may be excreted in the urine (*glycosuria*). This level, known as the *renal threshold for glucose*, is not usually exceeded in healthy individuals. Occasionally, with a lower threshold and after a high carbohydrate meal, some spillage of glucose into the urine may occur normally. A blood sugar level below normal is known as *hypoglycemia*; a level above the normal range is known as *hyperglycemia*.

Glucose released into the circulation for distribution to the body tissues serves as the major source of energy. Glucose may be completely oxidized to carbon dioxide and water in response to physiologic demands for energy. Energy for muscular work is obtained from high-energy phosphate bonds (as in such compounds as adenosine phosphates and creatine phosphate). These compounds are capable of yielding immediate energy on demand and restoring themselves to their previous high-energy states by acquiring the energy liberated by the oxidation of glucose to carbon dioxide and water inside the muscle cell and by the oxidation of fatty acids by muscle. In this main pathway (known as the *Embden-Meyerhof-Parnas pathway;* Fig. 4-8), glucose is degraded into two molecules of pyruvic or lactic acid. With sufficient oxygen, lactic acid does not accumulate, and pyruvate is oxidized to carbon dioxide and water through the mechanisms of the *Krebs* or *citric acid cycle* (Fig. 4-9). Without sufficient oxygen (as during

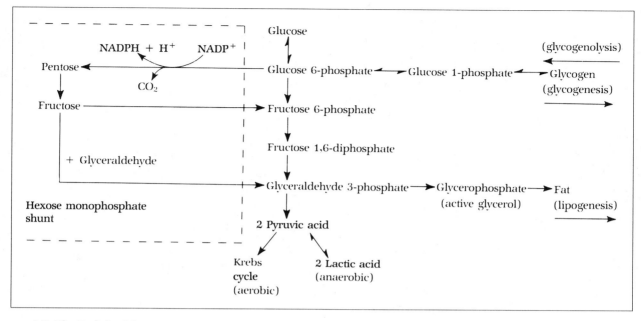

FIG. 4-8. The Embden-Meyerhof-Parnas pathway (glycolytic pathway). This is the initial pathway of glucose oxidation, and the crossroads for the interconversion of glucose with other nutrients. This series of reactions involves phosphorylation of glucose to form glycogen or proceeding down to glyceraldehyde to form fat. By metabolizing glucose to pyruvate, it leads into the final common pathway of energy production, the Krebs cycle.

continuous muscular exercise), lactic acid is formed in the working muscles as the product of the partial degradation of glucose (*glycolysis*) and diffuses into the circulation. The lactic acid is gradually withdrawn from the bloodstream by the liver and converted into glycogen.

Glucose is the only fuel acceptable to red blood cells and the kidney medulla, and although the central nervous system, including the brain, is capable of utilizing ketone bodies (the intermediate products of fatty acid degradation), it has a definite requirement for glucose. Because about one-fifth of the total basal metabolism takes place in the brain, with proportional glucose requirements, a fall in blood glucose is accompanied by neurologic signs of mental confusion, as seen with insulin overdose. Without oxygen (anaerobic conditions), glucose is the only potential energy source, but when oxygen is present, some tissues (e.g., skeletal muscle and heart) can utilize fatty acids and ketone bodies. The liver, which is enzymatically suited to the production of glucose, oxidizes fatty acids for energy metabolism in preference to glucose. The presence of some glucose is necessary for the normal oxidation of fats. In the absence of glucose or when it is severely restricted, fat is oxidized faster than its intermediate products can be metabolized by the body. The accumulation of the incompletely oxidized products of fatty acid degradation (ketones) leads to ketosis. Because some tissues in the body have an absolute requirement for glucose, a complex set of metabolic controls exists for the maintenance of adequate glucose levels and for the continuous distribution of glucose to these systems in adaptation to varying dietary and hormonal conditions.

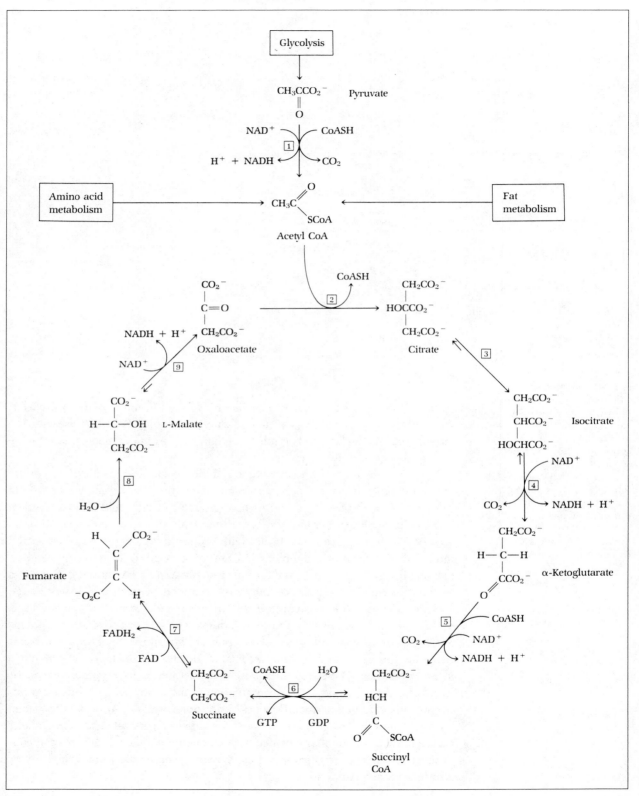

Storage as Glycogen

Excess glucose is converted in the liver into insoluble glycogen, the storage form of glucose in the body. This process (*glycogenesis*) is reversible (*glycogenolysis*); glycogen is mobilized as needed to maintain an optimal blood sugar level. Skeletal, cardiac, and smooth muscles maintain their own stores when at rest or under minor work loads. About 100 gm can be stored in the liver, and about 200 to 250 gm in cardiac, skeletal, and smooth muscles. Glycogen in muscle cannot be mobilized to regulate or replenish the blood sugar level; it can only be used for muscle tissue needs. Glycogen is also found in almost every organ, but in smaller quantities. The amount of glycogen stored in liver and muscle is influenced by the nature of the diet and the amount of exercise. Stores are progressively depleted during continuous and violent exercise. Cardiac muscle tenaciously guards its diminishing reserves of glycogen, preferentially utilizing blood glucose to furnish energy for its muscular contraction.

Conversion to Other Compounds

FAT. Because there is a limit on the amount of glycogen that can be stored within the tissues, excess quantities are converted to fatty acids (*lipogenesis*) and stored as triglycerides in fat depots. There seems to be no upper limit to storage in this manner. The process itself requires glucose.

OTHER CARBOHYDRATES. Glucose may also be converted to ribose and deoxyribose for the synthesis of nucleic acids; mannose, glucosamine, and galactosamine, which form parts of the mucopolysaccharides and glycoproteins; glucuronic acid, also involved in the mucopolysaccharides and in detoxification reactions; galactose, a component of the glycolipids; and the disaccharide, lactose, secreted in milk.

AMINO ACIDS. The nonessential amino acids derive their carbon skeletons from glucose or its metabolites.

SYNTHESIS AND RELEASE OF GLUCOSE

The main and initial source of blood glucose is glycogen, after galactose and fructose conversions have been utilized. Liver glycogen is the first to be mobilized; then muscle glycogen may be converted to lactic acid and then to glucose by the liver. Even if all stores could be utilized, the total body glycogen could supply the body's energy requirements for only about 12 hours. The oxidation of fatty acids contributes indirectly by providing energy for the formation of carbohydrates from noncarbohydrate sources (*gluconeogenesis*). The glycerol component of lipids, about 10 percent of the total fat molecule, can be converted to glucose. The major contributor for the synthesis of carbohydrates from noncarbohydrates is the amino acid. About half of animal protein is capable of conversion to carbohydrate. The 14 amino acids that can be converted to carbohydrates are termed *glucogenic*. The major site of gluconeogenesis is the liver. Figure 4-10 presents a summary of carbohydrate metabolism.

FIG. 4-9. The Krebs or tricarboxylic cycle. This 10-step pathway is the final course that all nutrients involved in energy production must enter. It provides over 90 percent of the body's energy requirements. Acetylcoenzyme A (acetyl-CoA) and oxaloacetate combine to form citric acid; oxaloacetate provides the carbohydrate fuel to perpetuate the process. With each complete cycle, acetyl-CoA is degraded to energy, CO_2, and H_2O, plus another unit of oxaloacetate, and the cycle repeats itself. (From G. H. Schmid, *The Chemical Basis of Life: General, Organic, and Biological Chemistry for the Health Sciences.* Boston: Little, Brown, 1982.)

FIG. 4-10. The utilization of carbohydrates. (From R. T. Lagua, V. S. Claudio, and V. F. Thiele, *Nutrition and Diet Therapy* [2nd ed.]. St. Louis: Mosby, 1974.) Area within dashed lines occurs in bloodstream.

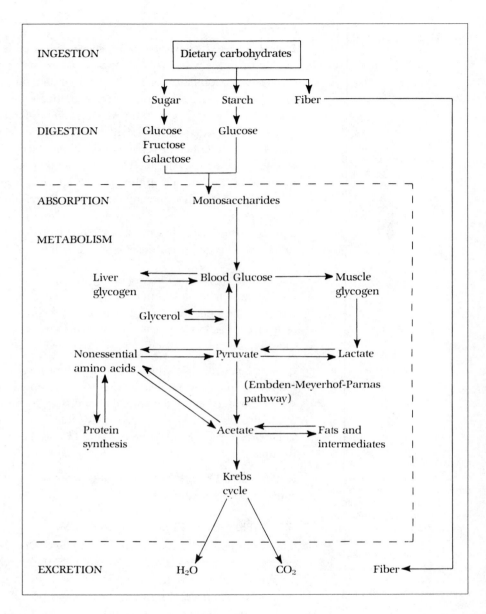

HORMONAL INFLUENCES ON CARBOHYDRATE METABOLISM

An increased concentration of blood glucose stimulates the release of *insulin*, the hormone produced by the beta cells of the islets of Langerhans in the pancreas. The only hormone known to lower the blood sugar level, insulin does so by facilitating synthesis of glycogen in the liver and muscles, inhibiting gluconeogenesis, aiding active transport of glucose across cell membranes, and promoting the conversion of glucose to fatty acids. Insulin shock or insulin reaction is the result of a very low blood sugar level caused by an overdose of insulin. Death

FIG. 4-11. Amino acids whose carbon chains can be utilized in the Krebs cycle for energy production.

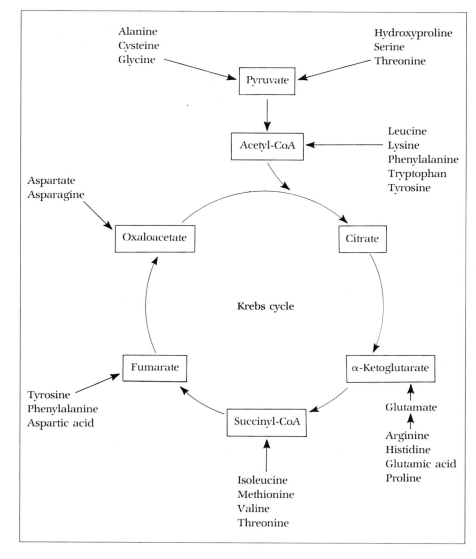

may occur if adequate glucose levels are not restored. Diabetes mellitus is thought to be caused by a deficiency of insulin.

Glucagon, another hormone secreted by the pancreas, increases the blood sugar level by stimulating the breakdown of glycogen in the liver. *Thyroid hormone* increases the rate of carbohydrate absorption from the gastrointestinal tract. The *steroid hormones* accelerate the catabolism of proteins, inducing glyconeogenesis. The *adrenocorticotropic hormones* (glucocorticoids, cortisol) are antagonistic to the action of insulin, thus preventing decreases in the blood sugar level. *Epinephrine* (adrenaline), which is released by the adrenal medulla during periods of stress, increases the rate of glycogen breakdown.

INTERRELATIONSHIP OF
CARBOHYDRATES, FATS,
AND PROTEINS

When any food, including carbohydrates, is supplied in the diet in excess of need, it is converted to fat and stored as such in the adipose tissue (lipogenesis). In the absence of adequate carbohydrate for energy production, fat and protein are mobilized from the body stores and metabolic pools, respectively. Without any dietary carbohydrates, as in uncontrolled diabetes mellitus, or when carbohydrates are not utilized effectively, fat (from dietary or fat depot sources) is the primary energy source. Fat is broken down to form active acetate (acetylcoenzyme A) and shorter-chain fatty acids, to be oxidized via the Krebs cycle to carbon dioxide and water. It is also broken down to glycerol and converted to glucose by the liver. In the absence of carbohydrate, fat is broken down so rapidly that the end products of incomplete fatty acid oxidation (ketones) accumulate. Since ketones are acidic, they disrupt the normal acid-base balance in the body, and acidosis develops (see Chaps. 5 and 10).

Proteins are also mobilized to provide energy when sufficient carbohydrate is lacking. The carbon chain of the protein molecule can be utilized in the Krebs cycle to produce energy (Fig. 4-11). Even a small amount of carbohydrate will spare protein from dietary or structural sources from being used for energy (*protein-sparing action of carbohydrates*). This effect is maximized if both protein and carbohydrate are ingested simultaneously.

References

1. Woodwell, G. M.   The energy cycle of the biosphere. *Sci. Am.* 223:124, 1970.
2. Paul, P. C.   Basic Scientific Principles: Sugars and Browning Reactions. In P. C. Paul and H. H. Palmer (eds.), *Food Theory and Applications.* New York: Wiley, 1972. P. 44.
3. Rosenau, J.   Food Processing. In F. Clydesdale (ed.), *Food Science and Nutrition.* Englewood Cliffs, N.J.: Prentice-Hall, 1979. P. 47.
4. Maillard, L. C.   Action des acides amines sur les sucres: Formation des mélanoidines par vois méthodique. *Compt. Rend.* 154:66, 1912.
5. Cori, C. F.   Mammalian carbohydrate metabolism. *Physiol. Rev.* 11:143, 1931.
6. Kretchmer, N.   Lactose and lactase. *Sci. Am.* 227:71, 1972.

Suggested Readings

Amerine, M. A.   Wine. *Sci. Am.* August 1964.
Biale, J. B.   The ripening of fruit. *Sci. Am.* May 1954.
Bolin, B.   The carbon cycle. *Sci. Am.* 223:124, 1970.
Bollenback, G. N.   Sugars in health. *Cereal Foods World* 26:213, 1981.
Brown, L. R.   Human food production as a process in the biosphere. *Sci. Am.* 223:160, 1970.
Crapo, P. A.   Sugar and sugar alcohols. *Contemp. Nutr.* December 1981.
Hutchinson, G. E.   The biosphere. *Sci. Am.* 223:44, 1970.
Inglett, G. E.   Sweeteners: A review. *Food Technol.* 35:37, 1981.
Luke, B.   Lactose intolerance during pregnancy: Significance and solutions. *Am. J. Mat. Child Nurs.* 2:92, 1977.
Olson, J. M.   The evaluation of photosynthesis. *Science* 168:438, 1970.
Oort, A. H.   The energy cycle of the earth. *Sci. Am.* 223:54, 1970.

Paige, D. M., and Bayless, T. M. (eds.). *Lactose Digestion: Clinical and Nutritional Implications.* Baltimore: Johns Hopkins University Press, 1981.

Pancoast, H. M., and Junk, W. R. *Handbook of Sugars* (2nd ed.). Westport, Conn.: AVI Publishing, 1980.

Sanderson, G. R. Polysaccharides in foods. *Food Technol.* 35:50, 1981.

Sipple, H. L., and McNutt, K. W. (eds.). *Sugars in Nutrition.* New York: Academic, 1974.

Torres, A., and Thomas, R. D. Polydextrose and its applications in foods. *Food Technol.* 35:44, 1981.

Chapter 5

LIPIDS

The lipid contained in natural foodstuffs is important not only as a carrier of fat-soluble vitamins and for its essential fatty acid content, but also as a dietary substance of high energy value. It serves as an immediate and potential energy source, superior to carbohydrate and protein in providing more energy per gram (9 calories per gram for lipid, versus 4 calories per gram each for carbohydrate and protein), and in its storage in an almost anhydrous (without water) state as adipose tissue in the body. Some deposits of lipids serve as insulating material in the subcutaneous tissues; others provide padding to protect internal organs. Some lipids are uniquely found in high concentrations in tissues of the nervous system; not much is known of their functions. Certain compounds derived from lipids provide vital components of biologically active agents, such as the essential fatty acid arachidonic acid from which the prostaglandins are made. Compounds of lipid and protein (lipoproteins) are important cellular constituents, occurring in the cell membrane, in the mitochondria within the cell, and as carriers of lipid in the blood.

Classification, Structure, and Bonding

The *lipids* constitute a heterogeneous group of organic compounds originating in living matter that are insoluble in water but soluble in nonpolar solvents such as alcohol, ether, benzene, and chloroform. Lipids contain one or more *fatty acids* (a hydrocarbon with a carboxyl group attached) in the molecule (Fig. 5-1). The physical and chemical properties of lipids are largely determined by the number of carbon atoms in the fatty acid component and the presence, number, and orientation of carbon-carbon double bonds. Over 40 fatty acids are found in nature, and most contain an even number of carbon atoms. Most plant lipids contain *monounsaturated* (one double bond) and *polyunsaturated* (more than one double bond) fatty acids, whereas most animal lipids are saturated (have no double bonds). Lipids may be classified as simple, compound, or derived, according to their structure and chemical composition.

NOMENCLATURE AND BONDING

A common nomenclature used in describing the number of carbon atoms in the carbon skeleton and the number of double bonds (degree of saturation) is to separate the two numbers by a colon. An example is butyric acid, $C_{4:0}$, with a four-carbon-atom skeleton and no double bonds. A summary of the common fatty acids, including the length of their carbon chains and number of double bonds, is given in Table 5-1.

SATURATED FATTY ACIDS

Saturated fatty acids are those in which all carbon atoms are linked to hydrogen so that only single bonds exist. Those with carbon skeletons less than 10 atoms long are liquids at room temperature; those with skeletons more than 10 atoms long are solids. *Palmitic acid* (C_{16}) is widely distributed in nature and is the most

FIG. 5-1. Fatty acid structure (saturated).

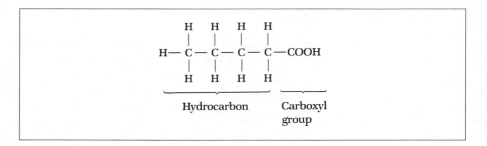

abundant saturated fatty acid in animal lipids, accounting for 10 to 50 percent of the total fatty acids in any fat. *Myristic acid* (C_{14}) and *stearic acid* (C_{18}) are also widespread saturated fatty acids; stearic is second only to palmitic in occurrence, present in up to 25 percent of beef fat. Shorter-chain and longer-chain saturated fatty acids (C_{12}, and up to C_{28}) do occur, but chains of 10 carbon atoms or less are rarely present in animal lipid. The saturated fatty acids are summarized in Table 5-2.

UNSATURATED FATTY ACIDS

Unsaturated fatty acids are those in which one or more double bonds exist within the carbon skeleton. Unsaturation alters certain properties of a fatty acid, including lowering its melting point and increasing its solubility in nonpolar solvents. All unsaturated fatty acids are liquids at room temperature. The two most abundant *monounsaturated* fatty acids found in nature are *oleic* and *pal-*

TABLE 5-1. Common fatty acids

Acid	Symbol
Saturated acids	
Butyric	$C_{4:0}$
Caproic	$C_{6:0}$
Caprylic	$C_{8:0}$
Capric	$C_{10:0}$
Lauric	$C_{12:0}$
Myristic	$C_{14:0}$
Palmitic	$C_{16:0}$
Stearic	$C_{18:0}$
Arachidic	$C_{20:0}$
Behenic	$C_{22:0}$
Monounsaturated acids	
Palmitoleic	$C_{16:1}$
Oleic	$C_{18:1}$
Erucic	$C_{22:1}$
Polyunsaturated acids	
Linoleic	$C_{18:2}$
Linolenic	$C_{18:3}$
Arachidonic	$C_{20:4}$

TABLE 5-2. Saturated fatty acids

Acid	Formula	Description
Acetic	CH_3COOH	Major end product of carbohydrate fermentation by rumen organisms
Propionic	C_2H_5COOH	An end product of carbohydrate fermentation by rumen organisms
Butyric	C_3H_7COOH	In certain fats in small amounts (especially butter); an end product of carbohydrate fermentation by rumen organisms
Caproic	$C_5H_{11}COOH$	Same as butyric
Caprylic (octanoic)	$C_7H_{15}COOH$	In small amounts in many fats (including butter), especially those of plant origin
Capric (decanoic)	$C_9H_{19}COOH$	Same as caprylic
Lauric	$C_{11}H_{23}COOH$	Spermaceti, cinnamon, palm kernel, coconut oils, laurels
Myristic	$C_{13}H_{27}COOH$	Nutmeg, palm kernel, coconut oils
Palmitic	$C_{15}H_{31}COOH$	Common in all animal and plant fats
Stearic	$C_{17}H_{35}COOH$	Same as palmitic
Arachidic	$C_{19}H_{39}COOH$	In peanut (arachis) oil
Behenic	$C_{21}H_{43}COOH$	In seeds
Lignoceric	$C_{23}H_{47}COOH$	In cerebrosides, peanut oil

Source: H. A. Harper, V. W. Rodwell, and P. A. Mayes, *Review of Physiological Chemistry* (17th ed.). Los Altos, Calif.: Lange, 1979. P. 113.

mitoleic acids. Oleic acid is the most widely distributed in nature, accounting for 30 percent or more of the total fatty acids. The *polyunsaturated* fatty acids, which contain more than one double bond, include *linoleic acid, linolenic acid,* and *arachidonic acid.* Linoleic acid, with two double bonds, occurs in many seed oils, including corn, peanut, cottonseed, and soybean. Linolenic acid, with three double bonds, is often found with linoleic acid, particularly in linseed oil. Arachidonic acid contains four double bonds and is found in small quantities with linolenic and linoleic acids, particularly in peanut oil. The percentage of various fatty acids in some common fats and oils is given in Table 5-3.

ESSENTIAL FATTY ACIDS

The polyunsaturated fatty acids cannot be synthesized in the body and are therefore considered *essential fatty acids.* Arachidonic acid may be made in the body if linoleic acid is supplied. Burr and Burr showed in 1929 [1] that there were essential acids for the growth and well-being of rats. They fed the animals a purified nonlipid diet with vitamins A and D added and observed a reduced growth rate, reproductive deficiency, scaly skin, necrosis of the tail, and lesions in the urinary tract. The deficiency syndrome was cured by the addition of linoleic, linolenic, and arachidonic acids to the diet.

TABLE 5-3. Fatty acids in fats and oils (approximate percentage of total fatty acids)

Fat or oil	Saturated (C_4–C_{12})	Myristic acid ($C_{14:0}$)	Palmitic acid ($C_{16:0}$)	Stearic acid ($C_{18:0}$)	Palmitoleic acid ($C_{16:1}$) and oleic acid ($C_{18:1}$)	Linoleic acid ($C_{18:2}$)	Other polyunsaturated fatty acids	Other fatty acids
Butter, cream, and milk	11	10	26	11	36	4	1[a]	0
Beef	0	3	29	21	44	2	0	0
Bacon and pork	0	1	26	12	50	10	0	0
Chicken	0	1	26	7	44	21	0	0
Fish oil	0	5	15	3	27	7	43[b]	0
Coconut oil	58	18	10	3	8	2	0	0
Palm oil	0	1	40	4	45	9	0	0
Cocoa butter	0	0	24	35	38	2	0	0
Rapeseed oil	0	0	3	1	16	14	9[a]	50[c]
Olive oil	0	0	13	3	71	10	0	0
Peanut oil	0	0	12	3	55	30	0	0
Sesame oil	0	0	9	5	40	43	0	0
Cottonseed oil	0	1	25	3	19	51	0	0
Corn oil	0	0	12	3	31	53	1	0
Soybean oil	0	0	10	4	24	53	7[a]	0
Sunflower seed oil	0	0	7	4	25	63	0	0
Safflower oil	0	0	7	2	15	72	0	0
Margarine	3	10	23	9	31	7	1	5[c]
Polyunsaturated margarine	2	1	12	8	22	52	1	0

[a] $C_{18:3}$ (linolenic).
[b] Long-chain polyunsaturated fatty acids (C_{20} and C_{22}).
[c] $C_{22:1}$ (erucic).
Source: Adapted from S. Davidson, et al., *Human Nutrition and Dietetics* (6th rev. ed.). Edinburgh: Churchill Livingstone, 1975. P. 76.

The functions of the essential fatty acids are diverse, but these substances are especially important in maintaining cell membrane structure and capillary wall integrity. Essential fatty acids are the structural lipids of the cell, including the mitochondrial membrane; they are also present in high concentrations in the reproductive organs. They occur in phospholipids and are required for the efficient transport and metabolism of cholesterol.

The deficiency syndrome has been produced in other experimental animals as well as in humans with diets restricted in essential fatty acids. In animals, the symptoms include poor growth, dermatitis, infertility, decreased resistance to stress, and impaired lipid transport. In humans, the skin symptoms and impaired transport have been noted. In humans consuming an ordinary diet no signs of deficiency have been reported, but infants receiving low-fat formulas have developed skin symptoms that were cured with the administration of linoleate. Also, in patients maintained for long periods on intravenous nutritional regimens (parenteral hyperalimentation), a deficiency of essential fatty acids has been reported. The prevention of a deficiency can be achieved by a very small intake of essential fatty acids, 1 to 2 percent of the total calories. Because this quantity is so easily obtained from most diets, deficiency symptoms are rarely seen. Currently there are no recommended dietary allowances for lipids or essential fatty acids.

REACTIONS OF THE DOUBLE BONDS

Unsaturated fatty acids may be hardened by the action of hydrogen in the presence of catalysts such as platinum, palladium, or nickel. This process, *hydrogenation*, converts unsaturated fatty acids into saturated fatty acids.

The double bonds of unsaturated fatty acids are also susceptible to *oxidation* by free radicals formed during metabolism or from exogenous agents. If a fatty acid is a part of a membrane when oxidized, oxidation results in the loss of some of the biologic properties of the membrane. This has been thought to be part of the process of aging. An *antioxidant*, a compound that accepts the free radical, thereby terminating the oxidation, is often used in food processing. The use of vitamin E as an antioxidant in vivo to minimize membrane damage by free radical oxidation, thereby slowing the aging process, has thus far been unsuccessful. (See Oxidative Rancidity on p. 90.)

IODINE NUMBER AND P/S RATIO

The ratio of dietary polyunsaturated to saturated fatty acids is often abbreviated as the *P/S ratio*. It has an influence on the serum cholesterol level and is therefore of interest in relation to coronary heart disease. The *iodine number*, another estimation of the degree of saturation, is the amount of iodine taken up by 100 gm of fat. It expresses the proportion of double-bond fatty acids in the chain: the higher the iodine number, the greater the degree of unsaturation (bonds available to react with the iodine). Coconut oil, composed mostly of saturated fatty acids, has an iodine number of 8 to 10; butter, 26 to 38; mutton tallow, 32 to 45; lard, 50 to 65; corn oil, 115 to 124.

ISOMERISM

Saturated or unsaturated fatty acids may be attached to a glycerol molecule. The unsaturated fatty acids may be in a linear conformation (*trans*) or bent at the position of the double bond (*cis*), as shown in Fig. 5-2. Unsaturated fatty acids exist naturally in the *cis* form, with their molecules bent back at each double bond. They cannot be packed closely together like the *trans* form and the long, straight chains of the saturated acids; hence the liquid state of unsaturated fatty acids and the solid state of saturated fatty acids. Polyunsaturated fatty acids in the *trans* form lack both essential fatty acid activity and the ability possessed by fatty acids in the *cis* form to lower the level of lipoproteins in the plasma.

CLASSIFICATION AND STRUCTURE

SIMPLE LIPIDS

Simple lipids are compounds of fatty acids with various alcohols. Fats, also termed *neutral fats*, are esters (compounds formed from an acid and an alcohol) of fatty acids with glycerol and are designated either monoacylglycerol, diacyl-

FIG. 5-2. *Cis* and *trans* isomerism. Unsaturated fatty acids have one or more rigid bends in the carbon backbone, contributed by the nonrotating double bond(s).

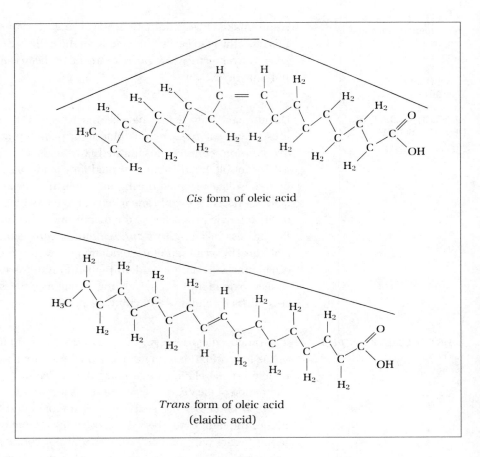

Cis form of oleic acid

Trans form of oleic acid
(elaidic acid)

glycerol, or triacylglycerol* depending on whether one, two, or three fatty acids are attached to the glycerol molecule. A molecule of water is lost at the addition of each fatty acid (Fig. 5-3). Triacylglycerols are the form in which fats chiefly occur, both in foodstuffs and in the fat deposits of most animals. Most fats consist not of a single triacylglycerol, but rather as a mixture. An *oil* is a fat in the liquid state. *Waxes* are fatty acid esters of alcohols other than glycerol. They are found in the cuticle of leaves and fruit and in secretions of insects, and may be mixed with very long chain hydrocarbons (C_{21-35}). They are of little importance to higher land animals or in human nutrition.

COMPOUND LIPIDS

Compound lipids are esters of fatty acids and glycerol combined with other chemical groups. *Phospholipids* are in this category. They contain phosphoric

---

*The International Union of Pure and Applied Chemistry (IUPAC) and the International Union of Biochemistry (IUB) have recently standardized terminology, designating monoglycerides, diglycerides, and triglycerides as monoacylglycerols, diacylglycerols, and triacylglycerols, respectively. The older terminology may still occasionally be used.

FIG. 5-3. The process of esterification (formation of monoacylglycerol). The solubility increases and the melting point decreases with a larger proportion of short-chain (less than 10 carbons) and un-saturated (double-bonded) fatty acid residues (R).

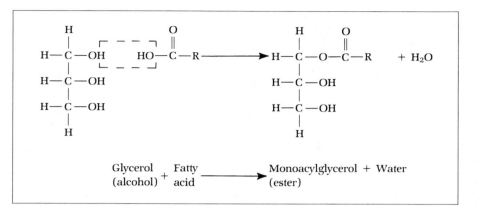

Glycerol (alcohol) + Fatty acid ⟶ Monoacylglycerol + Water (ester)

acid and a nitrogenous base in the place of one fatty acid radical. They are characterized by the large proportion of highly unsaturated fatty acids, including arachidonic acid, and constitute the next largest class of lipids in the body after triacylglycerols. As structural components of the cell wall and the mitochondria within the cells, the phospholipids are essential constituents of all living cells. They also function as metabolic intermediates in the transportation and utilization of fatty acids and constitute a readily mobilized and metabolized form of fatty acid reserve. *Glycophospholipids* are found mainly in the tissues and blood and, to a much lesser extent, in fat depots. They are part of the structure of cell membranes and transport fat within the body. *Lecithin* (phosphatidylcholine) is the main phospholipid in plasma. On hydrolysis, it yields choline, phosphoric acid, glycerol, and two molecules of fatty acid; choline is important in mobilizing fat from the liver. *Sphingomyelins*, composed of sphingosine, a complex amino alcohol, esterified with phosphorylcholine are found in large quantities in myelin sheaths in nerve tissue and in the brain. *Glycolipids*, including cerebrosides and gangliosides, are sphingosines complexed with galactose (a carbohydrate) and a high molecular weight fatty acid, with no phosphoric acid. They are important components of cell membranes found throughout the body. Other compound lipids include *sulfolipids*, *aminolipids*, and *lipoproteins*.

Specialized Structures and Compounds
LIPID BILAYERS

STRUCTURE

Most lipids are insoluble in water because of the predominance of nonpolar (hydrocarbon) groups. Fatty acids, some phospholipids, and sphingolipids contain a large proportion of polar groups, making them partly soluble in water and partly soluble in nonpolar solvents. These compounds (e.g., the phospholipid lecithin shown in Fig. 5-4) have an *amphipathic* structure, with a hydrophilic head and twin hydrophobic tails. The polar lipids become oriented at the interface of oil and water with the polar (hydrophilic) group in the water and the nonpolar (hydrophobic) group in the oil. A bilayer of polar lipids, as shown in

FIG. 5-4. The structure of lecithin. (Adapted from R. A. Capaldi, A dynamic model of cell membranes. *Sci. Am.* 230:26, 1974.)

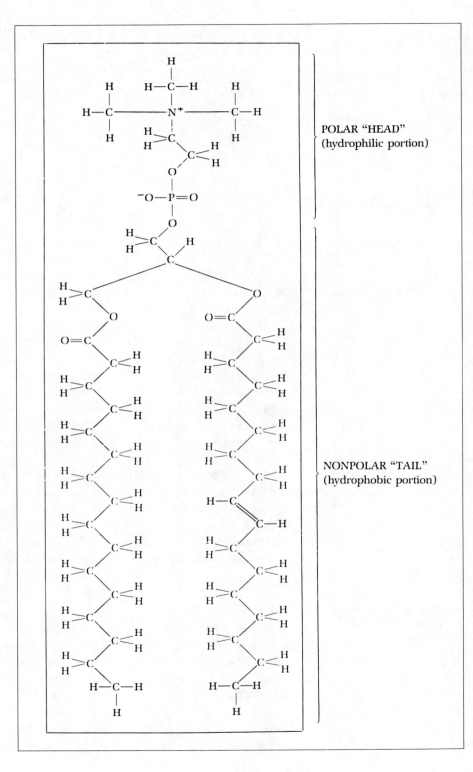

POLAR "HEAD" (hydrophilic portion)

NONPOLAR "TAIL" (hydrophobic portion)

FIG. 5-5. The structure of biologic membranes. This diagram shows a section of a bimolecular sheet formed by polar lipid molecules. (From G. H. Schmid, *The Chemical Basis of Life: General, Organic, and Biological Chemistry for the Health Sciences.* Boston: Little, Brown, 1982.)

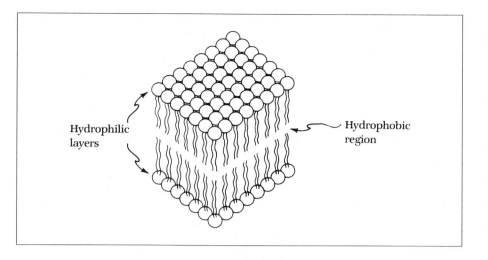

FIG. 5-6. Micelles
A. Diagram of a section of a micelle formed by polar lipid molecules.
B. Oil drop located in hydrophobic region of a micelle formed by soap molecules. Two micelles will not coalesce because of the repulsion between the negative charges on their surfaces. (From G. H. Schmid, *The Chemical Basis of Life: General, Organic, and Biological Chemistry for the Health Sciences.* Boston: Little, Brown, 1982.)

Fig. 5-5, is considered to be the basic structure of biologic membranes. When a certain concentration of polar lipids is reached, *micelles* are formed (Fig. 5-6A). Bilayers have self-healing properties.

SOAPS AND DETERGENTS

A *soap* is any salt of a long-chain fatty acid. The soaps of unsaturated fatty acids are more soluble in water than are those of saturated fatty acids. All detergents, including bile salts, contain both a hydrophobic (nonpolar) hydrocarbon structure and a hydrophilic (polar) group, as described above. The cleansing action of detergents and their ability to form stable emulsions depends on the trapping of lipid-soluble material in the interior of the hydrophobic portions of micelles (Fig. 5-6A). The formation of bile salts into micelles and the subsequent mixture

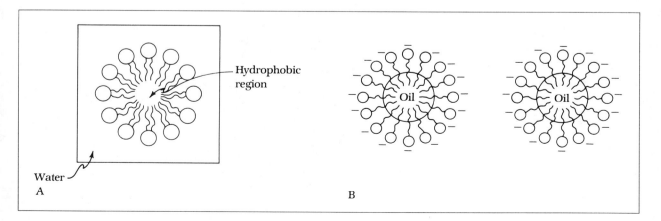

of these micelles with the products of fat digestion is important in the absorption of lipids from the intestine.

BIOLOGIC MEMBRANES

Cell membranes are the permeability barrier controlling the passage of water and solutes between the external and internal environments (e.g., between the intestinal lumen and the cells of the intestinal mucosa). The penetration of solutes is proportional to their solubility in lipids rather than to molecular size.

Singer and Nicolson [2] proposed the "fluid mosaic model" of the membrane—a mosaic of globular proteins in a phospholipid bilayer in a dynamic and fluid state. The hydrophilic portions of the layer are located on both surfaces in irregular coil configurations. The hydrophobic portions are within the membrane in the helical form. Two types of proteins are bound to the membranes: "peripheral" proteins, which can be removed without disturbing the integrity of the membrane; and "integral" proteins, extending into and through the membrane (Fig. 5-7). These proteins act as receptor sites for specific molecules or in the manufacture of substances needed by the cell.

STEROIDS

Members of this group of lipid compounds are derivatives of a completely saturated ring system, comprised of three cyclohexane rings in the nonlinear (phenanthrene) arrangement, and a terminal cyclopentane ring. This structure is shown in Fig. 5-8. All steroids are derived from the same basic ring structure; they are solid alcohols and as such can form esters with fatty acids. The large variety of steroid compounds can be grouped according to the number of carbon atoms at C-17. *Sterols* have compounds of 8 to 10 carbon atoms at C-17, with a total of 27 to 29 carbon atoms. The *bile acids* have 5 carbon atoms at C-17, with 24 carbons total. The *adrenocortical steroids* have 2 carbons at C-17, with 21

FIG. 5-7. The location of proteins in membranes. (From G. H. Schmid, *The Chemical Basis of Life: General, Organic, and Biological Chemistry for the Health Sciences.* Boston: Little, Brown, 1982.)

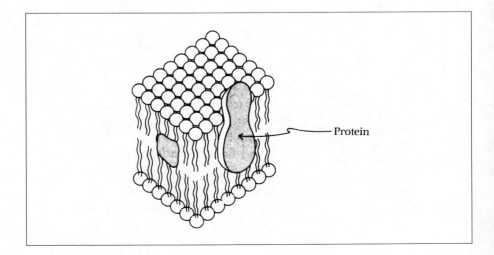

Protein

FIG. 5-8. Ring system of steroids. (A, B, C = phenanthrene; D = cyclopentane ring.)

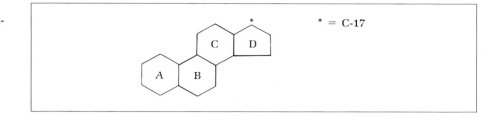

total, and the *estrogens* and *androgens* have no carbons at C-17, with 18 to 19 total.

STEROLS

Sterols are complex monohydroxyl alcohols found in both plants and animals. *Mycosterols*, the most important of which is *ergosterol*, are found in yeasts and fungus (ergot). Under the influence of ultraviolet light, ergosterol acquires antirachitic (antirickets) properties with the opening of ring B and conversion into vitamin D_2, ergocalciferol (Fig. 5-9). *Phytosterols* (plant sterols) include *sitosterol*, found in the oils of plants, especially wheat germ oil. *Cholesterol* is found only in animal tissue and is absent from foods of plant origin. It is a product of animal metabolism and is widely distributed in all cells of the body (see Cholesterol, below).

Cholesterol

Cholesterol is the only sterol in nature of any major significance in human nutrition. It is widely distributed, especially in nervous tissue, blood, and bile. It occurs both in the free form and esterified with fatty acids. Free cholesterol is the chief constituent of gallstones.

FUNCTIONS. The oxidation of cholesterol yields *7-dehydrocholesterol*, which possesses a conjugated pair of double bonds and is the sterol present in skin. When the skin is exposed to sunlight or ultraviolet radiation, the conjugated unsaturated B ring is ruptured, resulting in vitamin D_3 activity (Fig. 5-9). Cholesterol is also a precursor of bile salts and of the steroid adrenal and sex hormones.

Cholesterol facilitates the absorption of fatty acids from the intestine and their transport in the blood. By combining with the fatty acids to form cholesterol esters, they are made more soluble and emulsifiable than the fatty acid molecule alone.

METABOLISM. Found only in foods of animal origin, cholesterol is synthesized by the body. Acetic acid and acetoacetic acid are the precursors of the sterol molecule. They combine with coenzyme A and, through a long biosynthetic process, produce cholesterol. The major sites of cholesterol synthesis are the liver and intestinal mucosa. Active synthesis also occurs in the skin, muscle, heart,

FIG. 5-9. Cholesterol, ergosterol, and vitamin D.

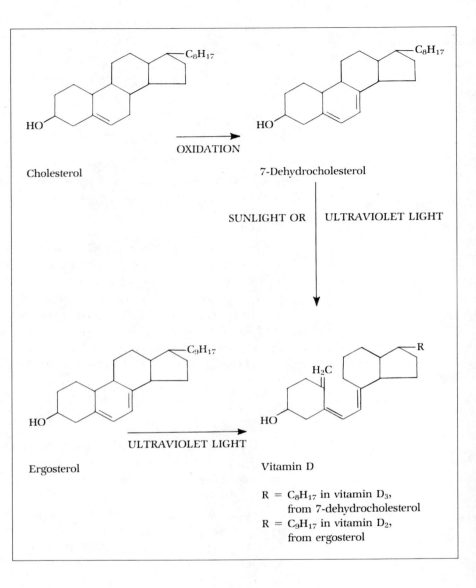

lungs, bone, spleen, red cells, kidneys, gonads, and adrenals. Cholesterol can also be synthesized by the arterial walls, as evidenced in atherosclerosis (see Chap. 40). These tissues produce their own supplies of cholesterol and draw on the plasma level only to a very limited extent. Synthesis and degradation occur simultaneously and continuously. The plasma level of cholesterol is influenced by the dietary intake and hepatic synthesis, as well as other factors that are still poorly understood, such as genetics. The rate of hepatic production (endogenous source) varies inversely with the dietary intake (exogenous supply). Hepatic synthesis is suppressed when the intake of dietary cholesterol is in-

TABLE 5-4. Changes in the plasma cholesterol level in selected diseases

Elevated (hypercholesterolemia)	Depressed (hypocholesterolemia)

1. Anemia due to acute hemorrhage	1. Anemia
	  a. Pernicious anemia
	  b. Hemolytic jaundice
	  c. Severe hypochromic anemia

2. Hypothyroidism	2. Hyperthyroidism

3. Hepatic and biliary tract disease
  a. Obstructive jaundice
  b. Biliary cirrhosis
	3. Hepatic disease (damage caused by)
	  a. Drugs
	  b. Hepatitis
	  c. Necrosis of the liver

4. Diabetes mellitus	4. Infection
5. Anesthesia (ether or chloroform narcosis)	5. Arthritis
6. Atherosclerosis	6. Celiac disease and sprue

	7. Terminal stages of disease
	  a. Congestive heart failure
	  b. Carcinoma
	  c. Acute pancreatitis
	  d. Pulmonary tuberculosis
	  e. Diabetes mellitus
	  f. Bacteremia, including bacterial endocarditis

creased. Generally, when the intake is very low, the plasma cholesterol level is even lower. Because the liver cell is the most important site in the formation of plasma cholesterol, impairment of liver cell function results in a decrease in total cholesterol levels. Table 5-4 outlines the changes in the plasma cholesterol levels in selected diseases.

Cholesterol is esterified in the intestinal wall, liver, and other tissues. The liver is the primary source of free cholesterol in the blood plasma, which is of particular importance in hepatic diseases. Free cholesterol released into the plasma forms part of the high-density lipoproteins. It can then be esterified and transferred to low-density lipoprotein moieties. These act as carrier vehicles for transporting cholesterol esters to the liver where free cholesterol is liberated. It can then be converted to bile acids (see below) or returned to the plasma to become part of the high-density lipoprotein.

CONVERSION AND EXCRETION. Cholesterol can be excreted through conversion to either neutral sterols or bile acids and release into the small intestine. About 10 to 20 percent of exogenous cholesterol is excreted as neutral sterols. Cholesterol is present in the liver and other tissues with small amounts of cholestanol (dihydrocholesterol). Together they are excreted through the intestinal wall and by the liver (in solution as micelles formed with bile salts and lecithin) into the small intestine. They mix with dietary cholesterol and may be partially reabsorbed from the lower ileum and recycled after a large meal; the unabsorbed portion is excreted in the feces. *Coprostanol*, the third neutral sterol, occurs in the feces as the result of the reduction of the double bond of cholesterol by bacteria in the intestines.

The remaining 80 to 90 percent of the exogenous cholesterol is converted by the liver to bile acids (cholic acid and derivatives) and excreted via the bile into the intestines. The majority of the bile acids are reabsorbed; the unabsorbed fraction is converted by intestinal bacteria into metabolites that are then excreted in the feces.

BILE ACIDS

The *bile acids* are steroids including *lithocholic acid, chenodeoxycholic acid, deoxycholic acid,* and *cholic acid,* the last of which is most abundant in human bile (Fig. 5-10). These acids are joined in amide linkages to the amino acids glycine and taurine as *glycocholic acid* and *taurocholic acid,* respectively. The salts of these conjugated bile acids are water soluble and are strong detergents.

ADRENOCORTICAL STEROIDS

Adrenocortical steroids include the glucocorticoids (e.g., cortisol), the mineralcorticoids (e.g., aldosterone), and the sex hormones (e.g., androstenedione) (Fig. 5-11). The adrenocorticotropic hormone (ACTH) stimulates adrenocortical hormone formation and results in a decrease in adrenal cholesterol content (see Cholesterol, p. 83).

ANDROGENS AND ESTROGENS

Androgens and *estrogens* include *testosterone,* synthesized in the testis, and *progesterone,* secreted by the ovary mainly from the corpus luteum (Fig. 5-12). Progesterone is essential for nidation (implantation) of the fertilized ovum and the maintenance of pregnancy. The cessation of its secretion at the end of the menstrual cycle triggers the onset of menstruation.

FIG. 5-10. Cholic and deoxycholic acids.

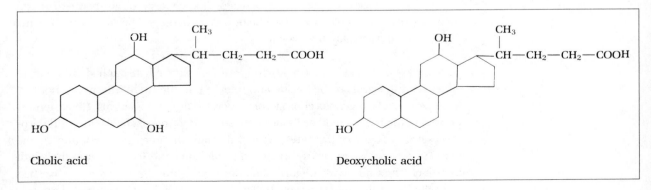

Cholic acid

Deoxycholic acid

FIG. 5-11. Corticosterone and aldosterone.

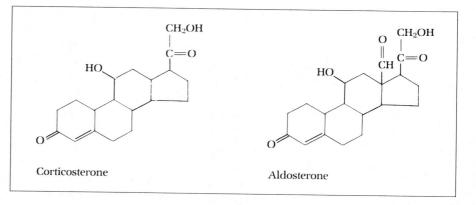

Corticosterone

Aldosterone

PROSTAGLANDINS

This group of fatty acid derivatives have a common structure containing 20 carbon atoms and are formed from essential fatty acids. Prostaglandins exhibit hormonelike activity and include some of the most potent biologically active substances known; they affect the nervous system, circulation, female reproductive organs, and metabolism.

They are produced, as needed, by the cell membrane. There is no storage reserve. The main source of the common essential fatty acid precursor, arachidonic acid, is the phospholipids, which constitute a principal component of the cell membrane. For this reason, it is thought that prostaglandins may play an important role in the regulation of membrane function.

Prostaglandins are agents for the regulatory functions of specialized cells. They regulate the activity of the smooth muscles of secretion, including endocrine gland secretions and blood flow. By stimulating contraction of the uterus, they induce labor at term or cause early termination of pregnancy. Because of this, they are used as agents for abortion and for inducing menstruation. Prostaglandins are present in amniotic fluid and in venous blood in women during labor

FIG. 5-12. Progesterone and testosterone.

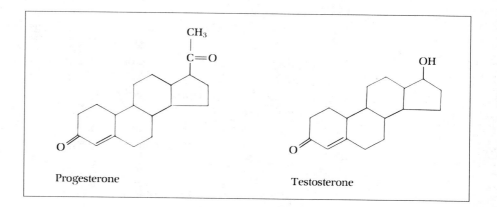

Progesterone

Testosterone

and play an important role after delivery by stimulating continued uterine contraction, clamping uterine vessels to prevent hemorrhage.

These substances can also inhibit gastric secretions (acid and pepsin) to prevent gastric and duodenal ulcers. Prostaglandins may serve to regulate gastric secretion under normal circumstances and thereby protect the stomach from ulceration. They relieve the symptoms of asthma by opening the airways to the lungs, improving the airflow by relaxing the smooth muscle of the bronchial tubes. By increasing the flow of urine and the excretion of sodium ions, prostaglandins regulate blood pressure. They can also relieve nasal congestion by widening the nasal passages by the constriction of blood vessels. Prostaglandins also influence the transmission of nerve impulses by blocking the release of norepinephrine in response to nerve stimulation (negative feedback mechanism).

Although the prostaglandins have a wide diversity of functions, their actions are nonspecific. While causing uterine smooth muscle to contract, they also cause gastrointestinal smooth muscle to contract as well, resulting in cramping and diarrhea.

Fats in Foods

Fats are mixtures of lipids and are present naturally in many foods. In the form of salad oils, frying fats, and shortenings, fats are commonly used in food preparation. In addition to contributing flavor, they enhance smoothness and texture, aid in emulsification, tenderize and aerate batter and dough, and serve as a heating medium. Some lipid-rich foods will be discussed at length in several chapters in Section III, so only foods that contain mostly fat will be covered here. The fat content of representative foods is given in Table 5-5.

ANIMAL FATS

Butter is made from the butterfat separated from cream by mechanical agitation (churning) or centrifugation. The churning process reverses the oil-in-water emulsion to a water-in-oil emulsion. According to federal regulations, butter must contain at least 80 percent butterfat; the other constituents include water, salt, and some natural components of milk. Butter is pasteurized to inactivate lipase and to destroy most of the organisms present. Butter contains both saturated and unsaturated fatty acids, about 60 percent and 40 percent, respectively. Oleic and linoleic acids are the most prevalent unsaturated fatty acids. Butterfat is the richest known natural source of butyric acid.

Lard, manufactured from the fatty tissue of hogs, varies in composition and general characteristics according to the type of feed. The fat is heat-rendered, with or without moisture, to separate it out and then modified by any of several methods, including bleaching, hydrogenation, and the addition of an emulsifier or antioxidant.

PLANT FATS

Margarine, made to simulate butter, is prepared by blending vegetable oils that have been hydrogenated to the desired consistency with pasteurized and cul-

TABLE 5-5. Fat content of representative foods

Percentage fat	Food
90–100	Salad and cooking oils, cooking fats, lard
80–90	Butter, margarine
70–80	Mayonnaise, pecans, macadamia nuts
50–70	Walnuts, dried unsweetened coconut meat, almonds, bacon, baking chocolate
30–50	Broiled choice T-bone and porterhouse steaks, spareribs, broiled pork chops, goose, cheddar and cream cheeses, potato chips, French dressing, chocolate candy
20–30	Choice pot roast, broiled choice lamb chop, frankfurters, ground beef, chocolate chip cookies
10–20	Broiled choice round steak, broiled veal chops, roast turkey, eggs, avocados, olives, chocolate cake with icing, French fried potatoes, ice cream, apple pie
1–10	Pork and beans, broiled cod, halibut, haddock, broiled chicken, crab meat, cottage cheese, beef liver, milk, cream soups, sherbet, most breakfast cereals
Less than 1	Baked potato, most vegetables and fruits, egg whites, consommé

Source: From G. E. Damon, *FDA Consumer.* February 1975 (HEW Publication No. 75-2026).

tured skim milk, salt, emulsifiers, preservatives, and color. Vitamins A and D may also be added, as may diacetyl for butter flavor and ground soybeans as part of the nonfat solids. Originally developed by the French chemist Mège-Mouries in 1869, margarine was manufactured to fill the butter shortage produced during the Franco-Prussian War. Like butter, margarine contains about 80 percent fat.

Vegetable oils are obtained from the seeds of corn, cotton, soybeans, and peanuts. The seeds are cleaned, hulled as needed, and then crushed; the oil is removed by solvent extraction, application of pressure, or a combination of methods. Olive oil is of two varieties: "virgin oil," which is expressed first under light pressure and not further refined; and "pure olive oil," which is solvent-extracted from the residue and pit kernels. Coconut oil is pressed from the dried pulp of the coconut. Vegetable oils undergo further processing to remove color pigments, free fatty acids, and odor-causing compounds. Some oils also are *winterized* to allow them to remain liquid during refrigeration. First the oil is chilled; then the solids are removed by filtration. Packaging vegetable oils in darkened glass containers protects them from light and reduces rancidity.

Vegetable shortenings are made by hydrogenating refined vegetable oils and then adding a monoglyceride-diglyceride emulsifier. The shortening is then chilled and whipped.

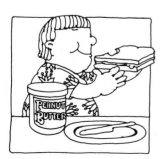

Peanut butter is made by grinding roasted peanuts and adding salt. Because of its high fat content (about 50%), it can sometimes be used as a substitute for other fats in cooking and baking.

**Digestion and
Metabolism**
ALTERATIONS IN FATS BY
COOKING AND OTHER
PROCESSES

MELTING POINT

The temperature at which a solid is changed to a liquid is its *melting point*. In fats, the melting point depends on the proportion of the fat that is present in the crystalline state. This proportion is influenced by several internal factors: (1) chain length, (2) degree of saturation of the component fatty acids, and (3) configuration at the double bonds of unsaturated fatty acids. Most oils are liquids at room temperature because of their high concentrations of unsaturated fatty acids. The melting point increases with increasing chain length and with increasing degree of saturation.

HYDROLYTIC RANCIDITY

During hydrolysis, the ester linkage between glycerol and fatty acid is broken, and one molecule of water is added (the reverse of the process shown in Fig. 5-3). Lipases, enzymes naturally present in such foods as nuts, whole grains, butterfat, and other fatty foods, catalyze lipid hydrolysis during storage. The accumulation of free fatty acids results in an off-flavor, termed *rancidity*. It is especially noticeable in foods such as butter that contain a high concentration of short-chain fatty acids, which are volatile at room temperature.

This same reaction, resulting in the accumulation of free fatty acids, occurs when frying fat is used repeatedly. Heat is the catalyst, and water is supplied from the moisture in the foods being fried. When fat is overheated, glycerol, freed by lipid hydrolysis, decomposes through dehydration. The decomposition product, *acrolein*, is a volatile, irritating compound in the acrid fumes emanating from overheated fat.

OXIDATIVE RANCIDITY (AUTO-OXIDATION)

The oxygen in air can combine with the double bond in unsaturated fatty acids to form a highly reactive peroxide linkage. Once initiated, this chain reaction is self-perpetuating. The reaction, catalyzed by light and metals, results in an off-flavor and rancidity. Excluding oxygen (by vacuum packaging) and light and reducing the catalytic activity of metal contaminants by the use of chelating substances or sequestrants are used commercially to prevent this spoilage. The use of antioxidants delays the process; some antioxidants occur naturally in lipid-containing foods, e.g., tocopherols (vitamin E) in vegetable oils. The antioxidant combines with the peroxide radical, terminating the process.

HYDROGENATION

The processing of highly unsaturated lipids with hydrogen under pressure and in the presence of a catalyst (usually nickel) results in the saturation of the carbon-carbon double bonds, known as *hardening*. This is the most common commercial method of converting liquid fats of plant origin into solid fats, such as lard substitutes, margarines, and solid shortenings. Some of the fatty acids are converted from the *cis* to the *trans* form by this process but can still be utilized by the body. The content of the essential fatty acid linoleic acid is reduced by this process. Excessive hardness would result from complete hydrogenation, so the process is carried only far enough to produce the desired consistency.

EMULSIFICATION

Fats are capable of forming *emulsions,* a liquid-in-liquid dispersion. This property is utilized in the homogenation of milk and the production of butter, ice cream, and mayonnaise. Lecithins, which contain glycerol, fatty acids, phosphoric acid, and choline, are often added in the processing of foods to facilitate emulsification. This ability of fats is also essential to their proper digestion and absorption.

DIGESTION

Fat is not digested in the stomach because the conditions there are not suitable for emulsification, which must precede digestion. Fat actually slows the emptying of the stomach, imparting a feeling of satiety after a meal rich in this substance. The inhibitory action on the stomach has been attributed to the hormone *enterogastrone* released when dietary fat enters the duodenum.

Most of dietary lipid is in the form of triacylglycerols and must be *emulsified* before digestion and absorption can occur. Conditions are suitable in the duodenum, where three substances together are needed to break down fat adequately: bile salts, fatty acids, and monoacylglycerols liberated by pancreatic lipases. *Lipases* hydrolyze triacylglycerol to fatty acids and glycerol. Since these enzymes require near-neutral pH, they are essentially inactive in the acidic environment of the stomach. Gastric lipase may be more important in infancy, since the gastric pH is higher and since the lipid of milk occurs in a highly emulsified state that facilitates attack by the water-soluble enzyme.

Lipid digestion occurs mainly in the small intestine. In the duodenum, the lipids come in contact with bile and pancreatic juice. Bile promotes the emulsification and solubilization of lipids through the action of the bile salts. Since lipids are insoluble in water, the enzymatic hydrolysis occurs only at the interface between the lipid droplet and the aqueous environment. The rate of hydrolysis is influenced by the area of the interface and the amount of emulsification. Pancreatic juice and bile are alkaline and help to neutralize the acidic gastric chyme. In the neutral environment of the duodenal lumen, the bile acids (mostly taurocholic and glycocholic acids) act as emulsifying agents, or detergents. Their action, combined with the churning of peristalsis, breaks down dietary lipid into progressively finer particles, facilitating hydrolysis. The products of the partial hydrolysis of fat, the soaps and monoacylglycerols, also act as detergents, supplementing the action of the bile salts.

The presence of gastric chyme in the duodenum triggers the hormonally controlled flow of pancreatic juice. An inactive precursor, or zymogen, of lipase becomes active in the intestinal lumen after a *colipase* (molecular weight 10,000) binds to it in the presence of bile salts. This lowers the optimal pH for enzymatic activity from 9 to 6. Pancreatic lipase splits neutral fats (triacylglycerols) into monoacylglycerols, diacylglycerols, glycerols, and fatty acids. Calcium ions in the small intestine have an accelerating effect on the rate of hydrolysis by pancreatic lipase. By forming insoluble soaps with liberated fatty acids, calcium prevents their inhibiting action on the enzyme, thus aiding hydrolysis. In addition to lipase, a group of *esterases*, including cholesterol esterase, are also present in the pancreatic juice. These enzymes preferentially catalyze the hydrolysis of short-chain fatty acid esters, as well as other fatty acid esters. Another zymogen produced by the pancreas is prophospholipase A, which is activated to phospholipase A in the presence of bile salts and calcium ions. This enzyme liberates lysophosphatidylcholine from lecithin (phosphatidylcholine). Lysophosphatidylcholine's detergent action aids in the emulsification of dietary lipids. Lecithin is present in the bile, contributing both precursors of lysophosphatidylcholine and other detergents. The resulting mixture of free fatty acids, monoacylglycerols, diacylglycerols, and triacylglycerols, emulsified by the bile salts and the soaps themselves, is then presented to the microvilli of the mucous membrane of the small intestine for absorption.

ABSORPTION

Fatty acids and monoacylglycerols pass as micelles into the cells of the mucous membrane, where further hydrolysis takes place. Within the cell, monoacylglycerol lipase continues the breakdown, and long-chain fatty acids (greater than 14 carbons) undergo reesterification into new triacylglycerols, partly characteristic of the animal species. During absorption, the resynthesis of triacylglycerol is accompanied by protein synthesis required for the formation of the lipoproteins of the *chylomicrons*, particles ranging from 0.1 to 0.6 μm in diameter. Chylomicrons provide the main transport vehicle for lipids from the alimentary canal. They are composed chiefly of triacyglycerols, with about 2% protein and small amounts of phospholipid and cholesterol. Because lipids are not soluble in water, they are carried in the blood attached to proteins as lipoproteins; these include chylomicrons, low-density and high-density lipoproteins, and free fatty acids bound to albumin. From the lymphatics of the small intestines, via the thoracic duct, the chylomicrons enter the systemic circulation via the right subclavian vein. Liberated glycerol and short-chain and medium-chain fatty acids (less than 14 carbons), because of their greater hydrophilic character, are absorbed in nonesterified form and pass directly to the liver via the portal vein. Of all the common dietary lipids, only those found in milk are rich in short-chain fatty acids; this is an important factor in infant nutrition. Generally, lipids that are liquid at body temperature are easily digested and absorbed. Lipids that melt above body temperature are poorly digested and absorbed, and fatty acids that are solids above body temperature will not be well absorbed unless combined with lipids that melt at lower temperatures. Ninety-five percent of most dietary fats are digested and absorbed by adults in quantities up to 100 gm per day. Greater quantities may also be as efficiently absorbed if the body is in need of additional energy. Under conditions of extreme cold or strenuous labor or exercise, diets high in fats provide the needed concentrated calories.

Chylomicrons enter and are cleared from the blood at about the same rate that they are formed in the intestinal wall. After the consumption of a large amount of fat, the plasma becomes milky with lipoproteins, with a maximum rise 2 to 4 hours after the meal. Because chylomicrons contain only a small amount of phospholipid and cholesterol, the plasma concentration of these lipids is raised only slightly by a fatty meal. The triacylglycerols are split from the chylomicrons by lipoprotein lipases in adipose tissue and muscle. The remaining components of the chylomicron are then taken up by the liver.

Bile acids do not enter the lymphatic circulation despite their association with lipid during its passage across the mucosal barrier. They are confined to the enterohepatic circulation, entering the portal blood, where they are removed by the liver and returned with the bile into the duodenum. Very little is lost from this recycling process, with only about 200 mg per day appearing in the feces.

MALABSORPTION

If bile is absent from the intestinal tract, as a result of severe liver dysfunction or biliary obstruction, lipid absorption is acutely impaired. The total lipid content of the feces is elevated, mostly as insoluble calcium salts of fatty acids. Together with the absence of bile pigments, these soaps result in characteristic "clay-colored" stools. The presence of more than 7 gm of fat daily in the feces indicates fat malabsorption and the diagnosis of *steatorrhea*. Excessive lipid in the stools may be the result of three types of imbalances: a deficiency of bile, a deficiency of pancreatic juice, or a defect in the intestinal mucosa. If fat malabsorption is caused by biliary insufficiency, it can be recognized by the presence of excessive amounts of digested but unabsorbed lipids in the stool, mostly in the form of soaps, as well as by the characteristic lack of bile pigment. Biliary insufficiency may result from obstruction of the biliary passages caused by a stone or neoplasm or severe diffuse liver disease. Steatorrhea as the result of pancreatic insufficiency is characterized by excessive amounts of undigested triacylglycerol in the stool. This type of steatorrhea occurs with cystic fibrosis of the pancreas or may result after total pancreatectomy. The third type of imbalance, steatorrhea caused by a failure of the active absorptive processes in the intestinal mucosa, is seen in children with celiac disease and adults with sprue. The lipid is predominately in the form of soaps. Because of their greater hydrophilic character, medium-chain triacylglycerols (MCT), especially those with chains 8 to 10 carbons long, are well digested and absorbed in the absence of bile salts. MCT are hydrolyzed more easily by pancreatic lipase than are other triacylglycerols and, once absorbed, go directly to the liver via the portal vein as fatty acids. For these reasons, they are often utilized in the diet therapy for malabsorption syndromes (see Chap. 38).

Other lipid-soluble substances may also be poorly absorbed. Signs of vitamin K deficiency in patients with biliary disease are promptly relieved by the oral administration of bile salts or by an injection (parenteral administration) of vitamin K. This is an especially important consideration when surgery is planned for these patients, since adequate vitamin K is vital to normal blood-clotting mechanisms.

PLASMA LIPIDS AND
LIPOPROTEINS

STRUCTURE

Supplying lipid to tissues as an energy source presents the problem of transporting a large quantity of hydrophobic material (lipid) in an aqueous environment. Nature's solution is to associate the more insoluble lipids with more polar ones such as phospholipids and then combine them with cholesterol and protein to form a hydrophilic lipoprotein complex. Many types of lipids are transported in the blood as lipoproteins: Triacylglycerols derived from intestinal absorption of fat or from the liver are transported in the blood as *chylomicrons* and *very low density lipoproteins* (VLDL); fat released from adipose tissue is in the form of free fatty acids bound to *albumin*; phospholipids are transported as *high-density lipoproteins* (HDL); cholesterol is carried as *low-density lipoproteins* (LDL).

The protein moiety of lipoproteins, known as the *apoprotein*, accounts for as much as 60 percent in some HDL and as little as 1 percent of chylomicrons. The larger lipoproteins, such as chylomicrons and VLDL, have a nonpolar lipid core surrounded by a more polar phospholipid, cholesterol, and apoproteins that make it soluble in the aqueous plasma.

CONCENTRATIONS

After a meal (postabsorptive state), normal blood plasma contains about 500 mg of total lipid per 100 ml. About 25 percent, or 125 mg, is triacylglycerol. Over 180 mg, or about 36 percent, is cholesterol. Two-thirds of the cholesterol is esterified with fatty acids and one-third is present as free sterol. An additional 32 percent, or 160 mg, of phosphoglycerides, including phosphotidylcholine, are also present. Free fatty acids bound to albumin account for 8 to 30 mg, or from 2 to 6 percent.

The concentration of cholesterol in plasma in healthy adults ranges from 140 to 300 mg per 100 ml. From this figure a good approximation of the LDL concentration can also be made, since cholesterol is carried in LDL. Plasma triacylglycerol concentration reflects VLDL, unless dietary fat has been consumed in the past few hours. Normal fasting levels of triacylglycerols range from 25 to 150 mg per 100 ml. Saturated fatty acids, especially $C_{14:0}$ and $C_{16:0}$, raise the plasma cholesterol concentration. Polyunsaturated fatty acids, both essential and others, tend to lower plasma cholesterol and triacylglycerol concentrations. See Chap. 40 for the classification and treatment of the cardiovascular diseases.

CLEARING FACTORS

Shortly after the absorption of fats, the mesenteric and thoracic lymph channels become distended with a milky fluid rich in triacylglycerols. Simultaneously, the discharge of chylomicrons into the venous blood results in a milky opalescence. An increased amount of lipid in the blood is termed *lipemia*; that which transiently follows the ingestion of fat, *absorptive lipemia*. *Lipoprotein lipases* in the blood appear during lipemia and catalyze the hydrolysis of triacylglycerols in chylomicrons and in lipoproteins. These enzymes are potent only in the presence of specific activating proteins (the high-density and very low density fractions) and acceptors of the liberated fatty acids (e.g., albumin). These free fatty acids, representing less than 5 percent of the total fatty acid present in the plasma, are metabolically the most active of the plasma lipids.

Lipoprotein lipases are also present in other tissues, including the heart, lungs, and adipose tissue. The enzymes are found in the capillary endothelium of these extrahepatic tissues and liberate free fatty acids before they can be assimilated. Within the tissues, free fatty acids are reesterified to triacylglycerol or oxidized as fuel. On hydrolysis, triacylglycerol yields fatty acids and glycerol, both of which are released into the plasma; the free fatty acids are bound to albumin. The liver, heart, kidneys, muscle, lungs, testes, brain, and adipose tissue can oxidize long-chain fatty acids and therefore utilize them as an energy source. The brain, however, cannot extract them from the blood. The liver, kidneys, intestine, lactating mammary glands, and brown adipose tissue (p. 98) can also utilize glycerol because of significant quantities of the necessary activating enzyme, *glycerol kinase,* present in their tissues.

HEPATIC METABOLISM

FATTY ACID INTERCONVERSIONS

The liver synthesizes triacylglycerols from fatty acids mobilized from adipose tissue, fatty acids derived from chylomicron remnants, and from carbohydrate entering from the intestine. Fatty acids are also obtained from the diet and from lipogenesis (the formation of lipid) by acetylcoenzyme A (acetyl-CoA) derived from carbohydrates and certain amino acids, although the primary source of carbon for the synthesis of fatty acids is carbohydrate. Glucose is the main source when the diet is rich in carbohydrates; during starvation and between meals, fatty acids are supplied from adipose tissue; and after a fatty meal, chylomicrons are utilized. When the caloric intake is in the form of fatty acids, they are deposited in adipose tissue as triacylglycerols. Fatty acids in the diet show a wide variation in the degree of saturation and chain length. Lipogenesis favors the formation of saturated over unsaturated fatty acids. A high carbohydrate diet will cause a "hardening" effect on depot lipid (adipose tissue fat), because of the more rapid synthesis of saturated than of unsaturated fatty acids.

The fatty acids produced by the liver are a composite that is both characteristic of the species and a reflection of the diet. This composite is achieved through the shortening and elongation of the carbon chain as well as the introduction of double bonds and their elimination by reduction. The shortening or lengthening of the carbon skeleton occurs by the gain or loss of two carbon atoms at a time. Saturation, the introduction of a double bond, may occur by anaerobic or aerobic pathways. Desaturation and elongation reactions occur primarily in the liver; fasting and diabetes mellitus inhibit this process. The availability of the initial substrate for fatty acid synthesis, acetyl-CoA, is increased by diets high in carbohydrate. The formation of acetyl-CoA from pyruvate is irreversible, making a net formation of fatty acids into carbohydrate impossible. In other words, it is not possible to form glucose from the breakdown of fatty acids. Under normal conditions, the synthesis and oxidation of fatty acids occur simultaneously, although at different rates.

LIPOTROPIC FACTORS

Fat leaves the liver as VLDLs, which, like the chylomicrons, are rich in triacylglycerols and have a high rate of turnover. The LDLs are derived from the intravascular degradation of VLDLs. Under normal circumstances, the liver contains only about 5 to 7 percent fat. As the result of poisons, disease, or certain dietary conditions, as much as 50 percent of the liver may be fat. This fatty infiltration results from a failure of the liver to dispose of endogenous lipids. Choline, part of lecithin, the principal phospholipid in the plasma lipoproteins, acts as a lipotropic factor, meaning it is capable of preventing this accumulation of fat. Choline is not a dietary essential and can be synthesized in the body in the presence of methyl (CH_3) groups supplied by the amino acid *methionine*. Most foods of animal origin supply choline, and most animal proteins contain methionine. The two most important dietary factors in the development of fatty liver are an excessive intake of ethyl alcohol and kwashiorkor (protein malnutrition). In the former, an increased hepatic synthesis of fatty acids is the cause; in the latter, insufficient amino acids for lipoprotein synthesis is the major abnormality [3] (see Chap. 34).

KETOSIS

Fatty acids are oxidized into two-carbon units complexed with *acetyl-CoA*. Two molecules of acetyl-CoA condense to form *acetoacetic acid*, which diffuses through the hepatic cell membranes to peripheral tissues, where it is reconverted to acetyl-CoA by dehydration and oxidized as an energy source.

From acetoacetic acid *acetone* is formed by chemical breakdown and *beta-hydroxybutyric acid* by enzymatic reduction. These three compounds are collectively termed *ketone* bodies and can readily be oxidized in muscle as fuel. Small numbers of ketone bodies are normally present in the blood and urine; *ketosis* results from excessive production of acetoacetic acid by the liver. Acetyl-CoA, formed in the liver, can be hydrogenated and utilized in lipid synthesis (anabolic pathway); it can be oxidized to oxaloacetic acid and pass into the tricarboxylic acid (Krebs) cycle, in which it is used as a source of energy (catabolic pathway); or it can be hydrolyzed and released into the blood, producing ketosis (hydrolytic pathway). The hepatic balance between the anabolic, catabolic, and hydrolytic enzymes competing for the available acetyl-CoA is delicate; ketosis results when the balance is in favor of the hydrolytic process.

In the absence of adequate carbohydrate to meet energy needs, as in fasting, starvation, and uncontrolled diabetes mellitus, the hepatic oxidation of triacylglycerols and production of acetoacetic acid exceeds the oxidative abilities of the peripheral tissues, so that excessive amounts of ketone bodies build up in the blood. The kidneys are not able to reabsorb all the ketone bodies; those excreted represent a loss of energy from the body. Because they are acids, ketone bodies must be excreted in the urine combined with a base, usually a sodium cation. This leads to a depletion of sodium and, later, of potassium, calcium, and other minerals as well. This also causes a depletion of the body's available base and results in *acidosis*, a lowering of the pH of the body fluids. The adverse effects of ketosis are secondary to the resulting severe acidosis. If unchecked, this condition can be fatal. If even a small amount of carbohydrate is present, 15 percent or more of the energy utilized, or 100 gm per day, ketosis does not occur. In diabetes mellitus, the administration of insulin slows the breakdown of lipid and restores carbohydrate metabolism to normal.

ADIPOSE TISSUE

Body lipid represents the body's largest reservoir of potential chemical energy, present in far greater quantities than available carbohydrate and in the most concentrated form in which energy can be stored. This form is ideal for mobile organisms: It has a high energy density and is in a relatively water-free state, compared with the heavily hydrated carbohydrate, which is stored with almost an equal weight of water, and which yields half the calories per gram as lipid. Body lipid is available in periods of restricted nutrition for the continuous energy-requiring processes necessary for the maintenance of life.

FUNCTIONS

The major portion of mammalian lipid is located subcutaneously (beneath the skin) and acts as an efficient insulator against excessive heat loss to the environment. This is exemplified in marine mammals, whose environments are both colder than body temperature and far better thermal conductors than air. In whales, this layer of fat serves two purposes: As a thick and continuous layer of subcutaneous tissue, *blubber*, it reduces heat losses to the environment; the depot of highly specialized lipid, *spermaceti*, allows the sperm whale to deliver blows of great force with its head.

STRUCTURE AND COMPOSITION

At least 10 percent of the body weight in the normal mammal is lipid, the majority of which is triacylglycerol. This lipid is found in all organs, as well as in certain depots of specialized connective tissue, the *adipose tissue*, where a large portion of the cytoplasm of the cells is replaced by droplets of lipid. Adipose tissue is composed of mesenchymal connective tissue cells (*adipocytes*). Stored within each is a single droplet of triacylglycerol. Protein accounts for about 2 percent and water about 10 percent of adipose tissue as cellular material and supporting tissue; the remaining 85 to 88 percent is fat (triacylglycerol). Adipose tissue is supplied by a capillary network as well as neuronal innervation from the autonomic nervous system. The lipid found in depots is richer in saturated fatty acids than that found in liver. Depot lipid is in the liquid state and is as saturated as possible. Since the more saturated the lipid the more energy is yielded during oxidation, it appears that depot lipid is the type richest in potential chemical energy while still remaining fluid at body temperature.

The composition of various adipose depots (chiefly triacylglycerol) is similar, regardless of anatomic location. Variations in the composition within a species may be induced by extremes of diet or of temperature. The composition reflects the origins of the fatty acids, from dietary lipids as well as carbohydrates. Prolonged feeding of diets rich in polyunsaturated fats leads to major increases in the unsaturated fatty acid content of the adipose tissue. The change in the composition may be seen earlier if the depot lipid is first depleted by a period of fasting followed by a diet rich in lipid of different physical properties from the original lipid.

METABOLISM

Lipid is transported to adipose tissue from the liver as VLDL or prebetalipoproteins and directly from the intestine as chylomicrons. At the luminal surface of the capillary endothelial cells of the adipose tissue, the triacylglycerols are hydrolyzed by lipoprotein lipases. The liberated free fatty acids then cross the endothelial cells into the adipose tissue cells. Once within the cells, the fatty acids are resynthesized into triacylglycerols. The assimilation and storage by adipose tissue is accomplished by its ability to abstract the fatty acids of triacylglycerol and free fatty acids from the circulation. The metabolism of carbohydrate enhances the process of esterification by supplying glycerol from glucose. The formation of fat by adipose tissue is chiefly controlled by the availability of insulin. This hormone increases the uptake of glucose by adipose tissue.

Depot lipid is in a continuous state of mobilization and deposition, with the total quantity being the result of the rates of these two processes. These rates are influenced by the amount of energy supplied at the last meal, the immediate energy needs of the tissues, and the amount of muscular activity. Adipose tissue has two major metabolic functions: to assimilate carbohydrate and lipids and their intermediates for fat synthesis and storage and to mobilize lipid as free fatty acids and glycerol. The regulation of appetite appears to be a control in the long-term balance of depot lipid, so that the total lipid content of the body does not change rapidly.

BROWN FAT

In many species of animals, another type of adipose tissue, containing high concentrations of glycogen (the storage form of carbohydrate) and a brown pigment, further helps them to adapt to exposure to cold. In addition to having the properties of regular adipose tissue, this specialized type of fat, termed *brown fat*, is metabolically active and functions in heat production. Brown fat is unique in containing many lipid vacuoles surrounded by *mitochondria*, the chemical "powerhouses" of the body that burn metabolic fuel, glucose, and fatty acids. The reddish brown color is from the iron-containing cytochromes of the mitochon-

FIG. 5-13. In newborn infants, a type of fat specialized for heat production is located between the shoulder blades, around the neck surrounding the subclavian and carotid vessels, behind the sternum, and around the kidneys and adrenal glands.

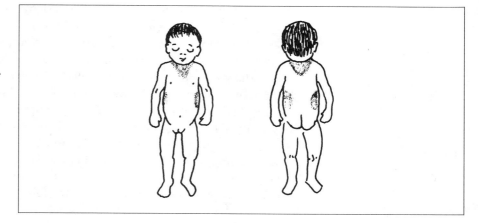

dria. The amount of this special tissue varies from one species to another, although it is increased with exposure to cold weather.

Humans do not have any brown fat and can increase heat production only by shivering or muscular exercise. Newborn babies, whose neuromuscular mechanisms have not yet been developed, cannot shiver to keep themselves warm. Although they do not have true brown fat, some of the adipose tissue over the shoulder blades and around the neck resembles brown fat (Fig. 5-13). These cells contain many small vacuoles of fat surrounded by many large mitochondria. The newborn baby responds to cold by generating heat through oxidation of the lipid content of these fat cells. Oxidation and phosphorylation are uncoupled, so that instead of conserving energy in the form of phosphate bonds (e.g., in adenosine triphosphate), energy is dissipated as heat, warming the body. This process, termed *nonshivering thermogenesis,* is an important mechanism of temperature control during the first few weeks of life in many species, including humans.

The lack of subcutaneous lipid during most of intrauterine life of the mammalian fetus is of interest in relation to the function of subcutaneous lipid during adult life. Because the fetus resides in a thermoregulated environment, protected from mechanical trauma by amniotic fluid and the maternal tissues, it requires little depot lipid. Unlike the adult, who eats only intermittently, the fetus does not require any long-term energy reservoir, since it is fed continuously across the placenta from the maternal circulation. Only shortly before delivery does the fetus acquire some depot lipid, and even then, very little.

HORMONAL INFLUENCES ON LIPID METABOLISM

Lipid leaves the adipose tissue for distribution to the tissues in the form of free fatty acids. They enter the blood from storage depots in adipose tissue to serve as fuel for the tissues. *Epinephrine, norepinephrine,* and *growth hormone* all cause a rise in the plasma free fatty acid level. During exercise, norepinephrine released in the adipose tissue is a physiologic stimulus for fat mobilization. Epinephrine and norepinephrine increase triacylglycerol hydrolysis and subsequent free fatty acid release from the adipose tissue for metabolism. Growth hormone also increases the rate of fat mobilization. It allows more nitrogen to be utilized for tissue synthesis by increasing the use of fat as a source of energy. The levels of growth hormone and *insulin* are similar after exercise and eating, respectively. They have analogous roles: Insulin is involved in storing energy consumed at a meal and growth hormone with utilizing energy from stores to meet the needs of physical activity and growth. An insufficient amount of insulin decreases fat synthesis and increases fat mobilization (see Ketosis, p. 96). Excess amounts of insulin inhibit fat utilization and stimulate fat synthesis. Insulin activates the clearing factor, *lipoprotein lipase,* which results in triacylglycerol hydrolysis and uptake of its products, fatty acids and glycerol, by adipose tissue.

References

1. Burr, G. O., and Burr, M. M.   A new deficiency disease produced by the rigid exclusion of fat from the diet. *J. Biol. Chem.* 82:345, 1929.
2. Singer, S. J., and Nicolson, G. L.   The fluid mosaic model of the structure of cell membranes. *Science* 175:720, 1972.
3. Davidson, S., et al.   *Human Nutrition and Dietetics* (6th ed.). Edinburgh: Churchill Livingstone, 1975. P. 81.

Suggested Readings

Babayan, V. K.   Medium chain length fatty acid esters and their medical and nutritional applications. *J. Am. Oil Chem. Soc.* 58:49A, 1981.

Bloch, K.   The biological synthesis of cholesterol (Nobel address). *Science* 150:19, 1965.

Bray, G. A.   "Brown" tissue and metabolic obesity. *Nutr. Today* 17:23, 1982.

Bretscher, M. S.   Membrane structure: Some general principles. *Science* 181:622, 1973.

Capaldi, R. A.   A dynamic model of cell membranes. *Sci. Am.* 230:26, 1974.

Fondu, M. (ed.).   *Lipids and Lipoproteins.* Basel, Switzerland: S. Karger, 1980.

Green, D. E.   The metabolism of fats. *Sci. Am.* January 1954.

Gutcho, M.   Edible Oils and Fats: Recent Developments. Park Ridge, N. J.: Noyes Data Corp., 1979.

Haslewood, G. A. D.   *Bile Salts.* London: Methuen, 1967.

Kuksis, A., and Mookerjea, S.   Choline. *Nutr. Rev.* 36:201, 1978.

Linolenic acid deficiency in man. *Nutr. Rev.* 40:144, 1982.

Pike, J. E.   Prostaglandins. *Sci. Am.* 225:84, 1971.

Rothfield, L. I. (ed.).   *Structure and Function of Biological Membranes.* New York: Academic, 1971.

Chapter 6

THE MINERAL ELEMENTS

About 4 percent of the human body is composed of mineral elements, those substances that remain as ash when the tissue is burned. Three-fourths of the mineral content of the body is made up of calcium and phosphorus, the main structural components of bone and teeth. The mineral elements are involved in a wide variety of functions ranging from hormonal activity (e.g., iodine in thyroxine) to oxygen transport (iron in hemoglobin). Minerals operate as catalysts in metabolic reactions and help to maintain fluid and electrolyte balance, osmotic pressure, the contraction of muscles, and the response of nerves to stimuli. They are a dynamic and vital part of the delicate balance of life.

This chapter discusses a variety of chemical elements by their function and amount present in the body: those elements present in the largest amounts (also termed *minerals*), and those present in small amounts (grouped together as "trace elements"). The electrolytes, the elements that maintain most control over fluid and acid-base balance, are discussed in Chap. 10. A summary of the body content and concentration of minerals and trace elements is given in Table 6-1.

Minerals
CALCIUM

DISTRIBUTION AND FUNCTIONS

The adult human body contains about 1200 to 1250 gm of calcium, 99 percent of which is bound in the hard matrix of bones and teeth. These structures provide both a rigid framework and a ready reserve of calcium to maintain a constant blood level. The calcium present in these structures is not static: The amount entering and leaving the bones equals about 700 mg per day. The amount of calcium found outside the skeletal structure is not more than 10 to 12 gm, or about 1 percent of the total body calcium, but this small amount has many vital functions. It acts as a catalyst for the conversion of prothrombin into thrombin in the process of blood clotting; it controls the integrity of intracellular cement substances and various cell membranes; it is necessary for the transmission of nerve impulses, the normal excitability of the heart and muscles, and the activation of many enzymes. Because the level of calcium in the blood affects so many diverse vital functions, its maintenance within a narrow range (9 to 11 mg/100 ml) is essential. This is accomplished by hormonal control [1]. About 60 percent of the blood calcium is ionized and about 40 percent is bound to serum proteins. A reduction in the blood calcium level results in the development of *tetany* (increased neuromuscular activity resulting in muscle spasms); an increase can lead to respiratory or cardiac failure as the result of impaired muscle function.

ABSORPTION

Calcium is absorbed by an active transport process, mainly in the upper small intestine, regulated by 1,25-dihydroxycholecalciferol, a metabolite of vitamin D produced in the kidney in response to low plasma calcium concentrations. The amount of calcium absorbed is therefore directly related and adjusted to body

TABLE 6-1. Body content and concentration of minerals and trace elements

Element	Body content	Plasma or serum concentration
Calcium	1000–1250 gm	9–10.5 mg/100 ml[a]
Chromium	6 mg	1–6 μg/100 ml
Cobalt	1 mg	4.3 μg/100 ml
Copper	100–150 mg	65–170 μg/100 ml
Iodine	20–50 mg	4–8 μg/100 ml
Iron	3–5 gm	80–160 μg/100 ml[b] 60–135 μg/100 ml[c]
Manganese	12–20 mg	4–20 μg/100 ml
Magnesium	20–35 gm	1.5–2.5 mEq/liter
Molybdenum	10–20 mg	1.4 μg/100 ml
Phosphorus (phosphate)	670 gm	3–5 mg/100 ml 4–7 mg/100 ml[d]
Sulfur	175 gm	0.7–1.5 mEq/liter
Zinc	1.4–2.3 gm	120 μg/100 ml

$$1 \text{ mEq (milliequivalent)} = \frac{\text{atomic weight (in milligrams)}}{\text{valence}}$$

[a] Higher in children.
[b] Males.
[c] Females.
[d] Children.

needs. About 30 percent of the calcium present in a mixed diet is normally absorbed by a healthy adult. The amount absorbed from individual foods ranges from 10 to 40 percent. Pregnant women and growing children absorb about 40 percent or more of the calcium from foods. With a limited intake of calcium, absorption becomes more efficient, especially when there is also an adequate amount of vitamin D.

Because calcium salts are more soluble in an acid medium, most of the absorption occurs in the duodenum. Achlorhydria (lack of normal gastric acid) and increased intestinal mobility both decrease absorption. Other factors hindering normal absorption include substances that form insoluble complexes with dietary calcium, such as phytic acid, oxalic acid, and free fatty acids. Phytic acid is an organic compound found in the outer layers of cereal grains. Oxalic acid is present in spinach, Swiss chard, beet tops, cocoa, and rhubarb. If the only food sources of calcium in an individual's diet are also high in these binding agents, the resulting absorption of calcium will be very poor [2]. Foods high in saturated fatty acids are likely to produce free fatty acids that will then combine with calcium to form insoluble complexes or soaps.

Factors increasing absorption include the presence of vitamin D, which facilitates the movement of calcium into the mucosal cells and increases absorption from the duodenum [3]; high protein diets, because of the action of specific amino acids, especially serine, arginine, and lysine; the presence of lactose, the disaccharide found exclusively in milk products; and an increase in acidophilic flora (that is, the lactobacilli), which lowers the pH, favoring absorption. The amount of calcium in proportion to phosphorus in the diet, the calcium-phosphorus ratio, also affects absorption. An excess of animal protein in the diet, which is high in phosphorus, can cause an imbalanced ratio and result in higher calcium requirements. To maximize absorption and minimize loss from bone, the calcium-phosphorus ratio should be between 2:1 and 1:2; the recommended dietary allowances (RDAs) are based on a ratio of 1:1.

METABOLISM

The level of calcium in the plasma is maintained within the narrow range of 9 to 11 mg per 100 ml. When the concentration begins to fall, the parathyroid gland secretes *parathormone,* which causes calcium to be released from bone, increases the reabsorption of calcium by the renal tubules, and increases the excretion of phosphates in the urine. Parathormone therefore restores the plasma calcium level while maintaining the proper calcium-phosphorus ratio in the blood. Another calcium-regulating hormone, *calcitonin,* has the opposite effect: It lowers the plasma calcium and phosphate levels. This is done by increasing absorption of calcium by bone and increasing the renal clearance of both calcium and phosphates. Together with vitamin D, parathormone and calcitonin maintain the plasma calcium level within narrow limits.

The maintenance of the plasma calcium level is more dependent on the bones than on the diet for a ready source of calcium. The calcium in the bones is constantly turning over, and in the healthy, fully grown adult, the rates of mineralization (addition of calcium to the bones) and demineralization (resorption of calcium from the bones) are equal. During periods of growth, the amount of calcium added to the bones exceeds that removed. When calcium needs exceed the dietary intake, the calcium from the bones is mobilized. Loss of up to 40 percent of the calcium may occur before it can be detected by x-ray, but by then the bones are fragile and fracture easily.

Bone itself is made up of organic and inorganic components. A gradual mineralization of the organic matrix gives bones their hardness; this process is termed *calcification* or *ossification.* Fetal bones begin to ossify during the second half of pregnancy, and by the first year there is sufficient mineralization to support the baby's weight as he or she begins to walk. The bones continue to grow in length and diameter during the first 20 years of life, so that by maturity they contain between 1000 and 1200 gm of calcium. The calcium-phosphorus ratio is important in ossification. The product of these two components of the ratio (in mg/dl) is normally 50 in children and 40 in adults. The product may be as low as 30 in persons with rickets. The role played by calcium in the development of teeth and factors influencing dental health are discussed in Chap. 28.

Most of the calcium eliminated from the body is excreted via the feces, with only a small amount in the urine. Most of the calcium present in the feces is that unabsorbed from the diet. Calcium losses in sweat range from 15 to 20 mg per day and may be higher during periods of strenuous physical exercise, even when dietary intakes are low.

RECOMMENDED DIETARY ALLOWANCES

The RDAs for calcium are given in Table 6-2. Although the World Health Organization recommends 400 to 500 mg per day for adults, indicating that there is no evidence of calcium deficiency in countries where this level of intake is common and that persons can maintain calcium balance with intakes as low as 200 to 400 mg per day, the Food and Nutrition Board of the National Research Council states that there are no advantages to such low recommendations.

During pregnancy, about 30 gm of calcium is mobilized for the calcification of the fetal skeleton, mostly during the last third of fetal life [4]. Calcium absorption is increased and calcium excretion decreased during pregnancy. Calcium is stored in the maternal skeleton in early pregnancy to be mobilized later when needed. About 300 mg per day above nonpregnancy levels is actually needed by the pregnant woman, but to provide for individual variation, 400 mg per day, for a total of 1200 mg per day for women over 18, is recommended. This is equivalent to the amount of calcium in about 4 oz of cheese, five 8-oz glasses of milk, or

TABLE 6-2. Recommended daily dietary allowances of mineral elements

Group	Age (years)	Calcium (mg)	Phosphorus (mg)	Magnesium (mg)	Zinc (mg)	Iodine (μg)
Infants	0.0–0.5	360	240	50	3	40
	0.5–1.0	540	360	70	5	50
Children	1–3	800	800	150	10	70
	4–6	800	800	200	10	90
	7–10	800	800	250	10	120
Males	11–14	1200	1200	350	15	150
	15–18	1200	1200	400	15	150
	19–22	800	800	350	15	150
	23–50	800	800	350	15	150
	51+	800	800	350	15	150
Females	11–14	1200	1200	300	15	150
	15–18	1200	1200	300	15	150
	19–22	800	800	300	15	150
	23–50	800	800	300	15	150
	51+	800	800	300	15	150
Pregnant*	—	+400	+400	+150	+5	+25
Lactating*	—	+400	+400	+150	+10	+50

*Allowances given for pregnant and lactating women are *in addition to* the normal allowance for women of a particular age.
Source: Food and Nutrition Board, National Research Council, *Recommended Dietary Allowances* (9th ed.). Washington, D.C.: National Academy of Sciences, 1980.

an 8-oz serving of yogurt. Maternal diets deficient in calcium, as well as in protein and calories, have been shown to produce decreased bone density in newborns [5].

The calcium content of breast milk is about 300 mg per liter; an average daily production of 850 ml results in about 250 mg of milk calcium [6]. To meet this need, 400 mg of calcium per day is recommended for the lactating woman in addition to her normal requirement. If milk production is higher, a greater allowance is needed.

Breast-fed infants receive about 60 mg of calcium per kilogram body weight and retain about two-thirds of this amount. Infants fed cow's milk formula receive about 170 mg per kilogram body weight but retain only 25 to 30 percent [6]. The breast-fed infant has less calcium available, but its needs are fully met. Children need two to four times as much calcium as adults per unit of weight. During periods of rapid growth (preadolescence and puberty), needs are increased to 1200 mg per day.

FOOD SOURCES

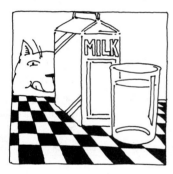

About 60 percent of the calcium intake in the United States is derived from milk and dairy products [7]. Ounce per ounce, milk and cheese are the richest sources of calcium in the diet. About 2 or 3 cups of milk per day for adults and 3 or 4 cups daily for children will meet calcium needs. Hard cheeses also provide a concentrated source of calcium. Cottage cheese and ice cream contribute smaller but still substantial amounts of calcium to the diet. Calcium is also found in such foods as mustard greens, turnip greens, kale, and collard greens. Spinach also contains considerable amounts of calcium but the presence of oxalates prevents much of the calcium from being utilized. Shrimp, clams, oysters, and salmon eaten with the bones also provide some calcium. When food sources of calcium cannot be taken, calcium salts such as calcium gluconate, lactate, sulfate, and carbonate may be prescribed by a health professional to supplement dietary intake. Although the calcium in organic or inorganic compounds is equally well utilized in the body, by substituting medicinal calcium for dietary calcium the body is deprived of the accompanying vitamins, protein, and other nutrients present in the foods.

RELATED DISEASES

A deficiency of calcium may result in abnormal calcification of bones and teeth in the young. A deficiency of calcium is not usually seen unless there is an accompanying lack of phosphorus and vitamin D. *Rickets*, characterized by faulty calcification of the bones caused by inadequate vitamin D, results from poor absorption of calcium and phosphorus. The clinical signs include stunted growth, bowing of the legs, enlargement of the wrists and ankles, and a hollow chest. *Osteoporosis*, the progressive demineralization of bone, most commonly in the elderly, was previously thought to be due to a deficiency of calcium. It has now been shown that high calcium intakes are not necessarily protective, nor are low intakes causative. The amount of bone present in old age may be more related to the amount present in early adult life and not to calcium intake [8]. Although osteoporosis is not directly related to calcium deficiency, it does appear to have some association with the mineral. Persons with this condition seem not to be able to adapt to a low dietary level of calcium. They may have an impaired absorptive mechanism or may continuously lose body calcium. Osteoporosis is a major problem in this country; more detail is presented in Chaps. 24, 27, 28, 33, and 35.

Tetany, caused by a decrease in the ionized serum calcium, is characterized by pain and severe, intermittent spasms of muscle. This condition may be seen in infants fed undiluted cow's milk (milk tetany). The phosphorus content of cow's milk is greater than that in breast milk, and the infant's kidneys are not able to clear the phosphate load fast enough. Phosphorus builds up in the blood, disturbing the normal calcium-phosphorus ratio, which results in tetanic muscular spasms. The *milk-alkali syndrome,* characterized by an elevated serum calcium level, is caused by excessive alkali therapy and large amounts of milk for extended periods for the treatment of peptic ulcer disease. When only large amounts of milk or nonabsorbable antacids are used, this syndrome does not occur.

PHOSPHORUS

DISTRIBUTION AND FUNCTIONS

Phosphorus accounts for about 1 percent of the total body weight, or about one-fourth of the total mineral matter. About 80 to 90 percent of the phosphorus is joined with calcium in the bones and teeth in a 2 : 1 ratio and, as a component of calcium phosphate, is constantly being deposited and liberated from the bone structure. The remaining 10 to 20 percent, unlike calcium, is present in all the living cells of the body as the phosphate ion. Phosphorus is a component of a wide variety of compounds and is involved in many metabolic reactions. For example, phosphorus is a component of the sugar-phosphate linkage in DNA and RNA, the substances that transmit genetic traits. As part of the phospholipids, phosphorus acts as a transporter of fat in the bloodstream, as well as being part of cell membranes and controlling the transport of substances in and out of the cell. Phosphorylation, the process by which phosphorus combines with glucose, is necessary for glucose absorption from the intestine, for glucose uptake by individual cells, and for resorption of glucose by the renal tubules. Monosaccharides are phosphorylated several times during their metabolic breakdown to yield energy. Phosphorus is involved in the storage and release of energy through the high-energy phosphate bonds of adenosine triphosphate (ATP) and adenosine diphosphate (ADP). Phosphates in the blood are an essential part of the body's delicate buffer system. Many of the B vitamins are active only when combined with phosphate. The serum phosphorus level is maintained between 3 and 5 mg per 100 ml in adults and 4 and 7 mg per 100 ml in children. The higher level in children indicates its vital role in cell metabolism. The serum phosphorus level is kept constant by the kidney and by the actions of vitamin D and parathormone.

ABSORPTION AND METABOLISM

The calcium-phosphorus ratio in the diet affects the absorption and excretion of both; an excess of either causes an increased excretion of the other. Normally, about 70 percent of dietary phosphorus is absorbed, compared with the 10 to 30 percent of dietary calcium. The factors influencing calcium absorption also apply to phosphorus, including enhancement by vitamin D and inhibition by binding agents (that is, iron, calcium, aluminum). Most of the phosphorus that occurs in foods is present in combination with other compounds. One of the first steps in the absorption of phosphorus is the splitting off of the phosphate by intestinal enzymes (phosphatases).

RECOMMENDED DIETARY ALLOWANCES

During periods of rapid growth, such as childhood, pregnancy, and lactation, the ratio of phosphorus to calcium in the diet should ideally be 1:1. In the normal adult diet, the intake of phosphorus usually exceeds that of calcium, and a wide range of ratios do not have any adverse effects. The Food and Nutrition Board suggests a phosphorus intake equal to that of calcium for all ages except infancy. Because the infant's kidneys cannot yet handle a high phosphate load, a calcium-phosphorus ratio of 1.5:1.0 is recommended to prevent the development of hypocalcemic tetany. This ratio is decreased to 1:1 by the first year of age. The RDAs for phosphorus are given in Table 6-2.

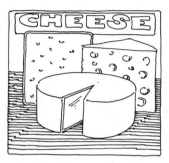

FOOD SOURCES

Phosphorus is present in nearly all foods; for this reason a dietary deficiency of this element is unknown. The distribution of phosphorus is similar to that of calcium, so an adequate intake of one generally assures a sufficient intake of the other. Milk and milk products are the best sources of phosphorus, and because of the presence of this element in all muscle cells, lean meats are also good sources.

RELATED DISEASES

In severe renal disease and in hypoparathyroidism, serum levels of phosphorus are high. As a result, the serum calcium level drops, which causes tetany. Low levels of phosphorus can result from malabsorption (in sprue or celiac disease) or bone disease (in rickets or osteomalacia). Hyperparathyroidism also results in low serum phosphorus levels because the excessive amounts of parathormone cause an abnormally high renal excretion of phosphorus. Muscle weakness is a symptom of low serum phosphorus, because of the lack of this element of cellular energy metabolism.

MAGNESIUM

DISTRIBUTION AND FUNCTIONS

Of the three major minerals in the human body, magnesium is present in the smallest amount, only about 20 to 35 gm. About 60 to 70 percent is complexed with calcium and phosphorus in bone; the remainder is present in the body fluids and concentrated within cells. The ratio of magnesium to calcium within cells is about 3:1. Whole blood contains about twice as much magnesium as does serum, since this element is concentrated in red blood cells. About 2 percent of the body's magnesium is found in the extracellular fluid. The serum level of this element ranges from 1.5 to 2.5 mEq per liter, with about 80 percent ionized and diffusible and the remaining 20 percent bound to serum proteins. Muscle contains more magnesium than calcium, since magnesium ions function as activators for many of the high-energy phosphate group transfer enzymes (that is, ADP to ATP, and ATP to a phosphate acceptor). As an essential element for humans, magnesium acts as a catalyst for numerous biologic reactions, maintains the electrical potential in nerves for the transmission of nerve impulses and in muscle membranes for muscle contraction, and is involved in active transport across cell membranes.

ABSORPTION AND METABOLISM

Many of the same factors influencing calcium absorption also affect magnesium. Factors that inhibit calcium absorption, such as the presence of excess fat, phosphates, and oxalic and phytic acids, also hinder magnesium absorption. Likewise, an acidic environment enhances both calcium and magnesium absorption. However, neither parathormone nor vitamin D influences the absorption, metabolism, or excretion of magnesium. About 40 to 45 percent of the magnesium present is normally absorbed from an average diet, mostly in the small intestine. With a high magnesium diet, the percentage falls; with a low magnesium diet, it is increased. Since calcium and magnesium compete for absorption sites in the intestinal mucosa, a high intake of one increases the requirements for the other. Magnesium and potassium are normally concentrated within the cell. Any changes in this balance produce neuromuscular irritability.

The body content of magnesium is controlled mainly by the kidneys, where it is filtered from the blood by the glomeruli and reabsorbed by the renal tubules. Almost all of the magnesium present in the feces represents unabsorbed dietary magnesium.

RECOMMENDED DIETARY ALLOWANCES

Because magnesium is needed for normal bone growth, the Food and Nutrition Board recommends liberal allowances for children and adolescents. Human milk contains about 40 mg per liter and cow's milk about three times that amount. The RDA is 350 mg for men and 300 mg for women. During pregnancy and lactation, the allowances for women are increased by 150 mg. The RDAs for magnesium are given in Table 6-2.

FOOD SOURCES

Magnesium is widely distributed in many foods; therefore dietary deficiency is rare. The richest sources of this element include cocoa, nuts, some seafoods, whole grains, dried beans, peas, and green leafy vegetables.

RELATED DISEASES

Since magnesium is slowly mobilized from bone, a deficiency or imbalance develops slowly and only if accompanied by a poor dietary intake and increased excretion. A lowered plasma level of magnesium causes an imbalance in the extracellular fluid, resulting in altered electrical potentials of nerve and muscle cells. Magnesium deficiency, therefore, causes *neuromuscular dysfunction,* as manifested by muscular hyperexcitability with tremors and convulsions, sometimes accompanied by behavioral disturbances. These symptoms are similar to those of hypocalcemic tetany, and may be differentiated by measuring blood levels of the two elements. Magnesium deficiency can occur with chronic alcoholism, cirrhosis of the liver, malnutrition, malabsorption, and diuretic therapy, and is usually due to impaired intake or absorption, or both. With high levels of magnesium, as when there is a decrease in urinary excretion, the therapy includes the administration of calcium gluconate.

SULFUR AND OTHER MINERALS

Sulfur is present in the cell protein in all cells of the body as the two sulfur-containing amino acids cysteine and methionine. It accounts for about 175 gm in the adult man. Sulfur is an essential element for all animal species, since they all require the sulfur-containing amino acids. It is an important component of the mucopolysaccharides, including chondroitin sulfate, which is found in tendons, cartilage, skin, and bones. Sulfur is also found in heparin, an anticoagulant; insulin; and many coenzymes, including thiamin, biotin, coenzyme A, and glutathione. It is an important component in intermediary metabolism and detoxification mechanisms.

The main sources of sulfur in the diet are the amino acids cysteine and methionine. Such foods as milk, meat, eggs, and legumes are good sources. The daily requirement for sulfur has not yet been established, but a diet adequate in methionine and cysteine should be adequate to meet the body's sulfur needs.

Many other elements have been shown to be essential, or possibly essential. Cobalt, vital for the production of vitamin B_{12}, is a human dietary essential. Nickel, tin, silicon, and vanadium have all been suggested as essential trace elements in human nutrition. Nickel may be important in the metabolism or structure of membranes. Tin and vanadium may influence lipid metabolism. Silicon may be a component of mucopolysaccharides and have a structural role in skin, bone, cartilage, and connective tissue.

Table 6-3 presents a summary of minerals.

Trace Elements

IRON

Iron is discussed at length in Chap. 7.

ZINC

DISTRIBUTION AND FUNCTIONS

The total body content of zinc ranges from 1.4 to 2.3 gm, widely distributed in all tissues. About 20 percent is present in the skin, with high concentrations also

TABLE 6-3. Summary of the major minerals

Element	Site of absorption	Primary functions	Interactions with other elements	Route of excretion	Dietary sources	Key terms
Calcium	Upper small intestine	Bone and teeth structure Blood clotting Nerve transmission Muscle excitability	Phosphorus	Gut	Milk, hard cheese	Vitamin D Tetany Parathormone Calcitonin Rickets Osteoporosis
Phosphorus	Upper small intestine	Bone and teeth structure DNA and RNA component Phosphorylation Energy transfer Part of buffer system Component of B vitamins	Calcium	Gut	Milk, meats	Vitamin D Parathormone
Magnesium	Small intestine	Phosphate group transfer Transfer across membranes Electrical potential in nerves and muscles	Calcium Phosphorus	Kidneys	Whole grains, cocoa, nuts, legumes	Neuro-muscular dysfunction
Sulfur	Small intestine	Component of teeth, skin, bones, cartilage Component of B vitamins		Gut	Milk, meat, eggs, legumes	Cysteine Methionine

found in the bones, teeth, liver, pancreas, kidneys, brain, prostate, and epididymis. Zinc is an essential element for normal growth and reproduction and has a beneficial effect on wound healing and tissue repair. This element is an essential component of many vital enzymes involved in most major pathways. In the retina of the eye, it is part of the enzyme (retinene reductase) required for the use of vitamin A. It is necessary for maintaining normal plasma concentrations of vitamin A and for mobilizing this vitamin from the liver. Zinc is also an integral component of carbonic anhydrase, which is responsible for the transfer of carbon dioxide, especially in red blood cells and the renal tubules. For this reason, the concentration of zinc in red blood cells is about 10 times that in serum. As a component of carboxypeptidase, the proteolytic enzyme that removes carboxyl groups from peptides to produce amino acids, zinc is also involved in protein metabolism. As part of the anaerobic oxidation of glucose, zinc is a part of the enzyme lactate dehydrogenase, which is essential for the conversion of pyruvic acid to lactic acid. Zinc also forms a complex with insulin, which increases the duration of action of insulin when given by injection. In the beta cells of the pancreas, the zinc-insulin complex helps store and release insulin as needed. The action of thymidine kinase, which is required for DNA synthesis and cell division, is depressed with zinc deficiency, which may explain the influence of this element on growth, repair, and reproduction.

ABSORPTION AND METABOLISM

About 40 percent of dietary zinc is absorbed, mainly in the small intestine, after which it combines with plasma proteins for transport to various tissues. Calcium and phytate in large amounts can inhibit zinc absorption by combining with it to form an insoluble complex. Unabsorbed zinc is eliminated via the gastrointestinal tract in the feces. Endogenous zinc, that which has entered the blood and tissues, is secreted into the small intestine in the pancreatic juice. Zinc is rarely excreted in the urine.

The most rapid accumulation and turnover of zinc is in the soft tissues, particularly the spleen, liver, kidneys, and pancreas. Large amounts of zinc are deposited in the bones but cannot be readily mobilized. There is a small pool of biologically active zinc with a rapid turnover. Because of this, a deficiency of zinc can quickly develop.

RECOMMENDED DIETARY ALLOWANCES

The turnover of zinc in the body has been estimated at about 6 mg per day. The average American diet contains between 10 and 15 mg of zinc. The RDA for adults is 15 mg per day, increasing for women by 5 mg and 10 mg per day, respectively, during pregnancy and lactation. During early lactation, the breast milk contains about 20 mg of zinc per liter; this amount falls to less than 2 mg per liter during latter lactation. The importance of zinc for fetal development has only recently been recognized, with additional zinc being required for the growth and development of the fetus and placenta. The RDAs for zinc are given in Table 6-2.

FOOD SOURCES

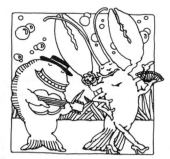

The availability of zinc in the average diet varies greatly. The zinc in meats, eggs, and seafoods, especially oysters, is better absorbed than that present in vegetable sources. The zinc present in whole grain products is not as well absorbed because of the grain's phytate and fiber content.

RELATED DISEASES

Because of the small body pool of biologically active zinc, a poor intake or increased demands can quickly lead to deficiency. Symptoms include loss of appetite, growth failure, skin changes, impaired wound healing, and decreased taste acuity. Zinc deficiency in humans has resulted in dwarfism and hypogonadism. In the Middle East this condition is fairly common and is considered to be due to the large amounts of phytate and fiber in the local bread, which bind most of the dietary zinc, and to intestinal infestations with hookworms and geophagia (the habit of eating dirt), both of which also interfere with the dietary absorption of zinc. Also in the Middle East, maternal zinc deficiency has been shown to cause severe congenital malformations of the central nervous system [9–11]. Impaired taste (*hypogeusia*) and smell (*hyposmia*) have been associated with zinc deficiency. Improved growth and wound healing has resulted from increased intakes in areas of marginal zinc nutrition. In many areas in the United States, the soil is zinc deficient and zinc must be added to the feeds of farm animals to prevent the development of zinc deficiency. Zinc deficiency can also develop with the excessive intake of alcohol, malabsorption syndromes, chronic renal failure, and the prolonged use of intravenous hyperalimentation without supplemental zinc. This element can be toxic at intakes of 2 gm or more, causing acute gastrointestinal irritation and vomiting; for this reason, it is sometimes used as an emetic. Excessive zinc intakes may aggravate marginal copper deficiency [12]. See Chap. 33 for more detail.

IODINE

DISTRIBUTION AND FUNCTIONS

The adult human body contains approximately 20 to 50 mg of iodine, required exclusively for the synthesis of the iodinated thyroid hormones. About one-third of the body's iodine is concentrated in the thyroid gland, with the remainder found in the muscles, skin, skeleton, and other endocrine tissue.

The only known function of iodine in the body is as a component of *thyroglobulin,* a protein-iodine complex of thyroid hormone. This hormone regulates the rate of oxidation within cells, and in doing so influences body temperature, the metabolism of all nutrients, physical and mental development, and the functioning of nervous and muscle tissue.

ABSORPTION AND METABOLISM

Iodine is present in foods as inorganic iodides and as organic compounds. During digestion, the iodine is split from the organic compounds and absorbed as inorganic iodide. It is transported in the blood as free iodide or as protein-bound iodine (PBI). This second type of iodine is sensitive to changes in thyroid activity, increasing during pregnancy and increased functioning of the thyroid gland, and decreasing with a fall in thyroid function. Measurement of PBI is used as a specific diagnostic tool to evaluate thyroid function.

The activity of the thyroid gland is controlled by thyroid-stimulating hormone (TSH), which is secreted by the anterior lobe of the pituitary gland. Low blood levels of thyroglobulin cause a release of TSH, which stimulates thyroid activity. A release of TSH causes an increased uptake of iodide by the thyroid gland, where the iodide is concentrated and oxidized into iodine to form part of diiodotyrosine, triiodothyronine, and thyroxine, which then become part of the thyroglobulin complex.

RECOMMENDED DIETARY ALLOWANCES

A daily intake of 50 to 75 μg, or 1 μg per kilogram body weight, is required to prevent the development of goiter. The adult allowance of 150 μg per day provides a margin of safety. The additional 25 μg and 50 μg for pregnancy and lactation cover the demands of the fetus and the amount of iodine excreted in breast milk. The RDAs for iodine are given in Table 6-2.

FOOD SOURCES

Seafood is a consistent, excellent source of iodine. Foods grown on soil that was once covered by the sea can also be valuable sources, but the effects of glaciers and weather have removed much of the iodine from the soil. Dairy products and eggs may also contribute some iodine to the diet, although their composition may vary with the iodine composition of the producing animal's diet. Some foods, termed *goitrogens,* have been shown to interfere with the use of thyroxine. They include peanuts, rutabagas, cabbage, cauliflower, and brussels sprouts. This effect is inactivated by cooking. Because the iodine intake was so low throughout the United States, enrichment of table salt (iodization) was begun in 1924. The current level of enrichment is about 76 μg per gram of salt [13]. About half of all table salt consumed in the United States is iodized. As a result, the incidence of goiter has fallen dramatically in this century. The distribution of the mean iodine intake in the United States is given in Fig. 6-1.

RELATED DISEASES

An inadequate intake of iodine in the diet causes the thyroid gland to enlarge (hypertrophy) to more efficiently utilize the iodine that is available. This hypertrophy of the thyroid gland is termed *goiter* (Figs. 6-2 and 6-3). Hypothyroidism, a condition that may result, causes subnormal body temperature and mental and

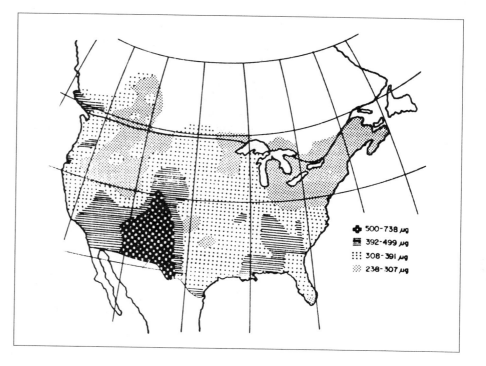

FIG. 6-1. Distribution of mean iodine intake in the United States. (From T. H. Oddie, D. A. Fisher, W. M. McConahey, and C. S. Thompson, Iodine intake in the United States: A reassessment. *J. Clin. Endocrinol.* 30:659, 1970.)

FIG. 6-2. This Guatemalan vendor has a large goiter. (Courtesy United Nations.)

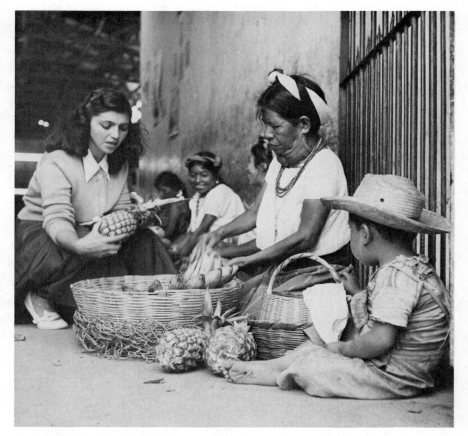

physical sluggishness. Other conditions, such as hyperthyroidism and cancer or inflammation of the thyroid, may also result in goiter. When the maternal diet is so low in iodine that it cannot supply the needs of the developing fetus, a condition termed *cretinism* results in the infant. Cretinism is characterized by a low basal metabolic rate and mental and physical retardation. Although some improvement can be seen when thyroid hormone is given early enough to the infant, any damage that has already occurred cannot be reversed.

Iodine intake in the daily diet has increased greatly in the past few decades to the point that the average intake may now be three to four times that recommended. No adverse effects have been reported from iodine intakes of up to 2000 μg per day in healthy adults and up to 1000 μg per day in healthy children [14]. Very high levels of iodine (10,000 to 200,000 μg per day) can cause goiter by reducing the amount of hormone released from the thyroid gland, as seen among some seaweed fishermen in Japan. Intakes between 200 and 500 mg/kg body weight/day produced death in experimental animals [15].

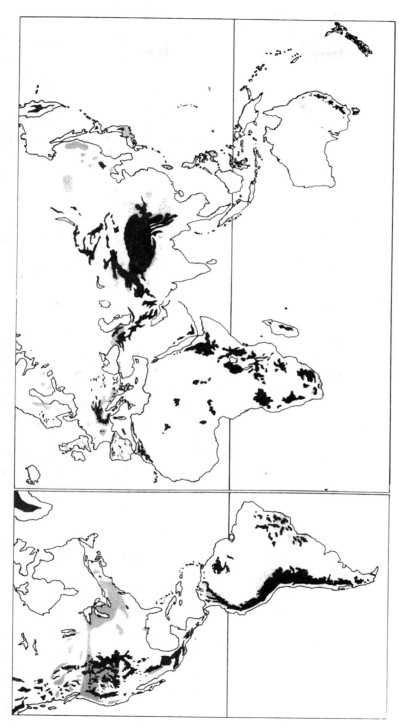

FIG. 6-3. Regions of endemic goiter (*hatching*). (Mountainous areas are shown in black.) (From *Scientific American, Human Nutrition.* San Francisco: Freeman, 1978.)

COPPER

DISTRIBUTION AND FUNCTIONS

The adult human body contains between 100 and 150 mg of copper, present in almost all tissues, but in the highest concentrations in the liver and brain. Copper is present in levels 5 to 10 times higher in the fetal liver than in the liver of an adult. This element is required for a variety of functions, including hemoglobin formation, normal bone development, maintenance of myelin within the nervous system, phospholipid synthesis, melanin pigment formation, and electron transport. As a component of a number of enzymes, copper is involved in fatty acid oxidation, purine metabolism, and energy production. *Hemocyanin,* a copper-protein complex in the blood of some invertebrates, functions like hemoglobin in oxygen transport.

ABSORPTION AND METABOLISM

Most dietary copper is absorbed from the stomach and small intestines. Between 80 and 95 percent of copper in the blood is bound to protein as *ceruloplasmin;* the remaining 5 to 20 percent is loosely bound to albumin and amino acids. Since copper exists only in a bound form, it is not readily excreted in the urine. Almost all of it is excreted via bile into the intestines and expelled in the feces.

DIETARY INTAKES

For copper and the remaining elements in this chapter, the Food and Nutrition Board has not yet established RDAs. Instead, the Board has issued estimated safe and adequate daily dietary intakes, as outlined in Table 6-4.

Tissue levels of copper remain constant in the adult. To allow for a margin of safety, a daily copper intake of 2 or 3 mg is recommended. As mentioned above, the fetus stores copper during gestation, with newborn hepatic levels being 5 to 10 times that found in the adult. These levels slowly decrease during the first year. Infants and children require between 0.50 and 0.10 mg/kg body weight/day

TABLE 6-4. Estimated safe and adequate daily dietary intakes of selected trace elements

Group	Age (years)	Copper (mg)	Manganese (mg)	Fluoride (mg)	Chromium (mg)	Selenium (mg)	Molybdenum (mg)
Infants	0–0.5	0.5–0.7*	0.5–0.7	0.1–0.5	0.01–0.04	0.01–0.04	0.03–0.06
	0.5–1.0	0.7–1.0*	0.7–1.0	0.2–1.0	0.02–0.06	0.02–0.06	0.04–0.08
Children	1–3	1.0–1.5	1.0–1.5	0.5–1.5	0.02–0.08	0.02–0.08	0.05–0.10
	4–6	1.5–2.0	1.5–2.0	1.0–2.5	0.03–0.12	0.03–0.12	0.06–0.15
	7–10	2.0–2.5	2.0–3.0	1.5–2.5	0.05–0.20	0.05–0.20	0.10–0.30
	11 +	2.0–3.0	2.5–5.0	1.5–2.5	0.05–0.20	0.05–0.20	0.15–0.50
Adults		2.0–3.0	2.5–5.0	1.5–4.0	0.05–0.20	0.05–0.20	0.15–0.50

*mg/kg body weight.
Source: Food and Nutrition Board, National Research Council, *Recommended Dietary Allowances* (9th ed.). Washington, D.C.: National Academy of Sciences, 1980. P. 178.

[16]. Infant formulas should furnish about 100 μg/kg body weight/day. Zinc and molybdenum are antagonistic to copper, so an increased intake of either of these elements also increases the requirement for copper.

FOOD SOURCES

The richest source of copper is oysters; other good sources include nuts, shellfish, liver, kidney, raisins, and dried legumes. Cow's milk is a poor source, with concentrations ranging from 0.015 to 0.180 mg per liter. Human milk contains between 1.05 mg per liter during early lactation and 0.15 mg per liter later.

RELATED DISEASES

Copper is intimately involved in iron metabolism; a deficiency of copper results in impaired release of iron into the plasma from ferritin stores in the intestinal mucosal cells (see Chap. 7). As a consequence of low plasma iron, hemoglobin synthesis is depressed and iron-deficiency anemia results. Although rare, nutritional copper deficiency can occur under a variety of circumstances. In newborns, it has been linked to prematurity, low birth weight, and maternal malnutrition [17]. The use of penicillamine in the treatment of rheumatoid disorders has been shown to have a chelating (binding) effect on copper, causing deficiency [18]. Long-term total parenteral nutrition with copper-deficient alimentation solutions has produced similar results. Low blood levels of copper have been observed in persons with kwashiorkor, sprue, malabsorption syndromes, and nephrotic syndromes. Bone disease may result from copper deficiency.

A rare inherited disease, termed *Menkes' kinky-hair syndrome,* results from impaired copper absorption from the intestines [19]. The clinical manifestations of this syndrome—depigmentation of the skin and hair, hypothermia, seizures, cerebral degeneration, and defective arterial walls—are all due to the impaired activity of copper-containing enzymes.

Wilson's disease, characterized by markedly reduced serum copper and ceruloplasmin levels, is not due to nutritional copper deficiency, but rather to abnormal hepatic copper storage and impaired ceruloplasmin metabolism. In this disease, most of the copper in the blood remains loosely bound to albumin and can therefore be transferred more readily to the tissues. In Wilson's disease, the liver and the lenticular nucleus of the brain contain abnormally large amounts of copper, and there is also an excessive urinary excretion of this element.

MANGANESE

DISTRIBUTION AND FUNCTIONS

Manganese is an essential element for many species, including humans. This element is a vital component of several enzyme systems involved in protein and energy metabolism, in the synthesis of mucopolysaccharides (cartilage) and glycoproteins (prothrombin), and in gluconeogenesis. Between 12 and 20 mg of manganese is present in the adult body, mainly in the liver and kidneys.

ABSORPTION AND METABOLISM

Manganese, like iron, is poorly absorbed, mostly from the small intestine. Mitochondria are the main sites of manganese uptake. Most of this element is excreted into the intestines via the bile; very little occurs in the urine.

DIETARY INTAKES

For adults, the Food and Nutrition Board suggests a range of 2.5 to 5.0 mg per day as providing a margin of safety. The introduction of solid foods to infants provides a higher intake of this element. Table 6-4 gives an estimated safe and adequate daily dietary intake of manganese.

FOOD SOURCES

Nuts, grains, legumes, soybeans, coffee, and tea are the best sources of manganese; fruits and vegetables are good sources. Meats, seafood, poultry, and fish are relatively poor sources.

RELATED DISEASES

Deficiency of manganese in animals results in poor reproductive performance, growth retardation, congenital malformations, abnormal formation of bone and cartilage, and impaired glucose tolerance. Evidence of manganese deficiency in humans has not yet been established. Manganese toxicity in humans has been reported, particularly among workers exposed to high concentrations of manganese dust in the air [20]. Excessive amounts of manganese accumulate in the liver and central nervous system, producing severe neuromuscular disturbances similar to those of Parkinson's disease.

FLUORIDE

DISTRIBUTION AND FUNCTIONS

Because of its protective effect against dental caries, fluoride (the ionized form of the element fluorine) has been accepted as a required nutrient. Fluoride normally accumulates as part of the hard structure of teeth and bones, although the amount varies with duration of intake and the age at which intake begins. It is most important during early infancy and childhood, because these are the periods of tooth development, but the caries-prevention activity remains through adulthood. A higher rate of fluoride uptake may be necessary during adulthood to maintain normal bone calcification [21]. Adequate fluoride intake during adulthood may decrease the incidence of osteoporosis, a defect in the maintenance of bone structure [22].

DIETARY INTAKE AND SOURCES

The geochemical environment strongly influences the fluoride content of foods grown in a particular area. Drinking water is the main source of fluoride. In areas of the country where the fluoride content of the water is less than 1 part per million (ppm), it is an advisable public health practice to add fluoride to the water (fluoridation). The safety and nutritional advantages of fluoridation, including a decrease in dental caries among children of 50 percent or more, have been clearly demonstrated [23]. The Food and Nutrition Board estimates that a safe and adequate intake of fluoride for adults is between 1.5 and 4.0 mg per day; for children 4 years and older, 1.0 to 2.5 mg per day; for toddlers ages 1 to 3, 0.5 to 1.5 mg per day; and 0.1 to 1.0 mg per day during infancy. Table 6-4 summarizes the recommendations.

RELATED DISEASES

A very high intake of fluoride during the period of tooth development causes a mottling and discoloration of the tooth enamel. High intakes can also cause increased bone density and calcification at points of muscle insertion. *Fluorosis,* caused by excessive fluoride intake, occurs only in geographic areas where the water contains high concentrations of fluoride, 10 to 45 ppm. In very large doses, fluoride can be toxic, inhibiting several magnesium-containing enzymes involved with phosphate metabolism and the citric acid cycle. See Chap. 28 for more detail.

CHROMIUM

This element is present at birth and is widely distributed in all tissues, although the total chromium content of the adult human body is less than 6 mg. Of the 2 to 5 percent of dietary chromium that is normally absorbed, most rapidly disappears from the bloodstream and is stored in the tissues. It is released from the tissues with the ingestion of glucose. It is thought to potentiate the action of insulin in promoting the utilization of glucose and may be involved in glucose tolerance.

Levels appear to decrease with age and in diabetes. Marginal deficiency states have been observed in old age, pregnancy, and protein-calorie malnutrition. The Food and Nutrition Board suggests a minimal daily requirement of 1 μg and an optimal adult intake between 50 and 200 μg (Table 6-4).

Good dietary sources of chromium include brewer's yeast, meat products, cheese, whole grains, and condiments. Leafy vegetables, polished rice, and table sugar are poor sources.

SELENIUM

Although recognized as an essential element for many animal species, selenium has not yet been clearly established as essential for humans. The best known biochemical function of this element is as part of the enzyme *glutathione peroxidase,* which protects vital components of the cell (e.g., membrane lipids and hemoglobin) against oxidative damage. It also may be involved in other important biologic processes, including immune mechanisms and mitochondrial ATP synthesis.

Selenium is widely distributed throughout the body, with highest concentrations found in the kidneys, liver, pancreas, and pituitary. The amount of selenium in foods is proportional to the soil content in the area where the food is grown. A level of selenium in excess of 5 ppm in foods is considered dangerous.

TABLE 6-5. Summary of trace elements

Element	Site of absorption	Primary functions	Interactions with other elements	Route of excretion	Dietary sources	Key terms
Zinc	Small intestine	Vitamin A metabolism; DNA synthesis; CO_2 transfer; Protein and glucose metabolism; Complexes with insulin	Copper; Calcium	Pancreatic and intestinal secretions (gut)	Meat, eggs, seafood	CNS malformations; Hypogeusia; Hyposmia
Iodine	Stomach and small intestine	Synthesis of iodinated thyroid hormones		Gut	Seafood, dairy foods, iodized salt	TSH; Thyroglobulin; PBI; Goiter; Cretinism
Copper	Stomach and upper gastrointestinal tract	Hemoglobin formation; Bone development; Phospholipid synthesis; Pigment formation; Myelin maintenance; Energy production	Zinc; Molybdenum	Bile (gut)	Oysters, nuts, raisins, shellfish, liver, kidney, legumes	Hemocyanin; Ceruloplasmin; Wilson's disease; Menkes' kinky-hair syndrome
Manganese	Small intestine	Synthesis of cartilage; Bone development; Lipid metabolism; Regulation of nervous irritability; Protein hydrolysis	Magnesium	Bile (gut)	Nuts, grains, legumes	Inhalation toxicity
Fluoride	Gut	Bone and tooth structure	Magnesium; Phosphorus; Calcium	Kidneys	Water	Fluoridation; Fluorosis
Chromium	Gut	Normal glucose tolerance; Potentiates insulin action		Kidneys	Meat, cheese, grains	
Selenium	Gut	Antioxidant; Immune mechanisms; ATP synthesis	Sulfur	Gut	Seafood, kidney, liver	Vitamin E
Molybdenum	Gut	Nitrogen fixation; Xanthine and aldehyde oxidation	Copper; Sulfur	Gut	Organ meats, grains, legumes	Teart

A level of 0.1 μg per gram of diet is considered adequate for optimal growth and reproduction, with 50 to 200 μg per day being safe and adequate for adults (Table 6-4). Toxicity occurs when the drinking water contains more than 2 μg per gram or the diet has more than 3 μg per gram. Good dietary sources include seafood, meat, liver, and kidney.

A syndrome termed *alkali disease* has been reported among cattle consuming feed high in selenium. The signs include lameness, stiffness, anemia, and emaciation. Concentrations in the range of 5 to 15 ppm have been shown to be toxic to animals. Deficiency occurs when the concentration is less than 0.02 to 0.05 μg per gram of diet.

Selenium has been found to cure some, but not all, of the deficiency symptoms produced in animals by vitamin E deficiency. It is thought that this is due to the similarity between the action of selenium and that of vitamin E as antioxidants. Sulfur is an antagonist to selenium in that it competes with this element for reactive sites in enzymes.

MOLYBDENUM

This element is an essential component of the enzymes xanthine oxidase, aldehyde oxidase, and sulfite oxidase, which are responsible for the oxidation of xanthines, aldehydes, and sulfites, respectively. Molybdenum is also present in nitrate reductase in plants and nitrogenase in microorganisms, where it functions in nitrogen fixation. Molybdenum is found in very low tissue concentrations throughout the body, with the highest levels found in the liver and kidneys.

Safe and adequate intakes for adults have been estimated to be between 0.15 and 0.50 mg per day (Table 6-4). Excessive intakes, between 10 and 15 mg per day, produce goutlike symptoms. The molybdenum content of foods varies with the concentration of the element in soil. Some good sources include organ meats, legumes, and whole-grain cereals.

In areas where the soil has a high molybdenum content, cattle have developed a syndrome called "teart," which is characterized by weight loss, brittle bones, and depigmentation. Molybdenum and copper compete for the same reactive sites, so an excess of molybdenum can cause symptoms of copper deficiency. When the intake of sulfate is increased, the excretion of molybdenum is increased.

A summary of the trace elements is given in Table 6-5.

References

1. Copp, D. H.   Endocrine regulation of calcium metabolism. *Annu. Rev. Physiol.* 32:61, 1970.
2. Singh, P. P., et al.   Nutritional value of foods in relation to their oxalic acid content. *Am. J. Clin. Nutr.* 25:1147, 1972.
3. Deluca, H. F.   Vitamin D: The vitamin and the hormone. *Fed. Proc.* 33:2211, 1974.
4. Pitkin, R. M.   Calcium metabolism in pregnancy: A review. *Am. J. Obstet. Gynecol.* 121:724, 1975.
5. Krishnamachari, K. A. V. R., and Iyengar, L.   Effect of maternal malnutrition on the bone density of the neonate. *Am. J. Clin. Nutr.* 28:482, 1975.

6. Food and Nutrition Board, National Research Council. *Recommended Dietary Allowances* (9th ed.). Washington, D.C.: National Academy of Sciences, 1980. P. 130.

7. United States Department of Agriculture. Dietary levels of households in the United States. Washington, D.C.: U.S. Government Printing Office, 1969.

8. Garn, S. M., Rohmann, C. G., and Wagner, B. Bone loss as a general phenomenon in man. *Fed. Proc.* 26:1729, 1967.

9. Cavdar, A. O., et al. Effect of nutrition on serum zinc concentrations during pregnancy in Turkish women. *Am. J. Clin. Nutr.* 33:542, 1980.

10. Cavdar, A. O., et al. Zinc deficiency and anencephaly in Turkey. *Teratology* 22:141, 1980.

11. Sever, L. E. Zinc and human development: A review. *Hum. Ecol.* 3:43, 1975.

12. Klevay, L. M. The ratio of zinc to copper of diets in the United States. *Nutr. Rep. Int.* 11:237, 1975.

13. Food and Nutrition Board, National Research Council. *Recommended Dietary Allowances* (9th ed.). Washington, D.C.: National Academy of Sciences, 1980. P. 149.

14. Taylor, F. Iodine: Going from hypo to hyper. *FDA Consumer* 15:14, 1981.

15. Select Committee on GRAS Substances. *Evaluation of the health aspects of potassium iodine as a food ingredient* (SCOG, S-39). Life Sciences Research Office. Federation of American Societies for Experimental Biology. Bethesda, 1974.

16. Cardano, A. The role played by copper in the physiopathology and nutrition of the infant and the child. *Ann. Nestlé* 33:1, 1974.

17. Karan, S., and Pathak, A. Systemic bone disease associated with low serum copper levels in preterm and low birth weight twin infants. *Indian Pediatr.* 12:903, 1975.

18. Multicentre Trial Group. Controlled trial of D(-)penicillamine in severe rheumatoid arthritis. *Lancet* 1:273, 1973.

19. Menkes, J. H., et al. A sex-linked recessive disorder with retardation of growth, peculiar hair, and facial, cerebral, and cerebellar degeneration. *Pediatrics* 29:764, 1962.

20. World Health Organization Expert Committee. Trace elements in human nutrition. *WHO Tech. Rep. Ser.* 532, 1973.

21. Shambaugh, G. E., and Petronic, A. Effects of sodium fluoride on bone: Applications to osteoporosis and other decalcifying bone diseases. *J.A.M.A.* 204:969, 1968.

22. Collier, D. R. Fluorine: An essential element for good dental health. *Contemp. Nutr.* October 1979.

23. Food and Nutrition Board, National Research Council. *Recommended Dietary Allowances* (9th ed.). Washington, D.C.: National Academy of Sciences, 1980. P. 170.

Suggested Readings

Altschul, A. M., and Grommet, J. K. Sodium intake and sodium sensitivity. *Nutr. Rev.* 38:393, 1980.

A primer on minerals. *FDA Consumer*. September 1974.

Arnaud, C. D. Calcium homeostasis: Regulatory elements and their integration. *Fed. Proc.* 37:2557, 1978.

Austin, L. A., and Heath, H. Calcitonin: Physiology and pathophysiology. *N. Engl. J. Med.* 304:269, 1981.

Copper intake and immune responses. *Nutr. Rev.* 40:107, 1982.

Cousins, R. J. Regulatory aspects of zinc metabolism in liver and intestine. *Nutr. Rev.* 37:97, 1979.

Dahl, L. K. Salt and hypertension. *Am. J. Clin. Nutr.* 25:231, 1972.

Danks, D. M.   Diagnosis of trace metal deficiency, with emphasis on zinc and copper. *Am. J. Clin. Nutr.* 34:278, 1981.

Dietary alteration of the trace element absorption. *Nutr. & the MD* June 1981.

Erdman, J. W.   Bioavailability of trace minerals from cereals and legumes. *Cereal Chem.* 58:21, 1981.

Experimental zinc deficiency in humans. *Nutr. Rev.* 37:76, 1979.

Fischer, P. W. F., Giroux, A., and L'Abbe, M. R.   The effect of dietary zinc on intestinal copper absorption. *Am. J. Clin. Nutr.* 34:1670, 1981.

Franey, P.   Copper and toxicity. *New York Times* Jan. 2, 1980.

Greeley, S., and Sandstead, H. H.   Zinc in human nutrition. *Contemp. Nutr.* April 1980.

Greger, J. L., Marhefka, S., and Geissler, A. H.   Magnesium content of selected foods. *J. Food Sci.* 43:1610, 1978.

Hair zinc in normal populations. *Nutr. Rev.* 40:74, 1982.

Hambridge, K. M.   Zinc and chromium in human nutrition. *J. Hum. Nutr.* 32:99, 1978.

Harland, B. F., et al.   Calcium, phosphorus, iron, iodine, and zinc in the "Total Diet." *J. Am. Diet. Assoc.* 77:16, 1980.

How trace elements in water contribute to health. *WHO Chron.* 32:382, 1978.

Inhibition of zinc absorption by inorganic iron. *Nutr. Rev.* 40:76, 1982.

Iron deficiency secondary to copper depletion. *Nutr. Rev.* 40:82, 1982.

Kay, R. G.   Zinc and copper in human nutrition. *J. Hum. Nutr.* 35:25, 1981.

Lee, C. J., Lawler, G. S., and Johnson, G. H.   Effects of supplementation of the diets with calcium and calcium-rich foods on bone density of elderly females with osteoporosis. *Am. J. Clin. Nutr.* 34:819, 1981.

Levander, O. A.   Selenium and human nutrition. *Contemp. Nutr.* November 1980.

Massry, S. G., Ritz, E., and John, H. (eds.).   *Phosphate and Minerals in Health and Disease. Advances in Experimental Medicine and Biology* (vol. 128). New York: Plenum Press, 1980.

McRae, M. P.   Foods high in potassium. *Hosp. Pharm.* 14:730, 1979.

Meadows, N. J., Smith, M. F., and Keeling, P. W. N.   Zinc and small babies. *Lancet* 2:1135, 1981.

Mertz, W.   Chromium: An essential micronutrient. *Contemp. Nutr.* March 1982.

Mertz, W.   The essential trace elements. *Science* 213:1332, 1981.

Mertz, W.   Mineral elements: New perspectives. *J. Am. Diet. Assoc.* 77:258, 1980.

Oberleas, D., and Harland, B. F.   Phytate content of foods: Effect on dietary zinc bioavailability. *J. Am. Diet. Assoc.* 79:433, 1981.

On the pathogenesis and clinical expression of Menkes' kinky hair syndrome. *Nutr. Rev.* 39:391, 1981.

Park, Y. K., et al.   Estimation of dietary iodine intake of Americans in recent years. *J. Am. Diet. Assoc.* 79:17, 1981.

Pekarek, R. S., et al.   Abnormal cellular immune response during acquired zinc deficiency. *Am. J. Clin. Nutr.* 32:1466, 1979.

Prasad, A. S.   Nutritional zinc today. *Nutr. Today* 16:4, 1981.

Prasad, A. S. (ed.).   *Trace Elements in Human Health and Disease.* New York: Academic, 1976.

Prohaska, J. R., and Lukasewycz, O. A.   Copper deficiency suppresses the immune response in mice. *Science* 213:559, 1981.

Ritchey, S. J.   Interrelationships among protein, zinc, and copper in human nutrition. *Cereal Chem.* 58:18, 1981.

Sandler, R. B.   Etiology of primary osteoporosis: An hypothesis. *J. Am. Geriatr. Soc.* 27:209, 1978.

Saver, G.   *Chromium in Nutrition and Disease.* New York: Alan R. Liss, 1980.

Seelig, M. S.   Magnesium requirements in human nutrition. *Contemp. Nutr.* January 1982.

Solomons, N. W.   On the assessment of zinc and copper nutriture in man. *Am. J. Clin. Nutr.* 83:856, 1979.

Solomons, N. W., and Jacob, R. A.   Studies on the bioavailability of zinc in humans: Effects of heme and nonheme iron on the absorption of zinc. *Am. J. Clin. Nurs.* 34:475, 1981.

The role of zinc deficiency in fetal alcohol syndrome. *Nutr. Rev.* 40:43, 1982.

Tracing elements grown into food. *FDA Consum.* 14:2, 1980.

Trapp, G. A., and Cannon, J. B.   Aluminum pots as a source of dietary aluminum. *N. Engl. J. Med.* 304:172, 1981.

Underwood, E. J.   Trace metals in human and animal health. *J. Hum. Nutr.* 35:37, 1981.

Vitamin D, calcium-binding protein and the intestinal transport of calcium. *Nutr. Rev.* 36:90, 1978.

Wright, A. L., et al.   Experimental zinc depletion and altered taste perception for NaCl in young adult males. *Am. J. Clin. Nutr.* 34:848, 1981.

Zinc deficiency in Crohn's disease. *Nutr. Rev.* 40:109, 1982.

Chapter 7

IRON

Iron is one of the most plentiful elements on earth, making up about 5 percent of its crust and an even greater part of its core. Iron was used to make tools and jewelry about 3000 B.C. The iron was probably from meteorites, since the Egyptians and Sumerians considered it to be the "heavenly metal." The mining and smelting of iron began about 1100 B.C. in Asia, Africa, and Europe. According to the Ebers papyrus, iron was first used as a medicine around 1500 B.C. to treat parasitic infections and a variety of other ailments. In the eighteenth century its presence was demonstrated in animal tissue, and blood was found to contain iron. Most of what is known about iron has been learned in this century, including its important interactions with other elements [1]. This chapter describes the functions, utilization, and sources of iron, and presents the human requirements for it. Iron deficiencies will be explored in greater depth in Chap. 41.

Function and Distribution

Iron plays a vital role in oxygen transport and energy production, and because of this, it is an essential element in the daily diet. Iron in the human body is almost exclusively involved in the uptake and release of oxygen at the cellular level. The average adult body contains about 4 gm of iron: 3 gm in active or functional form and about 1 gm in storage or transport form. Most of the active iron, as components of porphyrin, forms integral parts of hemoglobin, myoglobin, and the enzymes cytochrome, catalase, and peroxidase. The majority of this iron is found in the hemoglobin of red blood cells (erythrocytes). The hemoglobin molecule is composed of four polypeptide chains (two alpha and two beta), four protoporphyrin molecules, and four atoms of iron (see Fig. 3-6). Its purpose is to shuttle oxygen from the lungs to other tissues and to take carbon dioxide back from the tissues to the lungs. The hemoglobin molecule's ability to take up and release gases is dependent on the presence of iron; without iron, the molecule cannot function. Myoglobin works on a similar mechanism, but it takes up and releases oxygen only in the muscle. The cytochrome enzyme system functions in energy production. The distribution of iron-containing compounds in the human body is given in Table 7-1.

Absorption and Utilization

Iron is unique among mineral elements in that there is no physiologic mechanism for regulating its increased or decreased excretion. Iron balance is mainly controlled at the site of intestinal absorption. Absorption is influenced by the amount of iron already present in the intestinal mucosa, the amount and nature of iron in the diet, and compounds present in the food that increase or decrease the availability of iron for absorption.

Iron is absorbed only when needed, which prevents excessive storage of iron in the body. Ferrous, or oxidized, iron (Fe^{2+}) is better absorbed than is ferric, or reduced, iron (Fe^{3+}). Absorption is enhanced by an acid medium, which may

TABLE 7-1. Distribution of iron-containing compounds in the normal human adult

Compound	Total in body (gm)	Iron content (gm)	Percent of total iron in body
Iron porphyrins (heme compounds)			
Hemoglobin	900	3.0	60–70
Myoglobin	40	0.13	3–5
Heme enzymes			
Cytochrome c	0.8	0.004	0.1
Catalase	5.0	0.004	0.1
Other cytochromes			
Peroxidase			
Nonporphyrin iron compounds			
Siderophilin (transferrin)	10	0.004	0.1
Ferritin	2–4	0.4–0.8	15.0
Hemosiderin			
Total available iron stores		1.2–1.5	
Total iron		4.0–5.0	

Source: H. A. Harper, V. W. Rodwell, and P. A. Mayes, *Review of Physiological Chemistry* (17th ed.). Los Altos, Calif.: Lange, 1979. P. 585.

aid in the conversion of ferric to ferrous iron. Absorption is more efficient in the presence of ascorbic acid, sulfhydryl compounds, and other reducing substances. The efficiency of dietary iron absorption is also influenced by the form in which the iron is present and the foods with which it is eaten. Both fructose and ascorbic acid form soluble complexes with iron, enhancing absorption [2]. Phosphates, oxalates, and phytates form insoluble complexes with iron, preventing absorption. Iron from animal sources (primarily heme iron) is absorbed better than iron from vegetable sources (nonheme iron), although when both are eaten at the same time, absorption from vegetable sources is enhanced. Increased dietary fiber has been shown to result in decreased absorption of iron, zinc, and calcium [3]. Tea can inhibit the absorption of nonheme iron by the formation of insoluble iron-tannate complexes [4]. In patients with iron overload, such as those with thalassemia syndromes, tea has been found to produce a 41 to 95 percent inhibition of iron absorption [5]. During states of iron balance, about 10 percent of dietary iron is absorbed. This figure can increase by a factor of 2 or 3 during periods of iron deficiency. Iron absorption increases with need, such as during periods of rapid growth in infancy, childhood, and adolescence; during pregnancy; as a result of blood loss; and at high altitudes.

From the intestinal lumen, iron is absorbed in the ferrous (Fe^{2+}) oxidation state into the cells of the intestinal mucosa. Within the mucosal cells it is oxidized to the ferric (Fe^{3+}) form and then combines with a specific protein (apoferritin) to form an iron-protein complex, *ferritin*. When iron is needed by the body, ferritin gives up its iron component to the bloodstream: The ferric iron within the mucosal cell is reduced to the ferrous form and released. The apoferritin in the mucosal cell can then combine with dietary iron absorbed in the intestines. If all the mucosal cells are saturated (their apoferritin components have been changed to ferritin), no further iron will be absorbed. In the bloodstream, the released ferrous iron is reoxidized to ferric iron, which then combines with another specific protein compound to form *transferrin*, the transport form of iron in which it is carried to various tissues. Most of the iron in the bloodstream is utilized by the bone marrow to synthesize hemoglobin, although some is used by other tissues in the formation of enzymes (Fig. 7-1). Over 50 years ago it was discovered that copper was required for the synthesis of iron into hemoglobin and the cytochrome enzymes; copper may also be essential for the release of iron from ferritin [6].

Of the 3.5 to 4.0 gm of iron present in the adult human body, about one-fourth, or 1 gm, is stored, mainly in the liver and spleen. Other storage iron is found within cells as part of an iron-protein complex, *hemosiderin*. These forms are readily mobilized when iron is needed.

Red blood cells take about 7½ days for complete development and last about 120 days. After that time, they are broken down and the iron efficiently conserved. New hemoglobin is synthesized to replace that broken down in maturing red blood cells. Normal losses of iron occur daily in sweat, hair, desquamated (sloughed) epithelial and mucosal cells, and urine. Menstrual losses, pregnancy, blood donations, and injury with bleeding add to iron losses.

Requirements and Recommended Allowances

Because iron is efficiently conserved and reutilized in the body, the daily physiologic requirements are small. The average healthy man loses about 1 mg per day; women lose an additional 0.5 mg per day, the amount of iron in menstrual losses averaged over 1 month. Assuming an average availability (absorption) of 10 percent of dietary iron, an allowance of 10 mg per day is recommended to provide for the retention of 1 mg per day in men and postmenopausal women. For women of childbearing age, the allowance is set at 18 mg per day to meet the additional demands imposed by menstrual iron losses. Pregnancy increases iron needs to about 3.5 mg per day; these additional needs cannot be met by diet alone, so supplemental iron (30 to 60 mg per day) is recommended. During lactation, iron losses are about 0.5 to 1.0 mg per day, and continued supplementation is recommended for at least 2 or 3 months after delivery to help replenish iron stores depleted by pregnancy. Normal, full-term infants can maintain hemoglobin levels with an iron intake of 1 mg/kg/day, starting at about age 3 months. Infants weighing less than 2500 gm at birth require 2 mg/kg/day, starting soon after birth. Children and adolescents must maintain their hemoglobin levels and increase their total iron mass during periods of growth. An additional 0.8 to 1.0 mg per day is needed to maintain normal hemoglobin levels for these age groups [7]. A summary of the recommended dietary allowances of iron for various age groups is given in Table 7-2.

Dietary Sources of Iron

Iron is present in foods in one of two forms: *heme* or *nonheme* iron. Forty percent of all iron in animal tissues is considered to be heme iron; the remaining 60 percent of iron in animal tissues and all iron from vegetable sources is considered to be nonheme iron. Heme iron, which is actually the hemoglobin present in the animal tissue, is very well absorbed and not influenced by other dietary components present in the meal. Nonheme iron is much less well absorbed and is greatly influenced by other factors in the meal. It is mostly nonheme iron that is inhibited by phosphates, phytates, oxalates, and tea, as discussed earlier, and enhanced by ascorbic acid and the presence of heme iron.

FIG. 7-1. Metabolism of iron in the human. (From E. Selkurt [ed.], *Basic Physiology for the Health Sciences* [2nd ed.]. Boston: Little, Brown, 1982.)

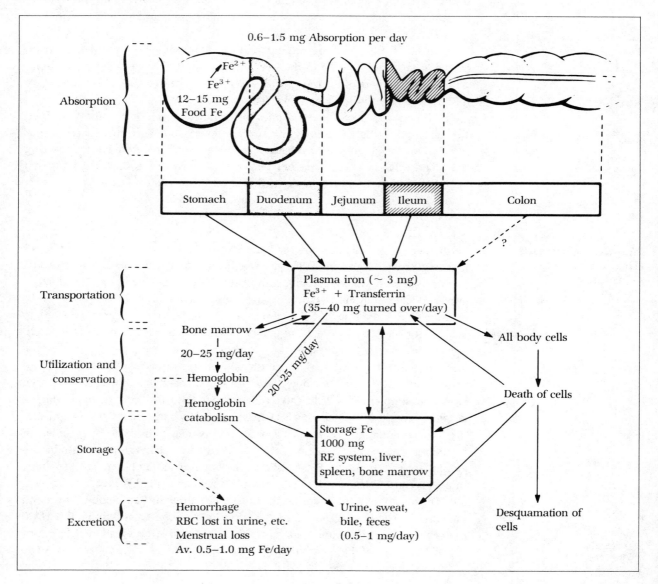

TABLE 7-2. Recommended daily dietary allowances of iron

Group	Age (years)	Iron (mg)
Infants	0.0–0.5	10
	0.5–1.0	15
Children	1–3	15
	4–6	10
	7–10	10
Males	11–14	18
	15–18	18
	19–22	10
	23–50	10
	51+	10
Females	11–14	18
	15–18	18
	19–22	18
	23–50	18
	51+	10
Pregnant		*
Lactating		*

*These needs cannot be met by diet alone; daily iron supplements of 30–60 mg/day are recommended.
Source: Adapted from Food and Nutrition Board, National Research Council, *Recommended Dietary Allowances* (9th ed.). Washington, D.C.: National Academy of Sciences, 1980.

The iron used to fortify foods is nonheme iron, and is therefore vulnerable to a variety of influences. In addition, when iron is added to a food it may react as a catalyst or reactant with chemicals within the food. In foods that contain sulfur compounds, the addition of iron may lead to the formation of black insoluble deposits or a gray appearance. Iron may also accelerate the oxidation (breakdown) of ascorbic acid and catalyze the oxidation of unsaturated lipids, leading to the development of off-flavors and the loss of vitamins A and E [8]. Because of these and many other problems, no increase in the level of iron enrichment is foreseen in the near future [9], and emphasis has been switched to increasing enhancing factors at the same meal, such as adding ascorbic acid and animal protein [10]. More about iron fortification is presented in Chap. 12. Table 7-3 lists the type and amount of iron in a variety of food sources.

Calculation of Available Iron

Previously, the recommended dietary allowances (RDAs) for iron were based on the assumption of an average of 10 percent iron absorption from the diet. For women in the childbearing years, the RDA has been 18 mg per day to meet the extra demands of this age group. Because the average diet consumed in this country furnishes about 6 mg of iron per 1000 calories, it has been difficult to meet these requirements by diet alone. Recent attempts at increasing the level of iron enrichment have been unsuccessful, so an alternative method has been

TABLE 7-3. Dietary sources of iron (mg)

Meats (40% heme iron, 60% nonheme iron)

Bacon, 3 strips (3 oz)	0.6	Kidney, 3 slices (3.5 oz)	9.5
Beef hamburger (4 oz)	3.3	Lamb chop (3.5 oz)	3.0
Beef, porterhouse (8 oz)	3.8	Liver, calf (2.5 oz)	9.0
Brains (3 oz)	2.0	Pork chop (3.5 oz)	4.4
Frankfurter (1.75 oz)	0.6	Spareribs (3.0 oz)	2.3
Ham, fresh (3.5 oz)	2.3	Sweetbread (3.5 oz)	1.2
Heart (1/3, 3.5 oz)	5.5	Veal cutlet (3.5 oz)	4.2

Fish and shellfish (40% heme iron, 60% nonheme iron)

Clams (3.5 oz)	3.4	Sardines (3.5 oz)	5.2
Crab (3.5 oz)	0.8	Scallops (3.5 oz)	3.0
Crayfish (3.5 oz)	1.5	Shrimp (3.5 oz)	2.0
Flounder (3.5 oz)	1.4	Snail, raw (3.5 oz)	3.5
Haddock (3.5 oz)	1.2	Tuna (3.5 oz)	1.9
Salmon (3.5 oz)	1.2		

Poultry and game (40% heme iron, 60% nonheme iron)

Chicken (3.5 oz)	1.5	Quail (3.5 oz)	3.8
Duck (3.5 oz)	5.8	Squab (3.5 oz)	1.8
Pheasant (3.5 oz)	3.7	Turkey (3.5 oz)	3.8

Legumes and vegetables (nonheme iron)

Beans, red kidney (3.5 oz)	2.4	Chickpeas (3.5 oz)	6.9
Beans, green lima (3.5 oz)	2.8	Dandelion greens (3.5 oz)	3.1
Beans, green snap (3.5 oz)	0.8	Fennel (3.5 oz)	2.7
Broccoli (3.5 oz)	0.8	Kale (3.5 oz)	2.2
Cauliflower (3.5 oz)	1.1	Lentils (3.5 oz)	2.1
Cabbage (3.5 oz)	0.4	Spinach (3.5 oz)	3.1

Dried fruits and nuts (nonheme iron)

Apricots (3.5 oz)	5.5	Almonds (3.5 oz)	4.4
Dates (3.5 oz)	3.0	Cashews (3.5 oz)	3.8
Figs (3.5 oz)	3.0	Peanuts (3.5 oz)	3.0
Prunes (3.5 oz)	3.9	Walnuts, black (3.5 oz)	6.0
Raisins (3.5 oz)	3.5	Walnuts, English (3.5 oz)	2.1

Cereals and cereal products (nonheme iron)

Barley (2 tbsp)	0.5	Oatmeal (1 cup)	1.7
Bulgar (2 tbsp)	1.0	Noodles (1 cup)	1.4
Farina (1 cup)	2.0	Wheat germ (3 tbsp)	2.6

Source: From C. F. Church and H. N. Church, *Food Values of Portions Commonly Used* (12th ed.). Philadelphia: Lippincott, 1975.

proposed by the Committee on Dietary Allowances, Food and Nutrition Board, National Research Council [7, 11]. By dividing the dietary iron into heme and nonheme compounds and evaluating the dietary factors that influence absorption, a more precise estimation of iron absorption can be made. This method provides a basis for increasing the amount of absorbable dietary iron by altering food selections at each meal. The calculation of absorbable iron is used in diet planning and in the evaluation of iron intake.

Two factors enhancing nonheme iron absorption include ascorbic acid and the quantity of animal tissue present in each meal. Depending on the amount of these two enhancing factors present, the availability (absorbability) of nonheme iron is classified as low, medium, or high.

Five variables are computed for each meal:

1. Total iron (values from food composition tables)
2. Heme iron (40 percent of total iron of animal tissues)
3. Nonheme iron (#1 minus #2)
4. Ascorbic acid (present in the meal)
5. The amount of meat, fish, or poultry present

Because of the interactions of dietary components with iron, the amount of absorbable iron must be calculated for each meal. Table 7-4 shows the availability of iron in different types of meals.

Iron Deficiency

A deficiency of iron causes *hypochromic anemia.* The number of red blood cells can be either normal or reduced, but the amount of circulating hemoglobin is below normal. Each red blood cell has a decreased content of hemoglobin and is pale. Because of the reduced hemoglobin content, the blood has a decreased oxygen-carrying capacity. The clinical features of iron-deficiency anemia include weakness, fatigue, and pallor. Iron deficiency can develop from a poor diet or chronic blood loss or both. Intestinal parasites, bleeding hemorrhoids, or peptic ulcer can also lead to iron depletion. If menstrual losses are heavy or pregnancies are spaced too closely, the iron stores of women can be depleted quickly. If these factors are combined with a poor diet or absorption, iron deficiency symptoms soon appear. Other dietary factors can also influence the development of reduced hemoglobin: insufficient protein, calories, B vitamins, or ascorbic acid.

The Food and Nutrition Board has found that there are four situations in which iron intake is frequently inadequate in the United States [7]:

1. During *infancy*, because of the low iron content of milk and because iron stores at birth are usually sufficient only for the first 6 months
2. During the periods of rapid growth in *childhood* and *adolescence*, because of the needs of the expanding iron stores
3. During the *female reproductive period*, because of menstrual losses

TABLE 7-4. Availability of iron in different meals

Type of meal	Percent absorption of iron present in meal	
	Nonheme iron	Heme iron
Low-availability meal <30 gm meat, fish, poultry <25 mg ascorbic acid	3	23
Medium-availability meal 30–90 gm meat, fish, poultry or 25–75 mg ascorbic acid	5	23
High-availability meal >90 gm meat, fish, poultry or >75 mg ascorbic acid or 30–90 gm meat, fish, poultry plus 25–75 mg ascorbic acid	8	23

Source: Adapted from E. R. Monsen, et al., *Am. J. Clin. Nutr.* 31:134, 1978.

4. During *pregnancy*, because of the increased maternal blood volume, demands of the fetus and placenta, and blood losses in childbirth

The detection and treatment of iron-deficiency anemia is discussed in detail in Chap. 41.

Iron Overload

The total amount of iron in the body can be increased by excessive iron intake, abnormalities in iron absorption, or parenteral (injection) administration of iron. It is difficult to overload with iron by food alone, because the intestinal mucosa is usually effective in preventing excessive absorption. However, excessive amounts of iron can sometimes overwhelm the body's ability to regulate iron balance. The South African Bantu consume a type of beer (kaffir beer) that is brewed in iron utensils, and iron overload is frequently seen among these people. Toxic intakes of iron have been reported in children and adults ingesting medicinal iron supplements. The lethal dose for a young child is about 3 gm; for adults it ranges between 200 and 250 mg per kilogram body weight [12]. Iron overload can also be caused by a defect in the mechanism that limits absorption by the intestinal mucosa. This condition, termed *hemochromatosis*, results in the deposition of iron in the parenchymal cells of the liver. In its advanced stages, it is characterized by graying pigmentation of the skin, poor liver function with enlargement and scarring, pancreatic infiltration with resultant diabetes, and myocardial disease resulting in heart failure.

References

1. Medcom, Inc. *Iron.* New York: Lakeside Laboratories, 1972.
2. Lynch, S. R. Ascorbic acid and iron nutrition. *Contemp. Nutr.* September 1980.

3. Reinhold, J. G., et al. Decreased absorption of calcium, magnesium, zinc and phosphorus by humans due to increased fiber and phosphorus consumption as wheat bread. *J. Nutr.* 106:493, 1976.

4. Disler, P. B., et al. The effect of tea on iron absorption. *Gut* 16:193, 1975.

5. de Alarcon, P. A., et al. Iron absorption in the thalassemia syndromes and its inhibition by tea. *N. Engl. J. Med.* 300:5, 1979.

6. Hart, E. B., et al. Iron in nutrition. *J. Biol. Chem.* 77:797, 1928.

7. Food and Nutrition Board, National Research Council. *Recommended Dietary Allowances* (9th ed.). Washington, D.C.: National Academy of Sciences, 1980. Pp. 138–140.

8. Problems in iron enrichment and fortification of foods. *Nutr. Rev.* 33:46, 1975.

9. No increase in iron fortification in offing. *J.A.M.A.* 239:1949, 1978.

10. The value of iron fortification of food. *Nutr. Rev.* 31:275, 1973.

11. Monsen, E. R., et al. Estimation of available dietary iron. *Am. J. Clin. Nutr.* 31:134, 1978.

12. Committee on Medical and Biologic Effects of Environmental Pollutants, National Research Council. *Iron.* Washington, D.C.: National Academy of Sciences, 1977.

Suggested Readings

Absorption of iron from breakfast foods. *Nutr. & the MD* May 1980.

Cooke, J. C., et al. Absorption of fortification of iron in bread. *Am. J. Clin. Nutr.* 26:861, 1973.

Cooke, J. C., and Monsen, E. R. Vitamin C, the common cold, and iron absorption in man. *Am. J. Clin. Nutr.* 30:235, 1977.

The correlation of serum ferritin and body iron stores. *Nutr. Rev.* 33:11, 1975.

Diet and iron absorption in the first year of life. *Nutr. Rev.* 37:195, 1979.

Frieden, E. The ferrous to ferric cycles in iron metabolism. *Nutr. Rev.* 31:41, 1973.

Inhibition of iron absorption in infants. *Nutr. & the MD* June 1981.

Inhibition of zinc absorption by inorganic iron. *Nutr. Rev.* 40:76, 1982.

Iron absorption and utilization in the elderly. *Nutr. Rev.* 37:222, 1979.

Lee, K., and Clydesdale, F. M. Effect of baking on the forms of iron in iron-enriched flour. *J. Food Sci.* 45:1500, 1980.

Lipschitz, D. A., Cook, J. D., and Finch, C. A. A clinical evaluation of serum ferritin as an index of iron stores. *N. Engl. J. Med.* 290:1213, 1974.

Martinez-Torres, C., Romano, E., and Layrisse, M. Effect of cysteine on iron absorption in man. *Am. J. Clin. Nutr.* 34:322, 1981.

Mertz, W. The new RDAs: Estimated adequate and safe intake of trace elements and calculation of available iron. *J. Am. Diet. Assoc.* 76:128, 1980.

Monsen, E. R. How to get more iron from the food you eat. *Nutr. & the MD* June 1981.

Sayers, M. H., et al. The effects of ascorbic acid supplementation on the absorption of iron in maize, wheat and soya. *Br. J. Haematol.* 24:209, 1973.

Solomons, N. W., and Jacob, R. A. Studies on the bioavailability of zinc in humans: Effects of heme and nonheme iron on the absorption of zinc. *Am. J. Clin. Nutr.* 34:475, 1981.

Chapter 8

THE FAT-SOLUBLE VITAMINS

Nutrition is a relatively new science, with most of the major discoveries having been made during this century. E. V. McCollum, one of the foremost discoverers of "accessory food factors," later to be called *vitamins*, stated that "in 1900 we were almost blind to the relation of food to health" [1]. At the turn of the century, deficiency diseases were widespread and common: Rickets affected the young and took the lives of many women during childbirth because of contracted pelvises. The fields of microbiology and biochemistry were just beginning. Although the relationships between essential food components, the vitamins, and health had been known empirically through folk medicine for hundreds of years, it was during the twentieth century, with the application of scientific research, that the physiologic action of these mysterious substances came to light.

This chapter covers the fat-soluble vitamins, grouped together on the basis of their solubility in fats (Fig. 8-1). Fat-soluble vitamins also share certain physiologic characteristics: They are absorbed along with dietary fats and stored in the body in moderate quantities. The water-soluble vitamins, also grouped by their solubility, are presented in Chap. 9.

Vitamin A

In 1913, McCollum and Davis of the University of Wisconsin and Osborne and Mendel of Yale University demonstrated that rats developed eye irritation and growth failure when fed a purified diet containing lard as the only dietary source of fat. When butterfat or egg yolk was added to the diet, growth resumed and the eye conditions improved. This discovery led to the determination that a fat-soluble substance, later called vitamin A, is important to eye function.

The source of all vitamin A is the carotenes synthesized by plants. Animals, including humans, convert the carotene in plants into vitamin A. Of nutritional importance are alpha, beta, and gamma carotene. Upon hydrolysis, alpha and gamma carotene yield one molecule of vitamin A; beta carotene yields two. Vitamin A is obtained in two forms in the diet: from preformed vitamin A (retinol) (Fig. 8-1A) and from *provitamin A carotenoids* (or vitamin A precursors). The most plentiful carotenoid in the diet is beta carotene.

FUNCTIONS

Vitamin A is important in maintaining the integrity of mucous membranes and normal vision in dim light. An early sign of vitamin A deficiency is impaired dark adaptation (night blindness). Prolonged deficiency leads to damage of the ocular tissues and blindness. Vitamin A is also essential for normal skeletal and dental development, the synthesis of hydrocortisone from cholesterol, and the stability of biologic membranes.

VISUAL PROCESS

In the retina of the eye there are two types of light receptors: *cones* for vision in bright light and for color vision, and *rods* for vision in dim light. The photosensi-

FIG. 8-1. Chemical structures of
the fat-soluble vitamins.
A. Vitamin A_1, $C_{20}H_{30}O$.
B. Vitamin D_3, $C_{27}H_{44}O$.
C. Vitamin E, $C_{29}H_{50}O_2$.
D. Vitamin K_1, $C_{31}H_{46}O_2$.

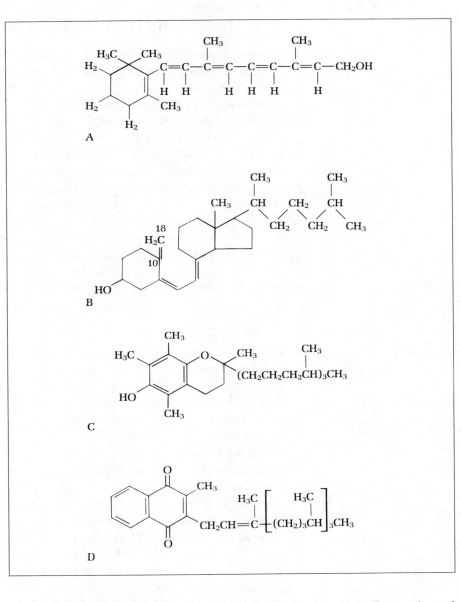

tive pigments in both of these receptors (*rhodopsin* or *visual purple* in rods, and
iodopsin or *visual violet* in cones) contain vitamin A plus different proteins.
When struck by light, the pigments are split apart into vitamin A and the constituent protein. In the dark, the pigments are regenerated at a speed dependent
on the blood level of vitamin A.

MUCOUS MEMBRANES

Vitamin A is also involved in the synthesis of components of mucus, including
mucoproteins and mucopolysaccharides. The integrity of the epithelium, partic-

ularly the membranes of the genitourinary, respiratory, and gastrointestinal tracts, and those lining the eyes and mouth are maintained by mucous secretions. When intact, the membranes confer resistance to bacterial invasion.

ABSORPTION AND METABOLISM

To become active, the provitamin A carotenoids must be converted into retinol during absorption through the intestinal wall. The hydrolysis of carotenes occurs in the mucosa of the small intestine. About half of the absorbed carotene is converted to vitamin A, and only one-fourth to one-sixth of the carotene present in foods is utilized. The absorption of vitamin A is facilitated by the presence of dietary fat, bile, thyroid hormone, and vitamin E. Mineral oil prevents the absorption of vitamin A and carotene and should therefore never be used as a substitute for fats in the diet nor taken as a laxative at mealtimes.

Vitamin A is both absorbed directly into the portal circulation and transported in chylomicrons through the lymph circulation to the thoracic duct where it enters the blood circulation to the liver. The majority of the body's vitamin A stores are in the liver; when they become depleted, the blood concentration of vitamin A drops.

RECOMMENDED DIETARY ALLOWANCES

Because of the poorer utilization of the provitamin A carotenoids as compared with retinol, the vitamin A allowances are now expressed as retinol equivalents [2]:

1 retinol equivalent = 1 µg retinol
= 6 µg beta carotene
= 12 µg other provitamin A carotenoids
= 3.33 IU vitamin A activity from retinol
= 10 IU vitamin A activity from beta carotene

The minimum requirement to prevent the development of deficiency symptoms for adults has been determined to be 500 to 600 µg retinol or twice as much beta carotene; larger daily intakes are needed to produce liver storage [2].

The average retinol content of human milk, about 49 µg per 100 ml, provides the basis for the recommended allowance for infants [2]. With an average daily intake of 850 ml, breast-feeding supplies about 420 µg of retinol. With the addition of solid foods at about 6 months of age, the allowance drops to 400 retinol equivalents (300 as retinol and 100 as beta carotene). The allowances for children and adolescents are based on average body weight and growth needs. The allowance levels off at adolescence and remains at the same level through adulthood. For adults, the recommended daily allowance (RDA) is set at 1000 retinol equivalents (or 5000 IU) for men and 800 retinol equivalents (or 4000 IU) for women. During pregnancy, the allowance is increased to 1000 retinol equivalents to allow for storage in the fetus. An even higher allowance (1200 retinol equivalents) is recommended during lactation to provide for the vitamin A secreted in the breast milk. Vitamin A is stored in the liver, and well-nourished

TABLE 8-1. Recommended daily dietary allowances of the fat-soluble vitamins

Group	Age (years)	Vitamin A (μg RE)[a]	Vitamin D (μg)[b]	Vitamin E (mg α-TE)[c]
Infants	0.0–0.5	420	10	3
	0.5–1.0	400	10	4
Children	1–3	400	10	5
	4–6	500	10	6
	7–10	700	10	7
Males	11–14	1000	10	8
	15–18	1000	10	10
	19–22	1000	7.5	10
	23–50	1000	5	10
	51 +	1000	5	10
Females	11–14	800	10	8
	15–18	800	10	8
	19–22	800	7.5	8
	23–50	800	5	8
	51 +	800	5	8
Pregnant[d]	—	+200	+5	+2
Lactating[d]	—	+400	+5	+3

[a] As retinol equivalents (RE). 1 RE = 1 μg retinol or 6 μg beta carotene.
[b] As cholecalciferol. 10 μg cholecalciferol = 400 IU of vitamin D.
[c] α-Tocopherol equivalents (α-TE). 1 mg D-α-tocopherol = 1 α-TE.
[d] Allowances given for pregnant and lactating women are *in addition to* the normal allowance for women of a particular age.
Source: From Food and Nutrition Board, National Research Council, *Recommended Dietary Allowances* (9th ed.). Washington, D.C.: National Academy of Sciences, 1980.

individuals have a 3-month supply. A summary of the RDAs is given in Table 8-1.

FOOD SOURCES

Most foods in the United States provide approximately half the total vitamin A activity as retinol and half as provitamin A carotenoids, with beta carotene comprising all the provitamin A. Fish-liver oils are the only concentrated animal sources of vitamin A. Also rich in this vitamin are milk, butter, cheese, liver, margarine, and egg yolk. The main source of vitamin A in the diet is from carotenes, which are widespread in deep green or yellow plants.

Vitamin A is stable at the usual cooking temperatures. Canning and freezing do not affect vitamin A activity, but this vitamin is rapidly destroyed by rancidity (oxidation) of fats. Table 8-2 gives dietary sources of vitamin A.

EFFECTS OF DEFICIENCY

Although vitamin A is present in a wide variety of available, low-cost foods, a deficiency of this vitamin is seen in the United States and many other countries. The deficiency may be due to poor dietary intake, incomplete absorption and metabolism (as in chronic diarrhea or with the use of mineral oil), abnormal fat metabolism (pancreatic disease), or hepatic disease.

A deficiency of vitamin A can cause night blindness (nyctalopia), the inability to see well in dim light, especially when entering a dark space from a bright

TABLE 8-2. Dietary sources of the fat-soluble vitamins

Vitamin	Source
Vitamin A and procarotenoids	High (10,000–76,000 IU/100 gm)
	Liver (beef, pig, sheep, calf, chicken)
	Liver oil (cod, halibut, salmon, shark, sperm whale)
	Carrots, mint, kohlrabi, parsley, spinach, turnip greens, dandelion greens, palm oil
	Medium (1000–10,000 IU/100 gm)
	Butter, cheese (except cottage), egg yolk, margarine, dried milk, cream
	White fish, eel
	Kidneys (beef, pig, sheep), liver (pork)
	Mangoes, apricots, yellow melons, peaches, cherries (sour), nectarines
	Beet greens, broccoli, endive, kale, mustard greens, pumpkin, sweet potatoes, watercress, tomatoes, leek greens, chicory, chives, collards, fennel, squash, chard
Vitamin D	High (1000 to 25×10^6 IU/100 gm)
	Liver oils (bonito, tuna, lingcod, sea bass, swordfish, halibut, herring, cod, sablefish, soupfin shark)
	Medium (100–1000 IU/100 gm)
	Egg yolk, margarine, lard, herring, salmon, mackerel, pilchards, sardines, shrimp, tuna, kippers
Vitamin E	High (50–300 mg/100 gm)
	Oil (cottonseed, corn, soybean, safflower, wheat germ)
	Margarine
	Medium (5–50 mg/100 gm)
	Oils (coconut, peanut, olive)
	Wheat germ, apple seeds, alfalfa, barley, dry soybeans, peanuts
	Chocolate, rose hips, yeast
	Cabbage, spinach, asparagus
Vitamin K	High (100–300 µg/100 gm)
	Cabbage, cauliflower, soybeans, spinach
	Pork, beef liver, beef kidney
	Medium (10–100 µg/100 gm)
	Potatoes, strawberries, tomatoes, alfalfa, wheat (whole, germ, bran), egg yolk

Source: *Handbook of Vitamins and Hormones* by R. J. Kutsky. Copyright © 1973 by Van Nostrand Reinhold Company. Reprinted by permission of Van Nostrand Reinhold Company.

light. This condition is particularly dangerous when driving at night because of the alternation of the glare of oncoming headlights with darkness. Night blindness occurs when there is insufficient vitamin A in the blood to quickly regenerate visual purple. Persons with alcoholic liver disease (cirrhosis) have frequently been found to have night blindness caused by hepatic damage affecting vitamin A release. The therapy for night blindness associated with cirrhosis includes vitamin A, zinc, and abstinence from alcohol [3, 4].

In the eye, the first symptoms of vitamin A deficiency include *photophobia*, sensitivity to bright light. With continued deficiency, the eyes and eyelids become inflamed. This is due to the impaired functioning of the lacrimal glands, whose function it is to wash away bacteria and keep the surface of the eye moist. When the cornea becomes dry, inflamed, and edematous, the condition is termed *xerophthalmia*. Permanent blindness results when infection leads to ulceration and softening of the cornea. This final stage is known as *keratomalacia*.

Another effect of vitamin A deficiency is *keratinization* of the epithelial tissues. This shrinking and degeneration of the skin increases susceptibility to infections of all membranes normally protected by mucus. *Follicular hyperkeratosis* is another skin change that occurs with vitamin A deficiency. The sebaceous glands become clogged, and the skin takes on a goosefleshlike appearance. It appears first on the thighs and upper forearms, then spreads to the back, abdomen, buttocks, and shoulders.

A deficiency of vitamin A may suddenly become apparent in children given skim milk for the treatment of kwashiorkor (protein-calorie malnutrition). The protein in the milk mobilizes the small stores of vitamin A from the liver, precipitating the signs of deficiency. Vitamin A supplements are therefore an important part of the treatment of kwashiorkor.

Animal studies have shown that vitamin A and its analogs can delay the appearance of tumors, retard their growth, and even cause them to regress. Human biochemical and epidemiologic studies suggest that cancers of epithelial origin may be caused by vitamin A deficiency, and that this vitamin may have a therapeutic and prophylactic role in this type of cancer [5, 6].

TOXIC EFFECTS

High intakes of vitamin A can be deleterious to adults and children. The daily intake of 3000 retinol equivalents (10,000 IU) by children or 15,000 retinol equivalents (50,000 IU) by adults may produce toxic effects [7, 8]. The symptoms and signs of vitamin A toxicity include drying and desquamation of the skin, anorexia, loss of hair, bone pain and fragility, and enlargement of the liver and spleen. The Food and Nutrition Board's Committee on Dietary Allowances recommends that adult intakes do not exceed 7500 retinol equivalents (25,000 IU) per day [2].

A summary of the features of vitamin A is given in Table 8-3.

Vitamin D

For the past six or seven hundred years, the empirical treatment for rickets, the bone disease caused by a deficiency of vitamin D, has been cod-liver oil. In 1919 Huldschinsky ameliorated rachitic symptoms in children with ultraviolet radiation. In 1925 McCollum named the antirachitic factor in cod-liver oil vitamin D, and by 1931 it had been isolated.

Vitamin D occurs in two forms, as vitamin D_2 (*ergocalciferol*), the chief vitamin D precursor found in plants, and as vitamin D_3 (*cholecalciferol*) (Fig. 8-1B), the main form occurring in animal cells and developing in skin on exposure to ultraviolet light. Vitamin D_2 is produced by ultraviolet irradiation of the plant

TABLE 8-3. Summary of the fat-soluble vitamins

Vitamin	Primary functions	Results of deficiency	Results of toxicity	Normal blood levels
A	Growth Production of visual purple Bone development Maintenance of membranes Maintenance of adrenal cortex Steroid hormone synthesis	Xerophthalmia Nyctalopia Keratomalacia Hyperkeratosis	Abnormal bone growth Decreased clotting time Anorexia Fatigue Bone and joint pain Nerve lesions	100–300 IU/100 gm
D	Bone growth Calcium and phosphorus absorption from intestine Maintenance of serum calcium and phosphorus levels	Rickets Osteomalacia Hypoparathyroidism	Calcification of soft tissues Anorexia Muscle weakness Diarrhea Polyuria	65–165 IU/100 ml
E	Normal growth Aids the intestinal absorption of unsaturated fatty acids Maintenance of membranes Biologic antioxidant	Degeneration of reproductive tissues and muscles Liver necrosis Anemia Increased excretion of creatine	Possible increase in blood pressure Interference with clotting and hemostatic mechanisms	1.11 mg/100 ml
K	Prothrombin synthesis in liver Growth Photosynthetic mechanisms Blood-clotting mechanisms	Hypoprothrombinemia	Possible thrombosis Vomiting Porphyrinuria	Not reported

sterol, ergosterol. The naturally occurring form of the vitamin in animal tissues, vitamin D_3, is formed by the action of sunlight on 7-dehydrocholesterol in the skin.

FUNCTIONS

Vitamin D is unique in several respects: It is a steroid and functions like other steroid hormones; it is not a dietary essential when there is adequate exposure to ultraviolet light; and it is the only vitamin known to be converted to a hormonal form [9]. Vitamin D plays a central role in the regulation of calcium and phosphate (phosphorus) metabolism by promoting their intestinal absorption and influencing the process of bone mineralization. A deficiency of vitamin D causes faulty mineralization of the bone matrix, resulting in *osteomalacia* in adults and *rickets* in children. It is thought that vitamin D exerts its antirachitic action by making the intestinal mucosa permeable to calcium and phosphorus and facilitating the active transport of calcium across cell membranes.

ABSORPTION AND METABOLISM

Vitamin D_3 is obtained from two sources: by intestinal absorption from the diet or food supplements, and from the conversion of 7-dehydrocholesterol in the skin by ultraviolet light (see Fig. 5-9) to previtamin D_3, which then slowly equilibrates to vitamin D_3. Before it can function, vitamin D_3 must be activated by hydroxylation by both the liver and the kidney. The initial conversion by the liver results in 25-hydroxycholecalciferol (calcidiol), the major circulating form of vitamin D_3. In the proximal tubule of the kidney, the second hydroxylation takes place, giving rise to 1,25-dihydroxycholecalciferol or *calcitriol*. This form is then transported to various sites, including bone, kidneys, and intestines, where the actions of vitamin D are initiated. These actions include the intestinal absorption of calcium and phosphorus; the mobilization of calcium from bone; and the renal reabsorption of calcium. The actions of vitamin D maintain calcium and phosphorus levels that, in turn, support normal mineralization of bone and neuromuscular activity. Liver damage, a decrease in bile salts in the gut, and a high pH all decrease the availability of vitamin D.

RECOMMENDED DIETARY ALLOWANCES

The amount of vitamin D formed by the action of sunlight on the skin is dependent on several variables, including the intensity of the sunlight, the length of exposure, and skin pigmentation. With deeper pigmentation, less active vitamin D is formed. For this reason, rickets is more common among dark-skinned children than among those with lighter skin pigmentation. Climates with seasonally limited sunlight or air pollution may not provide the amount of ultraviolet energy necessary for adequate formation of vitamin D in the skin.

Four hundred international units (10 μg) of vitamin D per day has been shown to promote optimal calcium absorption and enhance growth, although as little as 2.5 μg (100 IU) can prevent rickets and ensure adequate calcium absorption, satisfactory growth, and normal bone mineralization. The higher level is recommended for infants and children and should be provided in the diet or as a supplement since exposure to sunlight may not be adequate in this age group.

With a slowing and finally cessation of skeletal growth, the vitamin D allowance decreases to 7.5 μg (300 IU) for ages 19 through 22, and 5 μg (200 IU) for the later years. The adult allowances may be met by adequate exposure to sunlight, unless there are conditions preventing sufficient solar radiation, in which case dietary sources are necessary. During pregnancy and lactation, the vitamin D requirement is increased by 5 μg (200 IU) to allow for transfer across the placenta and into the breast milk, respectively [10]. A summary of the RDAs for vitamin D for all age groups is given in Table 8-1.

FOOD SOURCES

Vitamin D is stable through storage, processing, and cooking and is absorbed efficiently from the gastrointestinal tract. In the absence of bile salts, with a reduction in their availability, with pancreatic insufficiency, or with any other cause of fat malabsorption, there is also malabsorption of vitamin D. Such animal foods as eggs, liver, butter, and fatty fish naturally contain vitamin D. Pure milk is a poor source of the vitamin, but now most milk has been fortified with 10 μg (400 IU) of cholecalciferol per quart. Milk is an appropriate food for such fortification since it is a rich source of calcium and phosphorus and is consumed by growing children. Dietary sources of vitamin D are given in Table 8-2.

EFFECTS OF DEFICIENCY

A deficiency of vitamin D causes impaired intestinal absorption of calcium and phosphorus and faulty mineralization of the teeth and bones. Skeletal malformations result from the inability of the softened bones to withstand weight bearing. In children, this bone condition is termed *rickets* (Fig. 8-2). Rickets is more prevalent in northern areas; during the winter months; in dark, overcrowded sections of large cities; and among dark-skinned children. Other symptoms of rickets include delayed closure of the fontanelles (suture lines in the skull), especially in premature infants; projection of the sternum ("pigeon breast"); spinal curvature; bowing of the legs; and enlargement of the costochondral junctions (where the bone of the ribs joins cartilage) forming a "rachitic rosary" (Fig. 8-3).

In adults, this bone condition is termed *osteomalacia* and is caused purely by a lack of vitamin D and calcium. It is particularly prevalent among pregnant and lactating Oriental women, since their diets are traditionally low in these two

FIG. 8-2. Early skeletal deformities of rickets can persist throughout life. Bowlegs that curve laterally indicate that the weakened bones have bent after the second year, as the result of standing. If severe rickets occurs before the child walks, it produces a combination of bowed thighs and knock-knees. (Courtesy Dept. Medical Photography, Children's Hospital, Buffalo, N.Y.)

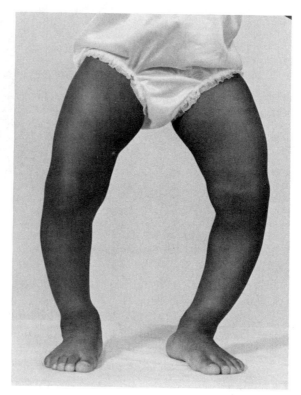

FIG. 8-3. This child exhibits the classic signs of rickets: large abdomen, big forehead, soft bones of the legs and vertebrae, and swelling of the wrists. (WHO photo.)

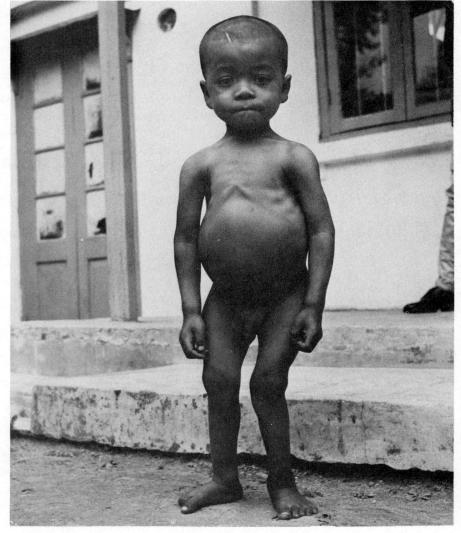

dietary essentials. Studies of these women suggest that pregnancy and lactation hasten skeletal demineralization and that adequate dietary calcium and vitamin D are vital, especially during late gestation and lactation, when calcium demands are greatest [11, 12].

Because vitamin D is also involved in neuromuscular activity, a deficiency of this vitamin can manifest as *tetany:* convulsions, muscle twitching, and sharp flexion of the wrist and ankle joints. This condition may result from parathyroid disease or from insufficient dietary intake or intestinal absorption of calcium or vitamin D.

As discussed in Chap. 28, vitamin D is important for the normal development and maintenance of the teeth. *Dental caries* are more prevalent among children with poor intakes of vitamin D, calcium, and phosphorus.

TOXIC EFFECTS

The precise toxic effects of the chronic high intakes of vitamin D are not known, but this is a potentially lethal vitamin. The symptoms of toxicity include polyuria (excessive urination) and nocturia (urination at night), weight loss, diarrhea, and nausea. With severe toxicity, calcification of the soft tissues, such as the blood vessels, heart, stomach, bronchi, and kidneys may occur. The Food and Nutrition Board recommends that intakes closely approximate the RDAs for adults and children and warns that daily doses of 1000 to 3000 IU per kilogram body weight are toxic [13].

A summary of the characteristics of vitamin D is given in Table 8-3.

Vitamin E
FUNCTIONS

Vitamin E's main action is as an antioxidant; it may be involved in the metabolism of glutathione and nucleic acids as well. Vitamin E supplementation in various experimental animals has been shown to substantially increase humoral immune response and disease resistance [14, 15].

In the rods of the pigment epithelium of the retina, there is a high concentration of unsaturated fatty acids. The retina also has a plentiful supply of oxygen for its unusually high rate of oxidative metabolism. The unsaturation of the fatty acids and the presence of oxygen and light are all known to enhance lipid peroxidation in the retina. The formation of *lipofuscin*, a yellow pigment, is correlated with polyunsaturated fatty acid oxidation. Lipofuscin accumulates in many tissues, especially the retina, with advancing age. The concentration of vitamin E in the rods of the retina protects the membrane lipids from auto-oxidation while retarding the accumulation of lipofuscin [16].

Most of the plasma vitamin E is carried on the lipoproteins (which account for the majority of the blood lipids). Any clinical or dietary condition that alters the plasma lipid levels also changes the vitamin E concentration. In newborn infants, the plasma levels of vitamin E are about one-third those of adults; in low-birth-weight infants it is even lower. Newborns, especially if premature, do not absorb vitamin E well, which contributes to the low levels. These may also be due to the lower concentration of plasma lipids in infants, inefficient placental transfer of the vitamin, or both. Within a few days the levels of vitamin E and the plasma lipids begin to rise, reaching normal childhood concentrations by 1 month of age. A deficiency of vitamin E has been reported among low-birth-weight infants fed commercial formulas with polyunsaturated fat and a low vitamin E content. The iron, vitamin E, and polyunsaturated fat content of commercial formulas should be carefully monitored, particularly when given to low-birth-weight infants. Although reports in recent years have suggested using supplemental vitamin E to prevent anemia and the respiratory and ophthalmologic complications of oxygen-enriched environments in premature infants, its value has not yet been proved [17].

ABSORPTION AND
METABOLISM

Both dietary fat and bile salts are required for the absorption of vitamin E across the intestinal mucosa. The vitamin is carried by the lymph circulation to the liver. All tissues in the body have some vitamin E, with the pituitary gland, testes, and adrenal glands having the highest concentrations.

RECOMMENDED DIETARY
ALLOWANCES

A series of compounds of plant origin, the tocopherols and tocotrienols, provide the vitamin E activity in foods. Alpha-tocopherol is the most powerful vitamin E compound, with beta-tocopherol, gamma-tocopherol, delta-tocopherol, and tocotrienols estimated to be 1 to 50 percent as biologically active as alpha-tocopherol (Fig. 8-1C) [18]. In a mixed diet, the amount of beta-tocopherol (in milligrams) should be multiplied by 0.5; that of gamma-tocopherol by 0.1; and that of alpha-tocotrienol by 0.3. When added to the amount of alpha-tocopherol (also in milligrams), the sum equals the total amount of *alpha-tocopherol equivalents*. When only alpha-tocopherol is reported, the amount should be increased by 20 percent (multiplied by 1.2) to allow for the other tocopherols that are present.

The vitamin E content of breast milk (2 to 5 IU, or 1.3 to 3.3 mg alpha-tocopherol equivalents per liter) causes a rise in the plasma tocopherols to adult levels within 2 or 3 weeks [18] and is therefore considered to be sufficient. With the introduction of solid foods and milk from ages 6 months to 1 year, an intake of this range is thought to be adequate. The vitamin E requirement increases with advancing body weight during childhood and levels off during adulthood. During pregnancy and lactation the increased caloric intake should be sufficient to provide for the additional vitamin E transferred to the fetus and secreted in the breast milk. A summary of the RDAs for vitamin E for the various age groups is given in Table 8-1.

FOOD SOURCES

Vitamin E is stable at high temperatures and under acid conditions but is readily oxidized in the presence of rancid fats, iron, or lead salts. Ultraviolet light also adversely affects vitamin E.

The vitamin E content of the diet varies with the amount and types of dietary fat consumed. The requirement for vitamin E increases with the intake of polyunsaturated fatty acids and is therefore related to the polyunsaturated fatty acid concentration of cellular structures. In the United States this does not cause any problems, since the main dietary sources of polyunsaturated fatty acids are also the best sources of vitamin E: vegetable oils, shortening, and margarines. Table 8-2 gives other dietary sources of this vitamin.

EFFECTS OF DEFICIENCY

The effects of vitamin E deficiency are highly variable from species to species. In humans, deficiency has been produced with long-term fat malabsorption and such malabsorption syndromes as cystic fibrosis, biliary atresia, and acanthocytosis. Laboratory findings in deficiency include increased fragility of the red blood cells (with resultant anemia caused by hemolysis), increased urinary excretion of creatine (caused by muscle breakdown and loss), and deposition of ceroid pigment in smooth muscles. Other effects of deficiency include degeneration of reproductive tissues and muscles, as well as liver necrosis.

TOXIC EFFECTS

Although vitamin E appears to be less toxic than vitamins A and D, the long-term effects of high intakes are not known. In adults, prolonged therapy can interfere with coagulation and hemostatic mechanisms; these effects have not been observed with vitamin E therapy of low-birth-weight infants [19]. Another possible toxic effect is an increase in blood pressure. See Chap. 33 for more detail about vitamin E toxicity.

The features of vitamin E are summarized in Table 8-3.

Vitamin K

In 1929 Dam reported that chicks fed a synthetic diet developed hemorrhagic conditions; by 1935 he had named vitamin K as the missing factor. In 1939 vitamin K was isolated and synthesized. Vitamin K exists in two forms naturally: as vitamin K_1 (phylloquinone) in green plants (Fig. 8-1D), and as vitamin K_2 (menaquinone) in animals and produced by intestinal bacteria. Menadione, vitamin K_3, is the synthetic form of this vitamin and is most commonly used clinically.

FUNCTIONS

This vitamin is necessary for the synthesis of prothrombin and other blood-clotting factors by the liver. A deficiency of vitamin K causes defective blood coagulation. Advanced liver damage, as caused by cancer or cirrhosis, causes prothrombin deficiency that cannot be alleviated by the administration of vitamin K. Other physiologic functions of this vitamin include electron transport, growth, and photosynthesis.

ABSORPTION AND METABOLISM

About half of the vitamin K present in the human liver is derived from green leafy vegetables, and about half is synthesized by the gut flora. Because it is fat-soluble, vitamin K requires the presence of bile for its absorption, which occurs mostly in the upper part of the small intestine.

DIETARY INTAKES

Because the intestinal bacteria synthesize this vitamin in normal persons, there are no specific recommended allowances. An estimated range of safe and adequate intake is given in Table 8-4.

FOOD SOURCES

Some excellent food sources of vitamin K include spinach, cauliflower, liver, and kidney. Table 8-2 lists dietary sources for this vitamin. It is heat stable but can be destroyed by acids, alkalis, and irradiation.

TABLE 8-4. Estimated safe and adequate daily dietary intake of vitamin K

Group	Age (years)	Vitamin K (μg)
Infants	0.0–0.5	12
	0.5–1.0	10–20
Children and adolescents	1–3	15–30
	4–6	20–40
	7–10	30–60
	11+	50–100
Adults		70–140

Source: Food and Nutrition Board, National Research Council, *Recommended Dietary Allowances* (9th ed.). Washington, D.C.: National Academy of Sciences, 1980. P. 178.

EFFECTS OF DEFICIENCY

A deficiency of vitamin K can be produced only by the elimination of dietary sources, by the suppression of the growth of the intestinal microflora by antibiotics, and with impaired lipid absorption, such as that resulting from the use of mineral oil as a laxative. A deficiency of this vitamin has also been reported in newborn infants before the establishment of intestinal flora (since the intestinal tract is sterile at birth). For approximately 1 week after birth the concentrations of prothrombin and other clotting factors are low, so vitamin K is frequently administered immediately after birth to prevent hemorrhage. The Committee on Nutrition of the American Academy of Pediatrics recommends that all formulas contain a minimum of 4 μg of vitamin K per 100 calories [20].

The characteristics of vitamin K are listed in Table 8-3.

References

1. McCollum, E. V. *A History of Nutrition.* Boston: Little, Brown, 1957. P. 421.
2. Food and Nutrition Board, National Research Council. *Recommended Dietary Allowances* (9th ed.). Washington, D.C.: National Academy of Sciences, 1980. Pp. 57–59.
3. Cirrhosis, abnormal dark adaptation and vitamin A. *Nutr. Rev.* 37:73, 1979.
4. Russell, R. M. Vitamin A and zinc metabolism in alcoholism. *Am. J. Clin. Nutr.* 33:2741, 1980.
5. Basu, T. K. Vitamin A and cancer of epithelial origin. *J. Hum. Nutr.* 33:24, 1979.
6. Vitamin A, tumor initiation and tumor promotion. *Nutr. Rev.* 37:153, 1979.
7. American Academy of Pediatrics. The use and abuse of vitamin A. *Pediatrics* 48:655, 1971.
8. Korner, W. F., and Völlm, J. New aspects of the tolerance of retinol in humans. *Int. J. Vitam. Nutr. Res.* 45:363, 1975.
9. DeLuca, H. F. Modern views of vitamin D. *Contemp. Nutr.* February 1981.
10. Kumar, R., et al. Elevated 1,25-dihydroxyvitamin D levels in normal pregnancy and lactation. *J. Clin. Invest.* 63:342, 1979.
11. Watney, P. J., and Rudd, B. T. Calcium metabolism in pregnancy and in the newborn. *J. Obstet. Gynaecol. Br. Commonw.* 81:210, 1974.
12. Liu, S. H., et. al. Calcium and phosphorus metabolism in osteomalacia: XI. The

pathogenetic role of pregnancy and relative importance of calcium and vitamin D supply. *J. Clin. Invest.* 20:255, 1941.

13. Food and Nutrition Board, National Research Council.   Hazards of overuse of vitamin D. Washington, D.C., 1974.

14. Nockels, C. F.   Protective effects of supplemental vitamin E against infection. *Fed. Proc.* 38:2134, 1979.

15. Sheffy, B. E., and Schultz, R. D.   Influence of vitamin E and selenium on immune response mechanism. *Fed. Proc.* 38:2139, 1979.

16. The effect of deficiency of vitamins E and A on the retina. *Nutr. Rev.* 38:386, 1980.

17. Bell, E. F., and Filer, L. J.   The role of vitamin E in the nutrition of premature infants. *Am. J. Clin. Nutr.* 34:414, 1981.

18. Food and Nutrition Board, National Research Council.   *Recommended Dietary Allowances* (9th ed.). Washington, D.C.: National Academy of Sciences, 1980. Pp. 64–67.

19. Safety of vitamin E therapy in low-birth-weight infants. *Nutr. Rev.* 39:121, 1981.

20. Committee on Nutrition, American Academy of Pediatrics.   Commentary on breast-feeding and infant formulas, including proposed standards for formulas. *Pediatrics* 57:278, 1976.

Suggested Readings

Carter-Dawson, L., et al.   Structural and biochemical changes in vitamin A-deficient rat retinas. *Invest. Ophthalmol. Vis. Sci.* 18:437, 1979.

Clemens, R. L., et al.   Increased skin pigment reduces the capacity of skin to synthesize vitamin D_3. *Lancet* 1:74, 1982.

DeLuca, H. F.   New developments in the vitamin D endocrine system. *J. Am. Dietet. Assoc.* 80:231, 1982.

DeLuca, H. F.   William C. Rose Lectureship in Biochemistry and Nutrition: Some new concepts emanating from a study of the metabolism and function of vitamin D. *Nutr. Rev.* 38:169, 1980.

DeLuca, H. F.   W. O. Atwater Memorial Lecture: The vitamin D system in the regulation of calcium and phosphorus metabolism. *Nutr. Rev.* 37:161, 1979.

DeLuca, H. F.   Vitamin D metabolism and function. *Arch. Intern. Med.* 138:836, 1978.

Farrington, K., et al.   Vitamin A toxicity and hypercalcemia in chronic renal failure. *Br. Med. J.* 282:1999, 1981.

Haussler, M. R., and McCain, T. A.   Basic and clinical concepts related to vitamin D metabolism and action. *N. Engl. J. Med.* 297:974, 1041, 1977.

Hittner, H. M., et al.   Retrolental fibroplasia: Efficacy of vitamin E in a double-blind clinical study of preterm infants. *N. Engl. J. Med.* 305:1365, 1981.

Horwitt, M. K.   Therapeutic uses of vitamin E in medicine. *Nutr. Rev.* 34:314, 1976.

Interactions among the fat-soluble vitamins. *Nutr. & the MD* March 1982.

Interaction between vitamin K_1 and fat absorption. *Nutr. Rev.* 34:314, 1976.

Lawson, D. E. M. (ed.).   *Vitamin D.* London: Academic, 1978.

Of vitamin A and polar bears. *Nutr. & the MD* May 1982.

Oski, F. A.   Vitamin E: A radical defense. *N. Engl. J. Med.* 303:454, 1980.

Peto, R., et al.   Can dietary beta-carotene materially reduce human cancer rates? *Nature* 290:201, 1981.

Roberts, H. J.   Perspective on vitamin E as therapy. *J. Am. Med. Assoc.* 246:129, 1981.

Rodriguez-Erdmann, R., Hoff, J. V., and Carmody, G.   Interaction of antibiotics with vitamin K. *J. Am. Med. Assoc.* 246:937, 1981.

Scriver, C. R., et al.   Serum 1,25-dihydroxyvitamin D levels in normal subjects and in patients with hereditary rickets or bone disease. *N. Engl. J. Med.* 299:976, 1978.

Sitrin, M., Meredith, S., and Rosenberg, I. H.   Vitamin D deficiency and bone disease in gastrointestinal disorders. *Arch. Intern. Med.* 138:886, 1978.

The effect of deficiency of vitamin E and A on the retina. *Nutr. Rev.* 38:386, 1980.

The vitamin D activity of milk. *Nutr. Rev.* 40:27, 1982.

Underwood, B. A.   Strategies for the prevention of vitamin A deficiency. *Food Nutr. Bull.* 2:11, 1980.

Vitamin D deficiency rickets, revisited. *Nutr. Rev.* 38:116, 1980.

Vitamin A toxicity; Vitamin E: therapy and toxicity; Vitamin K: deficiencies and interactions with vitamin E. *Nutr. & the MD* March 1982.

Chapter 9

THE WATER-SOLUBLE VITAMINS

The water-soluble vitamins are grouped together by virtue of their solubility in water. Like the fat-soluble vitamins, the water-soluble vitamins share many other features, including their excretion in the urine, their role in essential enzyme systems, and their need to be supplied in the diet daily since they are not stored in appreciable amounts.

Vitamin C

Vitamin C exists in two forms, as ascorbic acid and dehydroascorbic acid. Both are equally well utilized by humans, although most vitamin C is present as ascorbic acid (Fig. 9-1). Vitamin C is involved in a wide variety of metabolic functions, including the hydroxylation of the amino acid proline in the formation of collagen, the synthesis of epinephrine and anti-inflammatory steroids by the adrenal gland, white blood cell functions, and folic acid metabolism. The disease resulting from a lack of vitamin C, *scurvy*, is characterized by a weakening of collagenous structures and hemorrhaging. Scurvy plagued seagoing adventurers, particularly during the sixteenth and seventeenth centuries. Many remedies were recommended, but most were ineffective, with thousands of sailors dying from lack of vitamin C. In 1747 James Lind, a British physician, found that citrus fruit was a cure for scurvy. It was not until the 1800s that the British Navy began rationing lemons or limes on sailing vessels, from which the British sailors came to be known as "limeys."

At the beginning of the twentieth century true scientific work on vitamin C began, including experimentally produced scurvy in guinea pigs by the Norwegian scientists Holst and Frölich in 1907 and the isolation of the vitamin by Charles King of the University of Pittsburgh in 1932.

FUNCTIONS

The primary function of vitamin C is in the formation of collagenous intercellular substances. This vitamin is essential for the hydroxylation of the amino acids proline and lysine to hydroxyproline and hydroxylysine, components of collagen. Found in cartilage, bone, dentin, and vascular epithelium, collagen helps maintain body structure. Vitamin C is therefore important in wound healing and in responding to stress, injury, and infection.

Other functions of vitamin C include the conversion of folic acid to its active form, folinic acid; the synthesis of steroid hormones from cholesterol; the release of iron from transferrin; the reduction of ferric iron to ferrous iron in the gastrointestinal tract; the conversion of phenylalanine to tyrosine; and as an antioxidant.

ABSORPTION AND
METABOLISM

Vitamin C is quickly absorbed from the gastrointestinal tract and distributed in various tissues of the body. Highest concentrations are found in the adrenal gland, with appreciable amounts in such tissues as the kidneys, spleen, liver,

FIG. 9-1. Chemical structure of vitamin C (ascorbic acid).

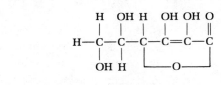

pancreas, thymus, and pituitary. Once the tissues are saturated, any excess vitamin C is excreted.

RECOMMENDED DIETARY ALLOWANCES

Many species are able to synthesize ascorbic acid from glucose and other simple sugars and therefore do not require it in the diet. Humans and four other species (monkeys, guinea pigs, Indian fruit bats, and red-vented bulbul birds) do not have this ability; for these species, vitamin C is an essential daily nutrient. The human requirement for this vitamin is based on the amount necessary to prevent or cure scurvy, the amount metabolized by the body daily, and the amount necessary to maintain adequate reserves [1, 2]. Many factors may alter the need for vitamin C. For example, environmental or emotional stress and exposure to elevated temperatures increase the daily requirement [2]. The ingestion of oral contraceptive agents and the use of cigarettes both lower plasma levels of vitamin C, but the importance of this is not yet clear.

For adults of both sexes, the recommended dietary allowance (RDA) is 60 mg. Because of new research, this level is higher than previously recommended (1974 and earlier) to permit the maintenance of a better body pool, to allow for vitamin C breakdown, and to take into account an absorption efficiency of 85 percent [1].

The recommendation of 35 mg per day for infants is based on the intake of the breast-fed infant. Human milk contains between 30 and 55 mg of vitamin C per liter, depending on the mother's diet, and breast-fed infants receive about 850 ml of milk per day. During the first week of life, newborns, especially if premature, may need additional vitamin C for the metabolism of the amino acid tyrosine, and an intake of 100 mg per day is recommended during this period [1].

Children have a higher vitamin C requirement than do adults, on a weight basis. For children up to 11 years of age, the allowance is 45 mg per day; for older children it is 50 or 60 mg per day.

During pregnancy and lactation, the need for vitamin C increases by 20 mg and 40 mg, respectively. A summary of the RDAs for all age groups is given in Table 9-1.

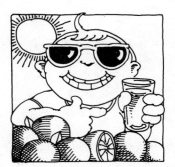

FOOD SOURCES

Vitamin C is present in a variety of fruits and vegetables, as outlined in Table 9-2. Fresh, frozen, or raw fruits and vegetables are the best sources of this vitamin. Dairy and meat products are poor sources. Vitamin C is easily destroyed by oxidation. Prolonged cooking at high temperatures and undue exposure to iron, copper, oxygen, light, alkali, and oxidation enzymes all accelerate the oxidation

TABLE 9-1. Recommended daily dietary allowances of the water-soluble vitamins

Group	Age (years)	Vitamin C (mg)	Thiamin (mg)	Riboflavin (mg)	Niacin (mg NE)[a]	Vitamin B_6 (mg)	Folacin (μg)	Vitamin B_{12} (μg)
Infants	0.0–0.5	35	0.3	0.4	6	0.3	30	0.5
	0.5–1.0	35	0.5	0.6	8	0.6	45	1.5
Children	1–3	45	0.7	0.8	9	0.9	100	2.0
	4–6	45	0.9	1.0	11	1.3	200	2.5
	7–10	45	1.2	1.4	16	1.6	300	3.0
Males	11–14	50	1.4	1.6	18	1.8	400	3.0
	15–18	60	1.4	1.7	18	2.0	400	3.0
	19–22	60	1.5	1.7	19	2.2	400	3.0
	23–50	60	1.4	1.6	18	2.2	400	3.0
	51 +	60	1.2	1.4	16	2.2	400	3.0
Females	11–14	50	1.1	1.3	15	1.8	400	3.0
	15–18	60	1.1	1.3	14	2.0	400	3.0
	19–22	60	1.1	1.3	14	2.0	400	3.0
	23–50	60	1.0	1.2	13	2.0	400	3.0
	51 +	60	1.0	1.2	13	2.0	400	3.0
Pregnant[b]	—	+ 20	+ 0.4	+ 0.3	+ 2	+ 0.6	+ 400	+ 1.0
Lactating[b]	—	+ 40	+ 0.5	+ 0.5	+ 5	+ 0.5	+ 100	+ 1.0

[a] As mg niacin equivalents (mg NE). 1 mg NE = 1 mg of niacin or 60 mg of dietary tryptophan.
[b] Allowances given for pregnant and lactating women are *in addition to* the normal allowance for women of a particular age.
Source: Food and Nutrition Board, National Research Council, *Recommended Dietary Allowances* (9th ed.). Washington, D.C.: National Academy of Sciences, 1980.

of vitamin C. Storage conditions and processing can also affect the vitamin C content. Since it is water-soluble, much of vitamin C is lost by leaching when fruits or vegetables are cooked in water. The slicing of produce increases the surface area exposed to leaching and releases oxidative enzymes. To retain maximum amounts of vitamin C, a minimum amount of water should be used, and cooking should be done for a short time in a covered pot. Steaming of fruits and vegetables also helps to retain a maximum amount of nutrients.

EFFECTS OF DEFICIENCY

A deficiency of vitamin C results in the faulty, defective formation of collagenous intercellular substances. This is manifested clinically as joint pain, poor growth, anemia, increased susceptibility to infection, and poor wound healing. *Scurvy*, the advanced form of vitamin C deficiency, results after several months of a diet lacking in vitamin C. The clinical findings include easy bruising (ecchymoses), bleeding of the gums, and petechial hemorrhages (pinpoint hemorrhages in the skin). The teeth become loose and eventually fall out. Even a slight injury causes excessive bleeding. Deterioration of the muscle and cartilage structure eventually occurs, leading to death.

Scurvy is rare among adults in the United States but is sometimes seen in infants during the second 6 months of life. Because of pain and tenderness in the thighs and legs, these children with *infantile scurvy* usually assume a position with the legs flexed for comfort and tend to move as little as possible (Fig. 9-2). They exhibit weight loss, fever, irritability, diarrhea, and vomiting. The gums are

TABLE 9-2. Dietary sources of the water-soluble vitamins

Vitamin	Source

Vitamin C	High (100–300 mg/100 gm)
	  Broccoli, brussels sprouts, collards, horseradish, kale, parsley, sweet peppers, turnip greens
	  Black currants, guava, rose hips
	Medium (50–100 mg/100 gm)
	  Beet greens, cabbage, cauliflower, chives, kohlrabi, mustard greens, watercress, spinach
	  Lemons, oranges, papayas, strawberries

Thiamin (B_1)	High (1000–10,000 µg/100 gm)
	  Wheat germ, rice bran, soybean flour
	  Yeast
	  Pork
	Medium (100–1000 µg/100 gm)
	  Gooseberries, plums, prunes, raisins, asparagus, beans, beet greens, broccoli, brussels sprouts, cauliflower, corn, peas, potatoes, oats, rice, peanuts, walnuts

Riboflavin (B_2)	High (1000–10,000 µg/100 gm)
	  Beef and calf kidney and liver
	  Chicken liver
	  Pork and sheep kidney and liver
	Medium (100–1000 µg/100 gm)
	  Avocados, currants, asparagus, beans, beet greens, broccoli, brussels sprouts, cauliflower, corn, peas, spinach, eggs, milk, cheese, oats
	  Bacon, beef, chicken, duck, lamb, fish

Niacin	High (10,000–100,000 µg/100 gm) (10–100 mg/100 gm)
	  Peanuts, rice bran
	  Liver (beef, calf, chicken, pork, sheep)
	  Heart (calf), kidney (pork, beef)
	  Rabbit, turkey, chicken
	  Tuna, halibut, swordfish
	Medium (1000–10,000 µg/100 gm) (1–10 mg/100 gm)
	  Avocados, dates, figs, prunes
	  Asparagus, beans, broccoli, oats, corn, kale, lentils, potatoes
	  Almonds, cashews, chestnuts, walnuts
	  Beef, veal, chicken, duck, lamb, fish

Vitamin B_6 (pyridoxine)	High (1000–10,000 µg/100 gm)
	  Liver, herring, salmon
	  Walnuts, peanuts, wheat germ, brown rice
	  Yeast, blackstrap molasses
	Medium (100–1000 µg/100 gm)
	  Bananas, avocados, grapes, pears
	  Barley, cabbage, carrots, corn, oats, peas, potatoes, turnips, spinach
	  Beef, lamb, pork, veal, fish
	  Butter, eggs

Folacin	High (90–300 mg/gm)
	  Liver, asparagus, spinach, wheat, bran, dry beans, yeast
	Medium (30–90 mg/gm)
	  Beef kidney
	  Lima beans, broccoli, corn

TABLE 9-2 (CONTINUED)

Vitamin	Source
	Almonds, filberts, peanuts, walnuts
	Barley, oats, rye, wheat
Vitamin B$_{12}$ (cyanocobalamin)	High (50–500 µg/100 gm)
	Lamb and beef kidney; lamb, beef, calf, and pork liver; beef brain
	Medium (5–50 µg/100 gm)
	Rabbit kidney; rabbit and chicken liver; beef, rabbit, and chicken heart; egg yolk
	Clams, sardines, salmon, crabs, oysters, herring
Biotin	High (100–400 mg/100 gm)
	Yeast, lamb liver, pork liver
	Medium (10–100 mg/100 gm)
	Wheat, rice, oats, barley
	Eggs, beef liver, chicken, mushrooms
	Cowpeas (black-eyed peas), chick-peas, lentils, soybeans, cauliflower, chocolate
	Mackerel, salmon, sardines
	Almonds, peanuts, pecans, walnuts, filberts, hazelnuts
Pantothenic acid	High (2–10 mg/100 gm)
	Beef, pork, sheep and chicken liver, lamb kidney
	Eggs
	Herring, wheat germ, bran, peanuts, dried peas, yeast
	Medium (0.5–2.0 mg/100 gm)
	Salmon, clams, mackerel
	Walnuts, broccoli, soybeans, oats, lima beans, cauliflower, peas, avocados, carrots, spinach, rice
	Beef, pork, chicken, lamb
	Mushrooms, wheat, cheese

Source: Adapted from R. J. Kutsky, *Handbook of Vitamins and Hormones*. Copyright © 1973 by Van Nostrand Reinhold Company. Reprinted by permission of Van Nostrand Reinhold Company.

swollen and bleed easily. Because of faulty bone calcification, the cartilage is weak, resulting in bone displacement. The ends of the long bones and ribs are enlarged as in rickets but are also tender.

The scurvy itself can be cured within a few days by the administration of 100 to 200 mg of vitamin C daily. The bone deformities and anemia resulting from scurvy, however, take much longer to correct.

TOXIC EFFECTS

High intakes of vitamin C have received much publicity and popular interest in recent years. Intakes in excess of 1 gm per day have been found by some investigators to decrease the frequency and severity of symptoms of the common cold [3, 4] while other investigators have not found this to be true [5].

Large doses of vitamin C have been shown to lower serum cholesterol levels in some patients [6] but not in others [7]. They have also been reported to increase the serum levels of the immunoglobulins IgA and IgM and complement component C3 [8].

FIG. 9-2. Child in scorbutic position. This is usually the first sign of scurvy. Because movement is painful, the scorbutic infant usually lies on its back.

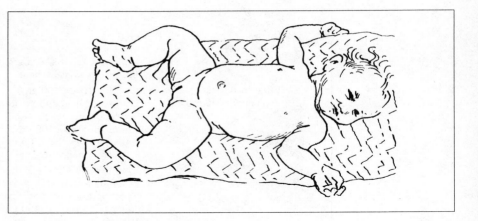

High doses of vitamin C are generally considered to be nontoxic, except for the gastrointestinal symptoms experienced by some individuals. Rebound scurvy has been observed in newborns whose mothers had taken large doses of vitamin C during pregnancy. Other findings have been reported, including impaired bactericidal activity of leukocytes, absorption of excessive amounts of iron, and vitamin C–induced uricosuria (urinary excretion of uric acid) with resultant kidney stone [9–11] formation. There is also a possibility of damage to the pancreas, resulting in decreased production of insulin. Many of the claims for intakes of large doses of vitamin C have not been substantiated, and since it may actually cause some adverse effects, the consumption of large amounts of this vitamin is not recommended.

The characteristics of vitamin C are summarized in Table 9-3.

Thiamin

Rice polishings and the vitamin thiamin have been associated for nearly 100 years. As early as 1897 Eijkman alleviated *beriberi*, a disease caused by thiamin deficiency, by the addition of rice polishings to the diet. In 1911 Funk isolated the dietary factor in rice polishings that cured beriberi and also coined the term *vitamin*. By 1926 the antiberiberi factor had been isolated from rice bran by Jansen and Donath. Williams synthesized the factor and named it thiamin in 1936. In areas of the world where rice is a staple food, beriberi has been epidemic for generations. The discovery and isolation of thiamin was therefore a major nutritional breakthrough with widespread public health implications. Thiamin in the diet is found in three forms: free, bound as in *cocarboxylase* (thiamin pyrophosphate), or in a protein-phosphate complex (Fig. 9-3).

FUNCTIONS

As cocarboxylase this vitamin is essential as a coenzyme in the metabolism of alpha-keto acids and alpha-keto sugars. Thiamin is also vital in key reactions in energy metabolism, especially carbohydrate metabolism, and therefore its requirement in the diet is related to energy intake. In carbohydrate metabolism, thiamin functions in the oxidative decarboxylation of pyruvic acid to form acetylcoenzyme A, which then enters the Krebs cycle. This is a vital step in metabolism and also requires several other cofactors, including pantothenic acid, nicotinamide-adenine dinucleotide (which contains niacin), lipoic acid, and magnesium ions. Within the Krebs cycle, thiamin is also involved in the oxidative decarboxylation of alpha-ketoglutaric acid to succinic acid. Cocarboxylase is a cofactor for the enzyme transketolase, which produces active aldehyde in the pentose shunt. Thiamin is also necessary for the synthesis of acetylcholine. In thiamin deficiency, nerve fibers are affected by the lack of acetylcholine, and the buildup of pyruvate, which directly impairs the functioning of neurons, may be the causative factor in anorexia and weakness.

ABSORPTION AND
METABOLISM

The bound forms of thiamin are split in the gastrointestinal tract during digestion and then absorbed mainly from the duodenum and jejunum. Very little thiamin is stored in the body, although the muscles, brain, kidneys, liver, and heart have higher concentrations than do other organs. Cocarboxylase is formed from the addition of two molecules of phosphate to thiamin by adenosine triphosphate (ATP). In the presence of magnesium ions, cocarboxylase can combine with a specific protein to form carboxylase, the active enzyme in a number of essential metabolic reactions. When thiamin intake is in excess of needs, it is excreted in the urine. When dietary intake is inadequate, tissue levels become depleted and urinary excretion falls.

RECOMMENDED DIETARY
ALLOWANCES

The thiamin allowance for adults of 0.5 mg per 1000 calories has been shown to prevent deficiency and to be compatible with health. Thiamin may be utilized less efficiently in the elderly, and therefore an intake of 1 mg per day is recommended even if the energy intake is less than 2000 calories per day. During pregnancy an additional 0.6 mg per 1000 calories is recommended, or about an additional 0.4 mg per day. To allow for the thiamin in breast milk plus the increased energy consumption during lactation, an additional 0.6 mg per 1000 kcal is recommended for these women, totaling to an additional 0.5 mg per day.

For infants, 0.3 mg per day is recommended, increasing to 0.5 mg per day during the second 6 months of life. The allowance steadily increases throughout childhood, paralleling increasing energy consumption. A summary of the RDAs for all age groups is given in Table 9-1.

FOOD SOURCES

Cereals and grains, particularly wheat germ, rice bran, soybean flour, and yeast, have the highest concentrations of thiamin. The enrichment and fortification of processed cereals and flours with thiamin and the other B vitamins has made a significant nutritional contribution to the American diet by practically eliminating deficiencies of these vitamins. (See Chap. 12 for more detail on enrichment

TABLE 9-3. Summary of the water-soluble vitamins

Vitamin	Primary functions	Results of deficiency	Results of toxicity	Normal blood levels
Vitamin C	Growth Healing Synthesis of bone, collagen, polysaccharides Maintenance of capillaries Absorption of iron Antioxidant	Perifollicular hemorrhage Poor wound healing Aching joints Ecchymoses, scurvy	Possible kidney stones Possible damage to pancreas with decreased insulin production Impaired white blood cell activity Excessive absorption of iron Rebound scurvy	0.5–1.0 mg/100 ml (plasma)
Thiamin	Pyruvate and carbohydrate metabolism Energy production Nerve activity Digestion Growth	Beriberi Retarded growth Nerve degeneration Fatigue Anorexia Weight loss Mental disturbances Muscular atrophy	Edema Tremors Tachycardia Fatty liver	1.3 µg/100 ml (serum)
Riboflavin	Part of respiratory enzymes Maintenance of epithelial, eye, and mucosal tissues	Angular stomatitis Glossitis Seborrheic dermatitis Photophobia, conjunctivitis	Paresthesia and itching (essentially nontoxic)	6.6 µg/100 ml
Niacin	Carbohydrate, lipid, and protein metabolism Photosynthesis	Pellagra Retarded growth Weakness Anorexia	Burning, itching skin Fatty liver	0.42–0.84 mg/100 ml

Vitamin	Function	Deficiency Symptoms	Toxicity	Blood Level
Vitamin B$_6$ (pyridoxine)	Protein, carbohydrate, and lipid metabolism Coenzyme in amino acid metabolism Erythrocyte formation Growth	Cutaneous lesions Anemia Convulsions	Limited toxicity (only at a 3 gm/kg dose)	11.2 µg/100 ml
Folacin	Amino acid metabolism Coenzyme in purine and pyrimidine metabolism Synthesis of choline	Pernicious anemia Macrocytic anemia Sprue Glossitis Leukopenia Thrombocytopenia	No toxicity reported	3.53 µg/100 ml
Vitamin B$_{12}$ (cyanocobalamin)	Coenzyme in lipid, protein, and nucleic acid synthesis Production of erythrocytes and leukocytes	Pernicious anemia Megaloblastic anemia Glossitis Sprue Spinal cord degeneration	General lack of toxicity	0.08 µg/100 ml
Biotin	Coenzyme in numerous reactions Growth and maintenance of skin, hair, nerves, bone marrow	Desquamation of the skin Lassitude Muscle pain Seborrheic dermatitis	Essentially nontoxic in humans	1.23 mg/100 ml
Pantothenic acid	Coenzyme in protein, lipid, and carbohydrate metabolism Porphyrin metabolism Acetylcholine production	Neuromotor disturbances Cardiovascular disorders Digestive disorders Weakness Infection	Essentially nontoxic in humans	19–32 µg/100 ml

FIG. 9-3. Chemical structure of thiamin (B₁).

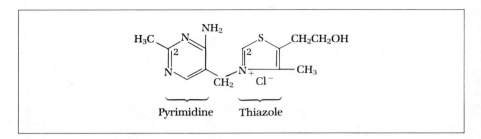

and fortification.) Pork is also especially rich in thiamin, as are a variety of fruits and vegetables, as outlined in Table 9-2.

Thiamin can be easily lost during cooking owing to its solubility in water, destruction in the presence of alkali, and sensitivity to prolonged exposure to heat. When rice is washed before cooking, losses may also be considerable. More thiamin is retained in "converted" than in regular rice because the processing distributes the water-soluble vitamins throughout the grain. As with vitamin C, fruits and vegetables should be cooked in a small amount of water in a covered pot for a short period of time for maximum thiamin retention.

EFFECTS OF DEFICIENCY

Beriberi, which is a Singhalese term meaning "weakness," is the disease produced by a deficiency of thiamin. Beriberi is frequently seen where refined rice is the dietary staple. It is characterized by a combination of neurologic, cardiac, and cerebral manifestations. This disease has been divided into three syndromes on the basis of the most common clinical features: *dry beriberi*, with predominantly neuromuscular symptoms; *wet beriberi*, with neuromuscular signs and edema; and *cardiac beriberi*, with cardiac decompensation. Usually the three forms overlap. The neuromuscular features include numbness and tingling of the legs and wasting and weakness of the muscles of the extremities. Mental depression may also be present. When accompanied by edema, the neuromuscular symptoms may also include loss of appetite, malaise, and generalized weakness.

Chronic alcoholism can also lead to thiamin deficiency. The disease produced is termed *Wernicke's syndrome*, and includes the triad of confusion, ataxia (incoordination of voluntary muscle action, particularly in walking), and ophthalmoplegia (paralysis of the oculomotor nerve), as well as other features related to degenerative changes in the central nervous system. The causes of thiamin deficiency in chronic alcoholism include an inadequate intake of thiamin, a decreased conversion of thiamin to the active coenzyme, decreased hepatic storage of the vitamin, inhibition by ethanol of intestinal thiamin transport, and impaired thiamin absorption [12].

Other groups at risk for developing thiamin deficiency include those on long-term hemodialysis or intravenous feeding and those with chronic febrile infections. Persons consuming a large amount of raw fish or tea, both of which contain thiamin antagonists (substances that bind thiamin and prevent its

FIG. 9-4. Chemical structure of riboflavin (B_2).

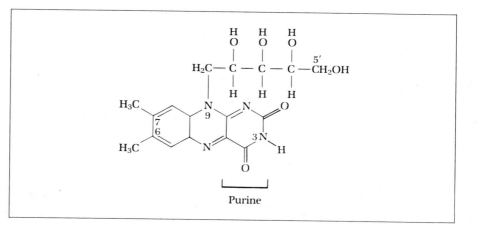

Purine

utilization in the body), are also at risk for developing a deficiency of this vitamin [13].

TOXIC EFFECTS

Humans have a limited toxic reaction to thiamin, starting at a dosage of approximately 125 to 350 mg per kilogram body weight [14]. The signs include edema, sweating, tremors, tachycardia (rapid heartbeat), fatty liver tremors, and vascular hypotension.

A summary of the characteristics of thiamin is given in Table 9-3.

RIBOFLAVIN

Over 100 years ago pigments with yellow fluorescence were discovered in such foods as egg white, liver, yeast, and heart. These pigments were called "flavins." In 1920 Emmett suggested the presence of several dietary growth factors in yeast concentrate, including a heat-stable component and vitamin B_1. In 1932 Warburg and Christian isolated a yellow enzyme, containing riboflavin, from yeast. During the next 3 years, Kuhn and his co-workers isolated pure riboflavin (also termed vitamin B_2 by the British Medical Research Council in 1927) from milk, identified its structure, and synthesized it. Riboflavin exists in several physiologic forms: free, in combination with phosphate, or in combination with protein and phosphate (Fig. 9-4). It is named riboflavin because of its structural similarity to the sugar ribose and its relationship to the flavins.

FUNCTIONS

In its phosphorylated form, as riboflavin phosphate or flavin mononucleotide (FMN) and flavin-adenine dinucleotide (FAD), riboflavin is an essential component of the flavoprotein coenzymes, which act as hydrogen acceptors (part of the respiratory enzyme system). Riboflavin is also involved in the oxidative degradation of short-chain fatty acids and the transfer of oxygen from plasma to the tissues. Riboflavin is a component of several oxidases, which oxidize amino acids and hydroxy acids to alpha-keto acids and catalyze the oxidation of purines.

Oxidative metabolism is dependent on an adequate supply of riboflavin. Maintenance of epithelial, eye, and mucosal tissues also require riboflavin.

ABSORPTION AND
METABOLISM

Riboflavin is rapidly absorbed from the upper part of the small intestine and then phosphorylated in the intestinal wall into its active form. Riboflavin is found in all cells of the body but is stored in large quantities in the liver and kidneys. With an increase in intake above needs, the vitamin is excreted by the kidneys. A reduction in supply quickly leads to reduced tissue levels and reduced urinary excretion.

RECOMMENDED DIETARY
ALLOWANCES

The Food and Nutrition Board recommends a daily intake of 0.6 mg per 1000 calories for persons of all ages. For those with a caloric intake of less than 2000 calories per day, a minimum intake of 1.2 mg per day is recommended. During pregnancy an additional 0.3 mg per day is needed; during lactation, an additional 0.5 mg. The daily requirement is increased by fever, surgery, hyperthyroidism, and malabsorption. The use of oral contraceptives may also increase requirements, but the data are inconclusive at present. The RDAs for all age groups for riboflavin are given in Table 9-1.

FOOD SOURCES

In the American diet, most of the daily riboflavin intake is from milk, meat, fish, poultry, and whole-grain or enriched cereal and cereal products. The richest sources of riboflavin are liver and kidney; fruits, vegetables, meats, and dairy products also make a substantial contribution. Dietary sources of riboflavin are given in Table 9-2.

Riboflavin is relatively stable to heat, acids, and oxidizing agents, but it can easily be destroyed by alkali. The pasteurization of milk destroys 10 to 20 percent of the riboflavin present. The baking of meats causes a riboflavin loss of about 25 percent, most of which is found in the drippings. Riboflavin is relatively insoluble, and therefore not much is lost by usual cooking procedures. The use of sodium bicarbonate (baking soda) to preserve the green color of vegetables is destructive because baking soda is alkaline.

EFFECTS OF DEFICIENCY

A deficiency of riboflavin is one of the most common deficiency diseases. The most characteristic sign is *cheilitis* or *angular stomatitis*, cracks in the skin at the corners of the mouth (Fig. 9-5). The condition starts with general pallor, then the corners of the mouth develop hyperkeratosis of the epidermis, ulceration, and inflammation, which lead to cracks or fissures. The tongue may develop a magenta hue because of inflammation, termed *glossitis*. Changes in the eyes including conjunctivitis, invasion of the cornea by blood vessels, and photophobia may also develop from riboflavin deficiency. A greasy, scaling dermatitis of the skin is also seen involving the genital area, nasolabial folds, cheeks, and ears.

Most cases of *ariboflavinosis* (riboflavin deficiency) are caused by an inadequate dietary intake. It is most common in the Orient, in areas where the economic standards are low, and among chronic alcoholics. The deficiency may

FIG. 9-5. Stomatitis in pernicious anemia. (From J. Judge, G. Zuidema, and F. Fitzgerald, *Clinical Diagnosis* [4th ed.]. Boston: Little, Brown, 1982.)

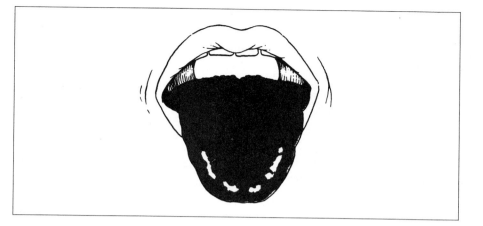

also be seen in severe gastrointestinal diseases that interfere with the absorption of riboflavin; in achlorhydria, hyperthyroidism, fever, or trauma; or during pregnancy or lactation.

TOXIC EFFECTS

Riboflavin is essentially nontoxic in man.

A summary of the characteristics of riboflavin is given in Table 9-3.

Niacin

The deficiency disease *pellagra*, caused by a lack of niacin, was first described in Italy in 1771. It was one of the leading causes of mental illness and death in the United States during the early part of this century. In 1867 Huber first synthesized nicotinic acid, and in 1914 Funk isolated it from rice polishings. It was not until 1915, however, that pellagra was shown to be caused by a nutritional deficiency. During that year Goldberger of the United States Public Health Service performed a classic dietary experiment with a dozen prisoners in the South. In return for their cooperation in eating a diet representative of that of the poorer classes in the southern states, they were promised release from prison. After a few weeks of black coffee, cornbread, cabbage, rice, collard greens, corn grits, syrup, sugar, and biscuits, the prisoners developed weakness, headaches, and abdominal pain; after about 5 months they developed the dermatitis typical of pellagra. From this experiment Goldberger concluded that pellagra was caused by a deficiency of some factor in the diet and suggested that the disease was related to one of the B vitamins. In 1937 Fouts cured pellagra with niacinamide.

Niacin is the term used for both nicotinic acid and nicotinamide or niacinamide. The latter occurs in animal tissues and is more soluble in water. Both are of equal biologic value (Fig. 9-6).

FUNCTIONS

As a vital component of two important coenzymes, *nicotinamide-adenine dinucleotide* (NAD, also known as coenzyme I) and *nicotinamide-adenine dinucleo-*

FIG. 9-6. Chemical structure of niacin.

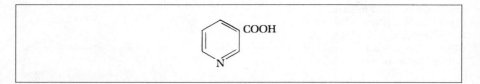

tide phosphate (NADP, also known as coenzyme II), niacin plays an essential role in the electron transport involved in cellular respiratory reactions. As a component of these coenzymes, niacin is involved in the metabolism of proteins, fats, and carbohydrates. In the Krebs cycle, NAD and NADP are part of dehydrogenation reactions; in the respiratory chain, hydrogen is transferred from NAD to FAD to cytochrome *c*. NADP is the hydrogen acceptor in the pentose shunt, forming NADPH (the reduced form of NADP), which is then used in the synthesis of fatty acids and cholesterol and the conversion of phenylalanine to tyrosine. Niacin is also involved in pigment metabolism, as well as photosynthesis.

ABSORPTION AND METABOLISM

Niacin is absorbed in the small intestine. As with the other B vitamins, body stores are limited, making adequate daily intake essential. Niacin is stored to some extent in the heart, liver, and muscles. An excess of niacin is excreted in the urine. A lack of this vitamin in the diet causes a marked reduction in its urinary excretion.

Tryptophan, an essential amino acid, is a precursor of niacin. The conversion, however, is dependent on an adequate supply of pyridoxine, vitamin B_6. A sufficient intake of tryptophan may compensate for a deficient level of niacin, but not for a total lack of the vitamin. Sixty milligrams of the precursor tryptophan may serve as the equivalent of 1 mg of niacin.

RECOMMENDED DIETARY ALLOWANCES

The allowance for niacin is related to the intake of tryptophan-containing foods. For adults the recommended allowance, expressed as niacin equivalents, is 6.6 niacin equivalents per 1000 calories, and not less than 13 niacin equivalents for caloric intakes of less than 2000 calories. For infants up to 6 months of age, the recommended allowance is 8 niacin equivalents per 1000 calories, of which two-thirds is derived from tryptophan. For children over 6 months of age and adolescents, the allowance is 6.6 niacin equivalents per 1000 calories. During pregnancy the allowance is increased by 2 niacin equivalents; during lactation, by 5 niacin equivalents. A summary of the RDAs for niacin for all age groups is given in Table 9-1.

FOOD SOURCES

The average diet in the United States contains 500 to 1000 mg or more of tryptophan daily and 8 to 17 mg of niacin or a total of 16 to 34 mg of niacin equivalents [15]. Proteins of animal origin contain about 1.4% tryptophan and are also among the richest sources of niacin; most vegetables contain about 1%

FIG. 9-7. Dermatitis of pellagra. (From C. Robinson, *Normal and Therapeutic Nutrition* [15th ed.]. New York: Macmillan, 1977.)

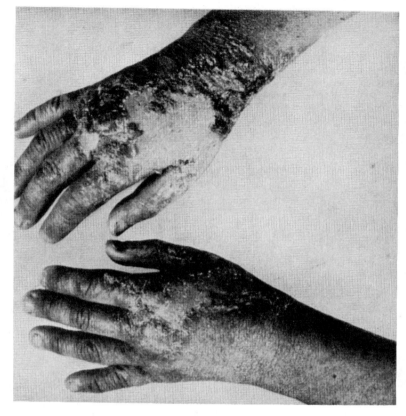

tryptophan and are moderately good sources of niacin (Table 9-2). The enrichment of grain products has done much to eliminate pellagra in this country.

Niacin is moderately soluble in hot water and only slightly soluble in cold water. It is stable under most conditions, including acid, alkali, light, heat, oxidation, and even boiling.

EFFECTS OF DEFICIENCY

The term *pellagra* is from the Italian words *pelle*, meaning "skin," and *agra*, meaning "rough." The clinical syndrome of this disease is classically identified by the three D's: dermatitis, diarrhea, and dementia. The dermatitis (skin changes) occurs symmetrically and is most severe on the areas exposed to sunlight. The skin initially becomes reddened and thickens, then shows signs of increased vascularization and scaling (Fig. 9-7). Changes that may interfere with normal eating also occur in the tongue. Diarrhea occurs as a result of lesions in the mucous membrane of the gastrointestinal tract. Pellagra also causes degeneration of the ganglion cells of the brain and the fibers of the spinal cord, resulting in dementia in advanced cases. Anorexia, weakness, and retarded growth are also common signs.

In many areas of the world pellagra caused by poor intake of niacin is seen; in other areas it may result from chronic alcoholism, gastrointestinal disturbances, pregnancy, hyperthyroidism, or other metabolically stressful conditions. The disease responds quickly to adequate oral supplementation with niacin.

TOXIC EFFECTS

Large doses of nicotinic acid have been shown to produce vascular dilation or flushing. Nicotinamide does not produce this effect. Intakes of 3 gm or more per day of nicotinic acid have been shown to increase utilization of muscle glycogen stores, decrease the level of serum lipids, and decrease the mobilization of fatty acids from adipose tissue during exercise [16]. Because of these effects, pharmacologic dosages have been used in some patients to protect against recurrent nonfatal myocardial infarction. Caution must be used at these dosages because of the various side effects, including abnormal biochemical findings, burning and itching of the skin, fatty liver, increase in arrhythmias, and gastrointestinal problems.

A summary of niacin's characteristics is given in Table 9-3.

Vitamin B$_6$

The existence of another B vitamin was suspected when in 1934 György cured a dermatitis in rats by a substance in yeast extract that was not vitamin B$_1$ or B$_2$. In 1938 Lepkovsky isolated a similar substance from rice bran extract. In that same year Keresztesy and Stevens isolated and crystallized pure vitamin B$_6$ from rice polishings. Pyridoxine was synthesized and its structure established in the years that followed. In 1945 pyridoxal and pyridoxamine were discovered, and by 1953 the human requirement for vitamin B$_6$ was identified.

Vitamin B$_6$ is actually a collective term for three naturally occurring pyridines that are functionally and metabolically related: pyridoxine, pyridoxal, and pyridoxamine. They all may occur in foods or in the tissues in their free form, combined with phosphate, or combined with phosphate and protein (Fig. 9-8).

FUNCTIONS

Vitamin B$_6$ is involved in a variety of metabolic processes. Pyridoxal phosphate, the active coenzyme form, plays a major role in amino acid metabolism. It is involved in transamination, the process by which a nonessential amino acid is formed by the transfer of an amino group from an amino acid to a keto acid. It is also involved in decarboxylation, the removal of a carboxyl group from amino acids, and transulfuration, the removal and transfer of sulfur groups from the sulfur-containing amino acids. Vitamin B$_6$ is also needed for the conversion of tryptophan to niacin; the formation of melanin; the breakdown of glycogen to glucose; the formation of the porphyrin ring, part of the hemoglobin molecule; the metabolism of unsaturated fatty acids; the synthesis of antibodies; and possibly bone development and the conversion of linoleic acid to arachidonic acid.

ABSORPTION AND METABOLISM

Very little is known about the absorption of vitamin B$_6$, but the vitamin is found mainly in the extracellular fluid. Concentrations of vitamin B$_6$ are relatively high

FIG. 9-8. Chemical structure of three forms of vitamin B_6.

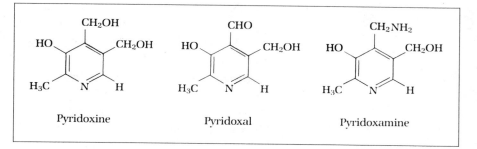

in leukocytes (white blood cells), nerve tissue, and the liver. Since this vitamin is water-soluble, very little is stored, and any excess is excreted in the urine as pyridoxic acid. With low intakes pyridoxic acid disappears from the urine. Therefore urinary levels of pyridoxic acid can be used as an indicator of intake.

RECOMMENDED DIETARY ALLOWANCES

The daily requirement for vitamin B_6 is directly related to protein intake: With a low protein diet less of the vitamin is needed; with a high protein diet, more. It has been suggested that a ratio of 0.02 mg of vitamin B_6 per gram of dietary protein be used in calculating the daily allowance [17]. Based on this ratio and the influence of protein intake, a daily allowance of 2.2 mg of vitamin B_6 is recommended for men and 2.0 mg for women. For infants, metabolic requirements are met if vitamin B_6 is present in a ratio of 0.015 mg per gram of protein, or 0.04 mg per 100 calories [18, 19]. The recommended allowance for infants less than 6 months of age is 0.3 mg; for those 6 to 12 months old, 0.6 mg. For children, the allowance is based on 0.02 mg of vitamin B_6 per gram of dietary protein. During pregnancy, the allowance is increased by an additional 0.6 mg per day, and by 0.5 mg per day during lactation. The RDAs for vitamin B_6 for all ages are given in Table 9-1.

FOOD SOURCES

Fish, poultry, and meats are good sources of this vitamin, as are walnuts, peanuts, wheat germ, brown rice, and blackstrap molasses. A variety of fruits, vegetables, and dairy products are moderately good sources of this vitamin (Table 9-2).

Vitamin B_6 is water soluble, sensitive to light, and destroyed in alkaline solutions. It is relatively stable to heat and acids.

EFFECTS OF DEFICIENCY

In adult humans, no clear-cut effects of primary vitamin B_6 deficiency have been observed. Vitamin B_6 deficiency can be induced, however, by the administration of vitamin B_6 antagonists or various drugs; by chronic alcoholism; or by malabsorption syndromes. The features of deficiency include seborrheic dermatitis, glossitis, cheilosis, angular stomatitis, peripheral neuropathy, and blood disorders. In infants, a lack of vitamin B_6 in formula may result in convulsions, weight loss, abdominal distress, nervous irritability, and vomiting.

Signs of vitamin B_6 deficiency have been reported in patients receiving isonicotine hydrazine (INH) for the treatment of tuberculosis. This drug acts as a vitamin B_6 antagonist, and the symptoms produced are corrected when supplements of B_6 are given. Also at risk for developing symptoms of vitamin B_6 deficiency are patients taking oral contraceptives, antihypertensive drugs, or levodopa (for Parkinson's disease).

TOXIC EFFECTS

This vitamin has limited toxicity in humans, although vitamin B_6 dependency can be induced.

The characteristics of vitamin B_6 are listed in Table 9-3.

Folacin

Investigators in the 1920s and 1930s were finding substances in such foods as yeast and liver that demonstrated unique properties. Folacin was another one of these "unknown" substances, found in yeast and used by Wills in 1931 to treat anemia. In 1939 Hogan and Parrott found that a similar substance in liver extract could prevent anemia in chicks. Folacin was named in 1941 by Mitchell, Snell, and Williams because of its prevalence in green leaves (*folium* is Latin for "leaf"). By 1946 the structure of folacin had been determined and folacin had been synthesized.

Folacin is the generic name for folic acid and related compounds. The chemical term for folacin and folic acid is *pteroylglutamic acid*, or *PGA*. Folic acid consists of three linked components: para-aminobenzoic acid (also termed *PABA* and sometimes classified as a B-complex vitamin), pteridine, and glutamic acid, an amino acid (Fig. 9-9). It may have from one to seven glutamate groupings and is therefore designated as monopteroylglutamate, tripteroylglutamate, or heptapteroylglutamate.

FUNCTIONS

Folacin is present in five different coenzymes. Their major function is in the transfer of one-carbon units from one compound to another. As such, folacin is involved in the synthesis of choline, DNA, RNA, and the amino acids methionine, serine, and glycine. It is also involved in the oxidation of phenylalanine to tyrosine. Folacin and vitamin B_{12} are vital in the production of red blood cells by the bone marrow. A deficiency of folacin therefore leads to impaired cell division and altered protein synthesis.

ABSORPTION AND
METABOLISM

All forms of folacin are equally well utilized in the body. More folacin is excreted in the urine and feces than is accounted for in the diet, which indicates that this vitamin is also synthesized by the intestinal flora. Most of the folacin present in the body is stored in the liver. Folic acid is converted to its biologically active form, folinic acid, in the liver. This conversion is aided by vitamin C.

FIG. 9-9. Chemical structure of folic acid.

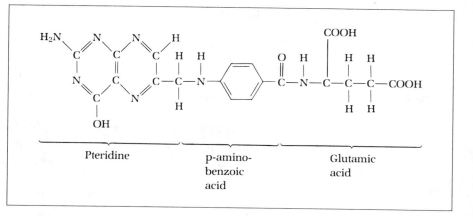

Pteridine   p-amino-benzoic acid   Glutamic acid

RECOMMENDED DIETARY ALLOWANCES

Because only 25 to 50 percent of dietary folacin is nutritionally available and 100 to 200 μg is needed daily to maintain tissue reserves, the RDA for adults is set at 400 μg of folacin daily. The daily requirement for infants is based on 5 μg per kilogram body weight, or 30 μg for infants under 6 months of age and 45 μg for those over 6 months. For older children the RDA is set at 8 to 10 μg per kilogram body weight. During pregnancy and lactation, the allowance for folacin is increased by 400 μg and 100 μg, respectively. A summary of the RDAs for folacin for all age groups is given in Table 9-1.

FOOD SOURCES

Folacin is found in a variety of foods in both the free and bound forms. The richest sources of folacin include liver, asparagus, spinach, wheat, bran, yeast, and dry beans. Almost all deep green leafy vegetables are also good sources of this vitamin (Table 9-2).

Folacin is only slightly soluble in water but is easily oxidized in an acid medium and by sunlight. Much of the folacin content of foods is lost by storage at room temperatures and by cooking.

EFFECTS OF DEFICIENCY

A pure deficiency of folacin is difficult to produce and usually is concurrent with vitamin C deficiency, the administration of a folic acid antagonist, or the addition of a high level of methionine to a diet already low in folic acid. The result of folacin deficiency is a characteristic anemia (macrocytic anemia). Folacin deficiency and its resultant anemia are sometimes seen in the elderly and among pregnant women because of poor diets, and in patients with malabsorption syndromes, leukemia, and Hodgkin's disease because of increased requirements for this vitamin. Various drugs, including oral contraceptives, antimalarials, and anticonvulsants, can interfere with folacin metabolism, thus causing deficiency. Other signs of folic acid deficiency include glossitis, leukopenia, and thrombocytopenia.

TOXIC EFFECTS

No toxic effects of folacin in humans have been reported.

Folacin's characteristics are summarized in Table 9-3.

Vitamin B₁₂

A treatment of pernicious anemia, a previously fatal disease, was suggested by Minot and Murphy in 1926. They suggested that eating large quantities of liver would control the anemia. Unfortunately, although their treatment was effective, the consumption of a pound or more of liver per day was impractical for most patients. The idea that the substance present in liver required another substance, present in normal gastric secretions, for absorption was proposed by Castle in 1944. It was believed that patients with pernicious anemia were lacking this second substance, termed *intrinsic factor*, and that only with the consumption of very large amounts of liver could some of it be absorbed by simple diffusion. By 1948 Smith and Parker had crystallized and designated the liver factor as vitamin B_{12}. In 1955 Hodgkin and his associates determined its structure (Fig. 9-10).

Vitamin B_{12} includes a group of cobalt-containing corrinoids known as cobalamins. The major forms found in plasma and tissue include methylcobalamin, adenosylcobalamin, and hydroxycobalamin. Cyanocobalamin is not nor-

FIG. 9-10. Chemical structure of vitamin B₁₂.

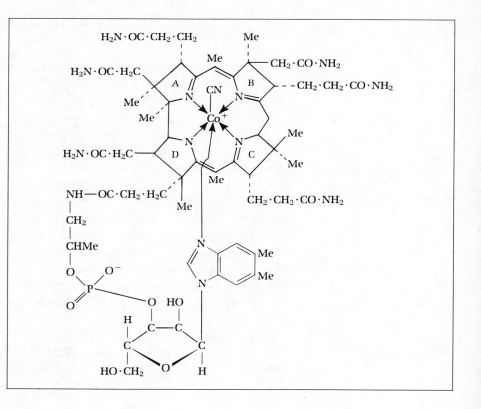

mally found in the body but is the most stable form of the vitamin and is therefore the form in which it is produced commercially. All of the above forms are biologically active. Vitamin B_{12} is an essential nutrient for all cells in the body, and growth is impaired when the supply of this vitamin is low or lacking.

FUNCTIONS

Vitamin B_{12} is required by all cells of the body, but particularly by those of the gastrointestinal tract, bone marrow, and the nervous system. Cobalamin-containing enzymes are involved in the transfer of single carbon units, such as the methylation of homocysteine to methionine. The conversion of methyl-malonylcoenzyme A to succinylcoenzyme A also involves the vitamin B_{12}– dependent transfer of single carbon units and is the common pathway for the breakdown of certain amino acids and fatty acids with an odd number of carbon atoms. Within the bone marrow, a vitamin B_{12} coenzyme is involved in the conversion of ribose nucleotides into deoxyribose nucleotides, an essential step in DNA synthesis. If DNA is not produced, the developing red blood cells increase in size but do not divide. As a result, macrocytes (large red blood cells) are released into the blood. Although they can transport oxygen, macrocytes have a fragile outer membrane and therefore a shorter life span than do normal red blood cells. Vitamin B_{12} is also involved in the synthesis of folacin and the production of leukocytes.

ABSORPTION AND METABOLISM

Vitamin B_{12} is absorbed through receptor sites in the ileum, mediated by a specific binding glycoprotein, Castle's intrinsic factor. Intrinsic factor is produced by glands in the stomach. Some absorption, about 1 to 3 percent, may also occur by simple diffusion [20]. In the ileum, in the presence of calcium, the vitamin B_{12} combined with intrinsic factor attaches to the receptor sites and the vitamin alone is transported across the intestinal cell and into the bloodstream; intrinsic factor remains in the intestine. Enough vitamin B_{12} is normally stored in the liver for 3 to 5 years.

RECOMMENDED DIETARY ALLOWANCES

Because vitamin B_{12} is recycled from bile and other intestinal secretions, it is unnecessary to consume this vitamin every day as a food or as a dietary supplement. Nutritional equilibrium can therefore be maintained in most healthy persons over a wide range of intakes. The RDA of 3.0 μg of vitamin B_{12} for adults allows for the maintenance of adequate vitamin B_{12} nutrition and substantial reserve body pool. The allowance for infants is based on the vitamin B_{12} content of breast milk, a reflection of maternal levels. For infants, the RDA is set at 0.5 μg per day, or 0.15 μg per 100 calories. During pregnancy and lactation, the RDA is increased by an additional 1.0 μg. Table 9-1 gives a summary of the RDAs for vitamin B_{12} for all age groups.

FOOD SOURCES

Vitamin B_{12} is found only in animal sources. Because of this, strict vegetarians may develop a dietary deficiency of this vitamin. The richest sources include lamb and beef kidney; lamb, beef, calf, and pork liver; and beef brain. Other good sources include heart, egg yolk, and a variety of seafood, as outlined in Table 9-2.

Vitamin B_{12} is stable to heat and only slightly soluble in water but is destroyed by strong acid or alkaline solutions. Little is lost with routine cooking procedures.

EFFECTS OF DEFICIENCY

A deficiency of vitamin B_{12} is usually caused by a defect in absorption rather than by dietary factors. Megaloblastic anemia caused by vitamin B_{12} depletion after total gastrectomy (surgical removal of the stomach) takes about 5 years or longer to develop. When intrinsic factor is not produced, vitamin B_{12} is not absorbed. As a result, the bone marrow cannot produce mature red blood cells and so releases the large, immature precursors (macrocytes) into the bloodstream instead. The symptoms of megaloblastic anemia (or pernicious anemia) include pallor, weight loss, anorexia, glossitis, sprue and, in the advanced stages, degeneration of the spinal cord.

TOXIC EFFECTS

No known toxic effects have occurred in humans.

A summary of the characteristics of vitamin B_{12} is given in Table 9-3.

Biotin

In the 1920s a substance in yeast that was essential for its growth was isolated and termed *bios*. In 1934 Lease and Parsons described a deficiency syndrome observed in chicks fed a diet including raw egg white. The symptoms were not seen when cooked egg white was used. By 1941 Williams and his coworkers had discovered the substance in raw egg white to be a glycoprotein that binds biotin, preventing its absorption from the gastrointestinal tract. This antivitamin, termed *avidin*, is inactivated by heat.

Biotin, a water-soluble, sulfur-containing vitamin, is widely distributed in nature and is an essential nutrient for many animal species. In both foods and tissues, it is usually complexed with protein.

FUNCTIONS

As a component of many enzymes, biotin is involved in carbohydrate and fat metabolism. Biotin is part of coenzymes involved in carboxylation (transporting carboxyl units), linking the metabolism of carbohydrate and fat, and fixing carbon dioxide in tissue (Fig. 9-11). It is also involved in protein metabolism through deamination reactions: The deaminases for threonine, aspartic acid, and serine all require biotin as a coenzyme. It is also vital to growth, maintenance of skin, hair, nerves, and bone marrow.

ABSORPTION AND METABOLISM

Because the urinary and fecal excretion of biotin exceeds the dietary intake, it is believed that the intestinal flora make a significant contribution. This vitamin is stored in minute amounts in the liver, kidneys, adrenals, and brain.

FIG. 9-11. Chemical structure of biotin.

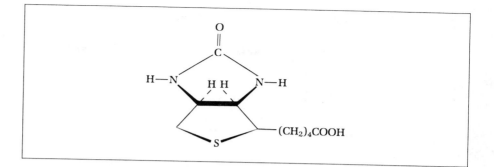

DIETARY INTAKES

Because of the intestinal synthesis of this vitamin, no RDA has been established. Table 9-4 lists estimated safe and adequate daily dietary intakes of biotin.

FOOD SOURCES

Biotin is widely distributed in foods. Liver and yeast are the richest sources; meats, some vegetables, seafood, and nuts are good sources (Table 9-2). There are wide differences in the availability of biotin from various foods. For example, it is well absorbed from corn and soybeans but is almost completely unavailable from wheat. It is therefore important to know both the chemical form (bound or unbound) and its content in a particular food.

Biotin is stable to acids, heat, and light but is affected by oxidizing agents and alkaline solutions.

EFFECTS OF DEFICIENCY

A deficiency of biotin has been documented in humans only after prolonged ingestion of raw egg whites. Recently biotin deficiency has also been seen as a complication of parenteral alimentation [21]. The signs and symptoms include scaly changes in the skin, muscle pains, anorexia, nausea, vomiting, glossitis, and mental depression. All signs and symptoms respond to biotin administration.

TABLE 9-4. Estimated safe and adequate daily dietary intakes of biotin and pantothenic acid

Group	Age (years)	Biotin (μg)	Pantothenic acid (mg)
Infants	0–0.5	35	2
	0.5–1.0	50	3
Children and adolescents	1–3	65	3
	4–6	85	3–4
	7–10	120	4–5
	11+	100–200	4–7
Adults	—	100–200	4–7

Source: Food and Nutrition Board, National Research Council, *Recommended Dietary Allowances* (9th ed.). Washington, D.C.: National Academy of Sciences, 1980. P. 178.

TOXIC EFFECTS

Biotin is essentially nontoxic in humans.

A summary of biotin's characteristics is given in Table 9-3.

Pantothenic Acid

In 1938 Williams isolated pantothenic acid from yeast and later from liver. Not much interest was shown in this vitamin until 1950 when Lipmann and coworkers found that pantothenic acid was a component of coenzyme A, a key regulatory substance for all of metabolism. The term *pantothenic acid* is derived from the Greek *pantothen*, meaning "from all sides, everywhere," indicating the distribution and importance of this vitamin in metabolism.

FUNCTIONS

Pantothenic acid has a vital function in the cellular metabolism of proteins, fats, and carbohydrates. As a component of coenzyme A, this vitamin is involved in the release of energy and the synthesis of fatty acids, steroids, cholesterol, acetylcholine, and the porphyrin ring of the hemoglobin molecule. The oxidation of fatty acids also requires pantothenic acid. Figure 9-12 shows the structure of pantothenic acid.

ABSORPTION AND
METABOLISM

Pantothenic acid is found in all living tissues, both animal and plant. It is synthesized in all cells but does not cross cell membranes. The highest concentrations of this vitamin are found in the heart, liver, brain, kidneys, and adrenal glands.

DIETARY INTAKES

The daily requirement for pantothenic acid is not yet known, but a daily intake of 4 to 7 mg for adults seems to be adequate. Table 9-4 outlines dietary intakes for all age groups.

FOOD SOURCES

As its name implies, pantothenic acid is widely distributed in many types of foods. The richest sources include liver, kidney, eggs, yeast, wheat germ, and dried peas. Other good sources are also listed in Table 9-2.

Pantothenic acid is water soluble and stable under ordinary cooking procedures, except in acid or alkaline solutions.

FIG. 9-12. Chemical structure
of pantothenic acid.

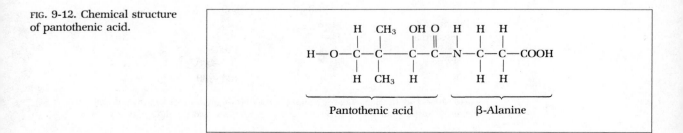

EFFECTS OF DEFICIENCY

Because of its presence in all living tissues, a deficiency of pantothenic acid is very difficult to produce. The clinical features of deficiency produced by a vitamin antagonist include fatigue, malaise, neurologic effects (numbness, muscle cramps, burning sensation of the feet), cardiovascular disorders, insomnia, gastrointestinal disturbances (nausea, abdominal cramping, epigastric burning), increased susceptibility to infection, and impaired muscular coordination, particularly in walking. Many of these features are also indicative of other B vitamin deficiencies and may mistakenly be treated unsuccessfully with another of the B vitamins.

TOXIC EFFECTS

This vitamin is nontoxic in humans.

The characteristics of pantothenic acid are summarized in Table 9-3.

References

1. Food and Nutrition Board, National Research Council. *Recommended Dietary Allowances* (9th ed.). Washington, D.C.: National Academy of Sciences, 1980. Pp. 73, 76.
2. Irwin, M. I., and Hutchins, B. K. A conspectus of research on vitamin C requirements of man. *J. Nutr.* 106:823, 1976.
3. Pauling, L. The significance of the evidence about ascorbic acid and the common cold. *Proc. Natl. Acad. Sci. U.S.A.* 68:2678, 1971.
4. Karlowski, T. R., et al. Ascorbic acid for the common cold: A prophylactic and therapeutic trial. *J.A.M.A.* 231:1038, 1975.
5. Coulehan, J. L., et al. Vitamin C and acute illness in Navajo school children. *N. Engl. J. Med.* 295:973, 1976.
6. Ginter, E., et al. Effect of ascorbic acid on plasma cholesterol in humans in a long-term experiment. *Int. J. Vitam. Nutr. Res.* 47:123, 1977.
7. Peterson, V. E., et al. Quantification of plasma cholesterol and triglyceride levels in hypercholesterolemic subjects receiving ascorbic acid supplements. *Am. J. Clin. Nutr.* 28:584, 1975.
8. Prinz, W., et al. The effect of ascorbic acid supplementation on some parameters of the human immunological defense system. *Int. J. Vitam. Nutr. Res.* 47:248, 1977.
9. Stein, H. G., Hasan, A., and Fox, I. H. Ascorbic acid–induced uricosuria: A consequence of mega-vitamin therapy. *Ann. Intern. Med.* 84:385, 1976.
10. Cook, J. D., and Monsen, E. R. Vitamin C, the common cold, and iron absorption. *Am. J. Clin. Nutr.* 30:235, 1977.
11. Shilotri, P. G., and Bhat, K. S. Effect of mega doses of vitamin C on bactericidal activity of leukocytes. *Am. J. Clin. Nutr.* 30:1077, 1977.
12. Hoyumpa, A. M. Mechanisms of thiamin deficiency in chronic alcoholism. *Am. J. Clin. Nutr.* 33:2750, 1980.
13. Vimokesant, S. L., et al. Effect of tea consumption on thiamin status in man. *Nutr. Rep. Int.* 9:371, 1974.
14. Kutsky, R. J. *Handbook of Vitamins and Hormones.* New York: Van Nostrand Reinhold, 1973. P. 42.
15. Food and Nutrition Board, National Research Council. *Recommended Dietary Allowances* (9th ed.). Washington, D.C.: National Academy of Sciences, 1980. P. 93.
16. Darby, W. J., McNutt, K. W., and Todhunter, E. N. Niacin. *Nutr. Rev.* 33:289, 1975.

17. Bureau of Nutritional Sciences, Department of National Health and Welfare. *Dietary Standard for Canada.* Ottawa, 1975.
18. Committee on Nutrition, American Academy of Pediatrics. Commentary on breast-feeding and infant formulas, including proposed standards for formulas. *Pediatrics* 57:278, 1976.
19. McCoy, E. E. Vitamin B_6 requirements of infants and children. In *Human Vitamin B_6 Requirements.* Washington, D.C.: National Academy of Sciences, 1978. Pp. 257–271.
20. Food and Nutrition Board, National Research Council. *Recommended Dietary Allowances* (9th ed.). Washington, D.C.: National Academy of Sciences, 1980. P. 114.
21. Mock, D. M., et al. Biotin deficiency: An unusual complication of parenteral alimentation. *N. Engl. J. Med.* 304:820, 1981.

Suggested Readings

Baker, S. J., and Mathan, V. I. Evidence regarding the minimal daily requirement of dietary vitamin B_{12}. *Am. J. Clin. Nutr.* 34:2423, 1981.

Bonjour, J. P. Biotin in man's nutrition and therapy: A review. *Int. J. Vitam. Nutr. Res.* 47:107, 1977.

Butler, W. M., Taylor, H. G., and Diehl, L. F. Lhermitte's sign in cobalamin (vitamin B_{12}) deficiency. *J.A.M.A.* 245:1059, 1981.

Colman, N., Hettiarachy, N., and Herbert, V. Detection of a milk factor that facilitates folate uptake by intestinal cells. *Science* 211:1427, 1981.

Coronary Drug Project Research Group. Clofibrate and niacin in coronary heart disease. *J.A.M.A.* 231:360, 1975.

Dietary fiber and vitamin B_{12} balance. *Nutr. Rev.* 37:116, 1979.

Food and Nutrition Board, National Research Council. *Folic Acid: Biochemistry and Physiology in Relation to the Human Nutrition Requirement.* Washington, D.C.: National Academy of Sciences, 1977.

Halsted, C. H. The intestinal absorption of folates. *Am. J. Clin. Nutr.* 32:846, 1979.

Heller, S., Salked, R. M., and Korner, W. F. Riboflavin status in pregnancy. *Am. J. Clin. Nutr.* 27:1225, 1974.

Horwitt, M. K., Harper, A. E., and Henderson, L. M. Niacin-tryptophan relationships for evaluating niacin equivalents. *Am. J. Clin. Nutr.* 34:423, 1981.

How vitamin C really works . . . or does it? *Nutr. Today* 1979.

Kallner, A., Hartman, D., and Hornig, D. Steady-state turnover and body pool of ascorbic acid in man. *Am. J. Clin. Nutr.* 32:530, 1979.

Levander, O. A., and Cheng, L. (eds.). *Micronutrient Interactions: Vitamins, Minerals, and Hazardous Elements.* New York: New York Academy of Sciences, 1980.

Levy, J. V., and Bach-y-Rita, P. *Vitamins: Their Use and Abuse.* New York: Liveright, 1976.

McCormick, D. B. Biotin. *Nutr. Rev.* 33:97, 1975.

Pauling, L. *Vitamin C, the Common Cold and the Flu.* San Francisco: W. H. Freeman, 1976.

Possible vitamin B-6 deficiency uncovered in persons with the "Chinese Restaurant Syndrome." *Nutr. Rev.* 40:15, 1982.

Ranum, P. M., Lowe, R. J., and Gordon, H. T. Effect of bleaching, maturing, and oxidizing agents on vitamins added to wheat flour. *Cereal Chem.* 58:32, 1981.

Rivlin, R. S. Hormones, drugs and riboflavin. *Nutr. Rev.* 37:241, 1979.

Rodriguez, M. S. A conspectus of research on folacin requirements of man. *J. Nutr.* 108:1983, 1978.

Roepke, J. L. B., and Kirksey, A.   Vitamin B$_6$ nutriture during pregnancy and lactation: II. The effect of long-term use of oral contraceptives. *Am. J. Clin. Nutr.* 32:2257, 1979.

Sanpitak, N., and Chayutimonkul, L.   Oral contraceptives and riboflavin nutrition. *Lancet* 1:836, 1974.

Sauberlich, H. E., et al.   Thiamin requirement of the adult human. *Am. J. Clin. Nutr.* 32:2237, 1979.

Skalka, H. W., and Prchal, J. T.   Cataracts and riboflavin deficiency. *Am. J. Clin. Nutr.* 34:861, 1981.

Tanaka, K.   New light on biotin deficiency. *N. Engl. J. Med.* 304:839, 1981.

The function of ascorbic acid in collagen formation. *Nutr. Rev.* 36:118, 1978.

Two signs of vitamin B$_{12}$ deficiency. *Nutr. & the MD* 7, 1981.

Chapter 10

FLUIDS, ELECTROLYTES, AND ACID-BASE BALANCE

Over billions of years, humans have evolved from ancestors that existed within the sea to land creatures that create their own internal environment, or "internal sea." The composition of this fluid must be kept constant within a narrow range to maintain the health and well-being of the individual. Mechanisms for regulating this internal sea, such as the kidneys and lungs, the buffer system of the blood, and thirst reflexes in the brain, have also evolved. The delicate interplay of these and many other systems allows humans to live on land while still functioning within a fluid and electrolyte balance.

In this chapter several important concepts will be presented that are vital to the understanding of the role and functioning of the internal sea: First, the concept of fluids and fluid compartments divided by various body membranes is presented. Next, the idea of solutes and electrolytes suspended in these fluids and their influence not only on fluid movement between compartments but also on overall health and well-being are discussed. Finally, the controls determining the composition and volume of the body fluids are described, and the concept of acid-base balance and its importance in nutrition and health are explained.

Water
DISTRIBUTION AND
FUNCTIONS

Water is an element vital to life, second in importance only to oxygen. It constitutes the most abundant compound in living cells, accounting for 65 to 90 percent by weight. Because of its polarity and hydrogen-binding capacity, water is an excellent solvent for many compounds. It is involved in many of the body's essential reactions, including hydrolysis during digestion and as the end product of glucose oxidation. Because of their solubility in water, it is a vehicle of transport of nutrients to cells and of wastes to the skin, gut, and lungs. It also serves as a dispersing medium and has a great influence on the functional and structural components of the cell. Because of its high heat of vaporization, water plays an important role in regulating body temperature through the evaporation of moisture from the skin and lungs. A 1 to 2 percent loss of total body water triggers thirst mechanisms, a loss of 10 percent constitutes a serious health hazard, and a 20 percent loss can cause death.

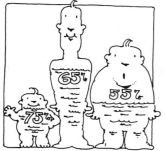

The total body water of an average adult is about 40 liters; about 15 liters is extracellular and about 25 liters intracellular. Infants have a total body water content of about 70 to 75 percent; lean adults, about 65 percent; and obese adults, 45 to 55 percent. All body tissues contain water, but the percentage varies greatly, from 5 percent in teeth to 80 percent in striated muscle.

FLUID COMPARTMENTS

The body can be divided into three major spaces, or *fluid compartments,* by the capillary walls and cell membranes. The majority of the body water (40 to 50 percent of the total body weight) is the *intracellular fluid,* that which exists within all body cells. The remaining *extracellular fluid* can be divided into the *intravascular* compartment (the blood plasma, 5 percent of the total body weight) and the *extravascular compartment* (the interstitial fluid, 10 to 20 percent of the total body weight) (Fig. 10-1).

The extracellular fluid includes the plasma; interstitial fluid and lymph; the fluid of dense connective tissue, cartilage, and bone; and transcellular fluids. The total blood volume is composed of the *plasma* and the cellular elements of the blood (erythrocytes, leukocytes, and platelets). The *interstitial fluid* bathes and surrounds the cells of the tissues. Water and most dissolved substances diffuse through pores in the capillaries, allowing the plasma and interstitial fluid to mix. This permits an exchange of nutrients and metabolic waste products. The fluid of *dense connective tissue, bone, and cartilage* does not readily exchange with the rest of the body water. The *transcellular fluids* include those fluids formed by the secretory action of specialized cells. Examples include the secretions of the salivary glands, pancreas, liver, and gallbladder and the products of the mucous membranes of the gastrointestinal and respiratory tracts.

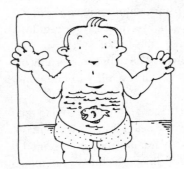

The most stable fluid is that of the intracellular compartment. The extravascular compartment is the most elastic, adjusting to permit the body to maintain homeostasis with variable fluid intake and losses.

FLUID INTAKE AND SOURCES

The body's need for water is met by several sources: the ingestion of water, water-containing fluids, and water-containing solid foods and the water resulting from the metabolic oxidation of foods. The oxidation of 100 gm of fat yields about 107 ml of water; 100 gm of carbohydrate, about 56 ml of water; and 100 gm of protein, about 41 ml of water. Most solid foods contain water, ranging from 95 percent in some fruits and vegetables to about 35 percent in breads; these foods account for much of the daily fluid intake. The average daily intake of water, including that formed in the body, is about 2500 ml. About 1200 ml is taken as water or beverages, another 1000 ml in solid foods, and the remaining 200 to 300 ml from the oxidation of foodstuffs ("metabolic water").

FLUID LOSSES

Fluids are lost from the body as urine by the kidneys, through evaporation from the skin and lungs, and as part of the feces (Table 10-1). The *obligatory* losses of water are those that are essential for the maintenance of physiologic equilibrium. In the kidneys, about 600 ml is required daily to dissolve the usual amount of wastes. With a decrease in the amount of solids to be dissolved (principally urea and sodium chloride), there is a corresponding reduction in the amount of obligatory water lost in the urine. A diet low in protein and high in carbohydrate reduces the formation of urea and thereby lowers obligatory losses.

The *insensible* water losses from the skin are fairly constant and are proportional to the surface area of the body. The evaporation of this water from the skin takes place constantly, which makes insensible water loss unnoticeable. It is one of the means by which body temperature is maintained. Infants have a greater surface area per unit of weight than do adults and are therefore more vulnerable to water losses from the skin and rapid changes in body temperature. Water lost

FIG. 10-1. Total body water composition. (From A. Plumer, *Principles and Practice of Intravenous Therapy* [3rd ed.]. Boston: Little, Brown, 1982.)

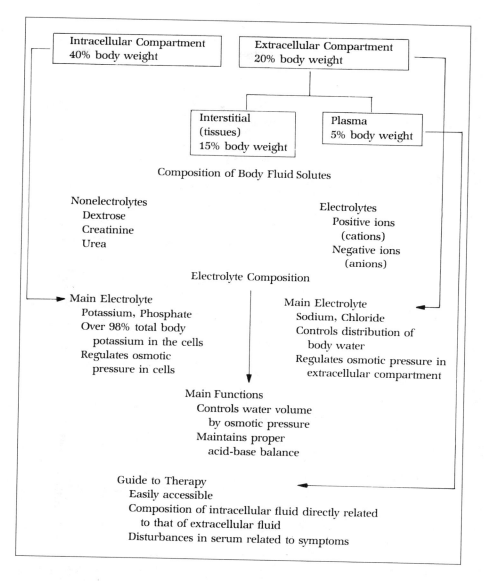

through visible perspiration varies from none in cool temperatures to several liters in warm temperatures by persons engaged in strenuous activity. When 1 to 2 percent of the total body water is lost, the kidneys compensate by excreting a more concentrated urine. Water lost via the lungs is proportional to the rate of respiration; any condition that increases respiration would therefore increase water loss.

MECHANISM OF THIRST

When as little as 1 to 2 percent of the total body weight is lost, thirst, the earliest sign of fluid depletion, results. The drying of the mucous membranes of the

TABLE 10-1. Daily losses of water

Route	Water lost (ml)
Feces	100–200
Urine	1000–1500
Lungs	250–400
Insensible perspiration	400–600
Visible perspiration	0–10,000

Source: Adapted from C. H. Robinson, *Normal and Therapeutic Nutrition* (14th ed.). Copyright © 1972 by Macmillan Publishing Co., Inc. P. 126.

lining of the mouth triggers the learned reflex of drinking. In addition, special cells in the hypothalamus of the brain, responding to changes in the osmotic pressure of the blood, give an unconscious signal to drink.

Under conditions in which body fluids are lost but only water is replaced, depletion of electrolytes may occur. Examples of this include heavy perspiration losses during hard physical labor in a hot climate and loss of electrolytes during illness, profuse vomiting, copious diarrhea, or gastric or intestinal suctioning. In all of these conditions, the replacement of fluids alone is not enough. The kidneys will compensate by excreting a dilute urine, while conserving the body's electrolytes.

REQUIREMENTS

The 24-hour water requirement is equal to the amount lost through the skin, kidneys, lungs, and bowel. Under normal conditions, thirst is an accurate indicator of fluid needs. With a minimum of physical activity, an absence of perspiration, and a low protein, low solute diet, an adult would require about 1.5 liters of water per day from food, beverages, and metabolic oxidation.

RELATED DISEASES

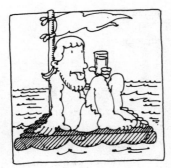

One of the classic problems of fluid and electrolyte balance is that of the castaway at sea. If he does not drink the salty sea water, he will die of dehydration and heat stroke or exposure. But what is the problem if he *does* drink sea water? The human kidney can concentrate urine to a maximum sodium chloride content of about 2 percent. Sea water contains about 3.5% sodium chloride. Therefore for every 100 ml of sea water the castaway drinks, his kidneys would have to excrete 175 ml of urine to remove the 3.5-gm salt load. He would therefore have suffered a 75 ml loss of water, hastening his dehydration. If his kidneys did not clear all the excess salt from his body, then a higher than normal salt concentration in his body fluids would result, causing a greater thirst.

For a discussion of specific diseases altering fluid and electrolyte balance, see Chap. 42.

Electrolytes
DEFINITIONS AND TERMS

An *electrolyte* is any substance that dissociates into its component ions when dissolved in a fluid. An electrical current can be transmitted by a solution containing electrolytes. Substances vary in their degree of dissociation, with strong electrolytes being acids or bases that dissociate almost completely. *Cations* are electrolytes that carry positive charges and can donate electrons. *Anions* are electron acceptors and carry negative charges. In every solution (and each fluid compartment of the body) the total number of cations equals the total number of anions. Most frequently, the composition of a fluid is expressed in milliequivalents rather than in a unit weight per milliliter. A *milliequivalent* (mEq) is equal to the atomic weight of a substance (in milligrams) divided by its valence. By using this unit of measurement, concentrations of anions and cations can be most easily compared. For example, since any cation can combine with any anion, 1 mEq of sodium (a cation) can combine with 1 mEq of chloride (an anion), even though they have different atomic weights (23 and 35, respectively).

In the plasma, sodium is the major cation, with small, but important, contributions made by calcium, magnesium, and potassium. Chloride is the main anion in plasma, with smaller additions made by bicarbonate, proteinate, phosphate, sulfate, and organic acids. In the intracellular fluid, potassium is the major cation, with sodium, calcium, and magnesium also present. Phosphate is the major anion in the intracellular fluid; bicarbonate and proteinate are also present (Fig. 10-2). It is important to note that the total number of anions is

FIG. 10-2. The electrolyte composition of the plasma, the interstitial fluid, and the intracellular fluid (Org. ac. = organic acids).

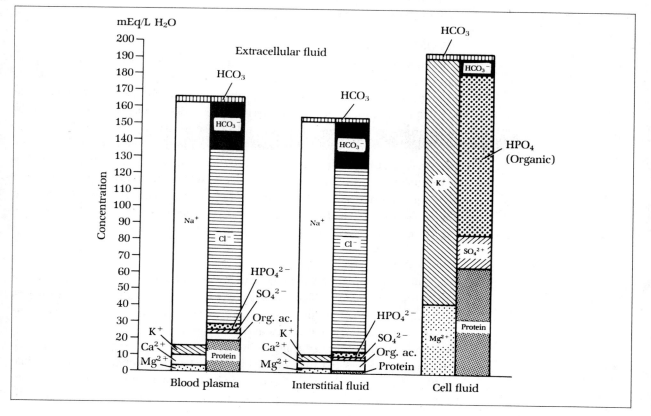

TABLE 10-2. Body content and concentration of electrolytes

Element	Body content (gm)	Plasma concentration (mEq/liter)
Chloride	85	98–106
Potassium	150	3.5–5.5
Sodium	63	136–145

always equal to the total number of cations in each fluid compartment, thereby maintaining osmotic balance. A summary of the body content and concentration of selected electrolytes is given in Table 10-2.

SODIUM

DISTRIBUTION AND FUNCTIONS

This element is the major cation (Na^+) in the extracellular fluid compartments of the body. In conjunction with chloride and bicarbonate, it is an important factor in the regulation of acid-base balance. Sodium acts to maintain the osmotic pressure of body fluid, thus protecting the body against excessive fluid losses. It also functions to preserve the normal irritability of muscle and the permeability of cells. About one-third of the sodium present in the body is in the inorganic portion of the skeleton. Most of the remaining two-thirds is in the extracellular fluids of the body.

ABSORPTION AND METABOLISM

Sodium is readily absorbed from the ileum; little is present in the feces, except in diarrhea. The kidneys are responsible for maintaining sodium homeostasis through the action of the hormone *aldosterone* (an adrenocortical steroid) on renal tubular functions. With a decrease in sodium intake there is a rise in aldosterone secretion and a resultant decrease in urinary excretion of sodium. The opposite occurs with an increase in sodium intake: The level of aldosterone decreases, causing an increase in urinary excretion of sodium. Extreme sweating can cause a considerable loss of sodium, and when 3 or more liters are required to replace sweat losses, extra sodium should be provided. Between 2 and 7 gm (34 to 120 mEq) of sodium per liter of extra water loss is suggested, depending on the severity of losses and the degree of acclimatization [1].

DIETARY INTAKES

The estimated safe and adequate daily dietary intakes of sodium are given in Table 10-3. For infants, the increase in lean body mass, composition of the feces, and cutaneous losses are the most important determinants of sodium needs. The minimum requirement for infants and young children is about 58 mg (2.5 mEq) per day; the recommended range is 92 to 184 mg (4 to 8 mEq) per day. Human milk contains about 161 mg (7 mEq) per liter, formulas range between 161 and 391 mg (7 to 17 mEq) per liter, and cow's milk about 483 mg (21 mEq) per liter. Adults can maintain sodium balance with little more than what is required by

TABLE 10-3. Estimated safe and adequate daily dietary intakes of electrolytes

Group	Age (years)	Sodium (mg)	Potassium (mg)	Chloride (mg)
Infants	0–0.5	115–350	350–925	275–700
	0.5–1.0	250–750	425–1275	400–1200
Children	1–3	325–975	550–1650	500–1500
	4–6	450–1350	775–2325	700–2100
	7–10	600–1800	1000–3000	925–2775
	11+	900–2700	1525–4575	1400–4200
Adults	—	1100–3300	1875–5625	1700–5100

Source: Food and Nutrition Board, National Research Council, *Recommended Dietary Allowances* (9th ed.). Washington, D.C.: National Academy of Sciences, 1980. P. 178.

infants. This low requirement reflects an absence of growth and minimal urinary and fecal losses.

FOOD SOURCES

The most common and concentrated source of sodium is table salt (NaCl); 2.5 gm of salt contain 1 gm of sodium (Fig. 10-3). Foods with added salt are high in sodium, as are bread, cheese, oysters, whole grains, milk, and dried fruits.

Sodium is found in nearly every food, including water, in some amounts, as well as in food additives. Careful inspection of food labels will indicate this. Consumer pressure on the food industry has resulted in more sodium labeling. See Chaps. 20 and 21 for more details.

RELATED DISEASES

Prolonged high intakes of sodium have been shown to be one of several factors associated with the development of *hypertension* (high blood pressure) [2]. For those with a family history of hypertension, a lowered intake of sodium (1 to 2 gm per day) is recommended (see Chap. 40).

Addison's disease, characterized by an increased loss of sodium due to adrenocortical insufficiency, requires the intake of high amounts of sodium just to maintain balance.

Excessive losses of sodium can also result from prolonged or severe vomiting or diarrhea. Just as fluid is retained with sodium retention, it is also lost with sodium depletion. Severe dehydration can result, manifested by a loss of skin turgor, softened eyeballs, muscle weakness, and cardiac arrhythmias.

POTASSIUM

DISTRIBUTION AND FUNCTIONS

This element is the principal cation (K^+) in the intracellular fluid, where it influences muscle activity, particularly that of cardiac muscle. Its concentration in the intracellular fluid is 30 times greater than in the extracellular fluid. This high level of intracellular potassium is essential for several metabolic functions, including protein synthesis by ribosomes. Within cells it also functions in main-

FIG. 10-3. Harvesting salt for export at the Elephant Pass salt works in Ceylon. (United Nations photo.)

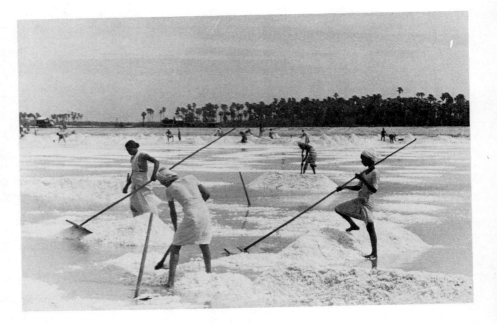

taining acid-base balance and osmotic pressure. Several enzymes require potassium for maximum activity.

ABSORPTION AND METABOLISM

Potassium is readily absorbed from the gut. Some potassium is secreted into the gut, as part of the digestive fluids, but is later reabsorbed. Very little of this element is lost in the feces. As with sodium, the kidneys provide the major regulatory mechanism for potassium excretion, under the influence of changes in acid-base balance as well as the activity of the adrenal cortex. *Hyperkalemia* (high blood potassium) will not occur, even after the ingestion or injection of large amounts of potassium, if kidney function is intact.

DIETARY INTAKES

The estimated safe and adequate daily dietary intakes of potassium are given in Table 10-3. In infants, an increase in lean body mass and fecal losses are the main determinants of potassium needs. Human milk contains about 500 mg (13 mEq) per liter, formulas have slightly more, and cow's milk contains 1365 mg (35 mEq) per liter. Adults can maintain potassium balance with intakes as low as infants, although the kidneys are not as effective at restricting potassium loss as sodium loss. The concentration of potassium in sweat is low (less than 390 mg, or 10 mEq, per liter) compared with that of sodium (25 to 30 mEq per liter).

FOOD SOURCES

The following are good sources of potassium: veal, chicken, beef and beef liver, pork, dried apricots and peaches, oranges, broccoli, and winter squash.

RELATED DISEASES

A deficiency of potassium occurs only when there is excessive loss through diarrhea, in diabetic acidosis, or with certain laxatives and diuretics. When blood glucose is converted to glycogen for storage, some potassium is stored with it. When a patient with diabetic acidosis is being treated with insulin and glucose, potassium is being drawn from the blood to be stored with the glucose, and *hypokalemia* (low blood potassium) can occur. Replacement of potassium should also be part of the treatment of this condition. A deficit of potassium can also occur in chronic wasting diseases, with malnutrition, prolonged negative nitrogen balance, and gastrointestinal losses. Potassium is stored with nitrogen as muscle protein, and when muscle is broken down the intracellular potassium is transferred to the extracellular fluid, where it is quickly removed by the kidneys. During rehabilitation from these diseases, diets should include both amino acids (protein) and potassium to ensure adequate retention. The signs and symptoms of hypokalemia include muscle weakness, irritability, paralysis, and tachycardia (rapid heart rate).

Sudden intakes above 12 gm (250 to 300 mEq)/sq m of surface area/day, or about 18 gm for an adult, may be fatal because they may cause cardiac arrest [1].

CHLORIDE

As a major anion (Cl^-) of the extracellular fluid and as a component of sodium chloride, this element (as chloride ion) is essential in fluid balance and regulation of osmotic pressure, as well as in acid-base equilibrium and the production of hydrochloric acid. The human body contains about 15 percent chloride, with highest concentrations being in the cerebrospinal fluid and the secretions of the gastrointestinal tract. The lowest concentrations are found in muscle and nerve tissue.

As a component of erythrocytes (red blood cells), chloride crosses the cell membrane to establish an equilibrium between the cell contents and the extracellular fluids to minimize fluid shifts. Chloride also enhances the ability of the blood to carry large amounts of carbon dioxide to the lungs and aids in potassium conservation.

Chloride in the diet exists almost exclusively as sodium chloride, and the intake of chloride is adequate as long as sodium intake is satisfactory. Human milk contains about 11 mEq per liter of chloride. Table 10-3 gives safe and adequate ranges of intake.

Any abnormalities in sodium metabolism will also result in derangements of chloride metabolism. When losses of sodium are excessive, as with profuse sweating, diarrhea, or certain endocrine disorders, there is an accompanying loss of chloride. When there is an excessive loss of gastric juice, the loss of chloride exceeds that of sodium, causing an increase in bicarbonate and resultant hypochloremic alkalosis.

The electrolytes are summarized in Table 10-4.

TABLE 10-4. Summary of electrolytes

Element	Site of absorption	Primary functions	Interactions with other elements	Route of excretion	Dietary sources	Key terms
Sodium	Ileum	Acid-base balance Cell permeability Normal muscle irritability	Chloride	Kidneys	Salt, milk, meat, eggs, vegetables	Aldosterone Hypertension
Potassium	Gut	Acid-base balance Osmotic pressure	—	Kidneys	Meats, dried fruits, vegetables	—
Chloride	Gut	Acid-base balance Production of hydrochloric acid	Sodium Potassium	Kidneys	Salt	—

Fluid Movement and Osmolarity

When a membrane between two fluid compartments is permeable to water but not to some of the dissolved solutes, it is termed a *semipermeable membrane*. When the concentration of the nondiffusible substance is greater on one side of the membrane than on the other, water passes through the membrane toward the side with the greater concentration of nondiffusible substance. This process of fluid movement caused by solute concentration is termed *osmosis*.

The internal membranes of the human body separating the three fluid compartments permit fluids to cross without difficulty but are impermeable to various solutes. The flow of fluid is affected by the *osmotic pressure* exerted by the solute (the amount of pressure required to exactly oppose osmosis). The osmotic pressure of the intracellular and extracellular fluids is due to dissolved solutes, most of which are ionized electrolytes. In the intracellular fluid, these include potassium, magnesium, organic phosphate, glycogen, nucleoproteins, proteins, nucleotides, and enzymes. In the extracellular fluid the ionized electrolytes include sodium, calcium, chloride, and bicarbonate. Sodium, the chief cation of the extracellular fluid, and potassium, the chief cation of the intracellular fluid, do not readily diffuse across cell membranes; therefore they exert a profound osmotic influence. Other factors, including active transport mechanisms, the competition of substances for carriers to transport materials across cell membranes, and hormonal and nervous controls, also influence the movement of water and solutes from one fluid compartment to another.

Unlike the relationship between the intracellular and extracellular solutes, there is a free exchange of all solutes between the blood and the extravascular fluid compartments. The plasma proteins, such as albumin, exert an osmotic effect, since they cannot diffuse across the capillary barrier. When the level of plasma protein drops, fluid moves from the blood to the interstitial spaces, causing the tissues to become swollen and waterlogged (*edema*). Plasma proteins are synthesized by the liver. The osmotic pressure exerted by these proteins prevents both the diffusion of fluid from the intravascular to the extravascular compartment and the excessive removal of water from the blood by the kidneys.

Renal Regulation
STRUCTURE

Each human kidney consists of about one million functional units, the *nephrons*. Each nephron is composed of a *glomerulus*, a group of capillaries surrounded by a capsule (*Bowman's capsule*); and a *tubule*, including the *proximal and distal convoluted tubules* and the ascending and descending *loop of Henle*. The nephrons empty into *collecting tubules* or *ducts* (Fig. 10-4). Blood flows to the kidneys via the renal artery, a branch off the abdominal aorta, into the glomerulus through an afferent arteriole, and away via an efferent arteriole, which then forms *peritubular capillaries* that surround the tubules. This anatomic arrangement permits the kidneys to form concentrated or dilute urine.

FUNCTION

The purpose of the renal filtration of the blood is to keep its composition and volume constant through osmotic pressure regulation and water, electrolyte, and acid-base balance. The production of urine allows the excretion of excessive solutes, electrolytes, and fluids, as well as the by-products of metabolism. The adaptive nature of renal function allows it to conserve or eliminate fluids and electrolytes as needed.

About one-fourth of the total cardiac output, or approximately 1200 ml every minute, is filtered through the glomeruli. This large blood flow is related to the kidney's function of removing metabolic wastes and excess fluid and electrolytes. The composition of the glomerular filtrate is the same as that of blood plasma, except that the filtrate does not contain any protein or large colloidal particles. In the glomeruli, selective reabsorption of water and certain solutes and selective secretion of other solutes occur. In the tubules, the concentration of various electrolytes and solutes is determined by *active transport* and *diffusion*. Active transport moves substances against concentration gradients and requires energy. In diffusion, substances move to equalize concentrations on both sides of a membrane, and no energy is required. In the distal convoluted tubule and the collecting duct, the action of antidiuretic hormone (ADH) is fundamental in regulating fluid volume and osmolarity. Also in the tubules, hydrogen ions are released from carbonic acid, where they combine with ammonia, produced by the tubules, to form the ammonium ion (NH_4^+). Bicarbonate ions are thus released back into the blood, maintaining the alkali reserve. Figure 10-5 shows how solutes and fluids move across membranes of the kidney tubules.

COMPOSITION OF THE URINE

The kidneys are able to excrete urine of varying specific gravity, from 1.008 to 1.035, depending on the amount of water and solutes present. About 70 gm of solids—mostly nitrogenous substances (predominantly urea), as well as some creatinine, ammonia, and uric acid—are excreted daily. Inorganic salts also present in the urine include sodium chloride and sulfate, chloride, and phos-

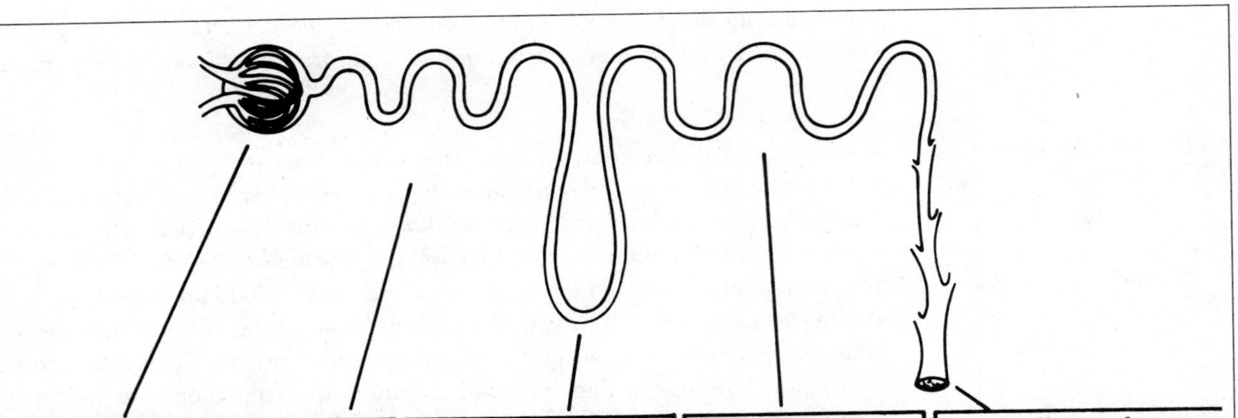

Glomerulus	Proximal tubule	Loop of Henle	Distal tubule	Collecting duct
Filtration	65% Na^+ and H_2O reabsorbed	Cl^- transport from ascending limb	Na^+, reabsorbed	Water reabsorbed in final concentrating operation
	ADH not required	Countercurrent establishes hypertonic interstitium	ADH required for H_2O reabsorption	ADH required
	All glucose, K^+, urate reabsorbed	Fluid leaves hypotonic	K^+ and urate secreted	Final adjustments in Na^+, K^+
	HCO_3^- reabsorbed		HCO_3^- reabsorbed	
	H^+ secreted		H^+ secreted	
	Fluid leaves isotonic		NH_3 secreted	
			Leaves hypotonic or isotonic	

FIG. 10-4. Major functions of each portion of the nephron (ADH = antidiuretic hormone). (From S. Papper, *Clinical Nephrology* [2nd ed.]. Boston: Little, Brown, 1978.)

phate salts of magnesium, calcium, and potassium. Normal values for 24-hour urine excretion are given in Table 10-5.

The daily obligatory fluid excretion by the kidneys is about 600 ml. With an increase in solid wastes to be excreted, such as when excess proteins from a high protein diet are deaminized, producing increased urea, the fluid needed for excretion is increased. Other situations causing increased obligatory fluid excretion include a high intake of salt and states of increased tissue catabolism (surgery, burns, fever, stress, infection).

Acid-Base Balance
DEFINITIONS

Acid-base balance reflects the hydrogen ion (H^+) concentration in the body fluids. Nutrients are transported in the blood as neutral, or near-neutral, substances. In contrast, the end products of metabolism are mostly acids, bases, and water. An *acid* is a substance that donates protons (H^+ ions), whereas a *base* accepts, or combines with, protons. A *weak acid* only slightly dissociates into H^+ and its other component; a *weak base* has only a mild affinity to combine with available H^+ ions. A *strong acid* dissociates almost completely, and a *strong base* combines readily with H^+ ions. Most of the carbon present in foods is

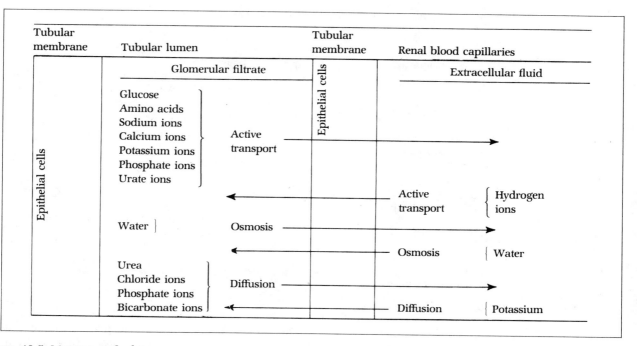

Tubular membrane	Tubular lumen		Tubular membrane	Renal blood capillaries
	Glomerular filtrate		Epithelial cells	Extracellular fluid
Epithelial cells	Glucose Amino acids Sodium ions Calcium ions Potassium ions Phosphate ions Urate ions }	Active transport →		
		←		Active transport { Hydrogen ions
	Water }	Osmosis →		
		←		Osmosis { Water
	Urea Chloride ions Phosphate ions Bicarbonate ions }	Diffusion →		
		←		Diffusion { Potassium

FIG. 10-5. Movement of solutes and fluids across membranes of the kidney tubules. (From M. Beyers and S. Dudas, *The Clinical Practice of Medical-Surgical Nursing* [2nd ed.]. Boston: Little, Brown, 1984.)

eventually oxidized to carbon dioxide and water and exists as carbonic acid (a weak acid) in solution. The sulfur in amino acids is metabolized to sulfuric acid, phospholipids and phosphoproteins to phosphoric acid, carbohydrates to lactic and pyruvic acids, lipids to keto acids, and proteins to amino acids. The metabolism of sodium and potassium results in the formation of cations of a strong base.

NEUTRALITY REGULATION   The hydrogen ion concentration (pH) of the extracellular fluid is normally maintained between 7.35 and 7.45 (a pH of 7.0 is exactly neutral). Maintenance of this narrow range is essential for normal body function and metabolism. The mechanisms that ensure strict pH regulation include *dilution*, the ability of the body fluids to *buffer* excess anions and cations, and the direct *excretion* of metabolites. Because the total volume of body fluid is so large (about 40 liters), an increase in carbon dioxide produced causes only a slight rise in the bicarbonate concentration. Thus dilution helps keep the pH constant. The second mechanism includes several substances, termed *buffers,* that combine with carbon dioxide and excessive hydrogen ions to help maintain the proper blood pH. The plasma proteins, including hemoglobin, phosphates, and carbonic acid, are important buffers. The direct excretion of metabolites is accomplished by the lungs and the kidneys. The lungs eliminate excess carbon dioxide; the kidneys, excess cations and anions.

On the basis of their influence on the pH of the urine, foods are classified as acid residue or base or alkali residue. On oxidation, meat, fish, eggs, cereal, and

TABLE 10-5. Normal values for 24-hour urine excretion

	Normal values
Calcium (usual diet)	100–250 mg
Chloride	100–250 mEq/24 hr (dependent on sodium reabsorption)
Hemoglobin and myoglobin	None
Osmolality	290 mOsm/kg water
pH	4.6–8.0 (average 6.0) (depends on diet)
Potassium	25–100 mEq/24 hr (dependent on sodium reabsorption)
Protein	
Qualitative	0
Quantitative	10–150 mg/24 hr
Sodium	80–180 mEq (varies with dietary ingestion of salt)
Glucose	0

Source: M. Beyers and S. Dudas, *The Clinical Practice of Medical-Surgical Nursing* (2nd ed.). Boston: Little, Brown, 1984.

many protein-rich foods leave an acidic residue of phosphorus, sulfur, or chlorine. The exception is milk, a protein-rich food that leaves a basic residue because of its calcium content. Most fruits and vegetables leave a basic residue rich in sodium, potassium, calcium, or magnesium. The exceptions to this rule include plums, prunes, and cranberries, owing to their large amounts of benzoic and quinic acids.

ACIDOSIS AND ALKALOSIS

An imbalance of acid and base in the body is caused by a loss or gain of acid or base. *Acidosis* is a condition caused by an increase in the hydrogen ion concentration, or a loss of base. The pH of the blood drops below 7.35. In *alkalosis*, there is an excess of base to above 7.45. *Respiratory alkalosis* or *acidosis* results from alterations in the normal pulmonary excretion of carbon dioxide. With decreased ventilation, as seen with pneumonia, lung cancer, or pulmonary edema, respiratory acidosis results. The kidneys attempt to compensate by excreting more hydrogen ions and synthesizing ammonia, which causes a return of bicarbonate (base) to the blood. With overventilation, as seen at high altitudes, with hysteria, and in fevers and infections, there is an excessive loss of carbonic acid. The kidneys respond by conserving hydrogen ions and decreasing ammonia production. *Metabolic alkalosis* or *acidosis* is caused by changes in the renal regulation of acid-base balance. Metabolic acidosis occurs with the production of ketones in uncontrolled diabetes mellitus and starvation, or the loss of bicarbonate and sodium in prolonged, acute diarrhea. The lungs attempt to compensate by increased ventilation. In metabolic alkalosis there is excessive loss of acid, as occurs with vomiting or gastric suctioning. Acid-base imbalances are summarized in Fig. 10-6.

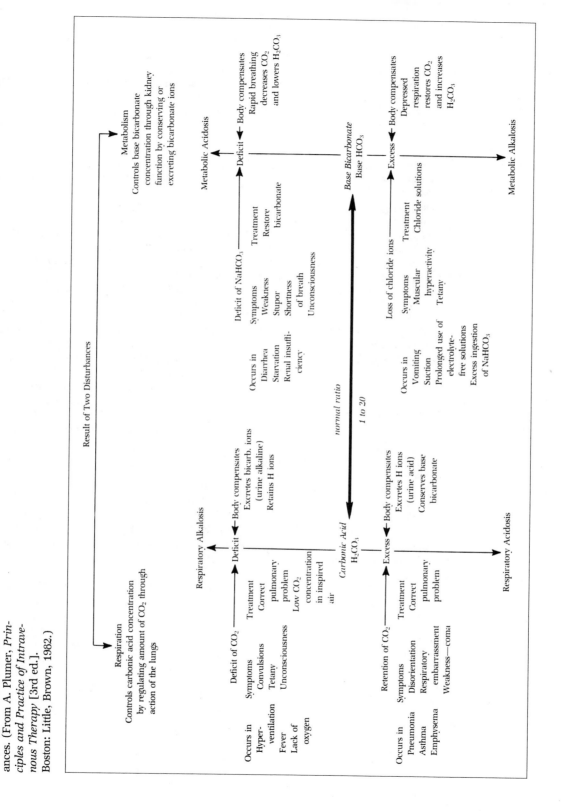

FIG. 10-6. Acid-base imbalances. (From A. Plumer, *Principles and Practice of Intravenous Therapy* [3rd ed.]. Boston: Little, Brown, 1982.)

References

1. Food and Nutrition Board, National Research Council. *Recommended Dietary Allowances* (9th ed.). Washington, D.C.: National Academy of Sciences, 1980. Pp. 170, 174.
2. Dahl, L. K. Salt and hypertension. *Am. J. Clin. Nutr.* 25:231, 1972.

Suggested Readings

A current prospective on the sodium issue. *Nutr. Policy Issues* no. 10, 1982.

Altschul, A. M., and Grommet, J. K. Sodium intake and sodium sensitivity. *Nutr. Rev.* 38:393, 1980.

Beauchamp, G. K., Bertino, M., and Moran, M. Sodium regulation: Sensory aspects. *J. Am. Dietet. Assoc.* 80:40, 1982.

Bloch, M. R. The social influence of salt. In N. Kretchmer and B. Robertson (eds.), *Human Nutrition.* San Francisco: W. H. Freeman, 1978. Pp. 120–129.

Crocco, S. C. The role of sodium in food processing. *J. Am. Dietet. Assoc.* 80:36, 1982.

Darby, W. J. Why salt? How much? *Contemp. Nutr.* June 1980.

Felver, L. Understanding the electrolyte maze. *Am. J. Nurs.* 80:1591, 1980.

Hill, M. Helping the hypertensive patient control sodium intake. *Am. J. Nurs.* 79:906, 1979.

Jacobson, M., and Liebman, B. F. Dietary sodium and the risk of hypertension. *N. Engl. J. Med.* 303:817, 1980.

Lane, H. W., et al. Effect of physical activity on human potassium metabolism in a hot and humid environment. *Am. J. Clin. Nutr.* 31:838, 1978.

Leung, H. K. Structure and properties of water. *Cereal Foods World* 26:350, 1981.

Luke, B. The clinical consequences of potassium loss. *Nurs. Drug Alert* 1:117, 1977.

McRae, M. P. Foods high in potassium. *Hosp. Pharm.* 14:730, 1979.

Shank, F. R., et al. Perspective of food and drug administration on dietary sodium. *J. Am. Dietet. Assoc.* 80:29, 1982.

Symposium on fluid, electrolyte, and acid-base balance. *Nurs. Clin. North Am.* 15:535, 1980.

The 1980 Report of the Joint National Committee on Detection, Evaluation, and Treatment of High Blood Pressure. *Arch. Intern. Med.* 140:1280, 1980.

Tuthill, R. W., and Calabrese, E. J. Drinking water, sodium and blood pressure in children: A second look. *Am. J. Public Health* 71:722, 1981.

White, P. L., and Crocco, S. C. (eds.). *Sodium and Potassium in Foods and Drugs.* Chicago: American Medical Association, 1980.

Chapter 11

PHYSIOLOGY OF THE GASTROINTESTINAL TRACT AND DIGESTION

The digestive system consists of the gastrointestinal tract and its associated glands. Its purpose is to obtain nutrients from ingested food for growth and maintenance of the body. *Digestion* is the process by which foods are broken down, both mechanically and chemically, into smaller molecules for assimilation (absorption) via the gastrointestinal tract. The physical, mechanical breakdown starts in the mouth, with the grinding of food by the teeth. This process is continued by the circular rings of muscle throughout the gastrointestinal tract, which subdivide and propel each bolus of food along.

The chemical breakdown of food is accomplished by a variety of specialized enzymes, digestive juices, and pancreatic, biliary, and hepatic secretions. The enzymes catalyze the hydrolysis of dietary proteins to amino acids, complex polysaccharides to monosaccharides, and lipids to monoacylglycerols, glycerol, and fatty acids. The chemical breakdown and absorption of nutrients occur mainly in the small intestine. In the large intestine mainly water is absorbed, making the remaining semisolid undigested contents more solid. William Beaumont, the famous American physician, was one of the first to describe gastric physiology in detail by his observations on Alexis St. Martin, a Canadian who had sustained a permanent gastric fistula (opening) as a result of a gunshot wound.

The physiology of the gastrointestinal tract and digestion is presented in this chapter. Refer to Fig. 11-1 as each stage in the digestive process is discussed. The absorption of proteins, carbohydrates, and lipids is discussed in detail in Chaps. 3, 4, and 5.

The Mouth and Esophagus

In the mouth, food undergoes several changes that prepare it for further digestion. Food is coarsely broken down to finer particles by the grinding and tearing action of the teeth. This first step can be inadequately or incompletely accomplished if the teeth are decayed or missing or if the soft structures of the mouth (gums, tongue, palate) are inflamed. At the same time, the food is moistened with *saliva*, which serves several purposes. Saliva has a physical function, lubricating food to facilitate swallowing. It also has a chemical function, since it contains the starch-splitting enzyme *ptyalin*, which hydrolyzes starch into dextrins and maltose.

The gastrointestinal tract is the body's first and major defense mechanism against foodborne infection. In the mouth, lymph follicles and the lingual tonsils on the surface of the tongue, as well as the palatine and pharyngeal tonsils in the pharynx, provide lymphatic defense against microorganisms.

SALIVARY DIGESTION

Saliva consists of about 99.5% water. About 1500 ml of it is secreted daily by three pairs of salivary glands in the oral cavity: parotid, submaxillary, and

FIG. 11-1. The gastrointestinal system. (From E. Selkurt [ed.], *Basic Physiology for the Health Sciences.* Boston: Little, Brown, 1975.)

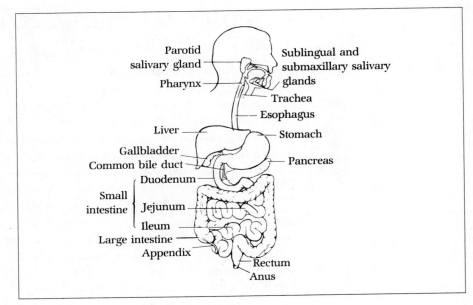

sublingual (Fig. 11-2A). In addition to acting as a lubricant, saliva is also a vehicle for the excretion of certain drugs, such as alcohol and morphine, and some inorganic ions, including iodine, calcium, bicarbonate, and potassium. Saliva is usually slightly acidic, with a pH of about 6.8, although it may vary on either side of neutrality. The enzyme ptyalin (also termed *salivary amylase*) can function only in a neutral or alkaline environment; it is inactivated by the acid pH of the stomach. Because food remains in the mouth for a relatively brief time, ptyalin contributes little to overall digestion. This enzyme is completely absent in some animal species.

Another enzyme also present in the mouth is *pharyngeal lipase,* which hydrolyzes triacylglycerols into free fatty acids, monoacylglycerols, and diacylglycerols. Its action begins in the throat and continues in the esophagus and stomach.

TASTE BUDS

While in the mouth, food comes in contact with the end organs for the sense of taste. The *taste buds* are located on papillae, or elevations, on the tongue and other parts of the oral cavity. There are three types of papillae on the tongue: fungiform, foliate, and circumvallate (Fig. 11-2B). Numerous mucous and serous glands provide a continuous flow of fluid over the taste buds so that new gustatory stimuli can be received and processed. Combined with the sense of smell, the sense of taste serves as a psychological stimulus for continued food intake and for stimulating the flow of gastric juices. The sensation of thirst is initiated by the drying of the mucous membranes of the mouth, and acts as a protective mechanism against dehydration.

FIG. 11-2.
A. Salivary system. (From R. D. Judge, G. D. Zuidema, and F. T. Fitzgerald, *Clinical Diagnosis*. Boston: Little, Brown, 1982.)
B. Distribution of gustatory papillae (taste buds) on the tongue.

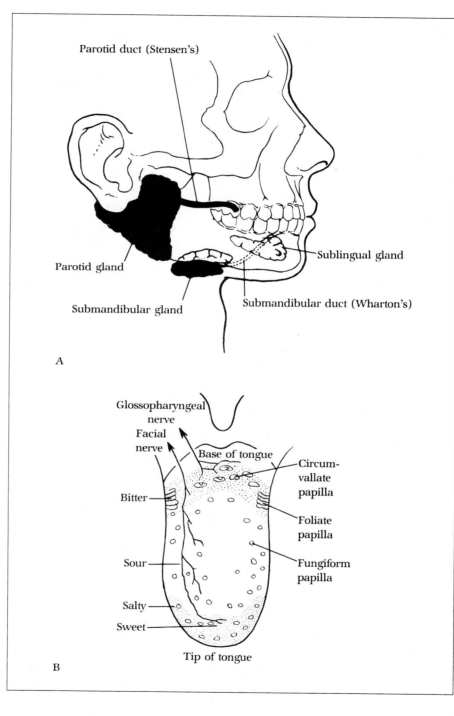

FIG. 11-3. Passage of a food bolus from the mouth through the pharynx and upper esophagus during a swallow. (From E. Selkurt [ed.], *Basic Physiology for the Health Sciences.* Boston: Little, Brown, 1975.)

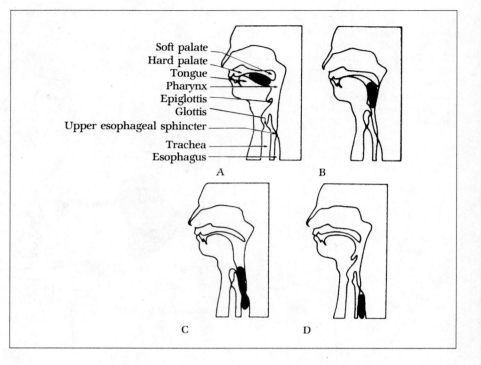

Soft palate
Hard palate
Tongue
Pharynx
Epiglottis
Glottis
Upper esophageal sphincter
Trachea
Esophagus

A   B   C   D

DEGLUTITION (SWALLOWING)

After the food has been completely masticated, reflex swallowing contractions propel each bolus of food from the back of the tongue downward through the pharynx into the upper part of the esophagus. At this point a peristaltic muscle wave moves it to the distal (lower) end of the esophagus, where the entrance to the stomach is guarded by the *cardiac sphincter,* a circular ring of muscle. The sphincter may open with the next peristaltic wave to permit the bolus of food to enter the stomach or wait to accumulate amounts from two waves (Fig. 11-3).

The esophagus is essentially a muscular tube whose function is to transport food from the mouth to the stomach. Mucus-secreting glands in the esophagus help to lubricate the food as it passes into the stomach. The cells lining the esophagus and the rest of the gastrointestinal tract are renewed every 3 to 5 days, which explains why this tract is so quickly affected by antimitotic drugs (those that interfere with cell division), such as anticancer drugs.

The Stomach
GASTRIC PHYSIOLOGY

This dilated segment of the gastrointestinal tract is divided into three sections: the upper *cardiac,* or *fundus, portion;* the large main body, the *body;* and the lower outlet, the *pylorus,* or *antrum* (Fig. 11-4A). The body is the site where the major portion of the gastric juices are secreted and most of gastric digestion occurs. The semisolid food that first enters the stomach spreads out to the periphery. Food eaten later remains in the center of the mass and continues to have a neutral pH;

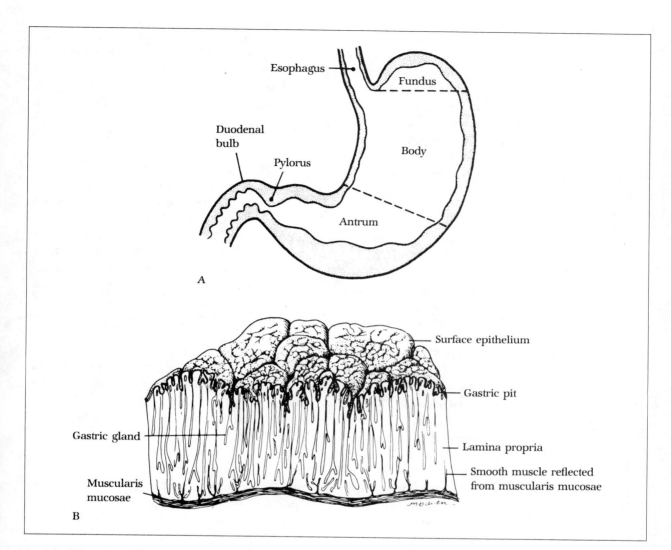

FIG. 11-4. Anatomy of the stomach.
A. Parts of the stomach. (From E. Selkurt [ed.], *Basic Physiology for the Health Sciences* [2nd ed.]. Boston: Little, Brown, 1982.)
B. The topography of the stomach lining and the appearance of the gastric mucosa when viewed in cross section at very low magnification. (From M. Borysenko, et al., *Functional Histology* [2nd ed.]. Boston: Little, Brown, 1984.)

there salivary digestion proceeds for 30 minutes or more. Gastric digestion begins in the outer layers (the food eaten first). Acidic gastric juices penetrate the food bolus, which is broken up by peristaltic waves originating at about the middle of the stomach and moving the food to the duodenum. As digestion progresses, the contractions increase in strength and depth.

The *pyloric sphincter*, a circular ring of muscle located at the lower outlet of the stomach, contracts with the approach of a peristaltic wave. After three or four waves, the sphincter opens to permit the *chyme*, the liquefied acid food mass, to pass into the duodenum. The pyloric sphincter serves two important purposes: First, it remains shut to allow the proximal part of the duodenum to change from an acid to a neutral pH. Second, it prevents the backflow (*regurgitation*) of the duodenal contents into the stomach.

The rate of gastric (and intestinal) digestion and secretions is influenced by the nature of the meal and by emotional states. Liquids pass through the stomach very quickly, but solids usually take 3½ to 4 hours. Fats have an inhibitory effect on gastric motility, proteins pass through faster, and carbohydrates faster still. Anxiety, excitement, fear, and depression can slow gastric motility, whereas anger and hostility can increase it. This is due to the gut's innervation by the autonomic nervous system, which is located between the muscle layers.

GASTRIC DIGESTION

The main function of the stomach is to initiate protein digestion as well as to add fluid to the ingested food. The cardiac portion of the stomach, located at the transition between the esophagus and the stomach, contains secretory glands that produce mucus and the enzyme *lysozyme*, which digests the cell walls of certain bacteria, thereby controlling the gastric flora. The body and fundus of the stomach contain gastric glands that secrete mucus, digestive enzymes, and hydrochloric acid (Fig. 11-4B). The neutral mucus secreted by the gastric mucosa serves several functions: It acts as a mechanical lubricant for the food bolus and protects the gastric mucosa against the acid digestive juices by its buffering effect. The pylorus contains pyloric glands, which also secrete the enzyme lysozyme and a hormone, *gastrin*.

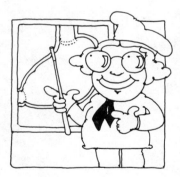

The initiation of gastric secretion is triggered by nervous or reflex mechanisms. Continued secretion is maintained by gastrin. Gastric juice consists of 97 to 99% water, plus the secretions of two specialized types of cells in the mucosa of the stomach wall. The *parietal cells* are the sole source of hydrochloric acid in the stomach, which maintains the optimum pH of about 1.5 (Fig. 11-5). Histamine, secreted by the gastric mucosa, and gastrin stimulate the production of hydrochloric acid. The acid environment of the stomach inhibits or destroys many microorganisms normally present in foods, as part of the body's defense mechanism against foodborne infection. Lymph nodes beneath the intestinal mucosa of the ileum, known as *Peyer's patches*, also protect against bacterial invasion. The parietal cells are also the site of production of *intrinsic factor*, a glycoprotein that binds to vitamin B_{12} and is required for its absorption by the ileum.

The principal digestive action in the stomach, the hydrolysis of proteins, can occur only in an acid environment. *Pepsinogen*, the inactive precursor (zymogen) of the proteolytic enzyme *pepsin*, is formed and secreted by the *chief cells*, the second type of specialized cells present in the gastric mucosa. This zymogen is converted to the active version of the enzyme by the acidity of the gastric juice and by pepsin itself (autocatalytic). Because food remains in the stomach for a relatively brief period, dietary proteins are here broken down only to a mixture of polypeptides. *Gastric lipase*, also produced by the chief cells, exerts a lipolytic effect, hydrolyzing triacylglycerols to short-chain and medium-chain fatty acids.

The Small Intestine

After the chyme has passed through the pylorus, the pancreatic and biliary secretions change the pH of the food mass to alkaline, which is necessary for the

FIG. **11-5.** A possible mechanism for the gastric secretion of HCl. (From E. Selkurt [ed.], *Basic Physiology for the Health Sciences.* Boston: Little, Brown, 1975.)

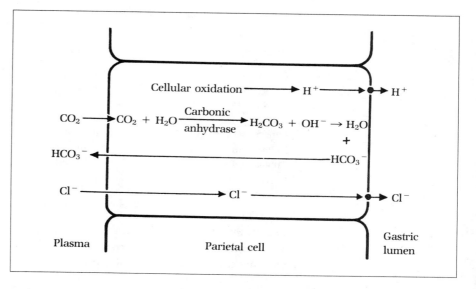

action of the enzymes contained within the intestinal and pancreatic juices. The long length of the small intestine, about 6 meters, permits prolonged contact between digestive enzymes and the food mass; therefore the majority of digestion and absorption occurs in this part of the gastrointestinal tract. The small intestine consists of three parts: the duodenum, the jejunum, and the ileum (see Fig. 11-1). Peristaltic movements continue to propel the chyme through the digestive tract.

The digestive secretions in the intestine come from the pancreas, the liver, and the glands of the intestinal mucosa (also called crypts or glands of Lieberkühn). The secretion of pancreatic digestive juices is under hormonal control and is triggered by the presence of food in the duodenum. The passage of the acidic chyme through the pyloric sphincter causes the production of *secretin, pancreozymin, hepatocrinin, cholecystokinin,* and *enterocrinin* by the duodenum. These hormones are secreted into the blood where they are carried to the pancreas, liver, and gallbladder. Secretin stimulates the pancreas to secrete a pancreatic juice rich in bicarbonate (alkaline) but low in enzymes. Pancreozymin also stimulates the pancreas but to secrete a fluid low in bicarbonate and rich in enzymes. Hepatocrinin stimulates the secretion of bile by the liver, and the contraction and emptying of the gallbladder is caused by the hormonal stimulation of cholecystokinin. Enterocrinin induces the flow of intestinal juice. The duodenal (or Brunner's) glands secrete an alkaline fluid that protects the duodenal mucous membrane from the effects of the acidic chyme and changes the intestinal contents to alkaline for optimum action of the pancreatic enzymes. A summary of the hormones controlling digestion is given in Table 11-1.

PANCREATIC SECRETIONS

Pancreatic juice has a water content similar to that of saliva, contains a number of organic and inorganic compounds, and has an alkaline pH of 7.5 to 8.0 or

TABLE 11-1. Hormonal control of digestion

Hormone	Target organ or compound	Effect
Gastrin	Stomach	Gastric secretions
Enterokinase (enteropeptidase)	Trypsinogen	Trypsin
Secretin	Pancreas	Pancreatic juice
Pancreozymin	Pancreas	Pancreatic enzymes
Enterocrinin	Small intestine	Intestinal juice
Cholecystokinin	Gallbladder	Bile release
Hepatocrinin	Liver	Bile secretion

higher. Since the majority of absorption and enzymatic digestion occurs in the small intestine, pancreatic juice is also rich in a variety of enzymes. Some of these enzymes are secreted as inactive precursors, or zymogens, such as trypsinogen and chymotrypsinogen, to be activated by factors and conditions in the small intestine.

The proteolytic (protein-splitting) enzymes found in pancreatic juice include *trypsin, chymotrypsin, carboxypeptidase A and B, ribonuclease,* and *deoxyribonuclease.* Trypsin attacks only specific linkages in the interior of the polypeptide chain, next to lysine or arginine residues. Secreted as the inactive precursor trypsinogen, it is converted into the active enzyme trypsin by the presence of enterokinase (also called enteropeptidase), which is secreted by the duodenal mucosa. Trypsin, in turn, converts the inactive zymogens chymotrypsinogen and procarboxypeptidase into the active enzymes chymotrypsin and carboxypeptidase, respectively. Chymotrypsin, like trypsin, attacks specific linkages in the interior of the polypeptide chain, those adjacent to methionine, tyrosine, tryptophan, or phenylalanine. Carboxypeptidase A and B, zinc-containing enzymes, split polypeptides into smaller peptides and amino acids by attacking the linkage next to the terminal amino acid containing a free carboxyl group. Ribonuclease and deoxyribonuclease split, respectively, ribonucleic and deoxyribonucleic acids into nucleotides.

The carbohydrate-splitting enzyme *pancreatic amylase* (also termed amylopsin), is similar in action to ptyalin (salivary amylase). It hydrolyzes starch to dextrins and maltose. The lipolytic (lipid-splitting) enzymes present in pancreatic juice include *pancreatic lipase, pancreatic esterase,* and *phospholipase A.* Pancreatic lipase hydrolyzes triacylglycerols to monoacylglycerols and fatty acids. Pancreatic esterase cleaves cholesterol esters to cholesterol. Phospholipase A, also activated by trypsin, hydrolyzes phospholipids from glycerophospholipids. This enzyme also hydrolyzes fatty acids off lecithin, forming lysolecithin. In acute pancreatitis, phospholipase may be activated within the pancreatic ducts (the pancreatic tissue itself), causing the destruction of pancreatic tissue and surrounding fat.

INTESTINAL SECRETIONS

The glands of Brunner and of Lieberkühn of the intestinal mucosa secrete an alkaline, enzyme-rich juice, or *succus entericus.* The secretion is under both mechanical and hormonal control. Stimulation of the walls of the intestine induces active secretion of intestinal juice, and the presence of acid chyme in the intestine causes the secretion of the hormone *enterocrinin* by the intestinal mucosa, which, in turn, directly activates the cells of the intestinal glands.

The digestive enzymes present in the intestinal juice include *peptidases* (aminopeptidases and dipeptidases), *phosphatases,* and *carbohydrases* (sucrase, maltase, and lactase). The peptidases are proteolytic enzymes that hydrolyze polypeptides into smaller peptides and amino acids. Aminopeptidase attacks the terminal peptide bond at the free amino acid end of the chain. Dipeptidase splits dipeptides into free amino acids. Phosphatases are enzymes that split phosphorylated compounds into inorganic phosphate and the organic component. The carbohydrases include the specific disaccharidases sucrase, maltase, and lactase, which hydrolyze sucrose, maltose, and lactose, respectively, into the monosaccharides glucose, fructose, and galactose.

FIG. 11-6. Left: A section of the small intestine showing two microvilli and two crypts. Right: Cross sections through a villus and a crypt of Lieberkühn. (From M. Borysenko, et al., *Functional Histology* (2nd ed.). Boston: Little, Brown, 1984.)

Specialized absorptive cells, containing a surface termed the *striated* or *brush border,* are important for the absorption of the metabolites that result from the digestive process. The brush border is composed of a layer of densely grouped microvilli, which increase the surface area of contact of the intestines with food (Fig. 11-6). The brush border is also the site of activity of the disaccharidases.

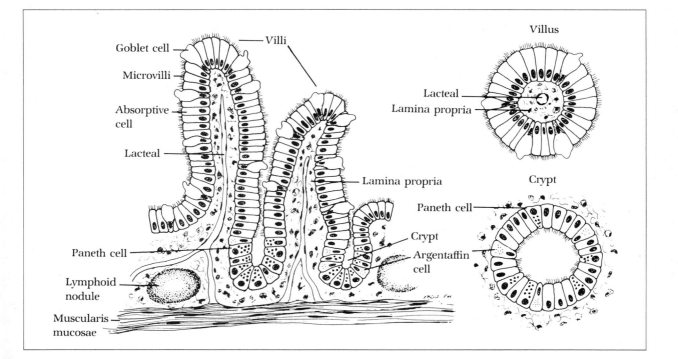

TABLE 11-2. Summary of the digestive process

Enzyme	Source of secretion and stimulus for secretion	Method of activation and optimal conditions for activity	Substrate	End products or action
Salivary amylase (ptyalin)	Salivary glands of mouth: Secrete saliva in reflex response to presence of food in mouth	Chloride ion necessary pH 6.6–6.8	Starch Glycogen	Maltose plus 1,6-glucosides (oligosaccharides) plus maltotriose
Pepsin	Stomach glands: Chief cells and parietal cells secrete gastric juice in response to reflex stimulation and chemical action of gastrin	Pepsinogen converted to active pepsin by HCl pH 1.0–2.0	Protein	Proteoses Peptones
Rennin		Calcium necessary for activity pH 4.0	Casein of milk	Coagulates milk
Trypsin	Pancreas: Presence of acid chyme from the stomach activates duodenum to produce secretin, which hormonally stimulates flow of pancreatic juice, and pancreozymin, which stimulates the production of enzymes	Trypsinogen converted to active trypsin by enterokinase of intestine at pH 5.2–6.0; autocatalytic at pH 7.9	Protein Proteoses Peptones	Polypeptides Dipeptides
Chymotrypsin		Secreted as chymotrypsinogen and converted to active form by trypsin pH 8.0	Protein Proteoses Peptones	Same as trypsin; more coagulating power for milk
Carboxypeptidase		Secreted as procarboxypeptidase, activated by trypsin	Polypeptides at the free carboxyl end of the chain	Lower peptides, free amino acids
Pancreatic amylase		pH 7.1	Starch Glycogen	Maltose plus 1,6-glucosides (oligosaccharides) plus maltotriose
Lipase		Activated by bile salts? pH 8.0	Primary ester linkages of fats	Fatty acids, monoacylglycerols, diacylglycerols, glycerol
Ribonuclease			Ribonucleic acid	Nucleotides

Source	Enzyme	Activators and/or optimum	Substrate	Products
	Deoxyribonuclease		Deoxyribonucleic acids	Nucleotides
	Pancreatic esterase	Activated by bile salts	Cholesterol esters	Free cholesterol plus fatty acids
	Phospholipase A		Phospholipids	Fatty acids, lysophospholipids
Liver and gallbladder	Bile salts and alkali	Cholecystokinin (a hormone from the intestinal mucosa) and possibly also gastrin and secretin stimulate the gallbladder and secretion of bile by the liver	Fats	Fatty acid–bile conjugates and finely emulsified neutral fat–bile salt micelles; Neutralize acid chyme
Small intestine: Secretions of Brunner's glands of the duodenum and glands of Lieberkühn	Aminopeptidase		Polypeptides at the free amino end of the chain	Lower peptides, free amino acids
	Dipeptidases		Dipeptides	Amino acids
	Sucrase	pH 5.0–7.0	Sucrose	Fructose, glucose
	Maltase	pH 5.8–6.2	Maltose	Glucose
	Lactase	pH 5.4–6.0	Lactose	Glucose, galactose
	Phosphatase	pH 8.6	Organic phosphates	Free phosphate
	Isomaltase or 1,6-glucosidase		1,6-glucosides	Glucose
	Polynucleotidase		Nucleic acid	Nucleotides
	Nucleosidases		Purine or pyrimidine nucleosides	Purine or pyrimidine bases, pentose phosphate

Source: P. A. Mayes, Digestion and Absorption from the Gastrointestinal Tract. In H. A. Harper, V. W. Rodwell, and P. A. Mayes (eds.), *Review of Physiological Chemistry* (17th ed.). Los Altos, Calif.: Lange, 1979. P. 247.

Between the absorptive cells are interspersed *goblet cells*, which produce acid glycoproteins to protect and lubricate the lining of the intestine. *Argentaffin cells*, present both in the stomach and intestines, secrete *5-hydroxytryptamine* (serotonin), which stimulates the smooth muscle layer of the gastrointestinal tract, increasing motility. A summary of the principal digestive enzymes is given in Table 11-2.

HEPATIC SECRETIONS

The liver has a central role in digestion and absorption, as well as in a wide variety of other complex functions. As the largest gland in the body, the liver is involved in carbohydrate metabolism (storage, ketone formation), protein metabolism (hormone production, amino acid breakdown), detoxification of drugs and toxins, and lipid metabolism, including the formation of bile. The liver's role in carbohydrate, protein, and lipid metabolism is discussed in detail in Chaps. 3, 4, and 5; only its function in producing bile is presented here.

Bile, composed of lecithin, cholesterol, bile acids, and bile pigments, is formed by hepatic cells and transported, via the hepatic duct, to the gallbladder, where it is stored between meals. In the gallbladder, the dilute biliary secretion is concentrated by the reabsorption of water. As mentioned above, the presence of food, especially fats, in the small intestine stimulates the production of the hormone *hepatocrinin* by the intestinal mucosa. This hormone in turn stimulates the secretion of bile by the liver. Another hormone, *cholecystokinin,* is also stimulated, causing contractions of the gallbladder and release of concentrated bile into the duodenum via the common (bile) duct. Pancreatic juices also mix with the bile, since they also enter into the duodenum via the common duct.

About 200 to 500 mg of bile acids is synthesized each day to replace daily losses in the feces. The daily output of bile is considered to be an accurate measure of the amount of cholesterol lost from the body, since it is the only important route of elimination from the body for this substance, and bile acids are considered to be the end products of cholesterol metabolism. Because cholesterol is insoluble in water, it must be incorporated into a lecithin-bile micelle (water-soluble complexes) (see Chap. 5 for details) for its elimination. When the concentration of cholesterol becomes too great, the excess precipitates as crystals, which then grow to form *gallstones.*

The primary bile acids found in bile include *cholic acid* (50 percent of total) and *chenodeoxycholic acid* (30 percent of total). Both are formed from a common precursor, which is derived from cholesterol. The action of intestinal bacteria (deconjugation and dehydroxylation) produces the secondary bile acids, *deoxycholic acid* (15 percent of total) from cholic acid, and *lithocholic acid* (5 percent of total) from chenodeoxycholic acid. Conjugation of the bile acids occurs in the liver, forming *glycocholic* and *taurocholic* acids. With the exception of lithocholic acid, which is insoluble, between 90 and 95 percent of the bile acids is reabsorbed in the ileum by an active transport process and then excreted again by the liver (the *enterohepatic circulation*) (Fig. 11-7). It has been estimated that the total bile pool of about 3.5 gm recycles twice per meal and 6 to 10 times per day via the enterohepatic circulation. The remaining 5 to 10 percent of the bile acids is unabsorbed and is eliminated in the feces. This small fraction is the major pathway for the elimination of cholesterol from the body. Each day the bile acid equivalent to that lost in the feces is produced from cholesterol by the liver so that the size of the bile acid pool remains constant.

Bile is needed for the emulsification of fats and their subsequent absorption. Without bile, as much as 25 percent of ingested fat would appear in the feces (*steatorrhea*); severe malabsorption of the fat-soluble vitamins would also result. Bile acids lower the surface tension of large fat globules and, in combination with the churning action of the small intestine, aid in their breakdown into progressively smaller globules. This breakdown creates a greater surface area for the action of the lipases. The absorption of partially hydrolyzed fat (monoacylglycerols and diacylglycerols), free fatty acids, and fat-soluble vitamins is dependent on the presence of bile acids. Bile emulsifies lipids, forming micelles from which lipids can be more easily absorbed. Bile has several other functions, including activating intestinal lipase and, since it is alkaline, helping to neutralize the acidic chyme from the stomach. Bile also acts as a vehicle of excretion, removing many drugs, toxins, and inorganic substances, such as mercury, zinc, and copper, from the body. The bile pigments *bilirubin* and *biliverdin* are breakdown products of hemoglobin and do not play a part in the digestive process. Bile provides a pathway for the excretion of these pigments.

The Large Intestine

The main functions of the large intestine include water absorption and production of mucus for lubrication. This latter function is accomplished by the mucus-secreting *goblet cells* located in the glands of Lieberkühn. As the terminal reservoir of the gastrointestinal tract, the large intestine absorbs the remaining digested food and actively reabsorbs excess fluid, making the semisolid intestinal contents more solid. In the large intestine bacteria degrade some materials resistant to previous digestion.

INTESTINAL FLORA

The gastrointestinal tract, sterile at birth, soon changes as a microbial population is established. In the breast-fed infant, *Lactobacillus bifidus* predominates; in the infant fed cow's milk formula, *L. acidophilus*. With the introduction of a more varied diet, the majority of organisms are from the genera *Diplococcus*, *Lactobacillus*, and *Streptococcus*. Other organisms present include *Escherichia coli* and *Bacillus subtilis*. A high carbohydrate diet increases the number of gram-positive, fermentative organisms; a high protein diet promotes the growth of gram-negative, putrefactive flora.

Bacterial fermentation and putrefaction produce a variety of gases (carbon dioxide, methane, hydrogen sulfide, nitrogen, and hydrogen) as well as lactic, acetic, and butyric acids. Intestinal bacteria may also decarboxylate (remove

FIG. 11-7. The enterohepatic circulation of bile salts as shown by the heavy solid arrows. The dashed arrow represents inhibition of bile salt synthesis. (From E. Selkurt [ed.], *Basic Physiology for the Health Sciences* [2nd ed.]. Boston: Little, Brown, 1982.)

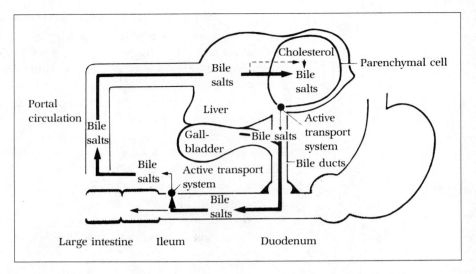

COO— from) many amino acids, producing toxic amines or other products (Table 11-3). The action of intestinal bacteria on nitrogenous substances can also produce considerable quantities of ammonia. Normally, this substance is absorbed and rapidly removed from the blood by the liver, but toxic levels may accumulate if hepatic function is impaired. High protein diets should therefore be used with caution in patients with severe liver disease, as they may lead to the development of ammonia intoxication.

In herbivores such as cows, the intestinal or ruminal bacteria permit the degradation and subsequent absorption of the polysaccharide cellulose, an indigestible component of the human diet. In addition, these bacteria may synthesize certain essential amino acids and vitamins. In humans, the intestinal flora does not have as much nutritional influence, although it does synthesize some vitamins, particularly vitamin K and possibly some B vitamins. Between one-fourth and one-third of human feces is composed of bacteria from the large intestine; the remainder includes material desquamated into the gastrointestinal tract, intestinal secretions, and unabsorbed food residues (fiber).

TABLE 11-3. Products of decarboxylation reactions by intestinal bacteria

Amino acid	Toxic amine or product
Lysine	Cadaverine
Arginine	Agmatine
Tyrosine	Tyramine
Ornithine	Putrescine
Histidine	Histamine
Tryptophan	Indole, skatole
Cysteine	Ethylmercaptan, methylmercaptan

Digestion involves the coordinated and rhythmic breakdown and absorption of a wide variety of foodstuffs. The activation and inactivation of enzymes and digestive juices, the changing pH, and the timed, self-protective measures to ensure the integrity of the lining of the gastrointestinal tract are all the end product of millions of years of evolution, resulting in the digestive process as it is known today. This chapter presented digestion as it normally occurs; in future chapters the influence of illness and disease on gastrointestinal functions will be explored.

Suggested Readings

Danielsson, H., and Sjövall, J.   Bile acid metabolism. *Annu. Rev. Biochem.* 44:233, 1975.

Davenport, H. W.   *A Digest of Digestion* (2nd ed.). Chicago: Year Book, 1978.

Davenport, H. W.   *Physiology of the Digestive Tract* (4th ed.). Chicago: Year Book, 1977.

Davenport, H. W.   Why the stomach does not digest itself. *Sci. Am.* 226:86, 1972.

Forker, E. L.   Mechanisms of hepatic bile formation. *Annu. Rev. Physiol.* 39:323, 1977.

Harvey, R. F.   Hormonal control of gastrointestinal motility. *Am. J. Dig. Dis.* 20:523, 1975.

Johnson, L. R. (ed.).   *Gastrointestinal Physiology.* St. Louis: Mosby, 1977.

Phillips, S. F., and Stephen, A. M.   The structure and function of the large intestine. *Nutr. Today* 16:4, 1981.

Schmid, R.   Bilirubin metabolism in man. *N. Engl. J. Med.* 287:703, 1972.

Walsh, J. H., and Grossman, M. I.   Gastrin. *N. Engl. J. Med.* 292:1324, 1975.

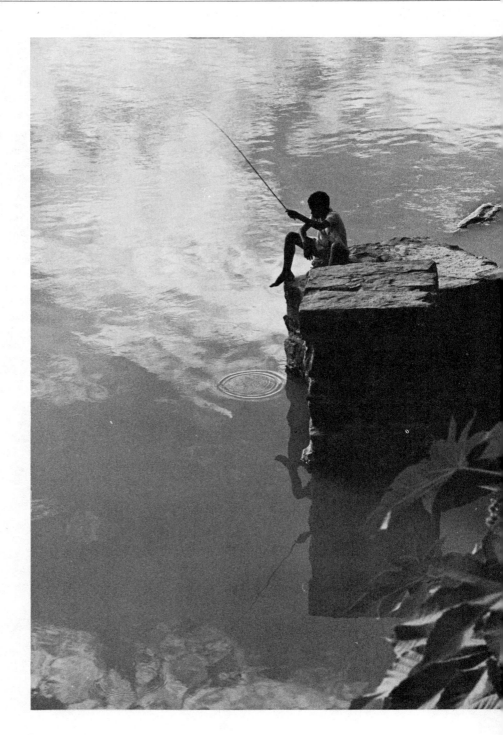

THE NATURE OF FOODS

It is important to have a sound knowledge of the nutritive value and nutrient availability of foods to effectively translate dietary recommendations and prescriptions into practical, useful information. In the following six chapters, the basic composition, structure, and nutritional value of the major food groups will be discussed. Since the nutrient content of foods is so dramatically affected by processing, cooking, and storage conditions, these elements of the food production process will also be considered.

Chapter 12

CEREALS AND CEREAL PRODUCTS

Grasses grown for their edible seeds are known as *cereal grains*. For at least 7000 years, cereal grains have provided the agricultural basis for civilization [1]. The special suitability of grain as a food staple stems from its structure: It contains both the embryo of a new plant and a food supply to nourish it. Like milk and eggs, cereal grains are part of a class of foods designed by nature for the nutrition of the young of the species [1]. These foods contain proteins, fats, carbohydrates, vitamins, and minerals—and come closer to providing an adequate diet than any other single group of foods. In addition to their high food value, cereal grains are also unique in their resistance to deterioration during storage. Cereal grains provide the cheapest source of food energy and constitute a large proportion of the world's calorie and protein intake. They remain at such a low cost because they can be grown in a variety of climates and soils, stored compactly, and transported long distances with little spoilage.

Structure and Composition

The cereal kernel is divided into three distinct portions: the pericarp, or bran layer; the endosperm, or inner portion; and the germ layer, which contains the embryo from which new grain develops (Fig. 12-1).

The *bran layer*, which comprises about 14 percent of the cereal kernel, contains mostly cellulose and some protein and minerals. This layer has three parts: an outer pericarp or epidermis; an inner pericarp; and a thin seed coat fused to the pericarp called the endocarp.

The *endosperm*, which makes up about 83 percent of the cereal kernel, is composed of starch granules embedded in a matrix (framework) of protein. The milling process separates the endosperm from the bran and germ layers. This is possible because the endosperm is more easily crushed than the other two layers. Free bran and germ are removed for other uses, including animal feed. The *aleurone* is an outer row of thick-walled cells of the endosperm, which is removed with the bran during the milling process. This layer does not contain any starch or gluten protein but does have a food reserve of oil and nongluten protein.

The *germ layer* is the richest part of the grain, but it is also the most unstable. Comprising about 3 percent of the cereal kernel, it is high in protein, sugar (mostly sucrose), minerals, and fats. Because of its high fat content, the germ layer is particularly susceptible to deterioration during storage. For this reason, the germ layer is usually removed during milling and sold separately. The germ layer is composed of two parts: the embryonic axis, which develops into the seedling; and the scutellum, which contains most of the thiamin of the kernel.

The milling of cereal grains, particularly wheat, produces several types of flour of varying protein content. Freshly milled flour, if permitted to age over a period of weeks or months, will improve in baking quality. To accelerate the maturing or aging process, chemical treatment is used after milling. Natural bleaching also accompanies aging, and this effect can also be duplicated and accelerated

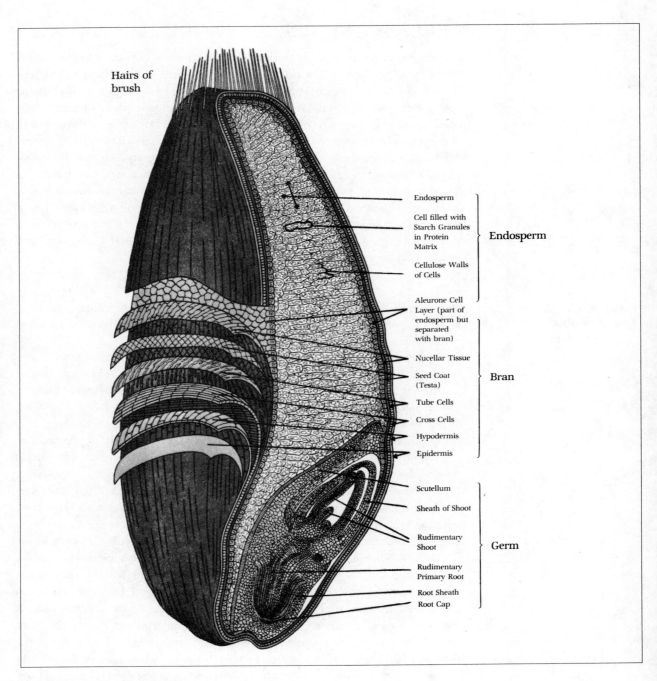

Hairs of brush

Endosperm

Cell filled with Starch Granules in Protein Matrix

Cellulose Walls of Cells

Endosperm

Aleurone Cell Layer (part of endosperm but separated with bran)

Nucellar Tissue

Seed Coat (Testa)

Tube Cells

Cross Cells

Hypodermis

Epidermis

Bran

Scutellum

Sheath of Shoot

Rudimentary Shoot

Rudimentary Primary Root

Root Sheath

Root Cap

Germ

FIG. 12-1. Structure of a kernel of wheat. (Courtesy Wheat Flour Institute and Kansas Wheat Commission.)

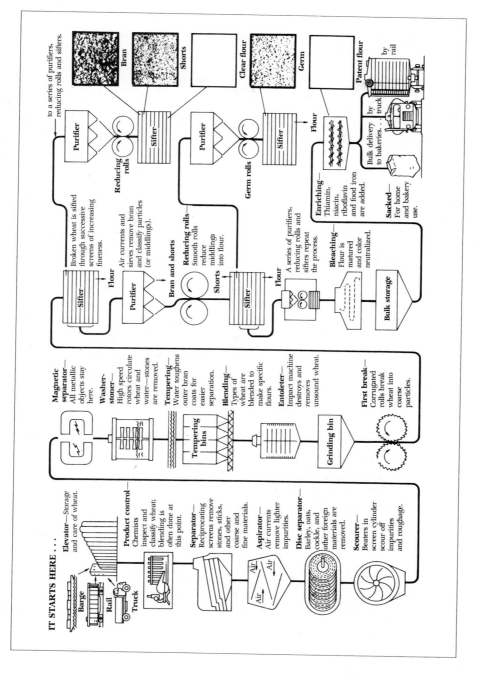

FIG. 12-2. The process of making flour. (Courtesy Wheat Flour Institute.)

IT STARTS HERE . . .

Elevator—Storage and care of wheat.

Product control—Chemists inspect and classify wheat; blending is often done at this point.

Separator—Reciprocating screens remove stones, sticks, and other coarse and fine materials.

Aspirator—Air currents remove lighter impurities.

Disc separator—Barley, oats, cockle, and other foreign materials are removed.

Scourer—Beaters in screen cylinder scour off impurities and roughage.

Magnetic separator—All metallic objects stay here.

Washer-stoner—High speed rotors circulate wheat and water—stones are removed.

Tempering—Water toughens outer bran coats for easier separation.

Blending—Types of wheat are blended to make specific flours.

Entoleter—Impact machine destroys and removes unsound wheat.

First break—Corrugated rolls break wheat into coarse particles.

Broken wheat is sifted through successive screens of increasing fineness.

Air currents and sieves remove bran and classify particles (or middlings).

Reducing rolls—Smooth rolls reduce middlings into flour.

A series of purifiers, reducing rolls and sifters repeat the process.

Bleaching—Flour is matured and color neutralized.

Bran and shorts

Shorts

to a series of purifiers, reducing rolls and sifters.

Bran

Shorts

Clear flour

Germ

Patent flour

Enriching—Thiamin, niacin, riboflavin and food iron are added.

Sacked—For home and bakery use.

Bulk delivery to bakeries . . .

by truck

by rail

215

by the use of chemicals. Gamma radiation is also used to eliminate insect infestation of wheat and flour. The total process of making flour is outlined in Fig. 12-2.

Nutritive Value
PROTEIN

Cereal grains provide incomplete proteins lacking in the essential amino acids lysine, threonine, or tryptophan. Combining grains with a complete protein such as milk helps bolster the protein content of the entire meal. The protein content, and therefore the baking quality, is affected by the fertility of the soil and by climatic factors, including temperature, rainfall, and sunlight. Soil fertility influences the amount of nitrogen available to the plant and therefore to the cereal grain. Excessive rainfall may cause leaching of nitrogen from the soil and a consequent decrease in the grain protein content.

Several different types of protein are found in cereal grains. *Albumins* are soluble proteins found in wheat and account for 6 to 12 percent of the total flour protein. They are high in tryptophan and contribute to the baking quality of flour through their pentosan content. *Globulins* are also soluble proteins and account for 5 to 12 percent of the total flour protein. Globulins are high in arginine and low in tryptophan.

Gliadin and *glutenin*, the major flour proteins found predominantly in wheat, are termed *gluten* proteins. Glutenin and gliadin combine to form gluten during dough formation. They have high concentrations of glutamine, asparagine, and proline. The gluten proteins are vital to the structure of bread that develops when the flour is hydrated and made into dough.

Gliadin has mostly intramolecular disulfide linkages, resulting in a protein with a compact shape and limited possible contact (see Structure and Bonding in Chap. 3). Glutenin has both intramolecular and intermolecular disulfide bonding (from its cystine components), which results in a more elongated structure and provides for more molecular interaction (Fig. 12-3).

Alone, neither gliadin or glutenin has the ability to form a good dough structure. The formation of gluten involves the breaking down of some disulfide bonds and the formation of new ones (Fig. 12-4). Gluten proteins provide a framework that will stretch during fermentation and coagulate during heating to form the ultimate structure and texture of bread.

FATS

The fats in cereal grains consist mainly of the fatty acids oleic acid and linoleic acid and lecithin. Most of the fats are located in the germ portion of the cereal grain, although 1 to 2 percent are in the endosperm.

CARBOHYDRATES

Cereal grains are an excellent source of energy, with calories derived mainly from starch and, to a much lesser extent, fat. While the main carbohydrate is starch, several other types are also present. *Cellulose* is the major component of wheat bran and is usually removed during milling. *Pentosans* (hemicellulose) are found in the cell walls and account for 2 to 3 percent of white flour. *Dextrins*

FIG. 12-3. Linear linkage of glutenin subunits. (From J. A. D. Ewart, Recent research on dough visco-elasticity. *Baker's Digest* 46[4]:22, 1972.)

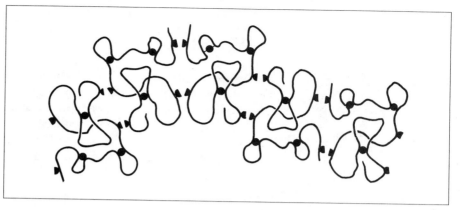

and other sugars account for less than 2 percent and may be present after grinding.

Starch is the major component of flour, accounting for 75 to 80 percent of its dry weight. Starch is a polysaccharide stored in the leukoplasts (plastids) of cereal seeds and certain roots and tubers (see Chaps. 4 and 13). There are two types of starch molecules: *amylose,* with a linear, or straight, chain of glucose units in alpha, 1-4 glycosidic linkage; and *amylopectin,* with highly branched chains in alpha, 1-4 glycosidic linkages and alpha, 1-6 linkages at branch points. The *starch granule,* the structural unit of starch, has a distinctive microscopic appearance for each plant source.

VITAMINS

Grains are good sources of the B vitamins but are almost completely lacking in vitamins A and D. Sprouted grains contain ascorbic acid, but otherwise grains

FIG. 12-4. Gluten is a combination of gliadin and glutenin. (From J. S. Wall and A. C. Beckwith, Relationship between structure and rheological properties of gluten proteins. *Cereal Sci. Today* 14:16, 1969.)

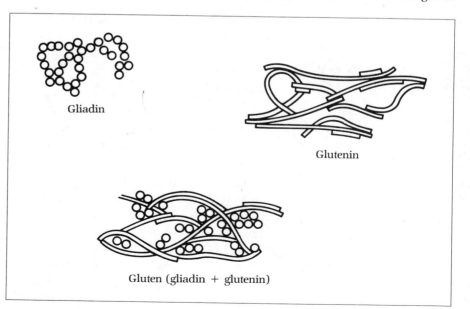

Gliadin

Glutenin

Gluten (gliadin + glutenin)

are poor sources of vitamin C. Yellow corn contains carotene, which is converted in the body to vitamin A. Processing grains destroys some vitamins, especially thiamin, which is unstable in heat.

MINERALS

The endosperm is about 0.37 percent minerals, although the more refined the flour, the lower the mineral content. Unmilled grains are rich in minerals, especially calcium, phosphorus, and iron, but in a form unavailable for absorption. They are chemically bound by the large quantities of fiber and *phytates* also present. During the milling process, the mineral content is greatly reduced. In unenriched flour, phosphorus and potassium are the major mineral components, followed by magnesium, calcium, and traces of sulfur, aluminum, and iron.

FORTIFICATION AND ENRICHMENT

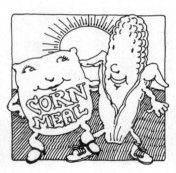

Enrichment of such cereal grain products as white flour and bread, breakfast cereals, cornmeal, rice, macaroni, spaghetti, and other pasta is required by law in many states and is optional in others. In establishing standards of identity, a set list of ingredients that may or may not be in a product [2], Congress has specified certain required and optional ingredients for cereals labeled *enriched*. Some of the required ingredients include thiamin, niacin, riboflavin, and iron; vitamin D and calcium are optional. Enriched flour contains iron and B vitamins at a level comparable with that found in whole wheat.

Fortified products contain one or more added nutrients, such as fluoride in water and iodine in salt, at higher levels than those normally present.

Fortification and enrichment have made important strides in improving the food supply and helping to eliminate deficiency diseases. See Chap. 19 for more detail.

A summary of the nutritive value of selected cereals is given in Table 12-1.

Types of Cereals and Flours

The principal cereals used in the United States are wheat, corn, rye, triticale, sorghum, barley, oats, buckwheat, and rice.

WHEAT

The United States grows about 20 percent of the world's wheat, mostly in the Midwest and upper Midwest (Fig. 12-5). Kansas grows more than any other state. Approximately 60 percent of the wheat in the world is grown in Eastern Europe.

The most used grain in the United States, wheat is classified as *hard* or *soft*, depending on the resistance of the endosperm to grinding. Hardness is a genetically determined quality and reflects the strength of the bonding between the starch and protein components. The greatest difference between flours of hard and soft wheat is in their baking qualities. Flour of hard wheat is especially well suited to making bread; flour of soft wheat, for cakes, pastry, and crackers. Flour of hard wheat contains a large percentage of high-quality gluten. *Durum* wheat is both high in protein and extremely hard. It belongs to a different species from

TABLE 12-1. Nutritive value of selected cereal grains

Food	Amount	Calories	Protein (gm)	Carbohydrate (gm)	Fiber (gm)	Fat (gm)	Iron (mg)	Thiamin (µg)	Riboflavin (µg)	Niacin (mg)	Ascorbic acid (mg)	Vitamin A (IU)	Vitamin D (IU)
Corn													
Cornmeal	¼ cup, dry	135	2.9	28.9	0.2	0.4	1.0	**162**	**96**	1.3	0	110	0
Corn grits	¼ cup, dry	145	3.5	31.2	0.2	0.3	1.2	**178**	**105**	1.4	0	120	0
Hominy grits	¼ cup, dry	131	3.3	28.4	0.2	0.2	1.0	**158**	**94**	1.3	0	0	0
Masa harina	⅓ cup, dry	135	3.4	28.0	0.9	1.5	1.6	**160**	**113**	1.8	—	—	—
Popcorn	1 cup, plain	54	1.8	10.7	0.3	0.7	0.4	—	17	0.3	0	—	—
Barley (Scotch)	2 tbsp, dry	87	2.6	19.5	0.2	0.2	0.5	23	13	0.6	0	—	—
Oatmeal	1 cup, cooked	148	5.4	26.0	0.5	2.8	1.7	**220**	**50**	0.4	0	0	0
Rice													
Brown	¾ cup, cooked	102	2.1	22.0	0.2	0.5	0.6	91	14	1.3	0	0	0
White	¾ cup, cooked	103	2.1	22.5	0.1	0.1	0.2	20	8	0.5	0	0	0
Wild	¼ cup (1 oz)	99	3.9	21.1	0.3	0.2	1.2	130	**180**	1.7	0	0	—
Wheat													
Farina	1 cup, cooked	140	3.8	29.6	0.2	0.3	2.0	**167**	**99**	—	—	—	—
Cream of wheat	1 cup, cooked	133	4.5	28.2	0.1	0.4	1.4	22	22	0.3	0	0	0
Bulgur (red)	2 tbsp	99	3.1	21.2	0.5	0.4	1.0	**80**	**40**	1.3	0	0	—
Cracked wheat	⅔ cup, cooked	92	2.9	20.4	0.7	0.6	1.0	**122**	**31**	1.0	0	0	0
Wheat germ	3 tbsp (1 oz)	102	7.4	13.1	0.7	3.1	2.6	**560**	**190**	1.2	0	0	—
Pasta													
Macaroni	1 cup, cooked	207	7.0	42.2	0.1	0.7	1.5	**250**	**140**	2.0	0	0	—
Egg noodles	1 cup, cooked	200	6.6	37.3	0.2	2.4	1.4	**220**	**130**	1.9	0	112	—
Spaghetti	1 cup, cooked	216	7.3	44.0	0.1	0.7	1.6	**260**	**150**	2.0	0	0	—

Note: Dashes indicate no significant data available. Boldface values are one-fourth or more of the recommended daily dietary allowance (1980) for that nutrient for the average woman aged 23–50.
Source: C. F. Church and H. N. Church, *Food Values of Portions Commonly Used.* Philadelphia: Lippincott, 1975.

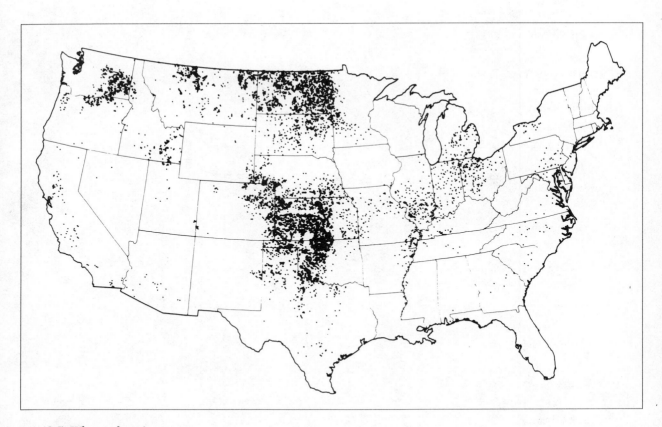

FIG. 12-5. Where wheat is grown in the United States. One dot = 10,000 harvested acres. Source: 1974 Census of Agriculture.

that of the common wheats. It is often used as a major ingredient in pasta because of its adaptability to the processes involved (see Macaroni Products, below).

Wheat is also classified as *spring* or *winter* wheat. Spring wheat is planted in the spring and harvested in the late summer and is usually hard. Winter wheat is planted in the fall, to allow for the development of a root system before cold weather, and harvested in the early summer. The advantage of winter wheat, which can be hard or soft, is higher yields.

The milling and processing of wheat produce several types of flour: *bread flour*, a hard wheat flour with 14% protein content; *family* or *all-purpose flour*, made from either hard or soft wheat, with a 10.5% protein content; *cake flour*, from soft wheat and having a 7.5% protein content; and *self-rising flour*, which is flour with salt and leavening agents added, for making quick breads. Two other wheat products are *bulgur* and *farina*. Bulgur is wheat that has been cooked and dried and had its bran partially removed. The kernels are cut to a fine, medium, or coarse consistency or left whole. Farina is made from wheat *middlings*, chunks of endosperm free of bran and germ. Middlings become flour when pulverized.

CORN

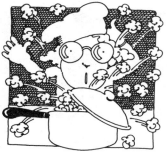

The second most used grain in the United States, after wheat, is corn. This grain is used in several forms as a nutritious staple in the American diet.

Cornmeal is made by grinding corn kernels to a coarse mixture. Because the high fat content of the germ portion rapidly becomes rancid during storage, cornmeal is usually processed by removing the bran and germ before the endosperm is ground. *Degerminated cornmeal* has less fat and more starch than does whole ground cornmeal. Although both white and yellow corn can be used to make cornmeal, yellow cornmeal contains more vitamin A in the form of carotene. Cornmeal can be cooked in water and served as porridge or cornmeal mush. With cheese and lard added, it is the Italian dish polenta.

In Central and South America, corn is soaked in an alkaline solution, which softens the kernel and liberates niacin. The corn is then rinsed, drained, dried, and ground into meal called *masa harina* and used to make tortillas, tacos, and enchiladas.

Grits are made by grinding corn to a coarse consistency. Hominy, a type of grits, is made from white corn.

Popcorn is corn kernels that have had their moisture decreased. When heated, the moisture in the endosperm expands 20 to 30 times its volume, causing it to pop open.

RYE

Rye is used mostly for the commercial manufacture of bread, to which it gives a distinctive flavor. Rye flour lacks the cohesive protein structure of wheat and is not improved with maturing agents. The protein in rye, which amounts to 9 to 16 percent, has poor gas-retaining qualities because it lacks strength. Bread made only from rye is more dense and compact than that made from wheat flour; often a combination of wheat and rye flours is used. Rye is grown in large quantities in the U.S.S.R. and Europe.

TRITICALE

This cereal grain is a hybrid produced from wheat and rye. Triticale combines the grain quality and disease resistance of wheat with the vigor and hardness of rye. Triticale flour is used in making breads, rolls, and pasta.

SORGHUM

Although not used extensively as a food in the United States, sorghum is the chief food grain in Africa and parts of China, India, and Pakistan. It is made into porridge, bread, or cakes, and can be fortified with soy and cottonseed proteins to improve its protein quality [3].

BARLEY

Because it lacks gluten, barley cannot be made into bread unless it is mixed with other flours (usually in a 1:5 ratio) [4]. This grain is used extensively in the United States in the production of malt. An enzyme present in sprouting barley changes starch to maltose. This maltose-rich barley is then roasted, dried, and used in the manufacture of alcoholic beverages or for food uses, such as malted milk.

OATS

Used mostly for breakfast foods, oats are very nutritious because they are made from the whole grain with only the bran removed. When combined with wheat flour, oatmeal is used in the preparation of breads and baked goods. Oat cereals include *groats*, *quick oats*, flakes made from particles of the whole groat; and *regular oats*, flaked whole groats. Oat cereals are high in incomplete protein, fat, carbohydrate, calcium, phosphorus, and iron; they also contain most of the B vitamins.

BUCKWHEAT

Buckwheat is used mainly in the United States in the manufacture of pancake flour. Buckwheat groats are also sold as a breakfast cereal.

RICE

More than 90 percent of the world rice crop is produced and consumed in Asia and on adjacent islands; rice provides more than one-half of the world's population with a low-cost food staple (Fig. 12-6) [4]. Rice is also cultivated in the United States. The varieties include long-grain, medium-grain, and short-grain. *Wild rice* is actually the seeds of a reedlike water plant rather than a true rice. Its high cost to the consumer is the result of its having to be harvested by hand.

In converting unprocessed brown rice to white, or polished, rice, a large amount of the protein, fat, minerals, and vitamins is lost. Methods have been devised to ensure maximum nutrient retention. Undermilled or "unpolished" rice does not have the customary white luster and is more prone to insect infestation and flour deterioration. Processing the rough rice by parboiling before milling increases vitamin retention; the result is known as *converted rice*. In this process, some of the B vitamins and minerals in the bran permeate the endosperm, thus increasing the nutrient content of the final milled product. Artificial enrichment of the grain is done by coating the rice with a solution of thiamin and niacin, allowing it to dry, and then applying a protective layer. Another layer of iron is applied in a similar manner. These coatings are resistant to washing, cooking, and storage losses. *Quick-cooking rice* is rice cooked to gelatinize the starch and then dried. The porous structure of the processed rice allows rapid rehydration.

Principles of Cereal Grain Cookery
CEREALS

The essential action involved in cooking cereals is gelatinization of the cereal starch. Water is absorbed as the starch gelatinizes, so adequate moisture is necessary to form a soft starch gel. Heat augments the penetration of moisture through the tough outer layer of the grains. Heat also produces steam that penetrates and disrupts the starch granules. The thickening of cereal as it cooks is the result of the release of soluble starch paste. Heating also affects flavor by causing a conversion of starch to dextrins and sugars. Although heat itself does not decompose the cell wall cellulose, it does soften it, making the cereal more palatable.

Grains must be cooked long enough to cook the starch, to form a starch paste or

FIG. 12-6. Rice harvest in Indonesia. (Courtesy United Nations/World Health Organization.)

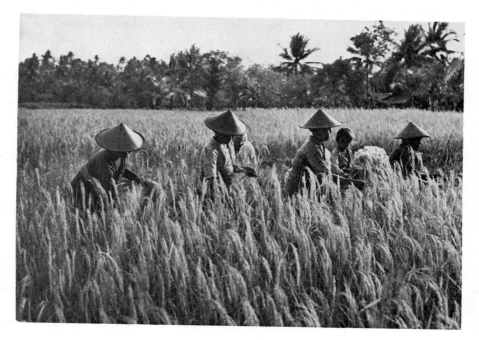

FIG. 12-6. Rice harvest in Indonesia. (Courtesy United Nations/World Health Organization.)

gel, and to develop the flavor, although short enough to prevent leaching of its water-soluble nutrients out into the cooking water.

BREADS

The formation of bread is the result of several physical and chemical reactions, including the breaking and reformation of disulfide bonds, the gelatinization of starch granules, the fermentation of yeast, and the expansion of gases by heat.

FACTORS CONTRIBUTING TO BREAD STRUCTURE
Flour

Flour, when hydrated, forms an elastic, cohesive network through the action of the gluten proteins as described above. The breaking of some disulfide bonds and the formation of new ones results in the development of *gluten*, the complex between gliadin and glutenin. Hydrophobic interaction, hydrogen bonding, and ionic bonding also contribute to dough development, although to a lesser degree. Gluten permits expansion during fermentation.

Starch

Starch granules become closely associated with the gluten proteins during mixing, which prevents an excessively cohesive structure. Starch embedded in the gluten matrix provides structural reinforcement. The *gelatinization* of the starch granules during baking contributes to the baked structure of bread.

Gelatinization is the change that occurs when starch is heated in water. When heat is applied, the moisture penetrates the layers of the grain, disrupting the hydrogen bonding in the crystalline starch granules. Some straight chains of amylose leave the granules, which increases the viscosity of the cooking solution. Gelatinization is maximal at the boiling point.

Acid, such as lemon juice, accelerates gelatinization because of hydrolysis of the granule surfaces, increasing surface permeability and rate of swelling. Sucrose retards the hydration of starch granules by competing for moisture. Unless the sugar concentration is very high, the retarding effect can be at least partially overcome by increasing the heating period.

Liquid

Liquid is essential for the hydration of flour proteins. Liquid also serves as a dispersion medium for yeast cells, sugar, and salt and is responsible for the partial gelatinization of starch during baking.

Yeast

The primary function of yeast in bread making is to provide carbon dioxide for leavening. Yeast contains the enzymes needed for carbon dioxide production from glucose. It also contains the enzymes maltase and sucrase, which hydrolyze maltose and sucrose, providing the glucose substrate. Yeast also makes an important contribution to the flavor of bread.

Sugar

In the proper amounts, sugar provides a substrate (glucose) for yeast fermentation. Without sugar, fermentation is slow. In excessive amounts, sugar can actually interfere with gluten development by competing with gluten proteins for moisture. When more sugar is added than needed for fermentation, the residual sugars participate in nonenzymatic browning (which gives the crust its brown color) during baking. Sugar also contributes flavor to the bread.

Shortening

This ingredient increases the volume of the loaf and improves the texture.

Salt

Salt provides a means of controlling fermentation. It has a retarding effect on yeast activity, achieved through an osmotic effect on yeast cells, and a stiffening effect on the dough. Salt also adds flavor.

THE BAKING PROCESS

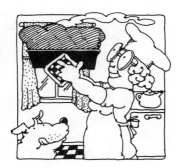

The rapid rise in volume during the first 10 to 12 minutes of baking is termed *oven spring*. The heat of the oven causes oven spring both by increasing the rate of fermentation and by causing the gases in the dough to expand. The action of the enzymes in the flour and yeast is first accelerated; then it is reduced when the enzymes are denatured with sufficient heat. Better oven spring is achieved with hard than with soft wheat flour, because of the gluten's ability to expand without breaking.

With continued baking, the gases leave the bread structure. The starch's granules gelatinize, receiving water from the gluten proteins. The gluten strands coagulate, forming the rigid structure of the bread.

The bread crust forms as the loaf dries and is a darker color because of the browning reaction. Milk helps produce a brown crust because its sugar (lactose) is not fermented by yeast.

Macaroni Products

Also termed *pasta* or *alimentary pastes*, macaroni is another type of food whose main ingredient is cereal grain.

The standard of identity established by the U.S. Department of Agriculture [2] for macaroni products specifies semolina, durum flour, or farina flour, alone or in combination, plus water as required ingredients. Optional ingredients include egg white solids (0.5 to 2.0 percent by weight of the finished product), disodium phosphate, and various seasonings. *Noodles* are macaroni products to which eggs have been added. Not less than 5.5 percent by weight of the total solids must be egg yolk solids. Noodles are usually enriched with B vitamins and iron.

Durum wheat is the most commonly used flour in making pasta because of its adaptability to the processes involved. *Durum semolina* (middlings of durum wheat, ground to a certain size) is used in most macaroni products. Durum has a characteristic yellow color from the carotenoid pigment xanthophyll. *Disodium phosphate* increases the alkalinity, enabling the starch grains to gelatinize faster.

References

1. Mangelsdorf, P. C.   Wheat. In *Human Nutrition.* San Francisco: Scientific American and W. H. Freeman, 1978. P. 70.
2. Code of Federal Regulations, *Title 21*, 1971.
3. Bookwalter, G. N., and Warmer, K.   Fortification of dry-milled sorghum with oilseed proteins. *J. Food Sci.* 42:969, 1977.
4. Peckham, G. C., and Freeland-Graves, J. H.   *Foundations of Food Preparation* (4th ed.). New York: Macmillan, 1979. P. 221.

Suggested Readings

AACC Committee on Dietary Fiber.   Collaborative study of an analytical method for insoluble dietary fiber in cereals. *Cereal Foods World* 26:295, 1981.
Barr, T. N.   The world food situation and global grain prospects. *Science* 214:1087, 1981.
Davis, D. R.   Wheat and nutrition. *Nutr. Today* 16:16 (part I); 16:22 (part II), 1981.
Dorn, P.   Pasta—twisted, bowed and shelled. *Cooking for Profit* 371:14, 1981.
Dutta, L., and Barua, J. N.   Evaluation of nutritional quality of some rice varieties grown in Assam. *Indian J. Nutr. Diet.* 15:42, 1978.
Erdman, J. W.   Bioavailability of trace minerals from cereals and legumes. *Cereal Chem.* 58:21, 1981.
Hoseney, R. C., and Seib, P. A.   Structural differences in hard and soft wheat. *Baker's Digest* 47:26, 1973.

Houston, D. F., and Kohler, G. O.   *Nutritional Properties of Rice*. Washington, D.C.: National Academy of Sciences, 1970.

Kasarda, D. D., Bernardin, J. E., and Nimmo, C. C.   Wheat Proteins. In Y. Pomeranz (ed.), *Advances in Cereal Science and Technology*. St. Paul: American Association of Cereal Chemists, 1976.

Kulp, K.   Physicochemical properties of starches of wheats and flours. *Cereal Chem.* 49:697, 1972.

Lachance, P. A.   The role of cereal grain products in the U.S. diet. *Food Technol.* 35:49, 1981.

Lee, K., and Clydesdale, F. M.   Effect of baking on the forms of iron in iron-enriched flour. *J. Food Sci.* 45:1500, 1980.

Mecham, D. K.   Flour proteins and their behavior in doughs. *Cereal Sci. Today* 17:208, 1972.

Miller, B. S. (ed.).   *Variety Breads in the United States*. St. Paul, Minn.: American Association of Cereal Chemists, Inc., 1981.

Oberleas, D., and Harland, B. F.   Phytate content of foods: Effect on dietary zinc bioavailability. *J. Am. Dietet. Assoc.* 79:433, 1981.

Schmidt, A. M.   New flour and bread enrichment standards. *Baker's Digest* 47:29, 1973.

Stenvert, N. L., and Kingswood, K.   The influence of the physical structure of the protein matrix on wheat hardness. *J. Sci. Food Agric.* 28:11, 1977.

Wendorf, F., et al.   Use of barley in the Egyptian Late Paleolithic. *Science* 205:1341, 1979.

Which cereal for breakfast? *Consum. Rep.* 46:68, 1981.

Chapter 13

FRUITS AND VEGETABLES

Fruits and vegetables are valuable components of the daily diet, contributing carbohydrate (in the form of sugar, starch, and fiber), vitamins, minerals, and trace elements, as well as unique and interesting flavors, textures, and colors. The same pigments, flavor-contributing substances, and structural components are found in both fruits and vegetables, but they differ in each unique combination. The substances contributing to the flavor of fruits and vegetables include pigments, sugars, organic acids (volatile and nonvolatile), mineral salts, sulfur compounds, and tannins.

Classification and Nutritive Value

Fruits and vegetables are the edible portions of plant tissue. Their nutritive value, color, flavor, and structure are influenced by the portion of the plant from which they are derived.

Grades based on such characteristics as shape, color, defects, and texture are established by the U.S. Department of Agriculture to be used in the purchase and sale of fruits and vegetables on the wholesale market [1]. The premium grades of fresh produce are U.S. extra fancy, U.S. fancy, and U.S. extra no. 1. The basic trading grades are U.S. no. 1 and U.S. no. 2. The greater price of higher grades is not always an indication of better quality or nutritive value but is more a reflection of supply and demand.

FRUITS

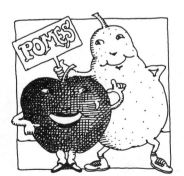

A *fruit* is the matured ovary of a flower, including its seeds and adjacent parts (Fig. 13-1). Fruits differ according to the kinds of flowers from which they originate. Such fruits as pears and apples come from a single blossom. An *aggregate fruit,* such as the strawberry, comes from a flower with many stamens and pistils. Pineapples and figs are considered *multiple fruits* because many flowers are collected together to form them. *Nuts* are also considered to be fruit, although the seed, rather than the fleshy pericarp, is the food portion. The nutritive value of selected fruits is given in Table 13-1.

One group of fruits, called *pomes,* is characterized by an enlarged, fleshy pericarp surrounding the seeds. Apples and pears are pomes and contain considerable amounts of ascorbic acid (vitamin C) and sugar. With storage, the sugar content increases and the vitamin content decreases. The unique flavor of pears is due to their citric acid and malic acid content.

Drupes are those fruits with a single seed surrounded by a fleshy pericarp, the edible portion. Fruits in this group include peaches, plums, apricots, nectarines, and cherries. Malic and citric acids give characteristic flavor to apricots and peaches; vitamin A is also found in large quantities in these fruits. All drupes are mild, natural laxatives because their indigestible fiber helps maintain good bowel tone and regular gastrointestinal functioning. In addition, plums (and dried plums, prunes) contain derivatives of hydroxyphenylisatin, a substance that stimulates the smooth muscle of the colon.

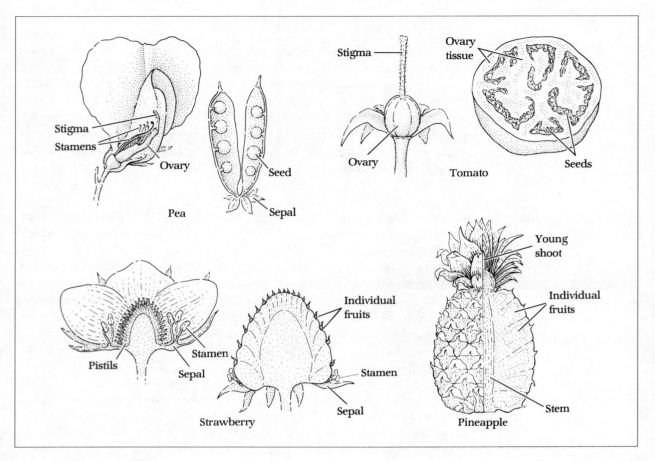

FIG. 13-1. Anatomy of flowers and developing fruits. All fruits are derived completely or in part from flowers. The pea is a legume—a type of dry fruit—while a tomato is a berry—a type of simple fleshy fruit. A tomato is an enlarged ovary. What we usually call berries, such as the strawberry, are in reality aggregate fruits. The fleshy part is derived from the flower stalk, and all the "seeds" are really fruits. Pineapples are multiple fruits, formed from the whole flower stalk. (From W. M. Laetsch, *Plants: Basic Concepts in Botany.* Boston: Little, Brown, 1979.)

Fruits in which seeds are contained within the layers of the pericarp are succulent and pulpy and are termed *berries.* Within this group are blackberries, blueberries, cranberries, grapes, and strawberries. Their flavor is derived from the nonvolatile acids malic acid and citric acid; tartaric acid also contributes flavor to grapes. The volatile benzoic acid is also found in cranberries and strawberries; acetic, capric, and formic acids are found in strawberries. As with most fruits, berries are sources of vitamin C, with strawberries being the highest in vitamin C, blackberries a fair source, and grapes a poor source.

The *citrus fruits* are among the best known and liked in the United States. All have a high content of vitamin C, and they are usually available all year. The citrus fruits include grapefruit, lemons, limes, and oranges. The colors of the rinds are produced by a combination of chlorophyll and carotenoids (see Pigments, below). Citric and malic acids, together with the pigments, contribute to the flavor of citrus fruits.

Another group of fruits, *melons,* is usually divided into the muskmelons—cantaloupe, honeydew, and casaba—and the watermelon. The flesh of muskmelons ranges from yellowish-white (casaba) and greenish-white (honeydew) to dark yellow or orange (cantaloupe). The watermelon contains the pigments lycopene and carotene, which give it its rich red color. Generally, the vitamin A content is greater with deeper orange color, as in the cantaloupe, but all melons provide good amounts of vitamin C and carbohydrate.

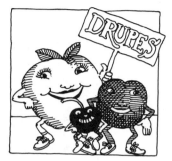

Other fruits include avocados, bananas, dates, figs, pineapples, mangoes, and papayas. Mangoes and papayas are especially rich sources of vitamin A. Avocados are one of the few fruits with a high fat content, which gives them a smooth, rich texture. Bananas are known as a good source of potassium and carbohydrate as well as a fair source of vitamins A and C. Dates are unique because of their very high carbohydrate content, almost 50 percent. Figs, which are high in potassium, are a very delicate fruit and are usually dried, canned, or preserved before being shipped. Pineapple contains the proteolytic enzyme *bromelin,* which is used in the preparation of meat tenderizers. For this reason, fresh pineapple is never added to gelatin salad, since this enzyme would impair the gelling process. In canned pineapple, which has undergone processing with heat, the enzyme has been denatured. Another protein-splitting enzyme, *papain,* is found in papaya; papain is used as a meat tenderizer and is added to beer for flavor.

VEGETABLES

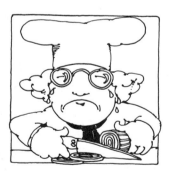

Vegetables, especially those that come from seeds, pods, tubers, and roots, contain more starch and less sugar than do fruits. Vegetables from the fruit, leaves, flowers, stems, and shoots of plants have a sugar content closer to that of fruits. Vegetables are especially rich in vitamins and minerals, although their nutritive value depends in part on the soil and climate in which they are grown. The same substances that contribute to the unique flavors of fruits are also found in vegetables; these include sugars, acids (volatile and nonvolatile), mineral salts, sulfur compounds, and tannins. The strong flavor of cabbage, turnips, onions, and brussels sprouts is a result of their volatile sulfur compounds. The color pigments found in fruits are also present in vegetables. Vegetables may come from any part of the plant and are therefore classified by the part from which they are derived. The nutritive value of selected vegetables is given in Table 13-2.

Root vegetables come from the enlarged root of the plant. White potatoes, sweet potatoes, yams, carrots, beets, turnips, parsnips, and rutabagas are the most common root vegetables. *Taproots,* such as beets, carrots, and parsnips, have an especially high sugar content. Sugar beets, a special variety, have a high sucrose content and are used in the manufacture of granulated sugar (see Chap. 4). The sugar in carrots is predominantly fructose; both sweetness and vitamin A content increase with the intensity of their color. *Tuber roots* include red and white potatoes, sweet potatoes, and yams. Red and white potatoes contain more starch, with only about 10 percent of their carbohydrate in the form of sugar. They also contain good amounts of vitamin C. Sweet potatoes have a high sugar and vitamin A content. Sweet potatoes and yams differ in color and sweetness, with yams being darker orange and sweeter.

TABLE 13-1. Nutritive value of selected fruits

Fruit	Amount	Calories	Protein (gm)	Carbohydrate (gm)	Fiber (gm)	Fat (gm)	Iron (mg)	Thiamin (µg)	Riboflavin (µg)	Niacin (mg)	Ascorbic acid (mg)	Vitamin A (IU)	Vitamin D (IU)
Pomes													
Apples	1 medium	87	0.3	21.7	1.5	0.9	0.5	**40**	**30**	0.2	6	140	—
Pears	½ medium	61	0.7	15.3	1.4	0.4	0.3	**20**	**40**	0.1	4	20	—
Drupes													
Peaches	1 medium	38	0.6	9.7	0.6	0.1	0.5	20	50	1.0	7	**1330**	—
Plums	2 medium	66	0.5	17.8	0.4	tr	0.5	**80**	30	0.5	—	300	—
Apricots	3 medium	51	1.0	12.8	0.6	0.2	0.5	30	40	0.6	10	**2700**	—
Nectarines	2 medium	64	0.6	17.1	0.4	tr	0.5	—	—	—	13	**1650**	—
Cherries (sour)	½ cup	58	1.2	14.3	0.2	0.3	0.4	**50**	**60**	0.4	10	**1000**	—
Berries													
Blackberries	⅝ cup	58	1.2	12.9	4.1	0.9	0.9	30	40	0.4	**21**	200	—
Blueberries	⅝ cup	62	0.7	15.3	1.5	0.5	1.0	**30**	**60**	0.5	14	100	—
Cranberries	1 cup	46	0.4	10.8	1.4	0.7	0.5	**30**	20	0.1	11	40	—
Grapes (Thompson)	½ cup	51	0.5	13.6	0.2	0.1	0.3	**40**	10	0.2	2	70	—
Strawberries	1 cup	56	1.0	12.6	2.0	0.8	1.5	**40**	**100**	0.9	**88**	90	—

	Portion												
Citrus fruits													
Grapefruit (pink)	½ medium	40	0.5	10.4	0.2	0.1	0.4	**40**	20	0.2	36	440	—
Lemons	1 medium	27	1.1	8.2	0.4	0.3	0.6	**40**	20	0.1	53	20	—
Limes	1 medium	28	0.7	9.5	0.5	0.2	0.6	**30**	20	0.2	37	10	—
Oranges	1 medium	73	1.5	18.3	0.8	0.3	0.6	**150**	**60**	0.6	**80**	**300**	—
Melons													
Cantaloupe	¼ melon	30	0.7	7.5	0.3	0.1	0.4	**40**	**30**	0.6	33	**3400**	—
Honeydew	¼ melon	33	0.8	7.7	0.6	0.3	0.4	**40**	**30**	0.6	23	40	—
Watermelon	1 slice (6 × 1½ in.)	156	3.0	38.4	1.8	1.2	3.0	**180**	**180**	1.2	**42**	**3540**	—
Other fruits													
Avocados	½ pitted	167	2.1	6.3	1.6	16.4	0.6	**110**	**200**	1.6	14	**290**	—
Bananas	1 small	85	1.1	22.2	0.5	0.2	0.7	**50**	**60**	0.7	10	190	—
Dates	10 medium	274	2.2	72.9	2.3	0.5	3.0	**90**	**100**	2.2	0	50	—
Figs	2 large	80	1.2	20.3	1.2	0.3	0.6	**60**	**50**	0.4	2	80	—
Pineapple	¾ cup	52	0.4	13.7	0.4	0.2	0.5	**90**	**30**	0.2	**17**	70	—
Mangoes	½ medium	66	0.7	16.8	0.9	0.4	**50.0**	**50**	**35**	1.1	—	**4800**	—
Papayas	⅓ medium	39	0.6	10.0	0.9	0.1	0.3	**40**	**40**	0.3	**56**	**1750**	—

tr = trace.

Note: All values are for raw, fresh fruit. Dashes indicate no significant data available. Boldface values are one-fourth or more the recommended daily dietary allowance (1980) for the average woman aged 23–50.

Source: C. F. Church and H. N. Church, *Food Values of Portions Commonly Used*. Philadelphia: Lippincott, 1975.

TABLE 13-2. Nutritive value of selected vegetables

Vegetable	Amount	Calories	Protein (gm)	Carbohydrate (gm)	Fiber (gm)	Fat (gm)	Iron (mg)	Thiamin (µg)	Riboflavin (µg)	Niacin (mg)	Ascorbic acid (mg)	Vitamin A (IU)	Vitamin D (IU)
Roots													
White potato	1 medium, baked	139	3.9	31.7	0.9	0.2	1.0	150	60	2.6	30	tr	—
Sweet potato	1 small, baked	141	2.1	32.5	0.9	0.5	0.9	90	70	0.7	22	8100	—
Yams (white)	½ cup, cooked	105	2.4	24.1	0.9	0.2	0.6	90	40	0.6	9	tr	—
Carrots	⅔ cup, cooked	31	0.9	7.1	1.0	0.2	0.6	50	50	0.5	6	10,500	—
Beets (red)	½ cup, cooked	27	0.9	6.0	0.7	0.1	0.4	30	30	0.3	5	17	—
Turnips	⅔ cup, cooked	23	0.8	4.9	0.9	0.2	0.4	40	50	0.3	22	tr	—
Parsnips	½ cup, cooked	66	1.5	14.9	2.0	0.5	0.6	70	80	0.1	10	30	—
Rutabagas	½ cup, cooked	35	0.9	8.2	1.1	0.1	0.3	60	60	0.8	26	550	—
Bulbs													
Garlic	1 bulb	2	0.1	0.4	tr	tr	tr	—	—	—	tr	—	—
Onion	1 small, raw	38	1.5	8.7	0.6	0.1	0.5	30	40	0.2	10	40	—
Leaves and stems													
Lettuce (iceberg)	3½ oz	14	1.2	2.5	0.5	0.2	2.0	60	60	0.3	8	970	—
Spinach	½ cup, cooked	21	2.7	3.2	0.5	0.3	2.0	60	130	0.5	25	7300	—
Kale	¾ cup, cooked	39	4.5	6.1	—	0.7	1.6	100	180	1.6	93	8300	—
Kohlrabi	⅔ cup, cooked	24	1.7	5.3	1.0	0.1	0.3	60	30	0.2	43	20	—
Brussels sprouts	⅔ cup, cooked	36	4.2	6.4	1.6	0.4	1.1	80	140	0.8	87	520	—
Cabbage	⅗ cup, cooked	20	1.1	4.3	0.8	0.2	0.3	40	40	0.3	33	130	—
Watercress	3½ oz, raw	19	2.2	3.0	0.7	0.3	1.7	80	160	0.9	79	4900	—
Dandelion	½ cup, cooked	33	2.0	6.4	1.3	0.6	1.8	130	160	—	18	11,700	—
Chicory	30–40 leaves, raw	20	1.8	3.8	0.8	0.3	0.9	60	100	0.5	22	4000	—
Escarole	4 large leaves, raw	20	1.7	4.1	0.9	0.1	1.7	70	140	0.5	10	3300	—
Collards	½ cup, cooked	29	2.7	4.9	0.8	0.6	0.6	140	200	1.2	46	5400	—

Turnip greens	⅔ cup, cooked	20	2.2	3.6	0.7	0.2	1.1	**150**	240	0.6	**69**	**6300**	—
Sorrel	½ cup, cooked	28	2.1	5.6	0.8	0.3	1.6	**90**	220	0.5	**119**	**12,900**	—
Beet tops	½ cup, cooked	18	1.7	3.3	1.1	0.2	1.9	**70**	150	0.3	**15**	**5100**	—
Celery	1 cup, raw	17	0.9	3.9	0.6	0.1	0.3	**30**	30	0.3	9	**240**	—
Asparagus	⅔ cup, cooked	20	2.2	3.6	0.7	0.2	0.6	**160**	180	1.4	**26**	**900**	—
Vegetable fruits													
Pumpkin	½ cup, canned	38	1.2	9.1	1.5	0.3	0.5	**30**	60	0.7	6	**7400**	—
Squash (winter)	½ cup, baked	63	1.8	15.4	1.8	0.4	0.8	**50**	130	0.7	13	**4200**	—
Tomato	1 medium, raw	33	1.6	7.0	0.8	0.3	0.8	**90**	60	1.0	**34**	**1350**	—
Okra	8–9 pods, cooked	29	2.0	6.0	1.0	0.3	0.5	**130**	180	0.9	**20**	**490**	—
Green pepper	1 large, raw	22	1.2	4.8	1.4	0.2	0.7	**80**	80	0.5	**128**	**420**	—
Cucumber	½ medium, raw	8	0.5	1.7	0.3	0.1	0.6	**15**	20	0.1	6	**125**	—
Eggplant	½ cup, cooked	19	1.0	4.1	0.9	0.2	0.6	**50**	40	0.5	3	**10**	—
Vegetable flowers													
Artichoke	1 large bud, cooked	44	2.8	9.9	2.4	0.2	1.1	**70**	40	0.7	8	**150**	—
Broccoli	1 large stalk, cooked	26	3.1	4.5	1.5	0.3	0.8	**90**	200	0.8	**90**	**2500**	—
Cauliflower	⅞ cup, cooked	22	2.3	4.1	1.0	0.2	0.7	**90**	80	0.6	**55**	**60**	—
Corn	1 medium ear, cooked	100	3.3	21.0	0.7	1.0	0.6	**120**	100	1.4	9	**400**	—
Pods and seeds													
Lentils	⅔ cup, cooked	106	7.8	19.3	1.2	tr	2.1	**70**	60	0.6	0	**20**	—
Beans													
White	½ cup, cooked	118	7.8	21.2	1.5	0.6	2.7	**140**	70	0.7	0	0	—
Kidney	⅖ cup, cooked	118	7.8	21.4	1.5	0.5	2.4	**110**	60	0.7	—	tr	—
Lima	⅝ cup, cooked	111	7.6	19.8	1.8	0.5	2.5	**180**	100	1.3	**17**	**280**	—
Snap	1 cup, cooked	31	2.0	6.8	1.2	0.2	0.8	**90**	110	0.6	**15**	**675**	—
Yellow	1 cup, cooked	22	1.4	4.6	1.0	0.2	0.6	**70**	90	0.5	**13**	**230**	—
Peas, green	⅔ cup, cooked	71	5.4	12.1	2.0	0.4	1.8	**280**	110	2.3	**20**	**540**	—
Sprouts													
Mung bean	3½ oz, raw	35	3.8	6.6	0.7	0.2	1.3	**130**	130	0.8	**19**	20	—
Soybean	1 cup, raw	46	6.2	5.3	0.8	1.4	1.0	**230**	200	0.8	13	**80**	—

tr = trace.

Note: Dashes indicate no significant data available. Boldface values are one-fourth or more of the recommended daily dietary allowance (1980) for that nutrient for the average woman aged 23–50.

Source: C. F. Church and H. N. Church, *Food Values of Portions Commonly Used*. Philadelphia: Lippincott, 1975.

Specialized stems holding a food reserve are *bulbs.* Among the most common bulbs are garlic, onions, chives, shallots, and leeks. Although used mainly for seasoning, some bulbs are a good source of vitamin C. The strong odors and flavors of this group of vegetables are due to the presence of sulfur compounds, which evaporate during cooking, leaving a milder flavor.

Plants in which the *leaves* or *stems* provide a reservoir of food make up another group of vegetables. Among the most common leaves and stems are lettuce, spinach, kale, kohlrabi, brussels sprouts, cabbage, greens, celery, and asparagus. As a group, leaf and stem vegetables are good sources of calcium, vitamins A and C, riboflavin, and thiamin; they are generally low in carbohydrate. The calcium in spinach may be in the bound form because of the presence of oxalates, which would reduce its availability as a nutrient.

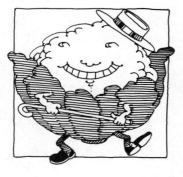

Among the vegetables classified as *vegetable fruits* are pumpkin, squash, tomato, okra, peppers, cucumbers, and eggplant. As a group, they are generally low in calories and high in minerals. Pumpkin and squash provide good sources of vitamin A, riboflavin, thiamin, calcium, magnesium, iron, and phosphorus. With storage, the starch content of both is changed to sugar. Tomatoes and peppers are excellent sources of vitamin C.

Another group of vegetables, classified as *vegetable flowers,* have small clusters of flowers on a stem, with fleshy scales. Vegetables in this group include artichokes, broccoli, cauliflower, and sweet corn. Both cauliflower and broccoli are types of cabbage in which flower buds are massed on short stalks. Sweet corn contains an oil that is often used in cooking for its mild, rich flavor.

Pods and *seeds,* also known as *legumes,* form another group of vegetables. Lentils, beans (string, navy, kidney, pinto, lima, and soy), and peas (black-eyed, cow, yellow, and green) are found in this group. Generally, vegetables that are pods or seeds are good sources of incomplete protein (containing some, but not all, of the essential amino acids; see Chap. 3). They provide good amounts of some B vitamins and trace minerals, particularly zinc and copper.

The last group of vegetables, *sprouts,* come from seeds that have been made to germinate. The most common sprouts are alfalfa, soybean, mung bean, fenugreek, and sunflower seed. The young shoots are very good sources of vitamin C and are often used as a garnish or salad ingredient.

Structure and Composition

The structure and composition of the plant cell is important in understanding the changes that occur in fruits and vegetables during ripening, storage, and cooking and the effects of these processes on color, flavor, texture, and nutritive value.

TYPES OF CELLS AND TISSUE

The texture of a fruit or vegetable is influenced by the proportion and arrangement of its various types of cells. Specialized cells within certain plants serve specific functions and comprise three distinct groups: dermal, ground or fundamental, and vascular.

The *dermal* cells include the *epidermis,* which provides mechanical protection for the plant. This outer layer of cells may be covered by a cuticle or additional layer of fatty material, such as *cutin*, a hydrophilic fatty acid polymer that limits water loss from the plant's surface. As some plants, such as the potato, mature, the epidermis is replaced by the periderm, a softer outer protective layer.

The *ground,* or *fundamental,* cells include parenchyma, collenchyma, and sclerenchyma cells. The *parenchyma* are specialized cells whose functions include photosynthesis, storage, and wound healing. The *collenchyma* are fibrous cells with walls thicker than those of the parenchyma. The collenchyma function as support tissue for growing plants and perform photosynthesis. *Sclerenchyma* are cells with woodlike walls that often contain lignin, a noncarbohydrate substance that resists the actions of bacteria, enzymes, and chemicals and does not break down or change under heat.

The two main cell types in the vascular system include *xylem* (which transports water) and *phloem* (which transports food); they also function in the storage of food and provide support.

CELL STRUCTURE

The plant cell itself is composed of several specialized organelles (Fig. 13-2). The *protoplasm* is the active, living part of the cell, on which all of its functions depend. The *nucleus* contains genetic material and is the regulator of the cell's metabolic activities. The *cytoplasm* is the undifferentiated part of the protoplasm surrounding the nucleus and forming a thin layer inside the cell wall. *Plastids*

FIG. 13-2. Structure of the plant cell. This schematic representation of a cell shows it as a box filled with strands of cytoplasm traversing the watery vacuole. The cytoplasmic strands are constantly changing, so a true representation of this cell would show a new pattern every second. (From W. M. Laetsch, *Plants: Basic Concepts in Botany.* Boston: Little, Brown, 1979.)

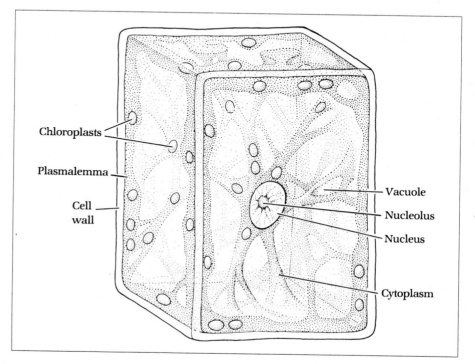

Chloroplasts

Plasmalemma

Cell
wall

Vacuole

Nucleolus

Nucleus

Cytoplasm

are organized bodies within the cytoplasm, and are of three different types: leukoplasts, chloroplasts, and chromoplasts. The *leukoplasts* lack pigment; their function is to produce and store food for the plant. In such starch-forming plants as potatoes, peas, and beans, these specialized cells are termed *amyloplasts.* *Chloroplasts* occur in green plants and contain chlorophyll in granules called *grana.* In plants with grana containing other than green pigment, such as xan-thophylls (yellow) or carotenes (orange), these specialized cells are designated *chromoplasts.* Other cellular components include the *mitochondria,* organelles in the cytoplasm with enzymes responsible for energy production; mitochondria are the site of oxidative reactions and the Krebs cycle [2]. The *endoplasmic reticulum* is a system of transport channels within the cell. *Vacuoles,* which are also found within certain plant cells, are spaces filled with a fluid called *cell sap,* and may contain pigments, dissolved sugars, salts, organic acids, or other com-pounds; it also stores food in a liquid form.

The *cell walls* provide elastic support and confining structure for the contents of the plant cell. In combination with the intercellular bonding material, the cell walls give mechanical strength to plant tissues. Cell walls are made of cellulose and hemicellulose. In some vegetables with a woody quality, lignin may also be present. Adjoining cells are held together by the intercellular layer or *middle lamella,* which is composed of one or more forms of pectin.

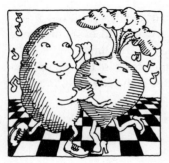

Cellulose, as discussed in the chapter on carbohydrates, is a polysaccharide composed of glucose units, as is starch. Unlike starch, however, in cellulose the glucose units are combined in beta glucosidic linkages, which makes them resistant to human digestive enzymes. The cellulose molecules are linked by hydrogen bonding and are combined in a crystalline arrangement of linear bundles called *fibrils.*

Hemicellulose, another cell wall component, is also made of polysaccharides of varying composition. It is insoluble in water but is readily hydrolyzed by alkali or dilute acid. The amount of hemicellulose is reduced by cooking [3], especially in water containing baking soda (alkali).

Lignin is a noncarbohydrate substance found in some plant cell walls that resists the actions of bacteria, enzymes, and chemicals. It does not break down or change during cooking [3]. Lignin accounts for as much as 50 percent of the dry weight of wood.

The middle lamella is composed of *pectin substances,* which include pectic acid, pectinic acid, pectin, and protopectin. *Pectic acid* is an acid derivative of galactose, is soluble in water, and contains an abundance of carboxyl (—COOH) groups, making it both acidic and capable of salt formation. *Pectinic acid* is similar to pectic acid except that some of the carboxyl groups are esterified with methyl (—CH$_3$) groups, which makes it even more water soluble. Like pectic acid, pectinic acid is capable of reacting with metallic ions to form salts. *Pectin* includes those pectinic acids capable of forming jelly with sugar and acid. *Protopectin* is the large, insoluble molecule from which pectin is formed by hydrolysis.

Plant cells do not fit together perfectly. The *intercellular spaces* that occur provide access for the cells to the external environment and permit an exchange of gases necessary for photosynthesis.

PIGMENTS

The bright, attractive colors of fruits and vegetables come from unique combinations of pigments, whose main classes are the chlorophylls, the carotenoids, and the flavonoids. The presence of color and its intensity is in part caused by *conjugated double bonds* in the pigment structure. Conjugated double bonds are double bonds separated by single bonds.

Chlorophyll, the green pigment in plants, is contained in the chloroplasts. It is present in the leaves because their large surface area is ideal for the exchange of gases and the absorption of sunlight necessary for *photosynthesis,* the process by which carbon dioxide and water are converted to sugar and light energy to chemical energy. (See the discussion of photosynthesis in Chap. 4 for more detail.) Chlorophyll is similar in structure to heme (in hemoglobin), in that both contain four pyrrole rings connected to form a porphyrin nucleus. Chlorophyll is affected by the acidity of the cooking medium and the time and temperature of cooking. The bright green color is best preserved if the vegetable is heated rapidly and cooked for a short time.

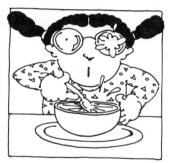

The *carotenoids* include several pigments with slightly different chemical structures. Located in the chromoplasts of plant cells, carotenoids are responsible for most of the yellow and orange and some of the red colors found in fruits and vegetables. They are insoluble in water but soluble in fats and organic solvents. For this reason, they are affected little by acid, alkali, length of cooking time, or volume of water. The color of the carotenoids is intensified with an increase in the number of double bonds. This is why *lycopene* is redder than *beta carotene,* and why *alpha carotene* is less orange than beta carotene. This is seen in the orange color of carrots, where beta carotene predominates, and in the red color of tomatoes, where lycopene is the main carotenoid. Other plants in which lycopene predominates include pink grapefruit, watermelon, and rose hips. Pigments from the carotenoid group are also found in pineapples, oranges, bell peppers, and paprika.

The water-soluble *flavonoids,* composed of two ring structures and a sugar group, are located in the cell sap of the plant cell. Derivatives of the flavonoid pigments are partially responsible for the flavor of certain foods, including citrus fruits. The presence of tanninlike substances in flavonoids in cider, wine, persimmons, bananas, chocolate, tea, and many fruits results in an astringent flavor when these substances react with proteins lining the mouth and in the saliva, decreasing lubrication. The flavonoids are also capable of chelating (binding with) metal ions, which makes these pigments valuable as antioxidants. As such, they bind free radicals and break the chain reaction in auto-oxidation (see Chap. 5). The flavonoids include two major groups of related compounds, the anthocyanins and the anthoxanthins.

The *anthocyanins* are the pigments responsible for the red, blue, pink, and

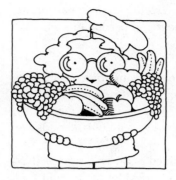

purple colors of fruits and vegetables. These pigments are found in such fruits and vegetables as raspberries, blueberries, Concord and other grapes, pomegranates, ripe gooseberries, strawberries, blackberries, radishes, red cabbage, and the skins of cherries, apples, plums, eggplants, peaches, and red potatoes. Because of the acidity of the anthocyanins, the color of foods with these pigments is not usually adversely affected by ordinary cooking. The pigments are more rapidly decomposed, however, by increases in temperature and pH, by enzymes, and by the presence of sugars, oxygen, ascorbic acid, and metals. In unlined cans, anthocyanins can combine with the metal, causing erosion, through which microbial invasion of the contents is possible. For this reason, foods containing anthocyanins are processed in enamel-lined cans.

The *anthoxanthins* include three structurally related compounds: flavones, flavonols, and flavanones. The pigments of this group, which range from pale yellow to almost colorless, occur alone in such vegetables as potatoes and yellow-skinned onions or in combination with other pigments, such as the anthocyanins. Derivatives of this group are found in asparagus, grapes, apples, citrus fruits, and tea. They are so widespread among fruits and vegetables that it is rare to find a plant without them. These pigments react with alkali or metal, especially iron and aluminum. Iron salts in tap water may react with anthoxanthin-containing fruits and vegetables to produce yellow brown discolorations. This is often seen in cooked white vegetables, including white potatoes (and sweet potatoes) and cauliflower.

Changes During Ripening

The ripening process, caused primarily by enzymes, brings fruits and vegetables to the peak of maturity, enhancing their quality. These enzymes continue to act even after the fruit or vegetable has ripened and cause it to spoil, with deterioration in texture, flavor, and nutritive value. The process can be viewed as changes in the following areas:

STRUCTURE

During ripening, the fruit or vegetable develops to its full size. The pulpy tissue surrounding the seeds becomes softer and more tender. The insoluble protopectins found in the cell walls of underripe fruit change to soluble pectic acid, resulting in reduced firmness and gelling qualities [4]. The demethylation (loss of methyl groups) of pectic substances also aids in the softening that accompanies ripening. An increase in water content also occurs.

COLOR

The color of the fruit or vegetable changes, with natural pigments (if present) predominating over the chlorophyll base of immature plants.

FLAVOR

In fruits, and to a lesser extent in some vegetables, the starch content changes to sugar, producing a mild, sweet flavor. The presence of tannins in some underripe fruits and vegetables is responsible for their astringent taste; with ripening and an increased water content, both tannins and organic acids are diluted, causing a milder flavor. The changes in pigments, sugar, and acid content also result in the full development of the plant's unique aroma.

NUTRITIVE VALUE

The starch content changes to sugar, especially in fruits, and the vitamin and mineral content increases. Under the proper conditions, the starch is hydrolyzed to sugar, mostly sucrose, glucose, and fructose. In peaches, the monosaccharides condense into sucrose as the fruit matures [5]. The organic acid content decreases as the sugar content increases with ripening. Fruits and vegetables are highest in nutritive value at the peak of maturity.

ARTIFICIAL RIPENING

Fruits and vegetables are often harvested early, while still firm, so that a minimum of the crop is lost from bruising. They are then artificially ripened [5] by carefully controlling the temperature and humidity of the surrounding air during storage and by using *ethylene gas*. By stimulating the fruit to respire by taking in oxygen and expelling carbon dioxide, the green pigment is discolored, which allows the other colors to develop. The permeability of the cell membrane is affected and the ripening process hastened.

Alterations During Cooking
STRUCTURE

Structural changes similar to those seen in ripening also occur during cooking. The cell walls become more permeable because of the transformation of the insoluble protopectins to soluble pectins in the presence of the plant's organic acids. Since the cell wall is held together by pectins, the cooked plant becomes soft. If fruit is cooked in sugar syrup, the water inside the cell is attracted to the more dense syrup. The water is replaced by sugar, which fills the dehydrated cells, with a firm, sweetened fruit the result. Moist heat will soften the cellulose, but the addition of sugar strengthens the cell wall structure. Vegetables are cooked when a specific amount of cell wall pectic acid has been solubilized, indicating a decreased adhesion between cells [6]. The presence of divalent ions (i.e., calcium, Ca^{2+}; magnesium, Mg^{2+}) helps minimize the loss of firmness that occurs with heating. By forming cross-links between carboxyl (—COOH) groups of pectinic acid molecules, these ions cause an increased rigidity of the cell wall [7]. Altering the acid content of the cooking medium also influences the cell wall integrity by inhibiting pectin-destroying enzymes. Cooking also denatures any proteins in the cytoplasm and cell membranes, with a resultant loss of their selective permeability. Water passes out of the cell by diffusion rather than osmosis, resulting in a loss of turgor, or crispness.

COLOR

The color changes that occur during cooking may be the result of an altered acid content or a reaction of the pigments with the cooking fluid or metals or both. The white and red pigments of vegetables are preserved if a small amount of dilute acid (that is, vinegar or lemon juice) is added to the cooking medium. The anthocyanins (the red and blue pigments) react with iron to form ferrous iron salts, causing brown discolorations. Many fruits and vegetables, such as raspberries, strawberries, peaches, and plums, are processed in coated containers to prevent their organic acids from reacting with the metal to produce metal salts and subsequent color change. Another solution to this problem is to package these foods in glass containers.

FLAVOR

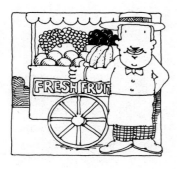

Alterations in the content of volatile and nonvolatile organic acids, sugar, tannins, minerals, and pigments in fruits and vegetables during cooking influences the flavor of the cooked plant. The volatile organic acids are heat labile (not stable in heat) and pass off easily from the cooking medium as vapor during cooking. The nonvolatile acids may pass off into the cooking liquid but are not lost as vapor. The reduction in the content of either type of acid results in the loss of some flavors. Short cooking periods and cooking in covered pans with little fluid will minimize these losses. The overcooking of sulfur-containing vegetables such as onions and members of the cabbage family (broccoli, turnips, kale, and brussels sprouts) make this undesirable flavor component more pronounced. The dilution of strong flavors, such as those in onions and cabbage, can be accomplished by cooking these vegetables uncovered in a fairly large amount of water. The addition of a small amount of dilute acid to the cooking medium will hasten the decomposition of the undesirable sulfur compounds.

NUTRITIVE VALUE

The greatest loss in nutritive value through cooking is in ascorbic acid content, through oxidation. This vitamin is unstable in heat; therefore most fruits and vegetables should be cooked only for short periods to retain maximum vitamin content. Losses are greater in fruits and vegetables cooked uncovered in large amounts of water than in those steamed or cooked covered in less water. Ascorbic acid is lost both through oxidation and from *leaching* out into the cooking medium. Short cooking periods, covering the food during cooking, and steaming it or cooking it in small amounts of boiling water are best for maximum retention of color, texture, flavor, and nutritive value.

References

1. U.S. Department of Agriculture. *Shopper's Guide to U.S. Grades for Food.* (Home Garden Bull. 58.) Washington, D.C.: U.S. Department of Agriculture, 1966.
2. Fahn, A. *Plant Anatomy* (2nd ed.). New York: Pergamon, 1979.
3. Kung, L. C. Complex carbohydrates of some Chinese foods. *J. Nutr.* 28:407, 1944.
4. Shewfelt, A. L., Paynter, V. A., and Jen, J. J. Textural changes and molecular characteristics of pectic constituents in ripening peaches. *J. Food Sci.* 36:573, 1971.
5. Peckham, G. C., and Freeland-Graves, J. H. *Foundations of Food Preparation* (4th ed.). New York: Macmillan, 1979. Pp. 160–161.
6. Hughes, J. C., Faulks, R. M., and Grant, A. Texture of cooked potatoes: Relationship between compressive strength, pectic substances and cell size of redskin tubers of different maturity. *Potato Res.* 18:495, 1975.
7. Campbell, A. M., Penfield, M. P., and Griswald, R. M. *The Experimental Study of Food* (2nd ed.). Boston: Houghton Mifflin, 1979. P. 169.

Suggested Readings

Berry, R. E.   Tropical fruits and vegetables as potential protein sources. *Food Technol.* 35:45, 1981.

Bressani, R., and Elias, L. G.   Improvement of the nutritional quality of food legumes. *Food Nutr. Bull.* 1:23, 1979.

Graham, H. D., and Negron do Bravo, E.   Composition of the breadfruit. *J. Food Sci.* 46:535, 1981.

Haytowits, D. B., Marsh, A. C., and Matthews, R. H.   Content of selected nutrients in raw, cooked, and processed legumes. *Food Technol.* 35:73, 1981.

Howard, R. A.   Captain Bligh and the Breadfruit. In N. Kretchmer and B. Robertson (eds.), *Human Nutrition.* San Francisco: Scientific American and W. H. Freeman, 1978. P. 98.

Hughes, R. E.   Fruit flavonoids: Some nutritional implications. *J. Hum. Nutr.* 32:47, 1978.

Labuza, T. P.   Effects of processing, storage, and handling on nutrient retention in foods: Effects of dehydration and storage. *Food Technol.* 27:20, 1973.

Matthee, V., and Appledorf, H.   Effect of cooking on vegetable fiber. *J. Food Sci.* 43:1344, 1978.

Nagy, S., and Shaw, P. E.   *Tropical and Subtropical Fruits: Composition, Properties and Uses.* Westport, Conn.: AVI Publishing, 1980.

Robinson, J. R. K.   Fruit in the diet of prehistoric man and of the hunter-gatherer. *J. Hum. Nutr.* 32:19, 1978.

Rockland, L. B., and Radke, T. M.   Legume protein quality. *Food Technol.* 35:79, 1981.

Salaman, R. N.   The Social Influence of the Potato. In N. Kretchmer and B. Robertson (eds.), *Human Nutrition.* San Francisco: Scientific American and W. H. Freeman, 1978. P. 115.

Wadsworth, G. R.   The use, dietary significance, and production of fruit. *J. Hum. Nutr.* 32:27, 1978.

Chapter 14

MILK AND MILK PRODUCTS

Designed for the nutrition of the very young of the species, milk is one of nature's most complete foods. It contains protein of high biologic value, essential fatty acids and fat-soluble vitamins, calcium in its most absorbable form, and a unique carbohydrate, lactose, which enhances the absorption and utilization of milk's minerals and proteins. The components of milk work synergistically toward their own unique optimum utilization.

Milk plays a central role in nutrition. The lactating mammary cell has been compared to the photosynthesizing cell of plants in its importance in sustaining life. Besides being important for its nutritional value, milk serves a vital commercial and economic role. The production, distribution, and sale of dairy products is the seventh largest industry in the United States, involving over 118 billion pounds of milk produced by over 15 million cows (Fig. 14-1) [1].

Throughout this chapter all references to milk will apply to cow's milk unless otherwise specified. For a discussion of human milk, see Chap. 26.

Composition and Nutritive Value

The composition of selected milks is given in Table 14-1. Milk contains many substances in very small quantities, ranging from 0.1 percent to parts per billion, including sugars, sugar phosphates, proteoses, peptones, fatty acids, amino acids, nitrogenous bases, gases, vitamins, and minerals. The most important components, however, are lipids, carbohydrates, and proteins.

LIPIDS

The lipid, or *butterfat,* content of milk is important for several reasons [2]. From an economic standpoint, butterfat plays an important role in determining the price of milk and milk products. It also serves as a carrier for fat-soluble vitamins and contains the essential fatty acids linolenic acid and arachidonic acid. The amount of butterfat present also influences the flavor of milk and milk products and therefore consumer acceptance.

The lipids in milk exist as minute droplets that under the proper conditions rise to the surface to form a layer of cream. The lipid droplet or globule consists of a membranous coat surrounding a core of pure glyceride. The lipid globule membranes, layers of phospholipid and protein, stabilize the lipid globules. The membrane surrounding the lipid globule is derived from the outer membrane of the lactating mammary cell at the time of secretion. The membrane includes some of the milk's cholesterol, phospholipids, glycolipids, and all of the vitamin A and carotene. It also includes some proteins and enzymes.

The principal fatty acids found in the glycerides of milk include oleic acid, palmitic acid, and stearic acid. Many others can be found in amounts of less than 1 percent. The lipid in cow's milk is unusual in its content of short-chain fatty acids, including caproic and butyric acids (the latter is unique to milk). These fatty acids are highly odorous and contribute to the flavor (and the development of off-flavors) of milk and milk products.

FIG. 14-1. Dairy calves grazing on farmland in Carroll County, Maryland. (U.S. Department of Agriculture–SCS photo by Tim McCabe.)

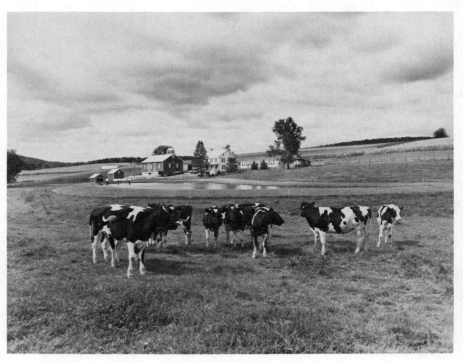

Other fat-soluble substances present in butterfat include carotene and xanthophyll, sterols, and the fat-soluble vitamins. Carotene and xanthophyll, which impart a yellowish color to milk, are derived from the feed the animal eats (vegetable matter) and are not synthesized by the animal. The sterols present include cholesterol, phospholipids, lecithin, and cephalin. The phospholipids include choline and phosphorus; lecithin contains choline. Oxidation of choline produces trimethylamine, a gas, which at ordinary temperatures produces a fishy odor.

CARBOHYDRATES

The disaccharide *lactose,* which is about one-fifth as sweet as table sugar, is the main carbohydrate found uniquely in milk. Trace amounts of glucose, galactose, and other sugars are also present. Lactose is not very soluble and may come out of solution during the heat treatment of condensed milk, imparting a grainy texture to the finished product (see Types of Milk, below). Lactic acid bacteria convert lactose to lactic acid in souring milk, giving it a characteristic flavor.

The evolutionary purpose of lactose may be to maintain the osmotic balance of the lactating cell, and to encourage certain desirable bacteria to thrive in the intestine [1]. Lactose is the main synergistic agent in milk, enhancing protein and mineral utilization. Because it is slowly hydrolyzed and absorbed, lactose promotes the proliferation of gastrointestinal flora, lowering the pH of the gut and aiding calcium absorption.

TABLE 14-1. Composition of selected milks, per 3½ ounces

Milk	Calories	Protein (gm)	Carbohydrate (gm)	Fiber (gm)	Fat (gm)	Sodium (mg)	Potassium (mg)	Calcium (mg)	Magnesium (mg)	Phosphorus (mg)	Iron (mg)	Thiamin (µg)	Riboflavin (µg)	Niacin (mg)	Ascorbic acid (mg)	Vitamin A (IU)	Vitamin D (IU)
Cow's	66	3.5	4.9	0	3.5	50	144	118	13	84	tr	33	172	0.1	0.8	139	—
Goat's	67	3.2	4.6	0	4.0	34	180	129	17	106	0.1	40	110	0.3	1.0	160	—
Human	77	1.1	9.5	0	4.0	16	51	33	4	14	0.1	10	40	0.2	5.0	240	—
Reindeer	234	10.8	4.1	0	19.6	157	159	254	—	198	0.1	—	—	—	—	—	—

Source: C. F. Church and H. N. Church, *Food Values of Portions Commonly Used.* Philadelphia: Lippincott, 1975.

LACTOSE INTOLERANCE

Sensitivity to milk's unique carbohydrate, lactose, is probably the most prevalent food allergy in the world [3]. Because it is a disaccharide, lactose must be broken down before being absorbed, since only monosaccharides are found in the blood. The enzyme *lactase,* located on the brush border of the small intestine, is responsible for hydrolyzing this sugar. When lactase is missing or reduced because of genetic defect, chronic disease, or nutritional insult, the undigested lactose is transported into the large intestine. The increased osmolarity caused by the presence of sugar in the bowel draws water from the surrounding tissues into the intestinal lumen. Bacteria normally present in the colon ferment the undigested lactose, producing organic acids, carbon dioxide, and hydrogen. All of these responses to lactose result in symptoms of intolerance in susceptible persons—abdominal cramps, bloating, diarrhea, and flatulence.

There are three main types of lactose intolerance. In the rare instance when lactase is absent at birth, it is considered an inborn error of metabolism and remains throughout life. The second form is often temporary, caused by inflammation or damage to the epithelial mucosa resulting from a disease. Upon recovery, lactase activity in these persons usually returns to normal. Chronic nutritional insults such as marasmus, kwashiorkor, parasites, infections, and diarrhea may result in permanent mucosal damage and impaired lactase activity.

The third, and most prevalent, type of lactose intolerance is known as racial intolerance or primary adult low lactase activity. It is most prevalent among Orientals, Jews, Africans, and cultures that never used dairy products in adulthood. This type occurs in late childhood after a normal infancy and early childhood. It is a decline in the level of lactase activity after the major skeletal growth spurt is completed. This type of intolerance is prevalent in the majority of the world's population.

PROTEINS

The proteins found in milk are of high biologic value, containing all the essential amino acids. The many proteins in milk may be divided into two groups: the casein fraction and the whey or serum protein fraction.

CASEIN

About 80 percent of the protein in milk is *casein*, combined mainly with calcium and phosphorus in the form of micelles suspended in solution. There are four distinct types of casein, differing in molecular weight and chemical characteristics: alpha, beta, gamma, and kappa. They comprise 50, 30, 5, and 15 percent, respectively, of the total casein content. Kappa casein uniquely contains the carbohydrate sialic acid, which makes it resistant to aggregation by calcium ions, unlike the other types of casein, and keeps the casein micelles from aggregating [1]. During the processing of milk to make cheese, the enzyme *rennin* is used to split off the peptide containing sialic acid from kappa casein, destabilizing the casein micelles, precipitating them out of solution, and thereby producing curds. The watery portion, the *whey*, is drawn off, and the curds are used to make cheese. The whey proteins, or *serum proteins*, remaining include *lactoglobulin* and *lactalbumin*.

WHEY PROTEINS

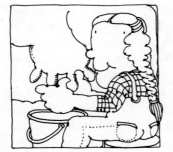

Lactoglobulin, like casein, is a protein unique to milk. It accounts for about 0.4 percent of the total milk content and is found in two common forms (A and B) and two uncommon forms (C and D). This protein contains a high proportion of the amino acid cysteine, which has a reduced sulfur group (—SH). On heating, the sulfur groups are released from the protein as hydrogen sulfide, giving cooked milk its distinctive flavor and scent. A factor present in lactoglobulin may cause milk to decrease the volume of yeast bread. This factor is inactivated by scalding the milk before adding it to the dough.

ENZYMES

The enzyme proteins in milk perform vital and unique roles. They incorporate fatty acids into glycerides and phospholipids, convert stearic acid into oleic acid, and can synthesize lactose from added glucose.

MILK ALLERGY

In most instances of cow's milk allergy, hypersensitivity is due to the protein component, specifically the presence of lactoglobulins and lactalbumins. Infants with this allergic reaction can usually tolerate formula prepared with evaporated milk, since the two offending proteins have been heat-denatured in processing. Goat's milk can also be tried, since its lactoglobulins and lactalbumins are of different molecular composition from those of cow's milk and may prove to be innocuous. One of the most serious side effects of milk sensitivity in infants is the occult loss of blood into the gastrointestinal tract, with resultant anemia. For further details on infant feeding, see Chap. 23.

VITAMINS AND MINERALS

Milk and milk products are good sources of both fat-soluble and water-soluble vitamins. The amounts of fat-soluble vitamins are proportional to the amounts found in the diet of the cow. The water-soluble vitamins present are independent of the diet, as they are synthesized by bacteria in the cow's rumen and other tissues.

Whole milk, cream, and products made from them are good sources of vitamin A. The content of this vitamin is highest during summer in milk from cows on green pastures. The amount varies with the amount of green food available to the cow. Carotene, the precursor of vitamin A, gives milk a yellowish tinge. The amounts of vitamin D vary also with the type of feed and the cow's exposure to sunlight. To ensure adequate intake of vitamin D, it is added to milk (about 400 IU per quart).

Milk is also an excellent source of riboflavin, found in the nonfat portion of the milk. This vitamin gives a greenish-yellow color to whey. Thiamin is also found in milk in fair quantities. Small amounts of ascorbic acid are also found in milk, but much of this unstable vitamin is lost during handling, storage, and pasteurization.

The mineral salts present in milk include chlorides, phosphates, citrates, sulfates, and bicarbonates of sodium, potassium, calcium, and magnesium. They are important because of their influence on the condition and stability of the proteins, especially the casein fraction. The trace elements, especially copper and iron, are important because of their influence in the development of off-flavors in milk and milk products. The chief mineral, calcium, is in the form of calcium phosphate, the most readily assimilable form, and in good quantities.

FACTORS INFLUENCING VARIATIONS IN COMPOSITION

The values given in Table 14-1 represent the average composition of cow's milk, but wide variations can and do exist for many reasons [2]. There are *inherited variations:* Different breeds of dairy cattle have characteristic differences in the composition of the milk they produce; additional variations exist between individual cows within a single breed. The *nutrition of the cow* affects the composition of the milk: Variations in the feed content of iodine, carotene, vitamin A, and some trace elements are reflected in the milk. The *season and the temperature* produce variations: Milk has a higher fat and protein content in the winter and in the summer; temperatures greater than 85°F (37°C) and below 40°F (18°C) cause an increase in the fat content. The *age of the cow* affects the fat content of the milk: Fat content decreases with increasing age. The *stage of lactation* also affects composition: Early in lactation, the milk contains more protein and minerals and less lactose than does later milk.

Sanitation, Processing, and Grading

The production and distribution of milk is under strict sanitary controls administered by local health departments. The main purpose of the controls is to ensure a safe milk, free from bacteria, toxins, and foreign substances. These controls also help produce milk that has a low initial bacterial count, high nutritive value, and good flavor and keeping quality [4]. Although the sanitary controls are not the same in every community, most states and cities follow the U.S. Public Health Service milk ordinance and code [5] as a guide.

PASTEURIZATION

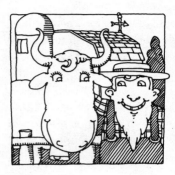

Milk cannot be marketed raw, or in an unprocessed state, because of the possibility of its carrying tuberculosis, diphtheria, typhoid, undulant fever, or scarlet fever bacteria. (Some states do allow raw milk to be sold if it has been certified.) Almost all fresh fluid milks are *pasteurized*, or heated for a specified time at a certain temperature. The primary purpose of pasteurization is to destroy all pathogenic bacteria and most of the nonpathogenic organisms. It also inactivates (denatures) certain enzymes that would produce off-flavors.

The two methods used in pasteurization are the flash method and the holding method. In the former, the milk is brought to 160°F (71°C) and held there for not less than 15 seconds. In the latter method, the milk is brought to 143°F (62°C) and held there for not less than 30 minutes. Both methods destroy the disease-producing bacteria and greatly reduce other, less harmful strains of bacteria.

By measuring the activity of phosphatase, a naturally occurring enzyme in milk, the adequacy of pasteurization can be measured. When this enzyme is denatured, or inactivated, the milk has been heated sufficiently also to destroy pathogenic organisms.

Pasteurization causes only small changes in the nutritive value of milk, including a slight decrease in the heat-labile vitamins thiamin and ascorbic acid. Since milk is not a good source of these nutrients to begin with, pasteurization is not destructive of any nutrients for which milk is a dependable source.

MILK GRADES

The basis for grading fresh milk is its bacterial count, with grade A having the lowest, although grades B and C are also wholesome and safe. According to the U.S. Public Health Service standards, the allowable bacterial counts per milliliter are as follows: grade A pasteurized, 30,000; grade A raw, 50,000; grade B pasteurized, 50,000; grade B raw, 1,000,000.

HOMOGENIZATION

By this process the lipid droplets in milk are reduced in size and stabilized in suspension so they do not separate out as a layer of cream. The milk is forced through small openings under pressure, which breaks the lipid globules up into smaller ones. *Homogenization* decreases the size of the lipid particles, increases their total number, and therefore increases their total surface area. This stabilizes the milk emulsion, preventing the lipid from rising to the surface.

Homogenization changes some of the qualities of milk: it becomes whiter, blander, and more viscous [6]. This process also requires an increase in cooking time because of the increased time needed for heat penetration. It produces a creamier product but one that tends to curdle more rapidly.

VITAMIN D FORTIFICATION

Irradiation of milk with ultraviolet light can transform the cholesterol compounds of milk into vitamin D (see Cholesterol in Chap. 5) but can also produce harmful toxisterols. For this reason, irradiation, once the primary fortification process, has been abandoned, and instead vitamin D is either added directly to the milk or the cows are fed irradiated feed. Usually, 400 IU of vitamin D is added per quart of milk.

Milk Products
TYPES OF MILK

As mentioned above, the butterfat content influences the flavor of milk and therefore consumer acceptance. Milk is also classified by its butterfat content, with *whole fluid milk* containing at least 3.25% butterfat. *Fluid skim milk* contains 0 to 0.5% butterfat and may be fortified with vitamins A and D. *Fluid low fat milk* contains 2% butterfat and 8.5 to 10% nonfat milk solids. *Chocolate milk* is made from whole milk, *chocolate drink* from skim milk, and *chocolate-flavored milk* from cocoa and whole milk.

CONCENTRATED MILKS AND CREAM

In *evaporated whole* and *skim milks* about 60 percent of the water is removed; they are then sealed and sterilized. They may be enriched with vitamin D. *Sweetened condensed milk* is made in a similar manner, except that it contains 44% sugar. *Dry milk* may be whole or nonfat. *Cream* includes heavy cream, with 36% butterfat, coffee cream (table or light) with 18 to 20 percent, and half-and-half, with 10 to 20 percent. *Sour cream* is light cream soured with lactic acid.

CULTURED MILKS

The sour flavor produced by bacterial breakdown of lactose into lactic acid gives cultured milk its distinction. The nutritive value of cultured, or fermented, milk is the same as the product from which it is prepared. The main cultured products used in the United States are buttermilk, yogurt, and acidophilus milk.

Buttermilk was originally made from the liquid remaining after butter was made from cream. It contains acid plus the phospholipid membranes that surrounded the fat globules before they were broken. Buttermilk is made today from pasteurized skim milk treated with a culture of lactic acid bacteria.

Yogurt can be made from skim, partly skim, or whole milk, and can be fortified with 3% nonfat dry milk. It is homogenized and then heated. The heat treatment involves holding at 180 to 185°F (82 to 85°C) for an amount of time and then cooling to 113°F (45°C). The cooked milk is then inoculated with a mixture of *Streptococcus thermophilus, Bacterium bulgarius,* and *Plocamo bacterium yoghouri* [4] and held for several hours at 106 to 108°F (41 to 42°C).

Acidophilus milk is made by inoculating milk with a culture of *Lactobacillus acidophilus.* It can be used therapeutically for enteric (intestinal) disorders to provide a change in bacterial flora.

Alterations During Cooking and Other Processing

Heat is the most important treatment milk receives during processing and food preparation. Prolonged heating adversely affects both flavor and odor. Heated milk forms a precipitate of albumin, which tends to scorch. When milk is heated

FIG. 14-2. Cheese making in a milk plant. (Courtesy Food and Agriculture Organization of the United Nations.)

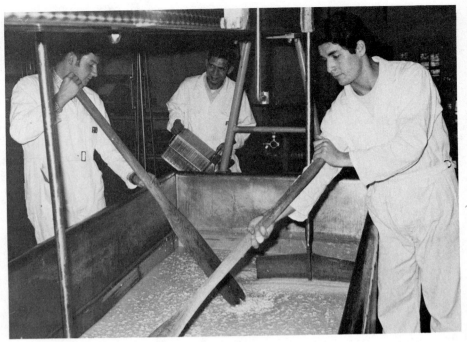

in an uncovered pan, a surface skin of coagulated proteins, fat, and minerals results from a drying of the top of the milk.

LIPIDS

The two processes that alter the lipids in milk are homogenization and churning. As discussed above, *homogenization* is the process by which the lipid globules are broken up and suspended in solution. *Churning* is the process of phase inversion, changing from an oil-in-water emulsion of cream to the water-in-oil emulsion of butter. With agitation, the lipid globules aggregate, forming butter.

CARBOHYDRATES

During heat treatment and storage, lactose participates in *Maillard-type (nonen-zymatic) browning reactions*. It undergoes *carmelization* under intense heating such as in sterilization. (See Chap. 4 for a description of these reactions.)

PROTEINS

Milk proteins can be coagulated by heat, acid, or the enzyme rennin. Heat-induced changes are responsible for the development of cooked flavor, brought about by the uncoiling of the protein structure so that the sulfhydryl groups (—SH) are more reactive and accessible. The formation of a gel or curdling both result from destabilization of the casein micelles. When added to heated milk, rennin brings about the clotting of casein. Boiling and an alkaline reaction retard the action of rennin, preventing clotting. The clots are gel-like and contain most

TABLE 14-2. Nutritive value of selected dairy products

Dairy product	Amount	Calories	Protein (gm)	Carbohydrate (gm)	Fiber (gm)	Calcium (mg)	Fat (gm)	Iron (mg)	Thiamin (μg)	Riboflavin (μg)	Niacin (mg)	Ascorbic acid (mg)	Vitamin A (IU)	Vitamin D (IU)
Whole milk	8 fl oz	159	8.5	12.0	0	**288**	8.6	tr	**70**	**420**	0.2	2	**340**	—
Skim milk	8 fl oz	88	8.8	12.6	0	**298**	0.2	tr	**100**	**440**	0.2	2	tr	—
Skim milk, fortified	8 fl oz	105	9.8	13.9	0	**359**	1.2	tr	**240**	510	2.5	—	**1000**	**100**
Evaporated milk	4 fl oz	165	8.4	11.6	0	**300**	9.5	0.1	**48**	**408**	0.2	1	**348**	—
Sweetened condensed milk	⅓ cup	321	8.1	54.3	0	**262**	8.7	0.1	**80**	**380**	0.2	1	**360**	—
Buttermilk, whole	8 fl oz	92	8.1	12.0	0	**293**	2.4	tr	**100**	**410**	0.2	2	100	—
Buttermilk, skim	8 fl oz	88	8.8	12.4	0	**296**	0.2	tr	**100**	**440**	0.2	2	tr	—
Nonfat dried milk	4 tbsp	103	10.0	14.6	0	**367**	0.2	0.1	**100**	50	0.3	2	8	—
Whole dried milk	4 tbsp	140	7.4	10.7	0	**252**	7.7	0.1	**80**	**400**	0.2	2	**316**	—
Butter	1 tbsp	100	0.1	tr	0	3.0	11.3	—	—	—	—	0	**462**	—
Cheese														
Cheddar	1 oz	112	7.0	0.6	0	**211**	9.1	0.3	8	**130**	tr	0	**370**	—
Cottage	3½ oz	106	**13.6**	2.9	0	94	4.2	tr	30	**250**	0.1	0	170	—
Cream	1 oz	105	2.2	0.6	0	17	10.6	0.1	6	60	tr	0	**430**	—
Gruyère	1 oz	115	8.1	0.5	0	**308**	8.9	0.3	2	**140**	0.1	0	**560**	—
Swiss	1 oz	104	7.7	0.5	0	**259**	7.8	0.3	3	**110**	tr	0	**406**	—
Cream														
Coffee	1 tbsp	32	0.4	0.6	0	16	3.1	tr	4	20	tr	tr	125	—
Half-and-half	1 oz	40	1.0	1.4	0	32	3.5	tr	9	50	tr	tr	140	—
Sour or cultured	1 oz	57	0.8	1.0	0	31	5.4	—	10	40	tr	0	**230**	—
Whipping	1 tbsp	45	0.4	0.6	0	13	4.7	tr	3	20	tr	tr	190	—
Ice cream (10% fat)	⅙ quart	174	4.0	18.7	0	131	9.5	0.1	**40**	190	0.1	1	**400**	—

tr = trace.

Note: Dashes indicate no significant data available. Boldface values are one-fourth or more of the recommended daily dietary allowance (1980) for that nutrient for the average woman aged 23–50.

Source: C. F. Church and H. N. Church, *Food Values of Portions Commonly Used.* Philadelphia: Lippincott, 1975.

of the calcium. Milk that has been curdled into curds and whey is termed *clobbered milk.* The curds are then pressed into cheese (Fig. 14-2).

When acid is added to milk, as in the preparation of cream of tomato soup, casein precipitates out of solution, forming casein salts and curdled milk. The resultant curd is soft, and most of the calcium remains in the whey.

NUTRITIVE VALUE

The nutritive value of milk and milk products is not greatly altered by processing, except for a reduction in some of the heat-sensitive vitamins, such as thiamin and ascorbic acid. The nutritive value of selected dairy products is given in Table 14-2.

References

1. Patton, S.   Milk. In N. Kretchmer and B. Robertson (eds.), *Human Nutrition*. San Francisco: Scientific American and W. H. Freeman, 1978. Pp. 89–93.
2. Paul, P. C., and Palmer, H. H. (eds.).   *Food Theory and Applications*. New York: Wiley, 1972. Pp. 564, 570.
3. Luke, B.   Lactose intolerance during pregnancy: Significance and solutions. *Am. J. Matern. Child Nurs.* 2:92, 1977.
4. Peckham, G. C., and Freeland-Graves, J. H.   *Foundations of Food Preparation* (4th ed.). New York: Macmillan, 1979. Pp. 260, 262.
5. U.S. Department of Health, Education and Welfare, Public Health Service.   *Milk Ordinance and Code* (Public Health Bull. 229). Washington, D.C.: Public Health Service, 1965.
6. Paul, P. C., and Palmer, H. H. (eds.).   *Food Theory and Applications*. New York: Wiley, 1972. P. 585.

Suggested Readings

Colman, N., Hettiarachchy, N., and Herbert, V.   Detection of a milk factor that facilitates folate uptake by intestinal cells. *Science* 211:1427, 1981.

Folate binder in milk may facilitate folate absorption. *Nutr. Rev.* 40:90, 1982.

Kon, S. K.   Milk and milk products in human nutrition. *FAO Nutr. Studies* 27:1972.

Kretchmer, N.   Lactose and lactase: A historical perspective (Memorial Lecture). *Gastroenterology* 61:805, 1971.

Kretchmer, N.   Lactose and Lactase. *Sci. Am.* 227:71, 1972.

Kroger, M.   Quality of yogurt. *J. Dairy Sci.* 59:344, 1976.

McCracken, R. D.   Lactase deficiency: An example of dietary evolution. *Curr. Anthropol.* 12:479, 1971.

Massiello, F. J.   Changing trends in consumer margarines. *J. Am. Oil Chem. Soc.* 55:262, 1978.

Morr, C. V.   Chemistry of milk proteins in food processing. *J. Dairy Sci.* 58:977, 1975.

Protective role of lipids in human milk. *Nutr. & the MD* January 1982.

Slattery, C. W.   Casein micelle structure: An examination of models (review). *J. Dairy Sci.* 59:1547, 1976.

Tamine, A. Y., and Deeth, H. C.   Yogurt: Technology and Biochemistry. *J. Food Prot.* 43:939, 1980.

The vitamin D activity of milk. *Nutr. Rev.* 40:27, 1982.

U.S. Department of Health, Education and Welfare, Public Health Services.   *Federal and State Standards for the Composition of Milk Products* (Handbook 51). Washington, D.C.: Public Health Service, 1971.

Webb, B. H., Johnson, A. H., and Alford, J. A. (eds.).   *Fundamentals of Dairy Chemistry* (2nd ed.). Westport, Conn.: AVI Publishing, 1974.

Chapter 15

EGGS

Like cereal grains and milk, eggs are a food designed by nature for the nourishment of the young of the species. Eggs therefore contain nearly all nutrients necessary to sustain growth and development. They also have a defense system against microbial invasion and are packaged in their own unique and ingenious container.

Eggs contain a wide variety of nutrients but are best known for their protein content. Used as the standard against which all other proteins are judged, egg protein is of the highest biologic value, with all the essential amino acids present in sufficient amounts.

The structure of the hen's egg is unique (Fig. 15-1). The outer coating is mostly calcium, which hardens during laying. Inside it contains a cushion of air (the air cell) that acts as a shock absorber. In addition, the yolk is surrounded by a membrane that thickens into cords at the points of attachment to the shell, serving to cushion and suspend the yolk and developing embryo, while still allowing them to revolve.

Structure and Composition

The *shell* comprises about 11 percent of the total egg and is composed mainly of calcium carbonate. The shell is granular, hard, translucent, and sufficiently porous to permit respiration of the developing embryo. The pores are filled with a thin layer of organic matter that prevents invasion by microorganisms [1]. The condition of the shell and the shell membranes influences the breaking strength, moisture and carbon dioxide loss, and susceptibility to microbial invasion of the egg.

Within the shell are two *membranes* that separate to form the *air cell* at the large (broad) end of the egg. The air cell forms as the egg cools and the contents contract after laying. On each side of the yolk are dense cordlike strands, the *chalazae*, composed mostly of mucin. They serve to anchor the yolk near the center of the egg and allow it to revolve. The yolk is surrounded by the *vitelline membrane*.

The *egg white*, or albumen, comprises about 58 percent of the total egg and is composed of several layers: a thin layer adjacent to the shell, a thick viscous layer within, and a thin layer surrounding the yolk and separated from it by the vitelline membrane.

The *yolk*, about 31 percent of the egg, is more concentrated than the egg white, having less water and more fat and protein. The yolk contains the nutritive material to support the growth and development of the maturing embryo. The *blastoderm* is the germinative portion of the fertilized egg, located on the uppermost surface of the yolk. In the unfertilized egg, it is termed the *blastodisc*. In fresh eggs, it tends to rise to the top of the albumen, which surrounds it.

FIG. 15-1. Structure of a hen's egg.

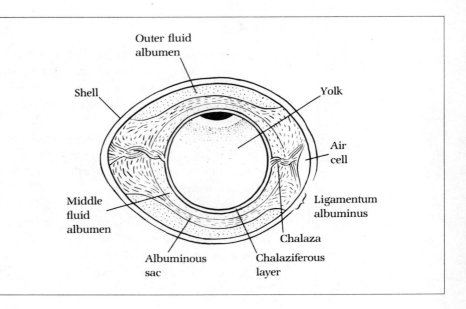

Nutritive Value
EGG WHITE

The egg white is composed of about 87.6% water, 10.9% protein, 1.1% carbohydrate, and traces of lipid. The presence of the small amount of carbohydrate causes brown discolorations when heated as the result of Maillard-type reactions between the sugar and proteins present (see Chap. 4). The proteins in eggs are of the highest biologic value, supplying all the essential amino acids needed for tissue growth, development, and repair. Milk protein, chiefly casein, ranks next highest. For this reason, egg protein is used as a standard against which all other proteins are compared.

The protein of egg white includes about 64% *ovalbumin,* a phosphoglycoprotein that when denatured by heat is an important structural component of baked products. Ovalbumin contains all of the sulfhydryl groups (—SH) in egg white. Denaturation by heat, agitation, or other denaturing agents is necessary to make these groups reactive.

Conalbumin, which accounts for about 12 percent of egg white protein, is characterized by its ability to bind divalent and trivalent metallic ions such as iron. This protein inhibits the growth of certain microorganisms that require iron. The complex of conalbumin with iron is more resistant than other proteins to denaturation by heat and chemical treatments. A pink color resulting from the reaction of conalbumin with iron is produced when egg white is in contact with iron during processing (e.g., iron utensils and pots) and disappears when conalbumin is denatured during heating. Conalbumin interacts with lysozyme to form a soluble complex.

Ovomucoid, a glycoprotein comprising about 12 percent of the egg white protein, is exceptionally heat stable. It is the inhibiting agent in egg white to the proteolytic enzyme trypsin.

About 8 percent of egg white proteins are *globulins*. This group of proteins is important for the foaming properties of egg whites. *Lysozyme,* one of the globulins, lyses certain microorganisms, contributing to the resistance of the intact egg to bacterial invasion. Lysozyme is relatively stable to most denaturing agents and conditions.

Ovomucin, another glycoprotein, comprises about 2 percent of the egg white protein. It contributes to the jellylike nature, or thickness, of egg white. Ovomucin and lysozyme may form a complex that is in part responsible for the thinning of egg white during storage (see Physiochemical Changes During Processing and Storage, below).

Avidin, about 0.05 percent of the egg white protein, binds the vitamin biotin and makes it biologically unavailable. Avidin is rendered inactive (denatured), however, by heat.

EGG YOLK

The egg yolk contains about 49% water, 16% protein, 32% fat, and traces of carbohydrate. Most of the proteins are lipoproteins, such as *lipovitellin* and *lipovitellenin.* Other proteins, such as *phosvitin,* a phosphoprotein, and *livetins,* water-soluble proteins containing sulfur, are also present.

The lipids in eggs, most of which are complexed with protein as lipoproteins, are concentrated in the yolk. The three types of lipids in the yolk are *triacylglycerols, phospholipids* (mostly lecithin and cephalin), and *sterols* (mainly cholesterol). Cholesterol is maintained in a colloidal state by the emulsifier lecithin.

MINERALS

The mineral content of the hen's diet is reflected in the concentration of minerals in the egg. Calcium is the most abundant mineral, but it is concentrated in the shell. In the yolk, phosphorus is most prevalent; other minerals present include calcium, magnesium, chlorine, potassium, sodium, sulfur, and iron. Most of the iron content of the egg is concentrated in the yolk. Minerals present in the greatest amounts in the egg white are sulfur, sodium, potassium, and chlorine; present in smaller amounts are phosphorus, calcium, magnesium, and iron. The sulfur present in the egg white reacts with silver utensils to form dark stains of silver sulfide.

PIGMENTS

The shell color, brown or white, is a breed characteristic and is not related to the egg quality. The egg white contains only the pigment *ovoflavin,* which gives a greenish-yellow cast. This is due to the presence of the vitamin riboflavin, the level of which is influenced by the hen's diet. The yolk contains pigments of the carotenoid group, primarily xanthophylls: reds, oranges, and yellows. The intensity of the pigmentation is influenced by the composition of the feed and its vitamin A content and very slightly by heredity. These pigments are derived from carotenoid-rich plants, such as corn, grass, and alfalfa. If hens are allowed free access to such plants, and thereby increase the level of dietary vitamin A, the eggs produced will have darker yolks.

Egg Quality, Grades, and Weights
QUALITY

Most marketed eggs are infertile; the quality of fertile eggs suffers as a consequence of embryo development. Although egg quality is determined mostly by inheritance, adding nutrients to the hen's feed can affect the egg's composition. Quality factors include both exterior and interior characteristics. Exterior factors include shell shape and texture, soundness, and cleanliness. Interior factors are evaluated by *candling*, the process of viewing an egg before a light source in a darkened room (Fig. 15-2). Factors evaluated include yolk centering and movement; clarity, firmness, and defects of the white; integrity of the shell and its normality; and the depth and regularity of the air cell. Marketed eggs are *sorted* (separated by size and grade); this classification benefits the consumer because it provides an indication of the internal quality of the egg.

GRADES

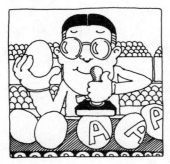

Eggs are sold commercially by weight and grade, two factors independent of each other. The grades and weights of eggs are based on standards established by the U.S. Department of Agriculture (USDA) [2]. Factors judged when grading include the height of the egg, centering of the yolk, and the viscosity of the egg white. The grades include AA (best for poaching and all cooking methods), A (not ideal for poaching, but fine for other methods), and B (good for scrambling or blended cooked foods). As the grade of the egg decreases, the size of the air cell increases, the white becomes thinner, and the yolk becomes more distinct in candling; the yolk from a lower grade egg also appears flattened and enlarged when the egg is broken from the shell. Eggs of any size may be of any grade, and all grades have the same nutritional value.

SIZES AND WEIGHTS

The size and weight classification for eggs is given in Fig. 15-3. When there is less than a 7¢ difference between sizes, it is more economical to buy the larger size. Medium and large eggs are assumed to be used for most recipes. Many factors influence egg size, including the size of the hen, the age at which she commences laying, the season of the year, the temperature of her environment, and the composition of her feed [3]. Eggs laid in winter retain their physical quality better than those laid in summer; eggs from younger birds have egg whites of greater volume when beaten [4].

EGG PRODUCT INSPECTION ACT

This act became law in 1970 and is administered by the Poultry Division, Consumer and Marketing Service, USDA. It ensures wholesome, unadulterated, and truthfully labeled egg products for the consumer. It provides for mandatory continuous inspection of plants processing egg products. Imported eggs must be inspected to meet the same standards as domestic eggs.

Physiochemical Changes During Processing and Storage
AGING AND STORAGE

Soon after the egg is laid, physical and chemical changes take place: The size of the air cell increases, the yolk enlarges and its membranes weaken, carbon dioxide is lost, the egg white becomes more alkaline and thinner, and the odor and flavor deteriorate. These changes may be retarded by proper handling, but

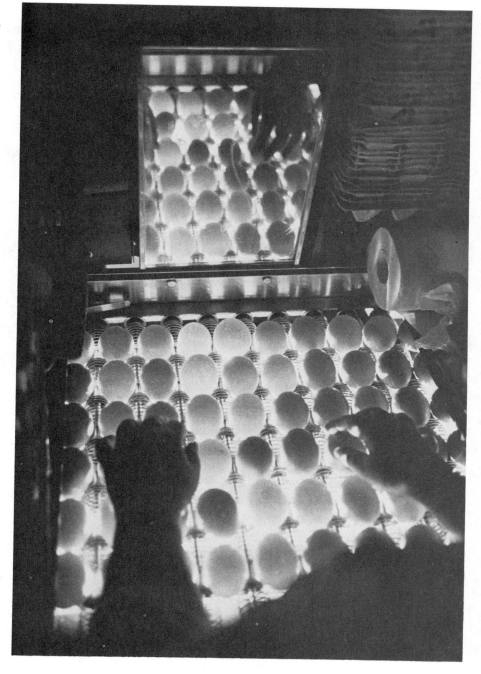

FIG. 15-2. Candling operation at a South Carolina egg farm. All eggs pass over a high-intensity light to allow experienced eyes to check their internal condition. (U.S. Department of Agriculture photo by David F. Warren.)

FIG. 15-3. Weight classes of eggs. Minimum weight is given in ounces per dozen. (U.S. Department of Agriculture photo.)

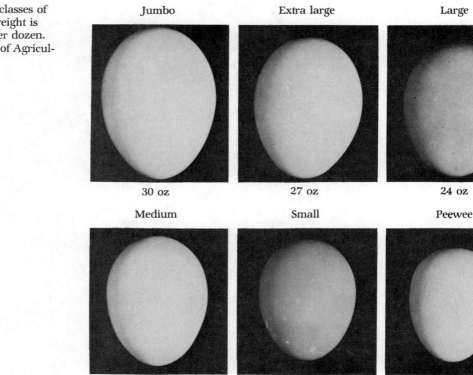

they cannot be prevented entirely. All these changes are influenced by temperature. Proper refrigeration can prolong the life of the egg up to 6 months.

For home care of eggs, a constant temperature is better than varying temperatures. The eggs should be refrigerated with the broad ends up, to prevent the movement of the air cell toward the yolk. Because they pick up odors and flavors from other foods by absorption through their porous shells, eggs should be stored covered. Eggs should not be washed before storage because the pores in the shell are filled with organic material that prevents invasion by microorganisms [1].

With age, the egg white becomes less viscous and more alkaline and tends to thin out. Fresh egg white is chemically neutral; with age, the loss of carbon dioxide turns it alkaline. The loss of carbon dioxide is influenced by storage temperature, time, and permeability of the egg shell. The decrease in viscosity of the egg white is caused by a lowering of the ovomucin content secondary to a reduction in disulfide bonds (S—S) [5]. The breaking of the S—S bonds is thought to be caused by the interaction of ovomucin and lysozyme and by alkaline hydrolysis of the disulfide bonds of ovomucin.

With storage, water passes from the white into the yolk, resulting in enlargement and decreased viscosity of the yolk and weakening of the vitelline membrane. The increased fluidity of the yolk, the decreased viscosity of the white, and the impaired mechanical support of the white cause a flattening of the egg when opened (a decrease in quality with age).

The air cell enlarges with age, as water evaporates during storage. Moisture loss is minimized by storing eggs at a relative humidity of 70 to 80 percent [6].

With age, the porosity of the shell increases. Deterioration in odor and flavor occur during storage, as flavors and odors are absorbed through the more porous shell. Infiltration by microorganisms is also more likely in older eggs, although the egg has natural defenses against microbial invasion even if the shell is penetrated. These include the shell membranes, an alkaline pH, the bacteriolytic enzyme lysozyme, the iron-binding protein conalbumin, and the biotin-binding protein avidin. Coating eggs with a thin layer of mineral oil helps retard some of the storage changes, but off-flavors that do develop may be more intense, since volatile flavor components do not diffuse from the egg.

PRESERVATION

The purpose of preservation is to minimize physiochemical deterioration and to prevent microbial spoilage. Preservation makes eggs available throughout the year. Several methods, including cold storage, freezing, pasteurization, and dehydration, are used to preserve eggs.

Cold storage usually consists of refrigeration at 29 to 30°F (-1 to -2°C) at humidities of 85 to 90 percent. *Freezing* keeps the growth of microorganisms to a minimum while still retaining the natural flavor. The eggs are taken out of the shell before being frozen at 0 to -20°F (-18 to -28°C). This process does not appreciably alter the physical characteristics of the egg white; the egg yolk does increase in viscosity (a gel structure forms). The addition of sugar, salt, and other substances effectively limits gelation of the egg yolks during freezing. Freezing is used mostly by large food industries.

Federal law regulates the processing of eggs. To ensure the destruction of potentially pathogenic microorganisms, particularly *Salmonella,* all liquid, frozen, and dried whole eggs, yolks, and whites must be *pasteurized* (heated to a certain temperature for a certain amount of time). See Chap. 19 for more detail.

Eggs may be *dehydrated* by removing 99 percent of the water present. This process conserves weight and space. The glucose is removed to prevent changes in color, flavor, and performance caused by the reaction between glucose and proteins.

Alterations During Cooking

The changes that occur in eggs during cooking are based on the ability of the proteins in the yolk and white to denature and coagulate when heated.

Denaturation is the rearrangement of the orderly alignment of the molecules in a protein, with a resultant loss of specific properties of the protein. The peptide chains of proteins are coiled and maintained by weak bonds between amino acid residues (side groups) along the chain. During denaturation, some of the weak forces are broken, allowing the peptide chain to uncoil, and new bonds are formed. The solubility of the protein decreases upon denaturation.

Coagulation is the entire process that results in a loss of solubility and a change from a liquid to a more solid state, usually caused by heat or mechanical agitation. Coagulation is partly responsible for the thickening effect of eggs in such foods as custards. Because of their differing protein composition, the temperatures at which the yolk and egg white coagulate also differ. Excessive heating causes the egg white to become tough and porous, lose water, and shrink. Because of its fat content, the yolk has less tendency to become tough; instead it becomes crumbly when heated excessively. The addition of sugar elevates the temperature of coagulation; salt lowers it.

Gelation is the formation of a gel structure by heat or cold. The addition of acid produces a firmer gel and lower coagulation temperatures. Prolonged heating with acid causes *peptization*, a breaking up of large molecules, with a resultant thinning of the gel structure.

The proteins in eggs attract and hold large amounts of water, making egg mixtures good *thickening* agents. Eggs are useful in thickening such foods as custards and puddings because the proteins are readily suspended in liquid, which results in gel formation.

The greenish color on the surface of the yolk of hard-cooked eggs is due to the formation of ferrous sulfide. On heating the sulfur from the egg white diffuses into the yolk and reacts with the iron there to form ferrous sulfide.

The egg yolk, which is itself an emulsion, is a good *emulsifying* agent for fats and water. It is used in the manufacture and preparation of mayonnaise, salad dressing, ice cream, cream puffs, and hollandaise sauce.

The *foam-forming* ability of egg whites is essential for the production of angel food cakes, meringues, divinity candy, soufflés, omelets, and sponge cakes. The egg white foam is a colloid of bubbles surrounded by denatured albumen. The denaturation, caused by the drying and stretching of the albumen with beating, stiffens and stabilizes the foam. The globulins contribute to viscosity and lower the surface tension. Acids (e.g., cream of tartar) increase the stability of egg white foams. Sugar delays the formation of foam by delaying surface coagulation; it also increases stability.

When the foam is incorporated into a mixture, it acts as a *leavening agent.* Upon heating, the air bubbles expand and the egg white film hardens.

Eggs are also used as *clarifying agents* and for *binding* and *coating.* When raw eggs are added to hot broths and coffee, they trap loose particles in the liquid as they coagulate, clarifying it. As the proteins coagulate in coatings, they bind the food in the desired form.

References

1. Vedehra, D. V.   Bacterial penetration of eggs. *Food Life Sci. Q.* 5:9, 1972.
2. U.S. Department of Agriculture.   Regulations governing the grading of shell eggs and United States standards, grades, and weight classes for shell eggs. *Federal Register Title 7*, Chap. 1, Subchap. C, Part 56, July 15, 1967.
3. Peckham, G. C., and Freeland-Graves, J. H.   *Foundations of Food Preparation* (4th ed.). New York: Macmillan, 1979. P. 238.

4. Paul, P. C., and Palmer, H. H. (eds.). *Food Theory and Applications.* New York: Wiley, 1972. P. 530.

5. Beveridge, T., and Nakai, S. Effects of sulfhydryl blocking on the thinning of egg white. *J. Food Sci.* 40:864, 1975.

6. Stadelman, W. J. Quality Preservation of Shell Eggs. In W. J. Stadelman and O. J. Cotterill (eds.), *Egg Science and Technology.* Westport, Conn.: AVI Publishing, 1973.

Suggested Readings

Childs, M. T., and Ostrander, J. Egg substitutes: Chemical and biological evaluations. *J. Am. Dietet. Assoc.* 63:229, 1976.

Eggs break the time barrier. *Rest. Insts.* 88:157, 1981.

Hasiak, R. J., et al. Effect of certain physical and chemical treatments on the microstructure of egg yolk. *J. Food Sci.* 37:913, 1972.

Hou, H. C. Egg preservation in China. *Food Nutr. Bull.* 3:17, 1981.

Navidi, M. K., and Kummerow, F. A. Nutritional value of Egg Beaters compared with "farm fresh eggs." *Pediatrics* 53:565, 1974.

Reinke, W. C., Spencer, J. V., and Trynew, L. J. The effect of storage upon the chemical, physical, and functional properties of chicken eggs. *Poult. Sci.* 52:692, 1973.

U.S. Department of Agriculture, American Marketing Service. *Egg Grading Manual* (Handbook 75). Washington, D.C.: Government Printing Office, 1975.

Chapter 16

MEAT

Over 800 million cattle worldwide provide humankind with a wide variety of services [1]. Over a third of these animals are engaged primarily in the physical tasks of plowing, hauling, and milling. As machines for converting vegetable matter into human food, animals are not particularly efficient. Beef steer convert less than one-twentieth of what they eat into food for human consumption; dairy cows less than one-sixth; and pigs, about one-fifth [1]. Cattle, however, can metabolize cellulose, a carbohydrate indigestible by the human gastrointestinal tract, because of microorganisms present in the bovine stomach. In this way, cattle can be utilized as intermediaries to process semiarid grasslands that could not otherwise be farmed, converting useless vegetation into milk and meat (Fig. 16-1).

Meat and meat products do contribute high-quality protein, minerals, and vitamins to the diet. The protein is well assimilated and contains all the essential amino acids needed for growth and development. Muscle meats are an important source of iron, phosphorus, zinc, and copper. Vitamin A, thiamin, and riboflavin are especially plentiful in liver, kidney, heart, and sweetbreads.

Besides yielding high-quality protein, cattle, sheep, and pork yield such valuable products as hormones and vitamin extracts, bone meal fertilizer, and high protein concentrates for livestock feeding. Meat holds a central position in the American economy: Meat packing is the largest of all American food industries [2].

Structure

Muscle meats have four components: muscle fiber, connective tissue, adipose tissue, and bone. The quality, grading, appearance, and acceptability of meat depend on the proportion contributed by each of these components in the structure of the meat.

MUSCLE TISSUE

This component gives meat its characteristic appearance. The lean portion of meat is composed of bundles of fibers, or *fasciculi*, held together with connective tissue. Surrounding the muscle is a connective tissue sheath, the *epimysium*. Surrounding the bundles is the *perimysium*; within the bundles, the individual fibers are enclosed in a connective tissue framework, the *endomysium*. The fibers increase in size as the animal grows, although they do not increase in number after the animal is born.

Muscle fibers are elongated, multinucleated cells, varying in size with amount of use and function. They are composed of myofibrils surrounded by the *sarcoplasmic reticulum,* a complex system of tubules and vesicles. Sarcoplasm, the material that fills the spaces between the myofibrils, contains many of the enzymes of muscle, as well as fat droplets, myoglobin, and glycogen. The fibers also contain mitochondria, the energy warehouse for the cell, and lysosomes, which contain most of the hydrolytic enzymes of the cell. These enzymes function

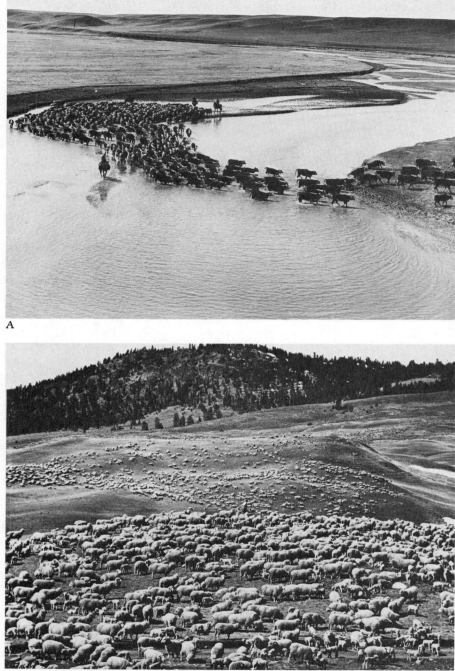

A

B

FIG. 16-1. Cattle, sheep, and pork all convert vegetation that is inedible by humans into milk or meat that contribute high-quality protein, minerals, and vitamins to the diet.
A. Cattle being rounded up and driven to summer pasture in Alberta, Canada. (Courtesy Food and Agriculture Organization of the United Nations [FAO].)
B. A herd of sheep grazing on a ranch in British Columbia (Courtesy FAO.)
C. A sow and piglets receiving their daily rations. (World Health Organization photo by T. Takahara.)

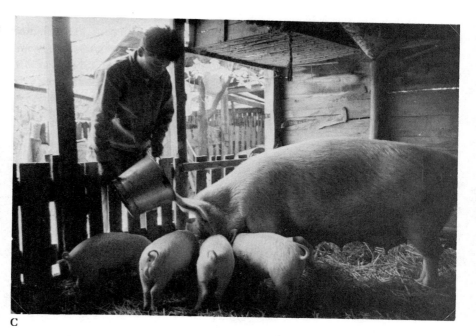

C

best under acid conditions of pH 4.5 to 5.5 [3]. The pH of 5.5 attained during the aging period after slaughter provides a favorable environment for the activity of these enzymes in tenderizing the muscle and producing flavor compounds (see Postmortem Changes, p. 271). The structure of muscles is shown in Fig. 16-2.

When the muscle fibers and bundles are small the meat has a finer texture and is of a better quality for eating. The grain of the meat is determined by the thickness of the muscle fibers, size of the fiber bundles, and the amount of connective tissue binding them together.

CONNECTIVE TISSUE

This component determines the tenderness of the muscle meat. As described above, it forms the walls of muscle fibers, binds them into bundles, and surrounds muscles as a membrane. It also makes up the ligaments and tendons.

ADIPOSE TISSUE

Otherwise termed *fat*, this component adds to the flavor and tenderness of the muscle meat. The pattern of distribution of fat throughout the muscle is termed *marbling* and is an important factor contributing to the flavor and tenderness of the muscle tissue. *Cover fat*, or *separable fat*, is the exterior layer of fat that helps muscle or lean tissue retain moisture and protects it from the action of microorganisms. The fatty deposits that occur within and between the muscles are influenced by species, breed, sex, age, level of nutrition, and individual animal differences.

BONE

This last component reflects the age of the animal: It is softer and has a reddish tinge in younger animals, and is flinty and white in older animals. The meat-

FIG. 16-2. Structure of muscle.

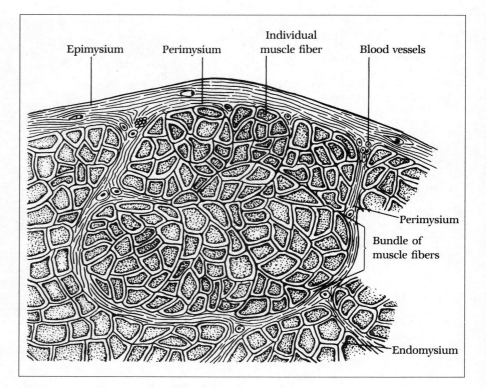

bone ratio is an important economic consideration for the consumer; a high ratio is most desirable. The shape of the bone is a useful guide in identifying various cuts of meats.

Nutrient Composition

The composition of the muscle tissue varies with the species, breed, age, type of feed, and length of time postmortem. Lean muscle is composed of approximately 75% water, 18% protein, 3% lipid, 1.6% nonprotein nitrogenous compounds, 1.2% carbohydrate and its metabolites, 0.7% inorganic salts, and traces of vitamins and other compounds.

PROTEINS

The protein in meats is of high biologic value, containing all essential amino acids. The amount of protein present is directly proportional to the amount of lean tissue; therefore as fat and bone increase, the amount of protein decreases. The principal proteins present include the contractile structures *actin* and *myosin;* the extracellular proteins abundant in connective tissue, *collagen* and *elastin;* the proteolytic enzymes present in the sarcoplasm (which are responsible for the increase in tenderness during aging or ripening); the oxygen-transporting components of the blood, *myoglobin* and *hemoglobin;* and the subcellular organelles, *mitochondria* and *lysosomes.* The nonprotein nitrogen present is found in such compounds as creatinine, free amino acids, and the metabolic nucleo-tides adenosine triphosphate (ATP), adenosine diphosphate (ADP), and adenosine monophosphate (AMP).

LIPIDS

Primarily present as neutral fat deposits, the lipid content of meat also includes that present within the muscle cells as lipoprotein and phospholipids. The adipose tissue of an animal appears late in its development. Fat cells begin to fill up with droplets of fat only after there is an excess of calories over the needs of the animal.

CARBOHYDRATES

The amounts of carbohydrate present vary with the state of nutrition of the animal and the recent activity of the muscle. The two forms present in meat include *glycogen,* the storage form of carbohydrate found mainly in the liver, and *glucose,* found mainly in the blood. As an intermediary product of carbohydrate metabolism, lactic acid is always present in the muscle and is increased after *rigor mortis* (stiffening of the muscle after slaughter) sets in.

MINERALS

The chief minerals present in meat are phosphorus, iron, and zinc. Potassium is concentrated in the muscle fiber, sodium in the fluid. The calcium present in the bones may also make a considerable contribution to the mineral content of the diet, depending on the method of cooking (e.g., meat bones used in soups, stews).

VITAMINS

Meat is an excellent source of the B vitamins thiamin, niacin, and riboflavin. Certain organ meats may also contribute substantial amounts of vitamins A, C, and D.

PIGMENTS

Eighty percent of the color of meat is due to the heme pigment in *myoglobin* and twenty percent to that in *hemoglobin.* Variation in color is caused by alterations in the chemical state of these pigments. Myoglobin holds oxygen in the muscles for contraction, and hemoglobin transports oxygen in the bloodstream. In organ meats and in muscles with a high oxygen demand, myoglobin is present in higher amounts and contributes to the more intense color.

Both pigments combine reversibly with oxygen, thereby supplying it to the tissues for metabolic processes. The heme portion of the two molecules is identical, the globins are different.

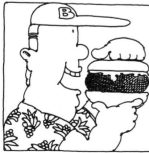

When meat is first cut and exposed to air, oxygen combines with myoglobin to produce *oxymyoglobin,* which is bright red; continued slow oxidation produces *metmyoglobin,* which is brownish-red (Fig. 16-3). The chemical change is due to the oxidation of the iron of myoglobin from the ferrous (Fe^{2+}) to the ferric (Fe^{3+}) state. In living tissue, myoglobin exists in equilibrium with its oxygenated form, oxymyoglobin. With cooking, oxymyoglobin is denatured, and the iron component is oxidized from the ferrous to the ferric state.

The pigments in fat are mainly carotenoids; the color varies from white to dark

FIG. 16-3. Pigment changes in red meat.

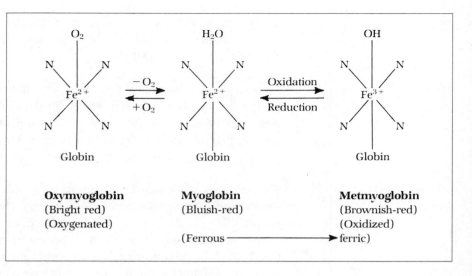

yellow, depending on the species, the breed, and the level of vitamin A in the feed.

The nutritive value of selected types of meat is given in Table 16-1.

Meat Quality, Grading, and Inspection
QUALITY

Many factors influence the eating quality and acceptability of muscle meats: the type and treatment of the live animal; slaughtering and carcass characteristics; the composition, structure, and function of the muscles; postmortem changes; cooking methods; processing treatments; and methods of preservation.

GENETIC INFLUENCES

Several factors associated with the living animal, including species, breed, sex, age, and weight, influence the amount and quality of the meat.

The major large animals used for food are cattle, sheep, and swine. Other mammals may provide major meat sources in other cultures. The amount and type of fatty acids deposited in the fat depots, as well as the location of the fat depots, vary with the *species*. The distribution of fat influences the firmness of the meat and the resistance of the fat to rancidity.

Variations by the *breed* of animal influence the yield of cuts, lean-fat ratio, intramuscular fat distribution (marbling), firmness of fat, and color, tenderness, and juiciness of cooked meat.

Among animals of the same species and breed, differences in sex, age, and weight play an important part. *Sex* differences in meat quality are in part due to the influence of hormones on the composition of the animals. Steer meat is usually more tender, flavorful, and juicier than bull meat; the differences become more marked with increasing age of the animals. With an increase in *age*, the

TABLE 16-1. Nutritive value of selected meats

Meat	Amount	Calories	Protein (gm)	Carbohydrate (gm)	Fat (gm)	Fiber (gm)	Iron (mg)	Thiamin (µg)	Riboflavin (µg)	Niacin (mg)	Ascorbic acid (mg)	Vitamin A (IU)	Vitamin D (IU)
Beef													
Frankfurter	1¾ oz	124	7.0	1.0	10.0	0	0.6	80	90	1.2	0	0	0
Hamburger	4 oz	224	**21.8**	0	14.5	0	3.3	136	153	**4.8**	0	0	0
Porterhouse steak	8 oz	242	**25.4**	0	14.7	0	3.8	100	120	**6.1**	0	0	0
Rib roast	8 oz	302	**28.4**	0	6.7	0	3.5	64	223	**4.2**	0	0	0
Veal													
Cutlet	3½ oz	277	**33.2**	0	15.0	0	4.2	122	**322**	**6.4**	0	0	0
Loin chop	3½ oz	421	**22.7**	0	35.9	0	2.9	139	211	**4.7**	0	0	0
Lamb													
Loin chop	3½ oz	302	**23.0**	0	22.5	0	3.0	172	271	**6.5**	0	0	0
Pork													
Bacon	3 strips	147	5.4	0.5	13.5	0	0.6	137	65	1.0	0	0	0
Ham	3½ oz	306	**32.9**	0	18.3	0	2.3	**578**	272	**4.5**	0	0	0
Loin chop	3½ oz	357	**29.4**	0	25.6	0	4.4	**1180**	190	**5.5**	0	0	0
Spareribs	6 ribs	246	**15.4**	0	20.0	0	2.3	**400**	150	2.8	0	0	0
Organ meats													
Brains	3 oz	106	8.8	0.7	7.3	0	2.0	196	221	**3.7**	15	0	0
Heart	⅓ heart	130	**20.3**	0.8	4.4	0	**5.5**	**278**	**694**	**5.7**	6	30	0
Kidney	3½ oz	169	**18.0**	1.1	9.7	0	**9.5**	178	**1989**	**3.8**	0	**1242**	0
Calves' liver	2½ oz	147	**16.2**	3.4	7.2	0	**9.0**	126	**2385**	**11.7**	15	**19,130**	**10**
Sweetbreads (thymus and pancreas)	3½ oz	184	**15.2**	0	13.2	0	1.2	40	**400**	3.1	44	17	0

Note: All values are after cooking. Boldface values are one-fourth or more of the recommended daily dietary allowance (1980) for the average woman aged 23–50.

Source: C. H. Church and A. Bowes, *Nutritive Value of Food Portions Commonly Used.* Philadelphia: Lippincott, 1975.

lean-bone ratio and fat-bone ratio increase, as does the amount of fat. The total moisture in the soft tissues decreases with age. Therefore, meat from young animals is different in tenderness, juiciness, yield, and flavor than meat from mature animals. Another reason for the quality difference may be the increased cross-linking of collagen (connective tissue) with age, which makes the tissue from older animals more resistant to the softening influence of heat.

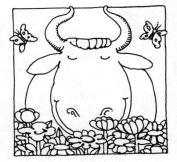

Animals are classified by age because of these different quality characteristics. The bovine (cattle) divisions are *veal* (less than 3 months of age), *calves* (3 to 8 months), *baby beef* (8 to 12 months), and *adult bovines*. The ovine (sheep) groupings are *milk lamb* (less than 3 months), *lamb* (less than 14 months), *yearling* (1 to 2 years), and *sheep* or *mutton* (over 2 years). Most pork is marketed at 6 to 7 months of age, and market classes are based on weight and sex rather than age. Especially with pork, the lighter weight groups have significantly better flavor and juiciness.

TREATMENT INFLUENCES

The type of feed and the amount of exercise can also influence the composition, and therefore the quality, of muscle tissue. *Feed* with a high energy content will yield meat with increased flavor, tenderness, and juiciness. A period of *starvation* will cause a decrease in the size of the muscle fibers, with a consequent increase in the percentage of connective tissue and tougher meat. The use of *estrogens* (e.g., stilbestrol) in the feed has various effects, depending on the species of animal. It increases the amount of connective tissue in lamb muscle but does not alter the flavor. Estrogens do increase the tenderness and juiciness of sheep meat. This female hormone decreases the amount of intramuscular fat in beef without loss in eating quality.

Exercise causes a reduction in the collagen content of muscle by a hypertrophy of contractile tissue without an increase in connective tissue. The result is enhanced tenderness.

GRADING

Federal grading and stamping of meat started in 1927. Official grade standards are published in the Federal Register. Grading of meat is optional but when used is of value to the consumer. Meat can be graded for either "quality," based partially on factors indicating the palatability of the lean muscle, including color, marbling, and firmness of both muscles and fat; or "cutability," the amount of edible lean meat and is stated as such. Meat packers pay for the services of a federal meat grader. The established grades of meat include prime, choice, good, standard, and commercial.

Factors on which grading is based include conformation, finish, and quality. *Conformation* is related to the bulk and general form of the animal—the relative development of the muscular and skeletal systems. The *finish* is related to the appearance of the fat and its distribution within the meat. A good finish is creamy fat evenly distributed throughout the lean meat. The third factor, *quality*, is related to the probable tenderness and palatability of the meat when cooked.

MEAT INSPECTION ACT

Every animal slaughtered in a meat-packing establishment engaged in interstate commerce is inspected by the Agricultural Research Service of the U.S. Department of Agriculture (USDA) under the *Meat Inspection Act* of 1906. This act requires federal supervision of the cleanliness, wholesomeness, and labeling of fresh and processed meat food products. The Meat Inspection Act guards the consumer against adulterated meat products, unsanitary conditions, and fraudulent practices. In 1967, this act was expanded to apply the same standards to meat products offered for sale within the state where slaughtered.

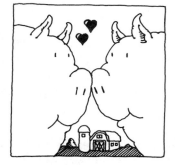

All inspections are made by trained veterinarians employed by the USDA and a few trained lay inspectors. The inspection itself consists of three parts. During the first part, the animals are inspected before slaughter (antemortem inspection); those that show any sign of disease are separated and tagged for special handling. The second part of the inspection occurs after slaughter, when each carcass, including the internal organs, is again inspected for any signs of disease. The third part includes the examination of processed meats such as bacon, lard, ham, sausage, and canned meat. Meats that pass inspection are marked with a round stamp on the wholesale cut stating that they have been inspected and approved.

PARASITES

Trichinella spiralis, a roundworm parasite, is thought to be the most dangerous worm parasite transmissible from domestic animals to humans. When present in sufficient numbers in a suitable host, these parasites produce an illness termed *trichinosis.* The main source of human trichinosis is infected pork eaten raw or after improper cooking. USDA regulations stipulate that all processed pork products prepared to be eaten without further cooking must have been subjected to temperatures sufficient to destroy all live trichinae. All parts must reach a minimum temperature of 137°F (58.5°C). Live trichinae can also be destroyed by cold (-15°C for 10 days).

Postmortem Changes

After slaughter, the carcass is cooled to just above freezing temperature for 2 or 3 days. During this period, physical and chemical changes in the composition of the meat caused by enzymes within the tissues and by microorganisms occur.

DEVELOPMENT OF RIGOR

During the first 8 hours after slaughter, the muscles of the animal become rigid (*rigor mortis*) because of the interaction of the muscle filaments actin and myosin as they slide past each other to form actinomysin. The fibers show dense nodes of contraction and areas of extreme stretching; the latter appear as breaks. The degradation of the muscle fibers, which continues through the aging process, may be caused by enzymatic hydrolysis. The change in muscle filament structure along with a drop in pH (see below) causes the muscles to lose their soft, pliable nature and become inflexible, rigid, and stiff. The term *rigor mortis* comes from the Latin, meaning "stiffness of death."

CHANGES IN pH

The cellular environment rapidly becomes anaerobic after slaughter since the cessation of blood circulation has cut off the oxygen supply. Glycolysis (the breakdown of glycogen to ATP) occurs until the carbohydrate supply is exhausted. The ATP then breaks down, with lactic acid as the end product (see Chap. 4 for more detail). Lactic acid accumulates in the muscles, lowering the pH from 7.0 or 7.2 in living tissue to about 5.5 after slaughter. The final pH depends on the amount of glycogen present in the muscle when the animal was slaughtered. If the glycogen supply is depleted by stress, starvation, or exercise immediately before slaughter, less lactic acid will be produced, and the ultimate pH will be higher. Beef of this type, termed *dark-cutting beef,* is brownish-red to purplish-black and sticky and gummy. Avoidance of antemortem stress and rapid chilling after slaughter minimizes this problem. The holding of meat for 48 hours after slaughter, known as *aging,* has a tenderizing effect. Aging is usually done at 0 to 1.5°C (32 to 35°F) to minimize microbial growth.

CHANGE IN QUALITY

When rigor first sets in there is a decrease in the quality of the meat; if cooked at this time it will be very tough. For this reason, all meats should be aged until rigor passes before being cooked or frozen. The improvement in flavor with aging may result from increased presence of free sugars, amino acids, or other compounds [4].

Tenderness

The tenderness of meat, which determines quality, consumer acceptability and, therefore, price, is influenced by many factors. The amount of *connective tissue* is directly related to the tenderness. The two types of connective tissue are collagen and elastin. Collagen hydrolyzes to gelatin at cooking temperatures, thus contributing to the tenderness of meat. Elastin is not broken down as readily. The intramuscular distribution of *fat* (marbling) increases tenderness, perhaps by separating connective fibers and making them more accessible to heat treatment.

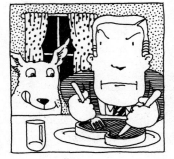

As stated earlier, *age* is an important factor in meat tenderness. Muscle from younger animals is more tender than that from older animals, because the tenderness of muscle decreases as the diameter of the muscle fiber increases, and the diameter of the muscle increases with age. Older animals also have increased connective tissue. In addition to age, *location* influences tenderness. The least-used muscles, such as in loin and rib cuts, are more tender than more fully developed ones, such as found in neck, chuck, and round cuts.

Treatments such as grinding and pounding, aging, and enzymes also influence meat tenderness. *Grinding* breaks and cuts muscle fibers and connective tissue; therefore ground meat can be cooked like more tender cuts. *Pounding* is used to tenderize meat, by tearing and breaking only the surface muscle fibers and connective tissue. *Aging,* as discussed previously, increases the tenderness of meat. When actinomysin is formed during rigor mortis, some of the muscle fibers contract as others are stretched. With continued aging the muscle softens, and breaks in the fibers thought to be caused by enzymatic action on the proteins can be detected. Additional *enzymes,* such as *papain* (found in the papaya), also aid the tenderizing process. These enzymes break down the outer covering of the muscle fiber, collagen, and elastin. Cooking deactivates (denatures) the enzymes.

Economic Aspects

The price of meat varies with market supply and demand, the cost of feed, and the quality and grade of the carcass. The protein value per pound of lean meat, regardless of grade, is about the same for beef, veal, pork, and lamb. The major differences are in the tenderness of the cut and the cooking method required to make the meat palatable.

The cost per pound should be evaluated in terms of proportion of bone and fat present; larger cuts of meat are generally more economical than individual portions. Organ meats are better buys because they have no waste in the form of bone or fat; they also have a high content of vitamin A, iron, and the B vitamins.

New uniform retail meat identity standards [5] have been developed to help end the confusion over the many popular and local names for a single cut of meat. The standard nomenclature is in effect for about 300 retail cuts of beef, pork, lamb, and veal. Figure 16-4 shows the retail cuts of meat for beef, veal, lamb, and pork.

Alterations During Cooking

The purpose of cooking meat before it is consumed is to improve its flavor, change its color, make it more tender, and destroy harmful organisms. Constant, low-temperature cooking improves palatability and appearance, while decreas-

FIG. 16-4. Seven basic cuts of meat, which may be applied to beef, lamb, veal, or pork. (Courtesy National Live Stock and Meat Board.)

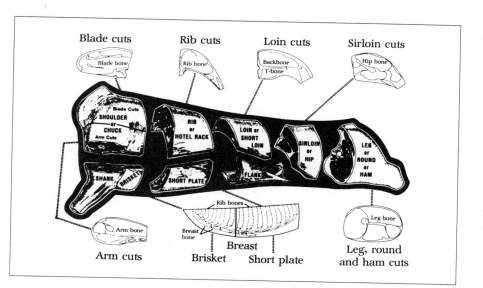

ing loss of weight and nutritive value. The heat-induced changes in meat are related to the composition of the meat and the method and extent of heating.

PHYSICAL AND CHEMICAL
CHANGES

When subjected to heat, the muscle proteins start to coagulate and toughen, collagen hydrolyzes and softens, and heat is conducted from the surface to the interior. Heat causes muscle fibers to harden and connective tissue to soften. Tender cuts contain little collagen and therefore decrease in tenderness during heating; less tender cuts become more tender during heating. Heat alters the selective permeability of cell membranes and accelerates the reaction rate of enzymes until the denaturation temperatures of the enzymes are reached.

COLOR CHANGES

The muscle pigment myoglobin and the blood pigment hemoglobin give meat its color. Meat changes color as it cooks as a result of the denaturing of the globin portion of the pigment molecule (see Fig. 16-3). Beef is the only meat that is acceptable when served bright red (rare). Lamb may be served medium rare (pink), but pork and veal are always served well done.

FLAVOR AND ODOR
CHANGES

Heat changes the flavor of meat by eliminating volatile substances, carmelizing carbohydrates, melting and decomposing fat, and coagulating and breaking down proteins. Characteristic flavors of various meats are due primarily to differences in fat composition.

References

1. Phillips, R. W.   Cattle. In N. Kretchmer and B. Robertson (eds.), *Human Nutrition*. San Francisco: Scientific American and W. H. Freeman, 1978. P. 81.
2. Peckham, G. C., and Freeland-Graves, J. H.   *Foundations of Food Preparation* (4th ed.). New York: Macmillan, 1979. P. 282.
3. Paul, P. C., and Palmer, H. H. (eds.).   *Food Theory and Applications*. New York: Wiley, 1972. P. 369.
4. Lawrie, R. A.   Chemical changes in meat due to processing: A review. *J. Sci. Food Agric.* 19:233, 1968.
5. *Uniform Retail Meat Identity Standards*. Chicago: National Live Stock and Meat Board, 1973. P. 1.

Suggested Readings

American Meat Foundation.   *The Science of Meat and Meat Products*. San Francisco: W. H. Freeman, 1971.
Bailey, A. G.   The basis of meat texture. *J. Sci. Food Agric.* 23:995, 1972.
Bourne, G. H. (ed.).   *The Structure and Function of Muscles*. New York: Academic, 1960.
Chang, S. S., and Peterson, R. J.   Symposium: The basis of quality in muscle foods. Recent developments in the flavor of meat. *J. Food Sci.* 42:298, 1977.
Giddings, G. G.   Symposium: The basis of quality in muscle foods. The basis of color in muscle foods. *J. Food Sci.* 42:288, 1977.
Huxley, H. E.   The mechanism of muscular contraction. *Science* 164:1356, 1969.
Jones, S. B.   Ultrastructural characteristics of beef muscle. *Food Technol.* 31:82, 1977.

Kang, C. K., and Rice, E. E.   Degradation of various meat fractions by tenderizing enzymes. *J. Food Sci.* 35:563, 1970.

Marsh, B. B.   The basis of tenderness in muscle foods. *J. Food Sci.* 42:295, 1977.

Meat Evaluation Handbook.   Chicago: National Live Stock and Meat Board, 1969.

Miller, R. W.   There's something to be said for never saying, "please pass the meat." *FDA Consum.* 15:24, 1981.

Murray, J. M., and Weber, A.   The cooperative action of muscle proteins. *Sci. Am.* 230:58, 1974.

Tiwar, N. P., and Kadis, V. W.   Microbiological quality of some delicatessen meat products. *J. Food Protect.* 44:821, 1981.

Chapter 17

FISH AND POULTRY

Both fish and poultry have received renewed attention in recent years. Because of their high proportion of polyunsaturated fatty acids and lower cholesterol and total fat content than red meats, both have been recommended for use in diets designed to prevent and treat cardiovascular disease, one of the leading causes of mortality in America.

Fish

Fish are valuable as a food source because of their high protein and mineral content and because they are generally low in fat, calories, and waste. Edible fish are grouped as either *shellfish* or *finfish*. Shellfish, which have an outer shell and no bones, include both mollusks and crustaceans; finfish have bony skeletons. Mollusks have hard, hinged shells and include oysters, clams, scallops, and mussels. Crustaceans have segmented crustlike shells and include lobsters, shrimps, and crabs. Most edible fish of both types come from salt water.

Anadromous fish are born in fresh water, swim to the sea for their adult life, and return to their birthplace to spawn. Such fish as salmon, sturgeon, smelt, and striped bass are anadromous.

STRUCTURE

Like other vertebrates, fish are composed of three types of muscle: smooth, cardiac, and skeletal. The bulk of the fish is made up of skeletal muscles. Myofibrils, the individual muscle fibers, are composed of the same proteins as those in muscle tissue from warm-blooded animals. The muscle fibers are shorter than those in meat or poultry and are arranged segmentally, separated by connective tissue. The ends of the fibers are embedded in sheets of connective tissue, the *myocommata*. When fish is cooked, the connective tissue sheets soften and gelatinize, freeing the coagulated muscle cells as "flakes."

COMPOSITION

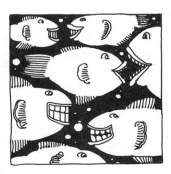

The composition of fish varies widely, mostly influenced by the amount of fat present. Fish average about 20% protein and 1.5% minerals. The moisture content of fish can vary from 66 to 84 percent; protein, 15 to 24 percent; fat, 0.1 to 22.0 percent; and minerals, 0.8 to 2.0 percent [1]. Such fish as cod, haddock, whiting, rockfish, and sole are very low in fat, less than 1 percent. Others, such as salmon, mackerel, lake trout, and butterfish, have almost 25% fat. Variation in composition may be caused by such factors as feeding, locality, size, age, and season. Differences in composition caused by seasonal variation may be related to the stage of sexual development and the feeding conditions. During the spawning period there is a decrease in fat and protein and an increase in moisture content in the muscles. During winter and spring there is a decrease in fat and free amino acids in muscle tissue, compared with the amounts in summer. Composition also varies with anatomic location: The head is richest in protein; the tail contains more fat and water than other parts. Like meat, fish muscles contain glycogen (carbohydrate). This nutrient represents a source of stored energy in the live fish. Shellfish generally have more carbohydrate and less fat than finfish.

A heavily pigmented, reddish muscle is present under the skin of many fish. This red muscle is a storehouse of fat, glycogen, and other metabolites and contains more B vitamins than does white muscle. Red muscle contains about 2% fat, compared with 0.7 to 0.8% for lighter muscle. The proportion of red-white muscle varies from species to species and from section to section in a fish.

Both salmon and lobster contain the red pigment *astacin*. Lobster turns red when boiled because of the stability of astacin and because the green and brown pigments on the shell of the live lobster are destroyed when heated, allowing the red pigment to predominate.

NUTRITIVE VALUE

FAT

The fat in fish is composed of many highly polyunsaturated fatty acids and some saturated fatty acids. Fish has a lower total fat content than an equivalent amount of poultry or meat. For these reasons, it is often used in therapeutic diets for diseases requiring modified fat and saturated fat intakes.

VITAMINS

The vitamin content of fish varies with the fat content. Salmon and halibut, with a high fat content, are good sources of vitamin A. These vitamins are also concentrated in fish liver oils and in fish viscera. All fish are excellent sources of the B vitamins thiamin, riboflavin, and occasionally niacin.

MINERALS

All fish are good sources of calcium, phosphorus, iodine and are fair sources of heme iron. Oysters are good sources of iron and copper. Unless they are cured in salt, most fish, except shark, are low in sodium—only slightly higher than in meat. Iodine, an element vital to normal metabolism, occurs more abundantly in saltwater fish than in any other food.

The nutritive value of selected fish is given in Table 17-1.

INSPECTION AND GRADING

The Fishery Products Inspection Program of the U.S. Department of Commerce's National Marine Fisheries Service is a voluntary program providing inspection and certification on a user-fee basis. The program applies the U.S. quality standards and specifications for fishery products and the standards of sanitary and operating requirements.

Oysters must bear a certificate showing that they have been produced in oyster beds that have passed inspection by health authorities.

POSTMORTEM CHANGES

The development and duration of rigor mortis is shorter in fish than in mammals. It starts about 1 to 7 hours after death. If fish are stored on ice, the duration

TABLE 17-1. Nutritive value of selected fish

Fish	Amount	Calories	Protein (gm)	Carbohydrate (gm)	Fiber (gm)	Fat (gm)	Iron (mg)	Thiamin (μg)	Riboflavin (μg)	Niacin (mg)	Ascorbic acid (mg)	Vitamin A (IU)	Vitamin D (IU)
Finfish													
Bass	3½ oz, baked	287	**23.6**	3.0	0	19.4	1.2	**70**	**160**	**3.5**	0	97	1
Bluefish	4 oz, baked	199	**32.8**	0	0	6.5	0.9	**140**	**130**	2.4	0	62	0
Butterfish	1¾ oz, fried	211	9.1	0	0	19.1	—	**27**	**32**	2.0	—	—	—
Catfish	3½ oz, raw	103	**17.6**	0	0	3.1	0.4	**40**	**30**	1.7	—	—	—
Caviar (sturgeon)	1 tsp	26	2.7	3.3	0	1.5	1.2	—	—	—	—	—	—
Cod	4 oz, broiled	162	**26.1**	0	0	5.0	0.9	**80**	**100**	2.8	—	170	—
Flounder	3½ oz, baked	202	**30.0**	0	0	8.2	1.4	**70**	**80**	2.5	2	—	—
Haddock	3½ oz, fried	165	**19.6**	5.8	0	6.4	1.2	**40**	**70**	3.2	—	—	—
Halibut	4 oz, broiled	214	**31.5**	0	0	8.8	1.0	**60**	**90**	**10.4**	—	**850**	—
Herring	3½ oz, broiled	217	**20.8**	0	0	14.2	1.2	14	**153**	3.3	0	130	—
Mackerel (canned)	3½ oz	180	**21.1**	0	0	10.0	2.2	**30**	**330**	**8.8**	0	30	—
Perch	3½ oz, raw	91	**19.5**	0	0	0.9	0.6	**60**	**170**	1.7	—	—	—
Rockfish	3½ oz, oven steamed	107	**18.1**	1.9	0	2.5	—	**50**	**120**	—	1	—	—
Salmon (canned)	⅖ cup	210	**19.6**	0	0	14.0	0.9	**30**	**140**	**7.3**	—	**230**	—
Sardines (canned in oil)	3½ oz	311	**20.6**	0.6	0	24.4	3.5	20	**160**	**4.4**	—	180	—
Trout	3½ oz, raw	101	**19.2**	0	0	2.1	—	**70**	—	—	—	—	—
Tuna (canned)	⅝ cup, drained	145	**25.2**	0	0	4.1	1.3	—	—	—	—	—	—
Shellfish													
Clams, soft	4 large or 9 small	82	**14.0**	1.3	0	1.9	3.4	—	—	—	—	—	—
Clams, hard	5 large or 10 small	80	**11.1**	5.9	0	0.9	**7.5**	—	—	—	—	—	—
Crab	3½ oz, steamed	93	**17.3**	0.5	0	1.9	0.8	**160**	**80**	2.8	—	**2170**	—
Lobster	¾ lb + 2 tbsp butter	308	**20.0**	0.8	0	24.9	0.7	**110**	**60**	2.3	0	**920**	—
Mussels	3½ oz	95	**14.4**	3.3	0	2.2	3.4	**160**	**210**	—	—	—	—
Oysters	5–8 medium, raw	66	8.4	3.4	0	1.8	**5.5**	**140**	**180**	2.5	—	**310**	—
Scallops	3½ oz, steamed	112	**23.2**	0	0	1.4	3.0	—	—	—	—	—	—
Shrimp	3½ oz, raw	91	**18.8**	1.5	0	0.8	1.6	20	30	3.2	—	—	—

Note: Dashes indicate no significant data available. Boldface values are one-fourth or more of the recommended daily dietary allowance (1980) for that nutrient for women ages 23–50.

Source: C. F. Church and H. N. Church, *Food Values of Portions Commonly Used*. Philadelphia: Lippincott, 1975.

of rigor is extended. Immediate slaughter after capture also extends rigor. With the onset of rigor, the appearance of lactic acid causes a decrease in muscle pH, by the mechanisms discussed in Chap. 16.

Postmortem changes are important determinants of the quality and characteristics of fresh and frozen fish. The size and condition of the fish, the type of feed, the amount of struggle, holding temperatures, physical handling, and time elapsed after death and before freezing all have an effect on postmortem changes [1].

For a full discussion of the postmortem changes in muscle tissue, see Chap. 16.

PURCHASING FISH

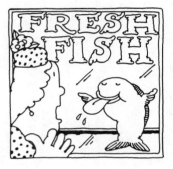

Fish is available throughout the year, not only in coastal areas, but in the interior as well.

FINFISH

In buying finfish, several qualities should be sought: The eyes should be bright, clear, and bulging; the flesh should be firm without traces of drying or browning; and the fish should not have any odor [2]. The fishy odor comes from deterioration of the fish by the oxidation of the polyunsaturated fats and by bacterial growth. Figure 17-1 shows the major food fish caught by fishermen on the Canadian coast.

SHELLFISH

Oysters sold in the shell must be alive when purchased, and the shells must be tightly closed. They may be kept under refrigeration for a short period before being eaten. Oysters are graded by size after being shucked (removed from the shell). They are found along coastal waters.

Clams may be embedded as deep as 50 feet along the coast; those close to the tidal zone can be dug up by hand or with rakes. Clams are sold alive in the shell or shucked. Hard-shell clams should be tightly shut; soft-shell clams may be partially open because of the long siphon extending to the interior.

Cape or bay *scallops* grow in shallow waters; sea scallops, in deeper waters. Scallops are capable of swimming freely in water, unlike oysters, clams, and mussels. They are sold shucked.

Crabs are produced mainly in the Chesapeake Bay area in the United States; Louisiana and Florida also produce some. Soft-shell crabs are molting hard-shell crabs. Soft-shell crabs are caught during the summer, hard-shell during the winter. Crabs must be alive when cooked and are steamed and picked by hand.

Lobsters come from the Atlantic coast, the largest proportion from New England. They are particularly expensive because of their limited number and

---

FIG. 17-1. Four of the ten main saltwater groups of fish commonly classified as having lean flesh. Other groups not pictured include cod, snapper, skate and ray, sea bass, rockfish, wolf fish, and uncommon market fish (such as the tilefish and monkfish). (Thomas L. Kronen, Courtesy National Marine Fisheries Service, Chicago.)

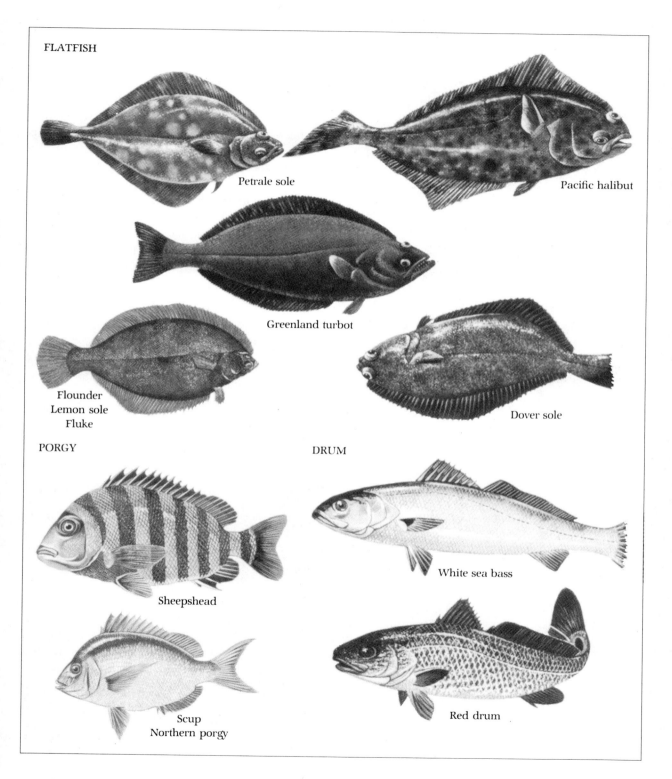

FLATFISH

Petrale sole

Pacific halibut

Greenland turbot

Flounder
Lemon sole
Fluke

Dover sole

PORGY

DRUM

Sheepshead

White sea bass

Scup
Northern porgy

Red drum

because they contain so little meat. They must be kept alive in seawater until cooked. If sold cooked, they will keep only a short period under refrigeration. A green sac, the lobster's liver, appears with cooking. Termed the *tomalley*, it is considered a delicacy. The red masses found in cooked lobster are the eggs of the female.

Shrimp are found mainly along the Atlantic coast and the Gulf of Mexico; Louisiana is considered the center of the shrimp industry. About half the catch is canned; the rest is frozen or marketed fresh or dried. Fresh shrimp are also termed *green shrimp;* the head and thorax are removed before packing.

PRINCIPLES OF COOKING FISH

The purpose in cooking fish is to develop its delicate flavor, coagulate the proteins, and break down the connective tissue. Because fish has so little connective tissue, it requires much shorter cooking times and lower temperatures than do poultry and meat. The use of acid, such as lemon juice, on raw fish will also coagulate the proteins; the acid will turn the raw fish white, and it can be served

FIG. 17-2. Trawling for fish in Canada. (Courtesy Information Services, Department of Fisheries, Ottawa; Food and Agriculture Organization of the United Nations.)

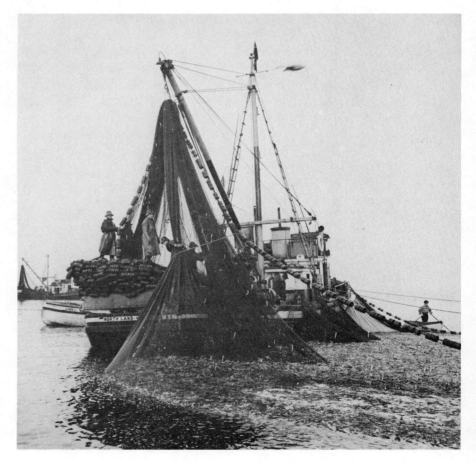

TABLE 17-2. Methods of cooking fish

Method	Description
À la meunière	Seasoned, floured, and sautéed in butter
Amandine	Baked with butter and almonds
De joughe	Baked with garlic, bread crumbs, and butter
En papillate	Enclosed in a sheet of oiled paper and oven heated
Florentine	Baked with spinach
Provençale	Baked with tomatoes, garlic, and onions

Source: G. C. Peckham and J. H. Freeland-Graves, *Foundations of Food Preparation* (4th ed.). New York: Macmillan, 1979. Pp. 347–348.

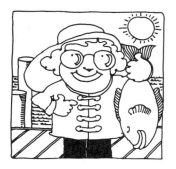

without cooking. Only fish that has been carefully inspected for parasites should be prepared in this manner.

Fish with a higher fat content, such as shad, salmon, bluefish, herring, swordfish, and mackerel, require little additional fat during cooking and may be prepared by dry heat: baking, frying, and broiling. Fish such as flounder, trout, bass, halibut, haddock, and cod contain very little fat and require additional fat during cooking. Shellfish may be eaten raw, plunged into simmering salted water, or steamed for maximum flavor retention. Table 17-2 lists terms describing methods of cooking fish.

Poultry

Poultry, as a class, includes chicken, turkey, duck, goose, Cornish hen, guinea hen, squab, and pigeon. Improved management practices during the past 20 years have resulted in better quality poultry and greater quantities of poultry produced. The use of certain antibiotics to prevent poultry diseases and to improve the nutritional status of the birds has led to the development of poultry with a higher percentage of palatable meat of superior quality than that of a few decades ago. Feeding small amounts of such antibiotics as tetracycline and penicillin has a growth-promoting effect on poultry. This enhanced growth is the result of the antibacterial action of the drugs on the intestinal tract, which improves the health and rate of growth of the birds. Some residues from the antibiotics are found in the liver and fat of the poultry.

COMPOSITION AND STRUCTURE

Poultry tissue does not differ from other muscle foods; the proteins in poultry are similar to those of livestock. The protein content of poultry is relatively high, ranging from 20 to 24 percent. The fat content ranges from 1 to 2 percent in breast meat to 4 to 5 percent in leg meat. Poultry fat has a high percentage of unsaturated fatty acids and a low cholesterol content. Because of its higher fat content, dark meat is usually more juicy but less tender than light meat.

The color of poultry is due to the presence of xanthophyll and carotene pigments in the diet. A diet rich in these pigments, including such foods as yellow

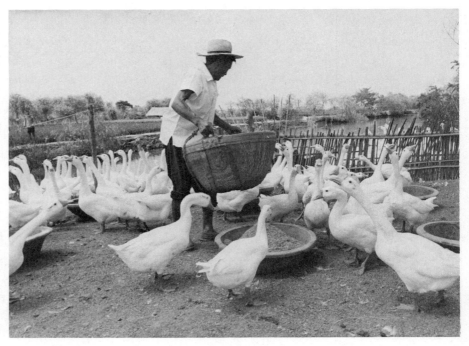

corn or gold marigold petals, will cause the fat of the bird to be deeper yellow, a characteristic preferred by consumers (Fig. 17-3).

The nutritive value of selected poultry is given in Table 17-3.

INSPECTION AND GRADING

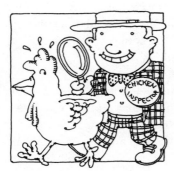

The Wholesome Poultry Products Act of 1968 is similar to the Meat Inspection Act: All poultry and poultry products sold in the United States must be inspected for sanitary conditions. This act requires inspection of sanitary conditions in plants engaged in interstate commerce; inspection of live poultry before slaughter for signs of disease; inspection of eviscerated poultry before further processing, also for signs of disease; and proper labeling of all inspected poultry. For poultry sold within the state where processed, individual states must provide inspection.

Inspected poultry is labeled with its class (Table 17-4), its net weight, the name of the packer or distributor, and the official inspection mark. Poultry products must also be prepared under inspection and labeled with the common name of the product; the net weight; the name of the packer or distributor; the official plant number; the inspection mark; and the ingredients, listed by their proportion in the product [2].

Grading (A, B, or C) is optional and is paid for by the processor. The qualities evaluated in establishing grade include conformation; fleshing; fat; freedom from pinfeathers, cuts, tears, and other flesh blemishes; and freedom from disjointed or broken bones.

TABLE 17-3. Nutritive value of selected poultry

Poultry	Amount	Calories	Protein (gm)	Carbohydrate (gm)	Fiber (gm)	Fat (gm)	Iron (mg)	Thiamin (µg)	Riboflavin (µg)	Niacin (mg)	Ascorbic acid (mg)	Vitamin A (IU)	Vitamin D (IU)
Chicken (broiler)	3½ oz, raw	151	**20.2**	0	0	7.2	1.5	**80**	**160**	**10.2**	0	0	—
Chicken (fryer)	3½ oz, raw	104	**23.3**	0	0	0.5	1.1	**70**	**90**	**10.5**	0	0	—
Duck (domestic)	3½ oz, raw	326	**16.0**	0	0	28.6	1.8	**100**	**240**	**5.6**	0	0	—
Guinea hen	3½ oz, raw	156	**23.1**	0	0	6.4	—	—	—	—	—	—	—
Pheasant	3½ oz, raw	151	**24.3**	0	0	5.2	3.7	—	—	—	—	—	—
Quail	3½ oz, raw	168	**25.0**	0	0	6.8	3.8	—	—	—	—	—	—
Squab (pigeon)	3½ oz, raw	279	**18.6**	0	0	22.1	1.8	**100**	**240**	**5.6**	0	—	—
Turkey	3½ oz, raw	268	**20.1**	0	0	20.2	3.8	**90**	**140**	**8.0**	0	tr	—

Note: Dashes indicate that no significant data available. Boldface values are one-fourth or more of the recommended daily dietary allowance (1980) for that nutrient for the average woman aged 23–50.

Source: C. F. Church and H. N. Church, *Food Values of Portions Commonly Used*. Philadelphia: Lippincott, 1975.

TABLE 17-4. Classification of common poultry

1. Chicken
   a. Rock Cornish game hen: young, immature chicken 5 to 7 weeks old
   b. Broiler or fryer: young, tender-meated chicken 9 to 12 weeks old
   c. Roaster: young, tender-meated chicken 3 to 5 months old
   d. Capon: male chicken less than 8 months old
   e. Hen, stewing chicken, or fowl: mature female chicken over 10 months old
   f. Stag: tougher male chicken less than 10 months old
   g. Cock or rooster: mature male chicken
2. Turkey
   a. Fryer-roaster: young, immature, tender-meated turkey of either sex less than 16 weeks old
   b. Young hen and Tom: male and female tender-meated turkeys less than 15 months old
   c. Mature or old turkey: turkey of either sex over 15 months
3. Duck
   a. Broiler or fryer duckling: tender-meated duck less than 8 weeks old
   b. Roaster duckling: tender-meated duck less than 16 weeks old
   c. Mature or old duck: tougher duck over 6 months old
4. Goose
   a. Young goose: tender-meated bird of either sex
   b. Mature or old goose: tougher goose of either sex
5. Guinea
   a. Young guinea: tender-meated bird of either sex
   b. Mature or old guinea: tougher guinea of either sex
6. Pigeon
   a. Squab: young, immature pigeon of either sex
   b. Pigeon: mature pigeon of either sex

Source: Adapted from P. C. Paul and H. H. Palmer (eds.), *Food Theory and Applications*. New York: Wiley, 1972. Pp. 495–498.

PROCESSING

The processing of poultry includes slaughter, bleeding, feather removal, evisceration, chilling, cutting into parts, packaging, and refrigeration or freezing.

Birds are killed by severing the carotid artery, which allows the heart to pump out most of the blood. Inadequate bleeding causes reddening of the skin. To facilitate feather removal, birds are scalded by immersion in water at temperatures ranging from 128 to 140°F (53°–60°C); if immersed in water that is too hot, or immersed too long, the poultry will be toughened [3]. Feathers are removed mechanically, although excessive beating to remove the feathers also has a toughening effect on the meat. Evisceration is done after the feathers are removed. The poultry is then chilled to 35°F (1.6°C). Aging at 40°F (4.4°C) for 24 hours (which coincides with the passing of rigor mortis) adequately tenderizes all muscles. Inadequate aging after slaughter causes toughness.

PRINCIPLES OF COOKING POULTRY

The purpose of cooking poultry is to develop the flavor, coagulate the proteins, break down connective tissue, and destroy harmful bacteria. Poultry is a source of *Salmonella* bacteria, which spreads from the bird's intestinal tract to the surface of the poultry with handling. Cooking to adequate temperatures destroys these bacteria, if present. Eating affected poultry that has been inadequately cooked results in salmonellosis (infection with *Salmonella*).

Low to moderate heat is best for cooking poultry. Young birds are more palatable when cooked with dry heat (roasted, broiled, fried, or braised); older poultry must be cooked with moist heat for maximum tenderness. In older birds with increased amounts of connective tissue, longer heating is needed to convert collagen to gelatin.

Poultry should be stuffed immediately before roasting to minimize the danger of bacterial growth. The stuffing should not fill the cavity completely, because stuffing swells as it cooks and would otherwise not cook completely. A temperature of 185°F (84°C) should be reached in the center of the stuffing to ensure adequate destruction of bacterial organisms.

References

1. Paul, P. C., and Palmer, H. H. (eds.). *Food Theory and Applications*. New York: Wiley, 1972. Pp. 510, 514.
2. Peckham, G. C., and Freeland-Graves, J. H. *Foundations of Food Preparation* (4th ed.). New York: Macmillan, 1979. Pp. 333, 342.
3. Paul, P. C., and Palmer, H. H. (eds.). *Food Theory and Applications*. New York: Wiley, 1972. Pp. 495–498.

Suggested Readings

Borgstrom, G. (ed.). *Fish as Food*. Vol. 1. New York: Academic, 1961.

Brackkan, O. R. Function of red muscle in fish. *Nature* 178:747, 1956.

Care and handling: Treat poultry like other high-protein menu items—with care and attention. *Rest. Insts.* 88:130, 1981.

Cipra, J. S., and Bowers, J. A. Flavor of microwave and conventionally reheated turkey. *Poult. Sci.* 50:703, 1971.

Duck: Special genetic programs produce ducks with less fat, more breast meat. *Rest. Insts.* 88:93, 1981.

Garcia, M. D., Lavern, J. A., and Olley, J. The lipids of fish. *Biochem. J.* 62:99, 1956.

Heine, N., Bowers, J. A., and Johnson, P. G. Eating quality of half-turkey hens cooked by four methods. *Home Econ. Res. J.* 1:210, 1973.

Institution's fish and shellfish purchasing and handling information. *Institutions* 87:73, 1980.

Johnson, P. G., and Bowers, J. A. Influence of aging on the electrophoretic and structural characteristics of turkey breast muscle. *J. Food Sci.* 41:225, 1976.

MacNeil, J. H., and Dimick, P. S. Poultry product quality. *J. Food Sci.* 35:191, 1970.

Seafood preparation and handling tips. *Institutions* 87:86, 1980.

Stansby, M. E., and Hall, A. S. Chemical composition of commercially important fish of the United States. *Fishery Industrial Res.* 3(4), 1967.

U.S. Department of Agriculture. *Poultry in Family Meals* (Home Garden Bull. 110). Washington, D.C., 1971.

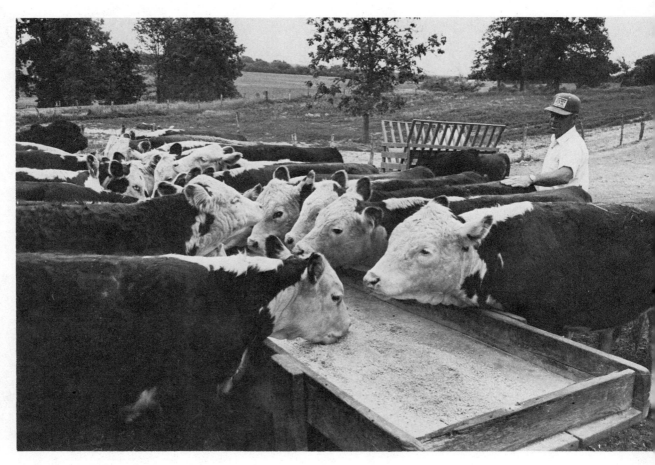

(Photo courtesy of U.S. Department of Agriculture.)

PRESERVING AND PROTECTING THE QUALITY OF FOOD

As long as human beings have existed, the supply of food and the numbers of persons able to survive have been directly related. In the earliest stages of their existence, humans lived as scavengers and predators, relying on what they could find or capture, at the mercy of natural circumstances. With the domestication of animals and the purposeful sowing and harvesting of grains and plants, humans were able to control and improve the food supply to meet the demands of a constantly growing population.

Since then, science has contributed to the many advances made in agricultural productivity, especially as much of the land available for food production has been taken over by growing cities and their suburbs. In the United States, where an abundance of food is produced, the distance between farmland and cities has presented a challenge in distribution—how to transport and distribute safely the food grown in agricultural sections to the people in densely populated cities. With every step in the long process of food production, the likelihood of spoilage or contamination is increased. As a result food preservation has become the focus of much scientific application today.

The fortification and preservation of the food supply has also become a major worldwide goal. The careful addition of vitamins and minerals to certain staples has proved to be an effective way of getting these needed nutrients into the normal daily diet.

In the United States, government agencies oversee both quality maintenance and improvement of food by imposing standards of quality, continually and scientifically checking on the safe use of additives and pesticides, and setting guidelines for labels of identity.

The next three chapters investigate more closely how foods can become contaminated and the mechanisms by which the quality of the food supply is protected and preserved.

Chapter 18

FOOD POISONING AND TOXICOLOGY

Food may become contaminated in many ways and at any point in the process of production and distribution. The carriers of foodborne or waterborne disease are of three main types: (1) pathogenic microorganisms such as bacteria, viruses, parasites, and protozoa; (2) manufactured chemicals (usually used for the purpose of preventing infestation or contamination but applied too close to harvesting or added in excessive amounts); and (3) food or animals that themselves are natural poisons.

Sources of Contamination

Fruits and vegetables can become contaminated during production on farms; seafood, in the aquatic environment. Meat can be contaminated if taken from diseased animals, if infected organs leak on meat surfaces, or if cross-contamination with animal feces occurs. Crops in storage may be damaged by molds. Eggs become contaminated during formation, from droppings, or while in contact with nesting material. Foods are also contaminated by environmental sources and by workers during handling and preparation in processing plants, food service establishments, and homes. The point in the food production, food processing, and food preparation processes at which contamination occurs depends on the natural sources of the pathogen or the source of the poisonous substance and on the opportunities for transfer.

The Nature of Microorganisms

The physical and chemical properties of foods make them vulnerable to the harmful action of microorganisms under favorable environmental conditions. Microorganisms, of course, may have beneficial effects on foods, as in the production of various antibiotics, cheeses, and pickles and the fermentation of compost. The harmful action of microorganisms on foods, however, may result in serious illness, such as typhoid, bacillary dysentery, streptococcal infections, salmonellosis, *Staphylococcus aureus* infections, staphylococcal food poisoning, and botulism. The serious side effects caused by these microorganisms are most often the result of their phenomenal growth rates. Bacteria consume more food per weight than any other biologic group and may release large amounts of metabolic by-products, including toxins, into the surrounding environment. They consume their own weight in food in a few minutes and can double their number and volume every half hour because their surface area is so large in relation to their size.

REQUIRED NUTRIENTS

All microorganisms require nitrogen, sulfur, and trace elements to live. They may or may not be able to synthesize specific vitamins needed for metabolism; most require one or more of the B vitamins. As a result, meat and meat products are an excellent growth medium for microorganisms because meat supplies amino acids (nitrogen, sulfur) and trace elements (copper, iron, calcium) and is rich in all the B vitamins. Other high protein foods also contain similar rich substrates for bacterial growth.

TEMPERATURE

The temperature of the environment or medium also influences both the rate and total amount of bacterial growth that can occur under ideal conditions. *Psychrophiles* ("cold-loving" organisms) can grow at temperatures as low as 0°C (32°F) or less but grow best at 15 to 20°C (56 to 68°F); *psychrotrophs* ("cold-feeding" organisms) can grow at below freezing temperatures of −7°C (19°F) but multiply fastest at about 15°C (56°F); *thermophiles* ("heat-loving" organisms) grow best at 45 to 60°C (113 to 140°F) [1]. The evolution of microorganisms has been such that some species have adapted to temperatures below the freezing point while others can grow and multiply at temperatures above boiling. Neither freezing nor boiling alone ensures complete destruction of all organisms.

ATMOSPHERIC ENVIRONMENT

Of all the gases present in the atmosphere, oxygen and carbon dioxide have the most influence on bacterial growth. *Aerobic* bacteria can grow only in the presence of free oxygen, whereas *anaerobic* bacteria can grow only in its absence. *Facultative anaerobic* organisms can grow in the absence or presence of oxygen. *Microaerophilic* bacteria grow best with minute amounts of oxygen but not with the amounts normally present in air. This explains why some microorganisms can grow and multiply deep inside airtight cans and jars, while others can survive only on the very surface of foods.

MOISTURE AND pH

Moisture is another factor that influences the type of organisms present and their ability to survive, grow, and multiply. The medium surrounding the bacteria must contain dissolved materials that can be used as food; it also must serve as a depository for waste products. The pH of the food and the moisture surrounding it influence the types of organisms that can survive. For centuries it has been known that adding salt or sugar or drying a food reduces the available moisture and improves the keeping qualities. These processes make the food more microbiologically stable.

The nutrient composition, moisture content, pH, and storage temperature all determine the types of microorganisms that cause spoilage or disease in a particular food. The factors that most often contribute to outbreaks of foodborne illness include inadequate refrigeration, lapse of a day or more between preparing and serving, handling by infected persons of foods that are not subsequently heat processed, inadequate time or temperature or both during heat processing, insufficiently high temperatures during hot storage of foods (that is, on steam tables), inadequate time or temperature or both during reheating of previously cooked foods, ingestion of contaminated raw foods or raw ingredients, cross-contamination, inadequate cleaning of equipment, obtaining foods from unsafe sources, and using spoiled leftovers [2]. Pathogenic bacteria often get into food preparation environments on contaminated raw foods, especially of animal origin. The bacteria are killed if the food is cooked long enough but contaminate the food handler's hands and the equipment used in processing, preparation, and storage. The food can be recontaminated after heating by coming into contact with the same worker or equipment if it has not been subsequently cleaned and sanitized.

Common Pathogenic Organisms
BACTERIA

SALMONELLA

The majority of infections caused by the ingestion of foods contaminated with pathogenic bacteria are due to organisms of the *Salmonella* species. About 200 different serotypes have been identified as pathogenic for humans. The symptoms of foodborne infection by all organisms in this group are similar: nausea and vomiting, abdominal cramps, diarrhea, headache, fever, and prostration. The symptoms are most severe and dangerous in infants and the aged. About 6 to 18 hours after the ingestion of the contaminated food are needed to produce appreciable populations of the pathogen. The illness usually has an abrupt onset after this asymptomatic incubation period and lasts only 1 or 2 days.

Most cases of salmonellosis involve large numbers of persons who all ate the same contaminated food, at a wedding dinner, restaurant, or church picnic, for example. Human carriers who act as food handlers are most often sources of infection. Insects can spread the pathogen from fecal sources to food. Unsanitary contaminated ingredients or utensils used in preparation can also spread the infection, as can improperly stored food contaminated with the excreta of infected rodents. Animals used for meat are major reservoirs of salmonellae. They become infected from feed or from an environment that has been contaminated by previous flocks or herds. Cross-contamination is another frequent source, especially from such raw foods as raw meat and poultry, eggshells, and unpasteurized egg products to cooked foods. Inadequate heating or reheating also contributes to the spread of this illness. These bacteria grow easily in moist foods of low acidity and may continue to be viable even in some dried foods. They are destroyed by usual cooking procedures and pasteurization but not by freezing.

SHIGELLA

This organism is usually transmitted through food or water that has been subjected to human contamination. Water and milk are most commonly associated with shigellosis. This foodborne illness is caused mainly by four species of *Shigella: S. dysenteriae, S. boydii, S. flexneri,* and *S. sonnei.* The symptoms include abdominal pain, fever, and diarrhea and usually last 48 to 72 hours.

VIBRIO PARAHAEMOLYTICUS

Infection with *V. parahaemolyticus* is a common food-poisoning syndrome in Japan associated with the consumption of raw fish and shellfish. These salt-tolerant bacteria are found in warm seawaters and are frequently isolated from raw seafoods. Causes of contamination include inadequate refrigeration; inadequate time or temperature during cooking; or the handling of raw then cooked foods, which recontaminates the cooked foods. Like salmonellosis, *V. parahaemolyticus* food poisoning is characterized by severe abdominal pain, nausea, vomiting, diarrhea, and fever.

ESCHERICHIA COLI

Normally found in the colon, this organism can contaminate foods when food handlers practice poor personal hygiene. It may also be found on meat and vegetable products and fresh produce. The incubation period for *E. coli* is from 7 hours to 4 days. The signs and symptoms include abdominal pain, nausea, vomiting, diarrhea, headache, and, in severe cases, fever.

CLOSTRIDIUM PERFRINGENS

Commonly found in the gastrointestinal tract and in the soil, *C. perfringens* produces a relatively mild weakness, abdominal pain, and diarrhea 8 to 18 hours after the ingestion of the contaminated food. These bacteria require certain amino acids and vitamins, which are present in meat and poultry, for growth. Small amounts of *C. perfringens* are common in raw meats, poultry, dehydrated soups and sauces, and raw vegetables and spices. During processing, foods can become contaminated by vegetative cells, or *spores*, which can survive boiling for 4 to 6 hours. In a protein-rich substrate, spores that survive cooking can germinate and multiply if these foods are stored for several hours at room temperature, in large pots in the refrigerator, or at 50°C (122°F) or below [2].

BACILLUS CEREUS

This is an aerobic, spore-forming bacterium commonly found in the soil, in vegetables, and in many raw and processed foods. It grows in moist, cooked, protein foods that are inadequately refrigerated. *B. cereus* is similar to *C. perfringens* with respect to the illness it produces.

TOXIN-PRODUCING BACTERIA AND MOLDS

BACTERIAL TOXINS
Staphylococcus

The most common type of food poisoning is the ingestion of a *toxin* produced by organisms of the genus *Staphylococcus*. These organisms are always present on human skin and are constantly discharged from the respiratory tract. Food handlers and homemakers are usually the main source of the organism, and most foods are contaminated by sneezing, coughing, and cutaneous infections.

Foods contaminated are those rich in protein; several amino acids and the vitamins thiamin and niacin are necessary for the growth of staphylococci and the production of the enterotoxin. High concentrations of sugar or salt and low moisture content inhibit the growth of many bacteria but not *Staphylococcus* [3]. Foods implicated in outbreaks of *Staphylococcus* food poisoning have usually been cooked, then cut, mixed, ground, or otherwise handled by carriers of the organism. The cooking has eliminated the presence of other bacteria, allowing the cooked food, when contaminated, to be an ideal medium for bacterial growth, especially if held at room temperature or refrigerated in such bulk as to retain heat for sufficient time. Staphylococci will grow in cream fillings, puddings, custards, hollandaise sauce, mayonnaise, and other starch, egg, and milk mixtures as well as in meats and meat-containing foods (e.g., chicken salad, ham salad). These organisms will grow rapidly and elaborate their enterotoxin within a few hours in fertile media if not properly refrigerated. Pasteurization can kill all staphylococci yet permit the extremely heat-resistant enterotoxins to survive, as evidenced by their presence in reconstituted powdered milk and powdered malted milk.

The toxin acts primarily on the gastrointestinal tract, and the onset of symptoms is rapid, since a preformed toxin is involved. Within 30 minutes to 3 hours after ingesting a contaminated food, acute nausea, vomiting, diarrhea, abdominal cramps, headache, and fever are experienced. The illness does not usually last more than 1 day and often lasts less than 6 hours.

Clostridium botulinum

Botulism, a rare form of food poisoning, is caused by the ingestion of a toxin secreted by various strains of *C. botulinum*. Unlike other food poisons, *C. botulinum* toxins produce neuroparalytic symptoms that prove fatal in 50 to 100 percent of cases. This is one of the most deadly biologic poisons known. The toxin is absorbed directly from the gastrointestinal tract and within 6 to 24 hours affects the nervous system, causing double vision, difficulty with speech and swallowing, and, when lethal, respiratory and cardiac failure in 3 to 6 days. An antitoxin has been developed for the known strains of *C. botulinum* but is of little value after advanced symptoms appear.

This organism, an anaerobic spore-forming bacterium, produces seven known types of toxins, designated A to G (the most common are types A, B, and E). The spores are widely scattered in soil and in offshore mud and waters throughout the world. Vegetables and fish are therefore most likely to become contaminated. It grows under anaerobic conditions in improperly sterilized preserved foods that have a nearly neutral or slightly alkaline pH. Types A and B, which are highly heat resistant, are major causes of botulism in canned meats and vegetables cooked in pressure cookers. Type E clostridia are destroyed at temperatures greater than 93°C (200°F). The toxin can be formed in foods at temperatures as low as 10°C (50°F) for types A and B and 3.3°C (38°F) for type E [4]. The tolerance to pH is influenced by temperature and type of food, but no strain can survive at a pH below 4.6.

Most cases of botulism are due to improperly sterilized home-preserved nonacid foods, especially corn and string beans. Boiling alone is not sufficient to complete sterilization of home-canned, low acid foods; a pressure cooker must be used to sterilize foods at 240°F (115.5°C) or more for appropriate periods, depending on the size of the container, the processing method, and the particular food. The toxin may be inactivated by boiling for about 15 minutes. Even though a particular jar or can may have supported growth of the organism, subsequent routine cooking may inactivate the toxin.

In the United States, all commercially canned nonacid foods are heat sterilized under pressure at temperatures exceeding the boiling point to ensure destruction of *C. botulinum* spores and therefore safety from botulism.

TOXINS FROM MOLDS (MYCOTOXINS)
Ergot

Ergotism is caused by the parasitic fungus of rye smut (*Claviceps purpurea*). The ergot is found in the fruiting body of the fungus, which is ground up with the grain and disseminated into the flour during milling. The consumption of bread made from such contaminated flour may result in severe or even fatal symptoms concentrated in the circulatory and central nervous systems. The symptoms are due to the vasoconstrictive action of the ergot. The latest epidemic of ergotism occurred in Russia toward the end of World War II, when tens of thousands of the starving rural population consumed unharvested grain that was heavily infested with the fungus.

Aspergillus flavus

This is a fungus that occurs on food crops when they are permitted to mold. The toxin from *A. flavus*, an aflatoxin, is often found on peanuts that have been improperly dried. This toxin has been found to be carcinogenic in rats. No immediate illness is caused in humans, although current research is investigating aflatoxin's carcinogenic potential. Commercial peanut products sold in the United States are free from the toxin, even if produced from contaminated nuts, because the aflatoxin is removed during the refining process.

OTHER PATHOGENIC ORGANISMS

VIRUSES

Infectious hepatitis is the most common viral infection spread by contaminated food. It may be spread by the consumption of contaminated food or water or by the blood of a carrier of the hepatitis virus. The incubation period ranges from 10 to 50 days, and the virus may be in the blood 2 to 3 weeks before the onset of symptoms.

PARASITES

Infection with parasites may be transmitted by food or water, or infected fish or shellfish. One of the most common parasitic infections is the result of muscle infestation with the roundworm *Trichinella spiralis;* the incidence of infection ranges from 9 to 20 percent in the United States. Dormant *T. spiralis* larvae are taken in by the consumption of infected pork that was insufficiently cooked to destroy the parasite. Symptoms include fever and generalized muscular tenderness after a 1- to 2-week incubation period, followed by edema of the eyelids, gastrointestinal symptoms, headache, retinal hemorrhages, sensitivity to light, sweating, and chills.

This infection can be prevented by the thorough cooking of all pork and the avoidance of uncooked pork products. The parasites can be destroyed in infected meat by heating to at least 160°F (71°C), by 30,000 rad of gamma radiation, or by freezing at 5°F (−15°C) for 20 days or more [5].

This parasite is widespread among pigs, owing mainly to the practice of feeding raw garbage, which is frequently contaminated with *T. spiralis* larvae. Some communities specify that hog raisers steam sterilize all garbage before it is used as feed.

PROTOZOA

Amebic dysentery is caused by *Entamoeba histolytica*, protozoa that may be transmitted by food and food handlers. They remain in the tissues of the intestinal tract and cause intermittent attacks until treated. A common complication is abscess of the liver.

Environmental Contamination
CHEMICAL CONTAMINATION

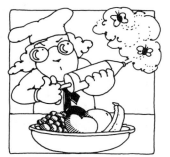

Contamination of food occurs when toxic and nontoxic chemicals escape into the environment. The contamination may be the result of low-level, long-term exposure to chemicals already present in the environment or high-level, short-term exposure from water disposal and industrial accidents. The federal responsibility for ensuring that food contaminants be kept at safe levels is divided among the Food Safety and Quality Service of the U.S. Department of Agriculture, the Food and Drug Administration (FDA) of the U.S. Department of Health and Human Services, and the Environmental Protection Agency. The Food Safety and Quality Service devises methods to ensure that toxic chemical residues are not present in meat, poultry, and egg products. The FDA ensures that the chemical residues in other foods and in animal feed are within safe limits and sets levels for contaminants that are unavoidably present. The Environmental Protection Agency regulates the use of pesticides; sets acceptable levels for those that might remain in food, animal feed, or livestock from intentional use; and governs the manufacture, use, and disposal of chemicals (covered by the Toxic Substance Control Act) that may present risks to the public health or the environment [6].

The FDA and the Food Safety and Quality Service periodically sample food products and test them for various pesticides and other chemicals. If excessive levels are found, these agencies must retrace the product through the food production and distribution system and isolate and remove the source of contamination. The cost of environmental contamination of food has recently been estimated at $282 million annually [6]. The true economic losses would probably be much higher if such factors as health costs and losses incurred by businesses, individuals, and government agencies were also included. The majority of the dollar losses are caused by polychlorinated biphenyls (PCBs) and polybrominated biphenyls (PBBs). These toxic chemicals belong to the chemical family of chlorinated hydrocarbons and are widely used in electrical capacitors and transformers and as additives in dyes, inks, pesticides, and plasticizers. Because their early use was extensive and uncontrolled, these substances have become persistent contaminants of food and the environment, especially freshwater fish. In the late 1960s PCBs were identified as food contaminants because of their presence as low-level environmental contaminants and their accidental leakage from equipment used in food processing equipment. In 1973 the FDA restricted the use of equipment containing PCBs in food plants and established acceptable levels of PCBs in certain commodities. Animal studies have shown that PCBs can cause reproductive difficulties, behavioral abnormalities, and cancer. Other chemicals in the chlorinated hydrocarbon family, including chlorophenothane (DDT), aldrin, endrin, and dieldrin, have been banned or restricted from use because they produce cancers, birth defects, or mutations in animals; they cause adverse side effects in species other than those for which they are intended; and they persist in the environment for long periods of time [6]. The current knowledge, use, and control of PCBs should be viewed in the light of the adverse health effects associated with related compounds.

CONTAMINATION WITH HEAVY METALS

The chronic ingestion of certain metals, including antimony, cadmium, selenium, lead, and arsenic, in foods can have toxic effects. These substances accumulate and are stored within the body, being incorporated into tissue structure. Cadmium will dissolve when in contact with acid-containing foods and is a strong emetic. Antimony, another emetic, has been used as a glaze on enameled vessels and pottery. Selenium has been found in toxic concentrations in cereals grown in certain areas in the United States. Mercury from industrial wastes enters the food cycle via microorganisms and plant life as methylated mercury ions and is concentrated in the food chain in fish. Lead poisoning is cumulative, and the onset is unnoticeable. The three major sources of lead ingestion are lead-containing paints on objects chewed by young children, the residues of sprays on edible crops, and enamel glazes and solders in cooking and food storage utensils [5]. Arsenic may be part of insecticidal sprays widely used on fruits and vegetables. This element can also be legally added to the diets of pigs and poultry, although a 5-day withdrawal period before slaughter is required to allow for its elimination from the animal's body. Arsenic in small doses has been shown to stimulate growth and improve feed efficiency, although the reasons remain unclear [7].

RADIOACTIVE CONTAMINATION

Radioactivity is a natural phenomenon that has been present since the creation of the universe. Some radioactivity is formed, decays, and disappears daily, and the soil, rocks, and atmosphere all contain radioactive matter. When a nuclear reactor malfunctions, or an accident involving the transport of radioactive materials or disposal of nuclear wastes occurs, or there is a fallout from testing a nuclear bomb, radioactive contamination of the food supply could result [8].

Besides monitoring food samples for pesticide residues, industrial chemicals, metals, and other contaminants, the FDA also checks for radionuclide levels. Routinely, as part of their "Total Diet Studies," the FDA analyzes samples of frequently eaten foods common to the American diet. In 30 cities around the country, field personnel shop for 117 individual food items, which are prepared and cooked as they would be for home consumption and then analyzed for chemical contaminants and radionuclide levels. Thus far, the radioactive levels have always been within safe limits.

In addition, the FDA has a "Radionuclides in Foods" program specifically aimed at monitoring levels of iodine 131, strontium 90, cesium 137, ruthenium 106, tritium, and potassium 40. This sampling and testing program was mobilized for extra duty in March 1979 with the malfunctioning of the nuclear reactor at Three Mile Island, Pennsylvania. Within 24 hours, samples of food, milk, and river and tap water were obtained; within 3 months, some 2100 samples had been checked for radioactive content. All samples were well below hazardous levels.

Imported foods including fish, cheese, and tea and coffee, because they are affected by surface contamination, are also routinely analyzed for radioactivity (Fig. 18-1).

Naturally Occurring Toxins

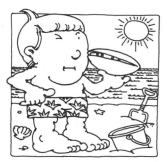

Depending on the amount ingested, a number of plants and animals will cause toxic symptoms. Such poisoning is most likely to occur among children who are more apt to eat unknown but attractive berries or leaves. Such plants include hemlock (coniine), jimsonweed (stramonium), foxglove (digitalis), monkshood (aconitine), and deadly nightshade (atropine). Some plants and animals are safe to eat only at certain times. In the early spring, the young white shoots of the pokeweed are edible, but later the green shoots may cause severe illness. The stems of the rhubarb are safe to eat, but the green leaves contain enough oxalic acid to cause illness. From June to October clams and mussels may feed on a poisonous unicellular marine organism (*Gonyaulax*) that produces a toxin similar to strychnine. Poisoning with this toxin is most common on the Pacific coast but is not restricted to this area. The consumption of clams and mussels during these months may result in acute poisoning. The signs and symptoms—tingling (paresthesia) around the mouth, nausea, vomiting, abdominal cramps, dizziness, incoordination, progressive paralysis, and finally death from respiratory paralysis—begin within 30 minutes.

Some types of sweet peas (vetches) (*Lathyrus sativus*) will cause *lathyrism* when eaten in large quantities. The signs include spastic paralysis of the legs with tremors and paresthesia. With prolonged consumption, bone deformities and rupture of blood vessels can occur. These plants survive droughts, and consequently there is an increased incidence of lathyrism during droughts when a large percentage of the population survives on vetches.

White snakeroot (richweed) poisoning is caused by drinking the milk of cows that pasture where the plant is plentiful. Commercial milk is pooled from many sources, so that toxic concentrations of the snakeroot toxin, tremetol, in processed milk is unlikely.

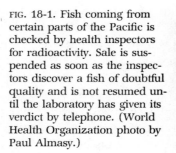

FIG. 18-1. Fish coming from certain parts of the Pacific is checked by health inspectors for radioactivity. Sale is suspended as soon as the inspectors discover a fish of doubtful quality and is not resumed until the laboratory has given its verdict by telephone. (World Health Organization photo by Paul Almasy.)

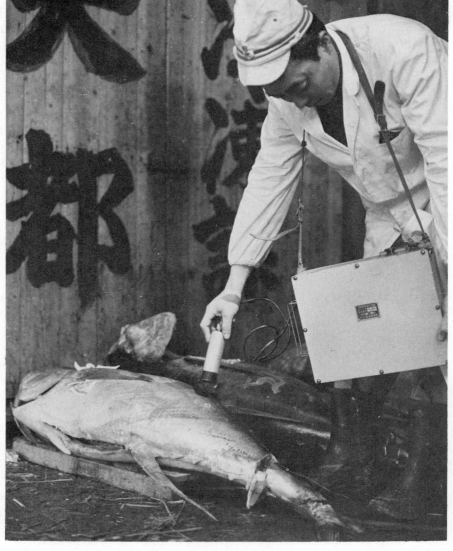

Favism is caused by the ingestion of fava beans or even exposure to the pollen of the blossoming plant by individuals with an inborn deficiency of glucose 6-phosphate dehydrogenase. The toxic substance in fava beans is unknown but causes severe hemolysis (destruction of red blood cells) with vomiting, diarrhea, and weakness. This inborn deficiency affects a large percentage of the population in Asia and the Mediterranean area.

In the raw state, pinto, soy, kidney, lima, and navy beans contain toxic substances including trypsin inhibitors and hemagglutinins. These substances are inactivated by roasting or normal cooking.

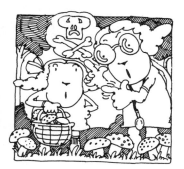

Specific botanical characteristics distinguish edible from poisonous mushrooms. Most cases of poisoning by mushrooms are due to two species of the genus *Amanita*: *A. phalloides* and *A. muscaria*. Rapid poisoning is caused by *A. muscaria*, which contains the toxin muscarine. The signs and symptoms, which occur within 1 to 2 hours, include vomiting, cramps, salivation, sweating, and collapse. Atropine is the antidote, and the mortality is low. Delayed poisoning is caused by *A. phalloides*. Abdominal pain, nausea, vomiting, and diarrhea occur 6 to 16 hours after ingestion; these are followed by extensive damage to the kidneys, liver, and central nervous system. The toxins are well absorbed before countermeasures can be taken; the mortality is 50 percent or higher.

Prevention of Food Poisoning

Most cases of food poisoning are caused by bacterial contamination. Strict sanitary handling of foods, adequate refrigeration, pasteurization of milk, inspection of meats, and pest control measures in food storage areas would greatly reduce the incidence of foodborne illness. The danger area for bacterial reproduction in foods is 50 to 120°F (10 to 49°C)—as little as 4 hours may suffice to permit growth, particularly in such an ideal medium as raw milk or ground meat. Inadequate refrigeration, time lapse between preparing and serving, and cross-contamination to utensils and surfaces are major factors responsible for infection.

References

1. Lechowich, R. V.   Food Microbiology. In F. Clydesdale (ed.), *Food Science and Nutrition: Current Issues and Answers.* Englewood Cliffs, N.J.: Prentice-Hall, 1979. Pp. 96–97.
2. Bryan, F. L.   Factors that contribute to outbreaks of foodborne disease. *J. Food Protection* 41:816, 1978.
3. Bryan, F. L.   Public health aspects of cream-filled pastries: A review. *J. Milk Food Technol.* 39:289, 1976.
4. Lechowich, R. V.   Food Microbiology. In F. Clydesdale (ed.), *Food Science and Nutrition: Current Issues and Answers.* Englewood Cliffs, N.J.: Prentice-Hall, 1979. P. 110.
5. Burton, B. T.   *Human Nutrition.* New York: McGraw-Hill, 1976. P. 464.
6. U.S. Comptroller General.   *Further Federal Action Needed to Detect and Control Environmental Contamination of Food* (Report to the Chairman, Committee on Appropriations, U.S. Senate). Washington, D.C.: Government Printing Office, 1980.
7. Lambert, M. R.   Arsenic: It's everywhere! *Prof. Nutr.* 13:5, 1981.
8. Lecos, C.   On guard against radioactive food. *FDA Consum.* 14:18, 1981.

Suggested Readings

Arnon, S. S., et al.   Honey and other environmental risk factors for infant botulism. *J. Pediatr.* 94:331, 1979.
Benedict, R. C.   Biochemical basis for nitrite-inhibition of *Clostridium* botulism in cured meat. *J. Food Protect.* 43:887, 1980.
Brown, L. W.   Commentary: Infant botulism and the honey connection. *J. Pediatr.* 94:337, 1979.

Bryan, F. L.   Current trends in foodborne salmonellosis in the United States and Canada. *J. Food Protect.* 44:394, 1981.

Bryan, F. L.   Epidemiology of foodborne diseases transmitted by fish, shellfish, and marine crustaceans in the United States. *J. Food Protect.* 43:859, 1980.

Bullerman, L. B.   Significance of mycotoxins to food safety and human health. *J. Food Protect.* 42:65, 1979.

Calabrese, E. J.   *Nutrition and Environmental Health: The Influence of Nutritional Status on Pollutant Toxicity and Carcinogenicity.* New York: Wiley, 1980.

Commoner, B., et al.   Formation of mutagens in beef and beef extract during cooking. *Science* 201:913, 1978.

Crocco, S. C.   Nitrosamines in beer. *J.A.M.A.* 245:968, 1981.

Crocco, S. C.   Potato sprouts and greening potatoes: Potential toxic reaction. *J.A.M.A.* 245:625, 1981.

Daun, H.   Interaction of wood smoke components and foods. *Food Technol.* 33:66, 1979.

De Paola, A.   *Vibrio cholerae* in marine foods and environmental waters: A literature review. *J. Food Sci.* 46:66, 1981.

Doull, J.   Assessment of food safety. *Fed. Proc.* 37:2594, 1978.

Doull, J., Klaassen, C. D., and Andur, M. O. (eds.).   *Casarett and Doull's Toxicology: The Basic Science of Poisons* (2nd ed.). New York: Macmillan, 1980.

Getoff, M. M.   Unsafe food practices in the kitchen. *J. Home Econ.* 70:45, 1978.

Graham, H. D. (ed.).   *The Safety of Foods.* Westport, Conn.: AVI Publishing, 1980.

Gray, J. I., and Morton, I. D.   Some toxic compounds produced in food by cooking and processing. *J. Hum. Nutr.* 35:5, 1981.

Gunby, P.   Botulism: Lingering puzzle. *J.A.M.A.* 245:1803, 1981.

Hanno, H. A.   Ciguatera fish poisoning in the Virgin Islands. *JAMA* 245:464, 1981.

Havery, D. C., Hotchkiss, J. H., and Fazio, T.   Nitrosamines in malt and malt beverages. *J. Food Sci.* 46:501, 1981.

Ivie, G. W., Holt, D. L., and Ivey, M. C.   Natural toxicants in human foods: Psoralens in raw and cooked parsnip root. *Science* 213:909, 1981.

Jay, J. M.   *Modern Food Microbiology* (2nd ed.). New York: Van Nostrand, 1978.

Larkin, E. P.   Food contaminants—viruses. *J. Food Protect.* 44:320, 1981.

Magos, L.   Mercury: An environmental and dietary hazard. *J. Hum. Nutr.* 32:179, 1978.

Rodricks, J. V.   Hazards from nature: Aflatoxins. *FDA Consum.* 12:16, 1978.

"Talc on rice" debate flares up again. *Food Eng.* 53:24, 1981.

U.S. Department of Health, Education and Welfare, Centers for Disease Control. *Foodborne and Waterborne Disease Outbreaks: Annual Summary 1975.* Atlanta: Centers for Disease Control, 1976.

Chapter 19

FOOD PRESERVATIVES AND ADDITIVES

The term *food additive* was introduced in legislation in 1958 and is defined by the U.S. Food and Drug Administration (FDA) as ". . . substances added directly to food, or substances that may reasonably be expected to become components of food through surface contact with equipment or packaging materials, or even substances that may otherwise affect the food without becoming part of it" [1]. Changing life-styles have resulted in an increased use of additives in our food supply. Americans have moved from farms to the cities, and as a result foods must be mass-produced, distributed over considerable distances, and stored for long periods. While improved standards of hygiene and improvements in food processing should have decreased the need for preservatives and additives, the movement of women from the home to the work place, as well as other factors, has instead created a greater demand for ready-made convenience foods and packaged foods, thus increasing the need for additives.

Nonfood substances have been added to food for centuries, but they have recently come under closer scrutiny because of the increase in their number, provoking the question, Are additives necessary and safe? The distinction between food ingredients and food additives is imprecise and somewhat arbitrary. Food additives may be classified by function: They are used for enhancing flavor, improving color, extending shelf life, and protecting the nutritional value of a food [2]. Additives are valuable, but not essential, in the manufacture of food. Without additives, many foods could not be offered for sale in their present form. To meet the increasing demands for food in undernourished areas and to keep up with the needs of the growing population, food additives, in many forms, will play an even bigger role in nutrition in the future.

Historic Perspective

From earliest times, foods have been preserved by heating, salting, drying, pickling, fermenting, and smoking and by incidental additives that resulted from cooking (e.g., metal ions from cooking utensils). Spices and condiments became important items in commerce as the art of flavoring and seasoning developed in ancient civilizations. To pass off an inferior item as a better one, or to dilute expensive items, products were often *adulterated*, or altered by the addition or substitution of another substance. Burned or roasted vegetable material and coloring substances were often used as additives; beer, wine, and bread were frequent victims of this process. The earliest food laws were aimed at controlling adulteration and fraud. Merchant guilds of the Middle Ages tried to protect the purity and reputation of their products.

Methods for evaluating the purity of products were limited before the major advances in organic chemistry during the middle of the nineteenth century. During the second half of the nineteenth century, however, national pure food laws were enacted to regulate the composition of food and the use of additives. Advances in organic chemistry also led to the production of new food additives, including synthetic flavorings, some of which proved to have more flavoring power than the analogous natural flavors.

The 1906 Pure Food and Drugs Act and the 1938 Food, Drug and Cosmetic Act gave the federal government the authority to remove adulterated and poisonous foods from the market. Not until 1958, with the Food Additives Amendment, and 1960, with the Color Additives Amendments, did the United States enact laws specifically regulating food additives. These laws shifted the burden of proof from the government, which formerly had to prove an additive unsafe, to the manufacturer, who must now prove it safe. The manufacturer must subject the proposed new additive to a battery of chemical tests to determine if it does what it is intended to do and must measure and analyze its presence in the finished product. The safety of an additive can be fully ensured only after it has been consumed in specified amounts by persons of all ages over a long period and it has been shown by toxicologic examination to have no harmful effects. Since humans cannot be used for testing, rats, mice, and dogs are usually used. Tests made with quantities of the additives far in excess of what would be used in food are made over short periods, for the lifetime of the animal, and often into succeeding generations. The animals are examined for the presence of tumors and for any change in growth, body function, tissue, and reproduction. The largest dose that produces no ill effects is reduced by a factor of 100 to determine an acceptable dose for humans. The "acceptable daily intake" is expressed in milligrams of the additive per kilogram of body weight.

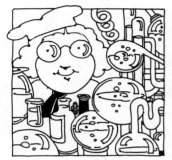

The Food Additives Amendment of the Food, Drug and Cosmetic Act contains the *Delaney clause,* which specifies that ". . . no additive shall be deemed safe if it is found to induce cancer when ingested by man or animals, or if it is found, after tests which are appropriate for the evaluation of the safety of food additives, to induce cancer in man or animals." This clause is *always* interpreted as meaning "zero tolerance" for additives that induce cancer.

Because testing is both time-consuming and costly, it is the desire of the food industry and many governments that test results be shared rather than have the test duplicated. The exchange of toxicologic data would allow the evaluation of the safety of more additives as soon as possible.

The Food Additives Amendment stipulates that two major categories of additives are exempt from testing: a group of some 700 substances "generally recognized as safe" (GRAS list) and "prior sanctional substances" that had been approved before 1958 by either the FDA or the U.S. Department of Agriculture. With further testing or new data, previously approved substances can be removed from these lists if demonstrated to be unsafe.

The Codex Alimentarius Commission of the United Nations Food and Agriculture Organization and the World Health Organization (WHO) have published a list of six general principles on the use of food additives:

1. The use of an additive is justified only when it has the purpose of maintaining a food's nutritional quality; enhancing its keeping quality or stability; making

the food attractive; providing aid in processing, packing, transporting, or storing food; or providing essential components for foods for special diets. The additive is not justified if the proposed level of use constitutes a hazard to the consumer's health, causes a substantial reduction in the nutritive value of the food, disguises faulty quality or the use of processing and handling techniques not allowed, or deceives the customer, or if the desired effect can be obtained by other manufacturing processes that are economically and technologically satisfactory.

2. The amount of additives should not exceed the level reasonably required to achieve the desired effect under good manufacturing practice.

3. The additives must conform with an approved standard of purity.

4. All additives, in use or proposed, should be subjected to adequate toxicologic evaluation, and permitted additives should be kept under observation for possible deleterious effects.

5. Approval of an additive should be limited to specific foods for specific purposes and under specific conditions.

6. The use of additives in foods consumed mainly by special groups of persons should be carefully evaluated before authorization.

Colorings

Colorings are used to give an appetizing appearance to food, to influence palatability, and to enhance flavor. Colors used in the food industry must not only produce the desired appearance but must also remain stable under conditions of manufacturing, storage, and preparation, including high processing temperatures and the action of acids.

Regulations on colors vary from nation to nation; they specify purity and restrict the types of foods to which the color may be added. The WHO has evaluated about 140 colors and published a short list of those deemed safe. The 1960 Color Additives Amendments to the Food, Drug and Cosmetic Act require that the FDA maintain a list of color additives that the agency has determined to be safe for the intended uses. Information about each color on the list includes its physical, chemical, or botanical identity; the products or kinds of products in which it may be used; the quantities allowed; and any other conditions of use the FDA considers necessary to protect the public health. The FDA also gives color additives simplified, official names consisting of the primary color and a number, preceded by the letters F, D, or C to designate the color's use in foods, drugs, or cosmetics. Some are also labeled *ext.* (for external use only), and a few, such as Citrus Red No. 2, have more explicit and specialized names.

Most color additives are obtained from coal. Most of the dyes used in products the FDA regulates are synthesized from a derivative of benzene called *aniline*. They are known as synthetic organic dyes or coal tar dyes because aniline was formerly obtained from bituminous coal, although presently it is manufactured from petroleum [3].

Color additives can be classified by whether or not they are regulated by the

FDA. Those that consist mainly of aniline derivatives are tested and certified by the FDA. Every newly synthesized batch of color additives subject to certification is analyzed by the FDA (batch certification) to determine how well it matches established standards. Color additives that consist of, or are closely related to, substances derived from vegetable, animal, or mineral products are exempt from certification requirements because the FDA does not consider batch certification necessary to protect public health. The FDA regulations do, however, specify the conditions and amounts in which these exempt color additives may be used in foods, drugs, and cosmetics and sets limits on impurities. Of the 25 exempt color additives permitted in foods, most are vegetable compounds, such as juices of edible fruits or vegetables, paprika, saffron, beet powder, and grape skin extract. Some are restricted to certain foods. Of the 28 exempt color additives permitted in drugs, most are derived from minerals: talc, bronze powder, copper powder, aluminum powder, mica, chromium hydroxide green. The list of permissible color additives for cosmetics is similar to that for drugs.

FDA-approved color additives are also grouped as "permanent" or "provisional." Those on the permanent list are assured safe by data the manufacturer has collected from tests in laboratory animals. Colors on the provisional list are those in use when the 1960 Color Additives Amendments were enacted that have not yet qualified for permanent listing because all the safety tests required by the FDA have not yet been completed.

The disclosure of colors used in a product is mandatory if it has been determined that their identification to the consumer is necessary to protect public health. Cosmetics manufacturers are required to list, on the label, the name of each color additive used.

In the event of unresolved safety questions or inability to prove safety, the FDA will ban the use of a color additive. An example of this was the withdrawal of FD&C Red No. 2 ("red dye no. 2") from the provisional list because its safety could not be proved. Researchers in Russia had reported that this color additive caused cancer in rats. During that same time, FD&C Red No. 4, used in maraschino cherries and drugs, and carbon black were taken off the provisional list, also because of unresolved safety questions. The FDA is reviewing all provisional and permanent color additives used in foods and internally taken drugs and hopes to abolish its provisional list when safety tests are completed for all colors. The permanent standing can be reversed if questions arise about a color additive's safety.

Consumers criticize the use of color additives by the food industry, arguing that the added colors contribute nothing to food safety or nutrition and are used only to give products better sales appeal. In addition, the use of color additives increases the cost of foods and can mislead consumers about the food's safety and value. The food industry maintains that it uses color additives because of consumer demand that food be aesthetically pleasing and appetizing. Much of the processing, packaging, storage, and preservation necessary to make food available would also cause it to be aesthetically unacceptable were it not for the use of color additives.

Fortification
INFLUENCE ON PUBLIC HEALTH

Fortification, the addition of nutrients to selected foods, has resulted in the virtual disappearance of rickets and pellagra and a substantial reduction in iodine-deficiency goiter in America, as well as an improvement in many other nutritionally related health problems. Fortification has been considered to be one of the great accomplishments of nutritional science, with its benefits ranking among the greatest medical discoveries of this century [4]. The goal of national and international nutrition policies is to make available to all people diets that meet all nutrient requirements. Until this ideal situation is achieved, fortification and enrichment (the replacement of nutrients lost in processing) provide a beneficial, practical, inexpensive, and effective method of closing the gaps in nutrient intake.

FACTORS AFFECTING THE NEED FOR FORTIFICATION

Factors in the geochemical environment may influence the need for fortification: Deficiencies in soil minerals in many areas of the world are reflected in low concentrations of trace elements and minerals in the drinking water, agricultural crops, and tissues of farm animals. An example of this is areas low in fluorine, where fluorine enrichment of drinking water benefits the dental health of children and the bone health of the middle-aged and elderly.

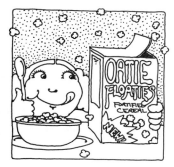

The availability and quality of the food supply also influences the need for enrichment and fortification programs. In areas where undernutrition and malnutrition are prevalent, the only real solution is to improve food production and distribution. This solution takes time and effort; in the interim, programs providing dietary supplements to increase nutrient intake can have immediate health benefits. This straightforward solution may not always be an effective answer, however. Since food plays a central role in culture and tradition, foods that are new to a society, or even foods that are substantially altered in form, may not be acceptable as substitutes for traditional foods. Thus, dietary supplements may have an effect opposite the intended and potentiate malnutrition. For this reason, food scientists are working on ways of improving the nutritional quality of food staples such as corn, rice, and wheat through hybridization and genetic manipulation, thereby maintaining the food in its accepted form.

The vitamin and mineral intake of a population can be compromised, even when an abundance of food is available at reasonable prices, because of trends in life-styles and eating habits. Improved technology has led to the mechanization of many physical chores and a reduction in energy expenditure during this century. A reduction in food intake has been necessary to avoid obesity but has led to widespread iron deficiency in the United States. A second trend that has been suggested is the dilution of the food supply with products that furnish substantial amounts of energy but no essential micronutrients [5]. Examples include the high consumption of refined sugars, which supply pure carbohydrates but no micronutrients (vitamins and minerals), and cereal products from highly processed white flour. Even when enriched, cereal products are not equivalent to the grain with respect to all essential micronutrients.

A fortification policy must be flexible, incorporating new knowledge of nutritional status and food technology. A recent policy revision by a subcommittee of the Food and Nutrition Board of the National Research Council reflects this, including zinc among the nutrients proposed for fortification, along with other changes in guidelines [6]. Five major areas should be considered in establishing fortification programs: (1) human requirements and nutritional status, (2) biologic availability, (3) interactions between nutrients, (4) the selection of a suitable carrier food for fortification, and (5) interactions between the fortifying nutrient and the carrier food [5].

HUMAN REQUIREMENTS AND NUTRITIONAL STATUS

When the human requirement for a micronutrient is known and sufficient data on its content in foods are available, an evaluation can be made of the national food supply as to whether abundant, sufficient, or marginal amounts of the micronutrient are available. If the micronutrient is abundant in the food supply, no fortification is necessary. If sufficient amounts are available, as with zinc, certain population groups may be at risk for marginal or deficient intake. Recent recommendations by the Food and Nutrition Board [6] for zinc fortification have already been implemented by most of the manufacturers of food for infants. The best example of the third case, marginal or insufficient availability, is iron. Although recommended intakes are based on sound scientific evidence, they are practically unattainable in the United States, especially for women. The present iron fortification program has increased the average intake of this element by 25 percent, but iron deficiency is still widespread.

BIOLOGIC AVAILABILITY

As stated by the Food and Nutrition Board, the micronutrients used in fortification must be physiologically available [6]. It is known, for example, that the different types of iron have different percentages of absorption and utilization (see Chap. 7). Therefore the type of compound used greatly influences its biologic availability. This is also true for a number of other trace elements, and research is contributing more knowledge in this area daily. Consideration of biologic availability is important if new fortification programs are to be effective.

INTERACTIONS BETWEEN NUTRIENTS

Before a food is fortified, it must be determined if fortification will lead to imbalances in the diet through interactions between macronutrients (carbohydrates, fats, and proteins) and micronutrients or between the vitamins and minerals themselves. An example is the calcium-phosphorus ratio, known to be important to bone health and which should ideally be about 1:1. Since the dietary intake of phosphorus exceeds that of calcium, fortification with calcium should be beneficial. An excessive intake of calcium, however, can reduce the biologic availability of zinc and iron. Another example is the known antagonism between copper and zinc. Marginal copper deficiency is aggravated by high levels of zinc; copper intake and status should be carefully evaluated before the initiation of a zinc fortification program. Another example is the interaction between selenium and heavy metals such as mercury and cadmium. Selenium has a protective influence against the effects of excessive exposure to these metals, and therefore fortification would offer a health benefit in a heavily contaminated environment, even though there may not be any overt indications of a deficient intake.

SELECTION OF A SUITABLE CARRIER FOOD FOR FORTIFICATION

The most important consideration in choosing a carrier food is its availability to the target population, the group particularly at risk of deficiency. For example, since the vitamin D requirements of adults are met by endogenous synthesis (exposure to sunlight), the fortification of a food such as milk, which is consumed by infants, children, and adolescents, with vitamin D is appropriate (Fig. 19-1). Such foods as salt and drinking water reach all of the population and are considered ideal carriers for fortification programs directed to all groups.

INTERACTIONS OF FORTIFICATION NUTRIENTS WITH CARRIER FOOD

Trace elements can be powerful catalysts, sometimes accelerating undesirable reactions and leading to off-colors, off-flavors, and off-tastes in the carrier food. The choice of the form of the fortifying nutrient therefore must take into account both nutritional and technologic considerations if the fortified product is to be acceptable to the public and contain the element in an available form.

Flavors

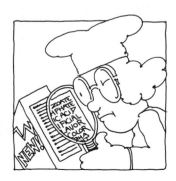

This group comprises the largest class of food additives: There are between 1100 and 1400 natural and synthetic flavors. Flavors pose the largest regulatory risk because there are so many, there is so little toxicologic data, and many natural flavors have been used for centuries. In this group are also the flavor enhancers, such as *monosodium glutamate* (MSG), a monosodium salt of glutamic acid, an amino acid. MSG has been linked with the "Chinese Restaurant Syndrome" (Kwok's disease), whose symptoms include tightening of the muscles of the face and neck, headache, and nausea. Many countries have restricted the use of MSG because of these side effects.

Current research is focusing on finding cheaper or more effective flavoring agents and flavor enhancers. Another need is for simulated food, for example, spun soybean proteins and dairy product substitutes, to imitate the complex flavor properties of traditional foods.

FIG. 19-1. Milk is an appropriate carrier food for vitamin D fortification since it is consumed mostly by infants, children, and adolescents, the groups who are most at risk for vitamin D deficiency. (U.S. Department of Agriculture photo.)

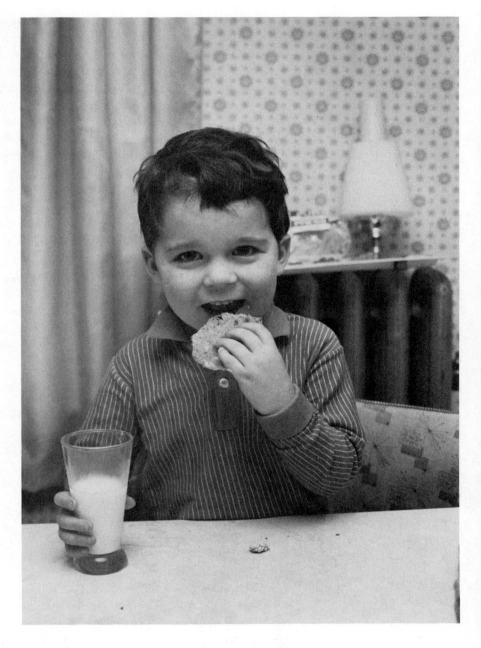

Preservatives

The purpose of this group of additives is to deter food spoilage by microorganisms. The World Health Organization estimates that about 20 percent of the world's food supply is lost to spoilage [2]. Physical and biologic processes such as freezing, heating, drying, refrigeration, curing, fermenting, and souring can also prevent or retard spoilage (Fig. 19-2). Some of these processes achieve only partial preservation. Additives, therefore, play an important role in keeping

FIG. 19-2. These women are judging jars of home-preserved food. Canning has become popular in urban areas as well. (U.S. Department of Agriculture photo by Fred White.)

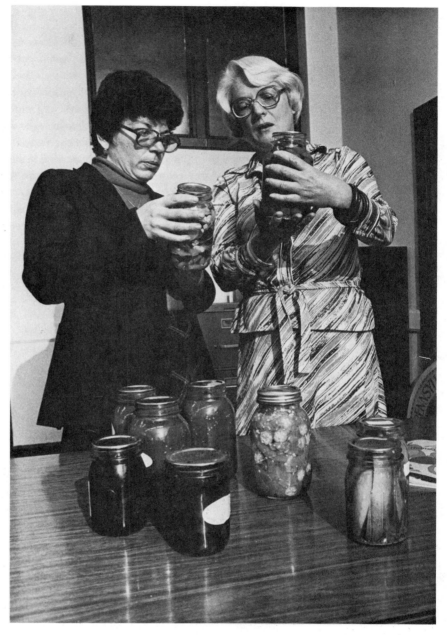

foods. Different types of preservatives are used depending on the type of food; the method of manufacture, packaging, and storage; and the kinds of microorganisms involved.

MOLD INHIBITORS

In baked products, which become stale and moldy quickly, such additives as sodium diacetate, acetic acid, lactic acid, monocalcium phosphate, sodium pro-

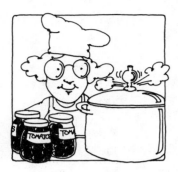

pionate, and calcium propionate are all effective in preventing the spread of spores and retarding spoilage. Sorbic acid and its salts prevent mold in cheese, syrup, and confections containing fruit or sugar. Margarine, fruit juice concentrates, juices, and pickled vegetables often contain benzoic acid and sodium benzoate as preservatives.

Sulfur dioxide is used in wine, fruit pulps, fruit juice concentrates, dried fruits, and vegetables to inhibit mold and discoloration. In countries where the wine consumption is high, there is concern over exceeding the acceptable daily intake of sulfur dioxide, 1.5 mg per kilogram of body weight. Half a liter of wine contains about 200 parts per million of sulfur dioxide, or about 100 mg, the acceptable daily intake for an average person. Studies in rats have shown that sulfite inhibits growth through the destruction of vitamin B_1. More work is needed to clarify the toxicity of sulfur dioxide and sulfites.

ANTIBIOTICS

Antibiotics have also been used as antimicrobial additives. One of the main drawbacks is that their liberal use in foods may produce resistant strains of pathogens, which would reduce the effectiveness of antibiotics in medicine, for which they are most important.

ANTIBACTERIALS

Smoke, spices, salt, and vinegar have been used since ancient times to prevent bacterial spoilage of foods. More recently such substances as benzoic acid and sorbic acid have been used successfully and safely in preventing bacterial spoilage. Sugar also prevents microbial spoilage, and its use in food processing has been steadily increasing. Salt is perhaps the oldest and most universally used food additive.

ANTIOXIDANTS

These compounds prevent rancidity that results from the oxidation of unsaturated fatty acids. Antioxidants are added to such fat-containing foods as margarine, biscuits, cooking oils, cereals, potato chips, salted nuts, soup mixes, and precooked meals containing meat, fish, or poultry.

The most widely used antioxidants include BHA (butylated hydroxyanisole), BHT (butylated hydroxytoluene), propyl gallate, octyl gallate, dodecyl gallate, and natural or synthetic tocopherols (vitamin E) alone or in combination. When combined with certain acids (ascorbic, citric, and phosphoric), the antioxidant effect is enhanced. Antioxidants inhibit certain carcinogens, as suggested by the decreased incidence of stomach cancer in the United States attributed in part to the addition of BHA and BHT to foods.

Packaging foods in transparent wrappings has led to the problem of discoloration on exposure to light. Ascorbic acid prevents discoloration in fruit juices, canned vegetables, frozen fruits, and cooked, cured meats. Many countries will allow the use of "natural" antioxidants, such as ascorbic acid (vitamin C) and tocopherols (vitamin E) only.

NITRITES AND NITRATES

Nitrates are normal components of plants found abundantly in such common vegetables as beets, celery, lettuce, carrots, and spinach. Bacteria in the soil oxidize ammonia from fertilizers to nitrites, then reduce nitrites to nitrates. Some of the nitrates are converted to nitrites by bacteria in the digestive tract; nitrites are also formed from nitrates in cooked vegetables standing at room temperature.

Nitrites can react with amines to form nitrosamines, which have been shown to be carcinogenic to laboratory animals at low dosages. This reaction can occur in the digestive tract and in the frying of bacon. For this reason, sodium nitrite, which fixes a red color in hams, frankfurters, and sausages, is under review. Other compounds, such as ascorbate and erythorbate have been suggested as substitutes for nitrites in the curing of meats. The main use of nitrites is to inhibit the growth of *Clostridium botulinum*.

Texture Agents

These additives include emulsifiers, stabilizers, and thickening agents. They are used extensively in preparing bread, pastry, ice cream, frozen desserts, whipped products, margarine, candy, soft drinks, and milk products. Texture agents permit oil to be dispersed in water, produce a smooth and even texture, and supply the desired body and consistency.

The first emulsifiers were either natural substances such as gums, alginates, and soaps or synthetic substances of fairly simple composition. Today, the most common emulsifiers and stabilizers are stearyl tartrate, glycerol esters, propylene glycol esters, monostearin sodium sulfoacetate, sorbitan esters of fatty acids, cellulose ethers, and sodium carboxymethylcellulose.

Thickeners include natural products such as agar, alginates, cellulose, starches, vegetable gums, dextrins, and pectin.

Miscellaneous Additives

Acids, alkalis, buffers, and neutralizing agents are also used in baked goods, soft drinks, chocolate, and processed cheese. Bleaching and maturing agents are used to develop flour for baked products. Sequestrants bind trace elements that may have contaminated the product during preparation, thereby preventing any oxidative activity. Humectants offset changes in humidity in the environment to which the food is exposed so that a desired level of moisture is maintained (e.g., in shredded coconut). Anticaking agents keep salt and powders free-flowing. Glazing agents make food surfaces shiny. Firming and crisping agents prevent flaccidity in processed fruits and vegetables and aid in the coagulation of certain cheeses. Release agents help food to separate from surfaces it touches during manufacture. Foaming agents and propellants make whipped toppings come out as foam; foam inhibitors have the opposite effect. Clarifying agents remove from liquids small particles of minerals that might otherwise turn them cloudy. Solvents act as carriers for flavors, colors, and other additives.

A summary of food additives and their uses is given in Table 19-1.

TABLE 19-1. Selected additives and their functions

Additive	Function	Additive	Function
Acetic acid	pH control[a]	EDTA (ethylenediamine-tetraacetic acid)	Antioxidant[d]
Acetone peroxide	Mat-bleach-condit[a]		
Adipic acid	pH control[a]		
Ammonium alginate	Stabil-thick-tex[a]	FD&C colors	
Annatto extract	Color[b]	Blue No. 1	Color[b]
Arabinogalactan	Stabil-thick-tex[a]	Red No. 3	Color[b]
Ascorbic acid	Nutrient[c]	Red No. 40	Color[b]
	Preservative[d]	Yellow No. 5	Color[b]
	Antioxidant[d]	Fructose	Sweetener[b]
Azodicarbonamide	Mat-bleach-condit[a]		
		Gelatin	Stabil-thick-tex[a]
Benzoic acid	Preservative[d]	Glucose	Sweetener[b]
Benzoyl peroxide	Mat-bleach-condit[a]	Glycerine	Humectant[a]
Beta-apo-8′carotenal	Color[b]	Clycerol monostearate	Humectant[a]
Beta carotene	Nutrient[c]	Grape skin extract	Color[b]
	Color[b]	Guar gum	Stabil-thick-tex[a]
BHA (butylated hydroxyanisole)	Antioxidant[d]	Gum arabic	Stabil-thick-tex[a]
		Gum ghatti	Stabil-thick-tex[a]
BHT (butylated hydroxytoluene)	Antioxidant[d]	Heptylparaben	Preservative[d]
Butylparaben	Preservative[d]	Hydrogen peroxide	Mat-bleach-condit[a]
		Hydrolyzed vegetable protein	Flavor enhancer[b]
Calcium alginate	Stabil-thick-tex[a]		
Calcium bromate	Stabil-thick-tex[a]	Invert sugar	Sweetener[b]
Calcium lactate	Preservative[d]	Iodine	Nutrient[c]
Calcium phosphate	Leavening[a]	Iron	Nutrient[c]
Calcium propionate	Preservative[d]	Iron ammonium citrate	Anticaking[a]
Calcium silicate	Anticaking[a]	Iron oxide	Color[b]
Calcium sorbate	Preservative[d]		
Canthaxanthin	Color[b]	Karaya gum	Stabil-thick-tex[a]
Caramel	Color[b]		
Carob bean gum	Stabil-thick-tex[a]	Lactic acid	pH control[a]
Carrageenan	Emulsifier[a]		Preservative[d]
	Stabil-thick-tex[a]	Larch gum	Stabil-thick-tex[a]
Carrot oil	Color[b]	Lecithin	Emulsifier[a]
Cellulose	Stabil-thick-tex[a]	Locust bean gum	Stabil-thick-tex[a]
Citric acid	Preservative[d]		
	Antioxidant[d]	Mannitol	Sweetener[b]
	pH control[a]		Anticaking[a]
Citrus Red No. 2	Color[b]		Stabil-thick-tex[a]
Cochineal extract	Color[b]	Methylparaben	Preservative[d]
Corn endosperm	Color[b]	Modified food starch	Stabil-thick-tex[a]
Corn syrup	Sweetener[b]	Monoglycerides	Emulsifier[a]
		MSG (monosodium glutamate)	Flavor enhancer[b]
Dehydrated beets	Color[b]		
Dextrose	Sweetener[b]	Niacinamide	Nutrient[c]
Diglycerides	Emulsifier[a]		
Dioctyl sodium sulfosuccinate	Emulsifier[a]	Paprika (and oleoresin)	Flavor[b]
			Color[b]
Disodium guanylate	Flavor enhancer[b]	Pectin	Stabil-thick-tex[a]
Disodium inosinate	Flavor enhancer[b]	Phosphates	pH control[a]
Dried algae meal	Color[b]		

TABLE 19-1 (CONTINUED)

Additive	Function	Additive	Function
Phosphoric acid	pH control[a]	Sorbitan monostearate	Emulsifier[a]
Polysorbates	Emulsifiers[a]	Sorbitol	Humectant[a]
Potassium alginate	Stabil-thick-tex[a]		Sweetener[b]
Potassium bromate	Mat-bleach-condit[a]	Spices	Flavor[b]
Potassium iodide	Nutrient[c]	Sucrose (table sugar)	Sweetener[b]
Potassium propionate	Preservative[d]		
Potassium sorbate	Preservative[d]	Tagetes (Aztec marigold)	Color[b]
Propionic acid	Preservative[d]	Tartaric acid	pH control[a]
Propyl gallate	Antioxidant[d]	TBHQ (tertiary	Antioxidant[d]
Propylene glycol	Stabil-thick-tex[a]	butyl hydroquinone)	
	Humectant[a]	Thiamin	Nutrient[c]
Propylparaben	Preservative[d]	Titanium dioxide	Color[b]
		Toasted, partially de-	Color[b]
Riboflavin	Nutrient[c]	fatted, cooked	
	Color[b]	cottonseed flour	
		Tocopherols	Nutrient[c]
Saccharin	Sweetener[b]	(vitamin E)	Antioxidant[d]
Saffron	Color[b]	Tragacanth gum	Stabil-thick-tex[a]
Silicon dioxide	Anticaking[a]	Turmeric (oleoresin)	Flavor[b]
Sodium acetate	pH control[a]		Color[b]
Sodium alginate	Stabil-thick-tex[a]		
Sodium aluminum sulfate	Leavening[a]	Ultramarine blue	Color[b]
Sodium benzoate	Preservative[d]		
Sodium bicarbonate	Leavening[a]	Vanilla, vanillin	Flavor[b]
Sodium calcium alginate	Stabil-thick-tex[a]	Vitamin A	Nutrient[c]
Sodium citrate	pH control[a]	Vitamin C (ascorbic	Nutrient[c]
Sodium diacetate	Preservative[d]	acid)	Preservative[d]
Sodium erythorbate	Preservative[d]		Antioxidant[d]
Sodium nitrate	Preservative[d]	Vitamin D (D_2, D_3)	Nutrient[c]
Sodium nitrite	Preservative[d]	Vitamin E (tocopherols)	Nutrient[c]
Sodium propionate	Preservative[d]		
Sodium sorbate	Preservative[d]	Yeast–malt sprout extract	Flavor[b]
Sodium stearyl fumarate	Mat-bleach-condit[a]	Yellow prussiate of soda	Anticaking[a]
Sorbic acid	Preservative[d]		

Anticaking = anticaking agents; leavening = leavening agents; mat-bleach-condit = maturing and bleaching agents, dough conditioners; pH control = pH control agents; stabil-thick-tex = stabilizers, thickeners, texturizers.

[a] These additives aid in processing or preparation. Emulsifiers help to distribute evenly tiny particles of one liquid into another and improve homogeneity, consistency, stability, and texture. Stabilizers, thickeners, and texturizers impart body and improve consistency or texture, stabilize emulsions, or affect the "mouthfeel" of food. Leavening agents affect cooking results—texture and volume. pH control agents change or maintain acidity or alkalinity. Humectants cause moisture retention. Maturing and bleaching agents and dough conditioners accelerate the aging process and improve baking qualities. Anticaking agents prevent caking, lumping, or clustering of a finely powdered or crystalline substance.

[b] These additives increase the appeal of foods. Flavor enhancers supplement, magnify, or modify the original taste or aroma of food without imparting characteristic flavors of their own. Flavors heighten natural flavor or restore flavors lost in processing. Colors give desired, appetizing, or characteristic color to food. Sweeteners make the aroma or taste of food more agreeable or pleasurable.

[c] These additives maintain or improve nutritional quality. Nutrients enrich (replace vitamins and minerals lost in processing) or fortify (add nutrients that may be lacking in the diet).

[d] These additives maintain product quality. Preservatives (antimicrobials) prevent food spoilage from bacteria, molds, fungi, and yeast; extend shelf life; or protect natural color or flavor.

Source: Adapted from P. Lehmann, *FDA Consumer* April 1979.

References

1. U.S. Department of Health, Education and Welfare, Public Health Service. *Some Questions and Answers About Food Additives* (DHEW Pub. No. [FDA] 74-2056). Washington, D.C.: 1974.
2. Kermode, G. O. Food Additives. In N. Kretchmer and B. Robertson (eds.), *Human Nutrition*. San Francisco: Scientific American and W. H. Freeman, 1978. Pp. 107, 110.
3. Hopkins, H. The color additive scoreboard. *FDA Consum.* 14:24, 1980.
4. Aykroyd, W. R. *Conquest of Deficiency Diseases: Achievements and Prospects* (WHO Basic Study No. 24). Geneva: World Health Organization, 1970.
5. Mertz, W. Fortification of Foods with Vitamins and Minerals. In N. Henry Moss and Jean Mayer, *Food and Nutrition in Health and Disease*. New York: New York Academy of Sciences, 1977. Pp. 153–159.
6. Food and Nutrition Board, National Research Council. *Proposed Fortification Policy for Cereal-Grain Products*. Washington, D.C.: National Academy of Sciences, 1974.

Suggested Readings

American Diabetes Association. Policy statement on saccharin. *Diabetes Care* 2:380, 1979.

Bannar, R. Canned wine. *Food Eng.* 53:63, 1981.

Banwart, G. J. *Basic Food Microbiology*. Westport, Conn.: AVI Publishing, 1979.

Batzinger, R. P., Ou, S.-Y. L., and Bueding, E. Saccharin and other sweeteners: Mutagenic properties. *Science* 198:944, 1977.

Bourland, C. T., et al. Space shuttle food processing and packaging. *J. Food Protect.* 44:313, 1981.

Bradley, H., and Sundberg, C. *Keeping Foods Safe*. Garden City, N.Y.: Doubleday, 1975.

Cassens, R. G., et al. Reactions of nitrite in meat. *Food Technol.* 37:46, 1979.

Farkas, D. F. New concepts for expanding and improving frozen preservation techniques. *Food Technol.* 35:63, 1981.

Fenner, L. Salt shakes up some of us. *FDA Consum.* 14:2, 1980.

Food fortifying: The balancing act. *FDA Consum.* 14:21, 1980.

Francis, F. J. Color the food naturally. *Prof. Nutrit.* 13:11, 1981.

Giddings, F. G., and Welt, M. A. Radiation preservation of food. *Cereal Foods World* 27:17, 1982.

Hickey, R. J., and Clelland, R. C. Hazardous food additives: Nitrite and saliva? (letter to the editor). *N. Engl. J. Med.* 298:1036, 1978.

Hopkins, H. Nitrites: Focusing on safety. *FDA Consum.* 12:9, 1978.

Hopkins, H. Speaking out on fortifying foods. *FDA Consum.* 12:18, 1979.

Irving, G. W. Safety evaluation of the food ingredients called GRAS. *Nutr. Rev.* 36:321, 1978.

Jacobson, M. F. *Eater's Digest: The Consumer's Factbook of Food Additives*, New York: Doubleday, 1972.

Lecos, C. W. Sugar: How sweet it is—and isn't. *FDA Consum.* 14:20, 1980.

Muller, H. G., and Tobin, G. *Nutrition and Food Processing*. Westport, Conn.: AVI Publishing, 1980.

National Academy of Sciences. *Technology of Fortification of Foods*. Washington, D.C., 1975.

Nickerson, T. A. Why use lactose and its derivatives in food? *Food Technol.* 32:40, 1978.

Pines, W. L., and Glick, N. The saccharin ban. *FDA Consum.* 11:10, 1977.

Problems in iron enrichment and fortification of foods. *Nutr. Rev.* 33:46, 1975.

Plain, J. M. Nitrates and nitrites in foods. *Food Nutr. Notes Rev.* 34:49, 1977.

Robach, M. C. Use of preservatives to control microorganisms in food. *Food Technol.* 34:81, 1980.

Rowley, D. B., and Brynjolfsson, A. Potential uses of irradiation in the processing of food. *Food Technol.* 34:75, 1980.

Saccharin: Where do we go from here? *FDA Consum.* 12:16, 1978.

Seligsohn, M. Is GRAS safe? *Food Eng.* 52:20, 1980.

Smith, J. L., and Palumbo, S. A. Microorganisms as food additives. *J. Food Protect.* 44:936, 1981.

Smith, M. V. Regulation of artificial and natural flavors. *Cereal Foods World* 26:278, 1981.

Smith, M. V., and Rulis, A. M. FDA's GRAS review and priority-based assessment of food additives. *Food Technol.* 35:71, 1981.

Stumpf, S. E. Social aspects of risk/benefit analysis of the food supply. *Food Technol.* 32:65, 1978.

Tannenbaum, S. R. Ins and outs of nitrites. *Sciences* 20:7, 1980.

Taylor, R. J. *Food Additives,* New York: Wiley, 1980.

The nutritive quality of processed foods: General policies for nutrient additions. *Nutr. Rev.* 40:93, 1982.

The value of iron fortification of food. *Nutr. Rev.* 31:275, 1973.

Watson, J. J. Development of food fortification. *Cereal Foods World* 26:662, 1981.

Yesterday's additives—generally safe. *FDA Consum.* 15:14, 1981.

Chapter 20

FOOD CONTROLS AND LABELING

The Need for Food Controls

Discoveries in food science and technology have led to the development of a wide diversity of foods and to the need for numerous food-related controls to protect the consumer. With industrialization and movement to the cities, people have become more dependent on growers, distributors, and manufacturers for the food supply.

Advances in organic chemistry, microbiology, food science, and many related fields have resulted in the development of new products, improvements in traditional ones, and a greatly increased variety of foods. Modern farmers use chemicals to fertilize and protect their crops and hormones to accelerate the growth of their livestock. Manufacturers use chemicals to improve the color, texture, and keeping quality of their products and may even use synthetic packaging materials. With the great increase in the type and variety of foodstuffs available, it soon became apparent that some type of control on quality and assurance of health safeguards were necessary. Combined with the surge of consumerism during the first half of the twentieth century, these developments led to the establishment of a series of food laws and amendments in the United States that have been regarded as models for other countries.

New chemicals and farming, manufacturing, and production methods have resulted in the ready availability of high-quality food year round throughout the United States. The food laws and amendments help ensure good manufacturing practice and protect against adulteration and dishonest labeling. This legislation aids both the food industry, by establishing guidelines and standards, and the consumer, by assuring quality and safety in the products offered for sale.

History
PURE FOOD AND DRUGS ACT

The first "pure food" law, the Pure Food and Drugs Act, was enacted in 1906. With the cooperation of women's groups, Harvey W. Wiley, who was then the chief chemist for the U.S. Department of Agriculture (USDA), was its main advocate through his writings and public appearances. Although it was the first law to provide protection and the strongest law of its kind, it soon became inadequate.

FOOD, DRUG AND COSMETIC ACT

As industrialization grew, the manufacture and distribution of food became increasingly complex. Pressure from consumer groups in the mid-1930s resulted in the passage of the Food, Drug and Cosmetic Act of 1938. This law retained the strong points of the 1906 law but broadened it to cover the new developments in the food industry and to strengthen enforcement provisions. The 1938 law has been amended several times to include current developments such as the use of food additives and pesticides. Basically, the law provides health safeguards and sanitary controls, requires label statements, and prohibits deceptions. Among other health safeguards, this act prohibits the sale of raw agricultural products with residues of pesticides in excess of established tolerances, the sale of food that is unsafe or injurious to health, the use of food colors that have not been certified as safe, and the use of food containers with any deleterious substances that may cause the contents to be harmful. The sanitary safeguards include the banning from sale of any food that is filthy, decomposed, or packed or held under unsanitary conditions. The sale of meat of diseased or contaminated animals is also prohibited. The prohibited deceptions include the sale of a food under the name of another food and the removal or substitution of a component of a food (e.g., whole milk may not be sold as such if part or all of the butterfat is removed). Food containers must be constructed and filled so as not to mislead the consumer about the amount of food in them. The Food and Drug Administration (FDA), an agency of the Department of Health and Human Services, is charged with enforcing this act and its amendments.

AMENDMENTS

Concern over residues of pesticides in food products and the widespread use of thousands of food additives led to the passage of the Pesticides Amendment in 1954, the Food Additives Amendment in 1958, and the Color Additives Amendment in 1960.

The purpose of the *Pesticides Amendment* was to provide safeguards in the use of pesticide chemicals and to minimize the hazards from their misuse. Safe tolerances for residues of pesticide chemicals on raw agricultural products were established. Under this law, a food may not be marketed if it contains a pesticide residue determined to be unsafe or if the amount present exceeds the established safe tolerance. Checks for residues on raw foods are made continuously. The detection of excessive residues necessitates the removal of a shipment of food from interstate commerce. Pesticide manufacturers submit data about the chemicals and the results of tests of the safety of the chemical and indicate a proposed safe tolerance to the government. The government then decides whether or not to accept the test results and sets a residue limit for that chemical. The Environmental Protection Agency issues permits for the use of pesticides and other chemicals in the environment and establishes tolerances for pesticides in foods. The Food Protection Committee of the Food and Nutrition Board (National Research Council) has reported that if the use of all pesticides were banned, the yield of many crops would be reduced 10 to 90 percent, forcing the price of available food to soar (Fig. 20-1) [1].

The *Food Additives Amendment* was enacted to ensure that the safety of chemicals used in processing foods is proven before use. The burden of proof of safety was transferred from the government to the manufacturer, who must submit detailed tests in support of the additive. This amendment, as well as the *Color Additives Amendment,* assuring safe food color additives, is discussed in detail in Chap. 19.

INSPECTION ACTS

The original pure food law of 1906 did not include meat and meat products but passed that same year was the *Meat Inspection Act,* enforced by the Meat Inspec-

FIG. 20-1. This plane is spraying crops infested with locusts. (Food and Agriculture Organization photo by Studios du Souissi, Rabat.)

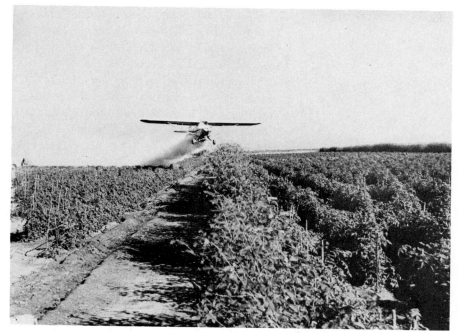

tion Division of the Agricultural Research Service of the USDA. With regulations similar to the Meat Inspection Act, the *Poultry Inspection Act* was passed in 1957. Both require the inspection of the animal products that enter interstate commerce, including animal inspection before slaughter, inspection of the carcass after slaughter for signs of disease, and examination of processed meat products. Inspection stamps are placed on meat that is determined to be safe and wholesome. Diseased meat is stamped "Inspected and Condemned" and must be destroyed.

In 1967 and 1968, respectively, the *Federal Wholesome Meat Act* and the *Federal Wholesome Poultry Products Act* were passed, giving the USDA authority to seize meat and poultry products that have become adulterated or misbranded after leaving official premises [2]. In 1970 the *Egg Product Inspection Act* became law, assuring wholesome, unadulterated, and truthfully labeled egg products for the consumer. It provides mandatory continuous inspection of plants processing egg products and is administered by the Poultry Division, Consumer and Marketing Service, USDA. See Chaps. 15, 16, and 17 for more detail.

Labeling

Some of the information provided on food labels may be required by the FDA, and some is included at the option of the manufacturer. Some of this information may be in the form of dates, codes, or symbols.

BASIC INFORMATION

In 1966 the *Fair Packaging and Labeling Act* was passed, supplementing the 1938 food, drug, and cosmetics law. This act authorized the FDA to establish requirements for labeling and packaging. Required on all food labels are the name of the product; the net contents or net weight, including the liquid in which the product is packed; and the name and address of the manufacturer, packer, or distributor. The ingredients must also be listed on the label of most foods. The ingredients are listed by descending weight. Colors and flavors do not have to be listed by name but may simply be stated as "artificial color" or "artificial flavor" or "natural flavor." The listing of artificial color is not required for butter, ice cream, or cheese. Current legislation, if passed, may require the listing of spices, colors, and flavors by specific names. Any other additives used in the product must be listed.

The only foods exempt from listing ingredients are those for which the FDA has set *standards of identity* [3]. These standards stipulate that all foods called a particular name (e.g., catsup, mayonnaise, white bread) contain certain mandatory ingredients, which then do not have to appear on the label. Optional ingredients may be added and should be so listed. A change currently under consideration is the mandatory listing of ingredients on standardized foods. There are about 275 foods with standards of identity; these include chocolate and cocoa products, cereal flours and related products, macaroni and noodle products, bakery products, milk and cream, cheese and cheese products, frozen desserts, salad dressing, mayonnaise, canned fruit and fruit juices, jellies and preserves, shellfish, canned tuna, eggs and egg products, vegetables and vegetable products, and margarine.

NUTRITION INFORMATION

Under FDA regulations, any food for which a nutritional claim is made or to which a nutrient has been added must have the nutritional content listed on the label. Many manufacturers put nutrition information on products even though they are not required to do so. The nutrition information given is the number of calories; the amount (in grams) of protein, fat, and carbohydrate; and the percentage of the U.S. Recommended Dietary Allowances (RDAs) of protein and seven vitamins and minerals (vitamins A and C, thiamin, riboflavin, niacin, calcium, and iron) per serving. The nutrition information is given per serving; the label tells the size of one serving as well as the number of servings per container. The manufacturer may also list the content of 12 other vitamins and minerals (vitamins B_{12}, D, and E; folic acid; phosphorus; iodine; magnesium; zinc; copper; biotin; potassium and pantothenic acid), cholesterol, fatty acid, and sodium at his option. Amounts are shown in grams rather than ounces. The U.S. RDA is an average of the recommendations for adults and children at least 4 years old and is the approximate amount of protein, vitamins, or minerals that should be included in the daily diet for good health. The nutrition information is listed as a percentage of the U.S. RDA; the total amount of food eaten in a day should supply the U.S. RDA of all essential nutrients. Future changes in these requirements may include mandatory expanded use of percentage labeling; required cholesterol labeling; and listing of the fat content by the specific fat or oil ingredient used in the product, the total quantity of sugars, and the total sodium and potassium content [4].

IMITATION VERSUS REAL

"Imitation" must be used on the label when a product is not as nutritious as the one it resembles or for which it is a substitute. If the new product is as nutritious as an existing one, it can be given another name rather than being called imitation; an example is the nutritionally equivalent egg substitute Egg Beaters.

COMMON OR USUAL NAME

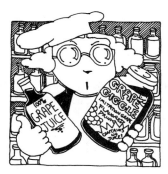

To give the consumer accurate information about what is in the package or container, the FDA has ruled that foods must have a "common or usual" name. For example, a grape juice drink that contains very little juice must use the name "diluted grape juice drink"; the percentage of juice it contains may also be required. The label required in this case might be "diluted grape juice beverage, contains 10 percent grape juice." Similarly, if a beverage does not contain any juice but appears to by its color or texture, the label must state that it contains no juice.

In packaged foods in which the main ingredient or component of a recipe is not included, the common name consists of each ingredient in order by weight (e.g., noodles and tomato sauce), identification of the food to be prepared from the package (e.g., lasagna), and a statement of the ingredients that must be added to complete the recipe (parmesan cheese, ricotta cheese, ground beef).

GRADES

The USDA provides official grading services for the food industry and approves sanitary facilities in processing plants whose products bear the USDA-approved label. Grades set by the USDA are based on qualities such as taste, texture, and appearance, and not on nutritional content. Milk and milk products with a grade A label have passed FDA-recommended sanitary standards and have the required levels of vitamins A and D.

CODE DATING

Code dating is for the manufacturer's information rather than the consumer's benefit. The code tells precise information about when and where the product was packaged. In the event that a product must be recalled for some reason, code dating allows it to be identified quickly and taken off the market. The secrecy of such dating has been the cause of much consumer concern, and several "underground" manuals have been published translating manufacturers' codes [5].

OPEN DATING

In response to consumer pressure for uncoded dating of products, some manufacturers use open dating. Although not required or regulated by the FDA, open dating helps consumers purchase food that is fresh and wholesome. Four kinds of open dating are commonly used:

1. *Pack date.* The date of processing or final packaging, the pack date tells the consumer how old the product is when it is purchased. The pack date is more

important in foods that spoil quickly than in canned products, which under dry, cool conditions have a long shelf life.

2. *Pull, or sell, date.* The last day of fresh sale is the pull date. This is the most commonly used dating and assures that quality is still at its peak. The sell date allows for some storage time in the home. Examples of foods with pull or sell dates include refrigerated fresh dough products, cold cuts, milk, and ice cream.

3. *Expiration date.* The expiration date is the final date of recommended use. Yeast, baby formula, and some canned goods may have expiration dates.

4. *Freshness date.* The freshness date is similar to the expiration date, but allows for some home storage. This is the date recommended for obtaining optimum product quality. The freshness date is frequently seen on baked products.

UNIVERSAL PRODUCT CODE   A small block of parallel lines of various widths with accompanying numbers, the universal product code is seen on many food labels and is unique to that product. Computerized checkouts can read the code and automatically ring up the sale. The universal product code also serves as an automated inventory system, telling management how much of a particular item is at hand, how quickly it is being sold, and when and how much to reorder.

SYMBOLS ON FOOD LABELS   A circled *R* signifies that the trademark used on the label is registered with the U.S. Patent Office. © means that the literary and artistic content of the label is protected against infringement under the copyright laws of the United States.

A circled *U* is a symbol whose use is authorized by the Orthodox Jewish Congregation of America for foods that comply with the Jewish dietary laws. A circled *K* signifies a food is "kosher," that is, it complies with the Jewish dietary laws and its processing has been under the direction of a rabbi.

None of these symbols is required by, nor is under the authority of, the FDA.

Enforcement of the Food Laws   The FDA enforces the food laws and amendments, employing teams of scientists, bacteriologists, chemists, biochemists, entomologists, pharmacologists, veterinarians, and physicians in Washington, D.C., and in the 18 district offices. Each office is equipped with laboratories capable of analyzing samples of foods under investigation.

Over 700 FDA inspectors make periodic visits to the factories, processing plants, warehouses, and packaging plants of about 60,000 manufacturers, packers, and distributors that process foods that enter interstate commerce or are imported. The inspectors check to see that the raw materials, manufacturing processes, storage and packaging practices, and plant sanitation comply with the food laws. Violations of the food laws are dealt with by the courts, which may impose fines or imprisonment or both. Injunctions may also be issued to prevent repetition of a violation. Notices of judgment such as the following are often published [6]:

Beans, white, small, canned, at Puerto Nuevo, Dist. P.R. Charged 8-20-79: while held for sale, the article was contained in swollen cans; 402 (a) (3). Default decree ordered destruction.

Cottonseed, at Anthony, Dist. N. Mex. Charged 10-20-78: when shipped by Monty Corbin, Gila Bend (Theba), Ariz., the article contained the added poisonous and deleterious substance aflatoxin (approximately 5,000 ppb); 402 (a) (1). Default decree ordered destruction.

Crabmeat, Shell Key, at Philadelphia, E. Dist. Pa. Charged 10-17-79: when shipped by Shell Key Packing Co., Baldwin, La., the article had been packed and held under unsanitary conditions; 402 (a) (3). Default decree ordered destruction.

Tomatoes, at Glendale, Dist. Ariz. Charged 11-30-79: when shipped by Agri Sales, Oceanside, Calif., the article contained the pesticide chemical acephate (approximately 0.22 ppm), and there was no tolerance or exemption for such pesticide in tomatoes; 402 (a) (2) (B). Default decree ordered destruction.

Other Food Agencies

The *Food Protection Committee,* a subcommittee of the Food and Nutrition Board, was established to study the uses of chemical additives and to assist other regulatory agencies in formulating principles and standardized procedures. It also acts as a clearinghouse for information on pesticides and other chemicals.

The *Public Health Service* is a division of the Department of Health and Human Services. It recommends sanitary codes and ordinances, does research to establish effective procedures to ensure a safe food supply, and during outbreaks of food poisoning conducts tests to determine the source and nature of the poisoning. The Public Health Service also has defined standards for milk production and quality that are the basis for the codes used in most states and certifies interstate milk shippers. See Chap. 14 for more detail.

The *Agricultural Research Service* (USDA) develops and improves methods of marketing and processing foods. This service is also responsible for inspecting food products at ports of entry to prevent the spread of foreign animal and plant diseases.

The *Consumer and Marketing Service* (USDA), in conjunction with farm, industry, and research groups, establishes grade standards to measure quality level in foods. It also provides a grading service to producers and distributors and can prevent the interstate sale of meat and poultry products that do not meet federal standards.

The *Food and Nutrition Service* has as its purpose the elimination of hunger and malnutrition in the United States through the administration of federal food programs. It helps schools and child-care institutions purchase food for breakfasts and lunches for children and administers such special programs as food stamps.

The *National Bureau of Standards* provides technical assistance in establishing measurements and performance standards. The *Office of Technical Services* limits the types and sizes of packages and cans manufacturers can use. It has no regulatory function relating to food.

The *Bureau of Commercial Fisheries* offers an official inspection service for all fishery products and promotes the consumer use of fish. The *National Marine Fisheries* regulates the grading standards for fish and fish products. These grades are not required by law, but do aid the consumer. The *U.S. Department of Commerce* establishes voluntary grades and standards for fish and shellfish, as provided for in the Fish and Wildlife Act of 1956.

References

1. Food Protection Committee, Food and Nutrition Board, National Research Council. *The Use of Chemicals in Food Production, Processing, Storage, and Distribution* (Pub. 887). Washington, D.C.: National Academy of Sciences, 1961.
2. New meat inspection laws for consumer protection. *Public Health Rep.* 84:214, 1969.
3. U.S. Department of Health, Education and Welfare, Food and Drug Administration. *Definitions and Standards of Identity for Food: Code of Federal Regulations, Title 21.* Washington, D.C., 1971.
4. Corwin, E. Telling more about the stuff in foodstuffs. *FDA Consum.* 14:4, 1980.
5. Helm, S. Blind dates: How long was that spinach in the can? *Village Voice*, p. 61, Jan. 21, 1980.
6. Notices of judgment. *FDA Consum.* 14:34, 1980.

Suggested Readings

A perspective on food legislation. *Nutr. Rev.* 39:413, 1981.

Ahlberg, S. Following the road to produce labeling. *School Food Serv. J.* 35:30, 1981.

Axelson, J. M. Labeling and food additives. *School Food Serv. J.* 35:32, 1981.

Bramsnaes, F. Maintaining the quality of frozen foods during distribution. *Food Technol.* 35:38, 1981.

Brody, J. E. Making some sense of nutrition labels. *New York Times* Jan. 2, 1980.

Brown, C. J. Revising the U.S. food safety policy: Government viewpoint. *Food Technol.* 33:61, 1979.

Clausi, A. S. Revising the U.S. food safety policy: An industry viewpoint. *Food Technol.* 33:65, 1979.

Darby, W. J. The nature of benefits. *Nutr. Rev.* 38:37, 1980.

de Figueiredo, M. P. Quality assurance of food safety. *Food Technol.* 35:58, 1981.

FDA's changing role in food safety. *FDA Consum.* 15:28, 1981.

Forbes, A. L. Revision of the food label. *Cereal Foods World* 26:661, 1981.

Hall, R. L., and Merwin, E. J. The role of flavors in food processing. *Food Technol.* 35:46, 1981.

Hkui, Y. H. *United States Food Laws, Regulations, and Standards.* New York: Wiley, 1979.

Hopkins, H. Toward more nutrition labeling. *FDA Consum.* 11:22, 1977.

IFT's Expert Panel on Food Safety and Nutrition: Open shelf-life dating of food. *Food Technol.* 35:89, 1981.

La Du, B. N., Jr. Analysis of the National Academy of Sciences Food Safety Report. *Food Technol.* 33:53, 1979.

Miller, S. A. Achieving food safety through regulation. *Food Technol.* 33:57, 1979.

Packard, V. S. *Processed Foods and the Consumer: Additives, Labeling, Standards, and Nutrition.* Minneapolis: Univ. of Minnesota Press, 1976.

Phillips, M. J.   An analysis of consumer demands for information on the frozen food label. *Food Technol.* 35:61, 1981.

Symons, H. W.   The frozen food label and consumer needs. *Food Technol.* 35:65, 1981.

The story of the laws behind the labels. *FDA Consum.* 15:32, 1981.

Vratanina, D. L.   Labeling: Understanding the issues. *School Food Serv. J.* 35:27, 1981.

Wodicka, V. O.   Risk and responsibility. *Nutr. Rev.* 38:45, 1980.

Part 3

NUTRITION IN HEALTH

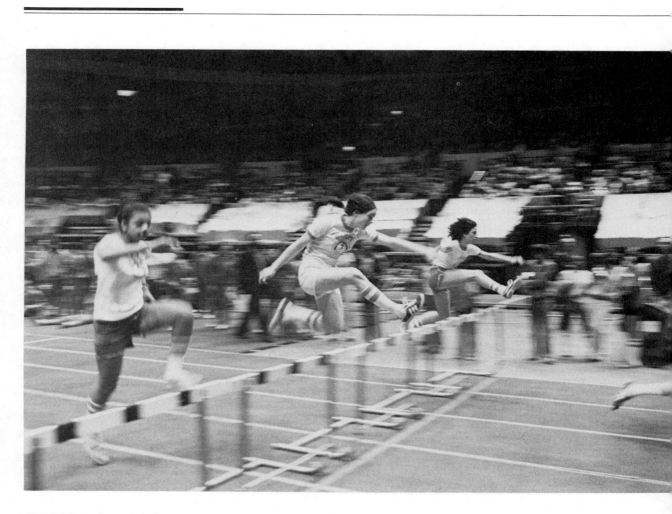

(1975) (Photo from United Nations/J. Isaacs.)

DIETARY OVERVIEW

Like any other field, the study of nutrition must be based on a set of standards and guidelines. These are presented in this section, Dietary Overview. The United States Dietary Goals are a series of recommendations based on the latest scientific findings correlating diet and disease. In very practical terms, these guidelines suggest changes in the daily diet that, hopefully, will ensure better health.

The chapter on Assessment and Evaluation of Nutritional Status presents the standards on which an individual's nutritional health is evaluated. A variety of methods are given, depending on the clinical setting and the resources at hand. These two chapters provide the foundation for the specialized chapters on diet through the life cycle and for the section on diet therapy.

Chapter 21

UNITED STATES DIETARY GOALS

Many health professionals have considered the past 100 years to be the first "public health revolution" whose enemy was the major infectious diseases. One of its goals was officially celebrated on October 26, 1979, 2 years after the last reported case of smallpox, signifying the global eradication of this disease. A second public health revolution, against many of the chronic diseases afflicting Americans, is now gaining momentum. Diet and prevention have become the cornerstones of this war. Diet has been cited as *the* most important contributor to disease prevention [1].

Nutrition plays an important role in an individual's susceptibility to disease. With infectious diseases, mortality is influenced by differences in nutritional status: *Deficiencies* have been found to increase morbidity and mortality. The problems seen with chronic diseases are the opposite: Morbidity and mortality are related to *dietary excesses*. It has become more and more evident in recent years that most of the major chronic diseases in America are directly or indirectly related to diet.

The leading causes of death are summarized in Table 21-1. Six of the eight leading causes—heart disease, cancer, cerebrovascular disease, diabetes mellitus, cirrhosis, and arteriosclerosis—have been linked to dietary habits. When the causes of death are viewed by age group and sex (Table 21-2), the cumulative effects of diet become even more apparent. While heart disease ranks as the number 6 cause of death in children aged 1 to 14 years, it moves to number 5 for those aged 15 to 34, to number 1 for men aged 35 to 54 and number 2 for women 35 to 54, and to number 1 for both men and women over 55. Accidents, cancer, congenital anomalies, homicides, and suicides are the leading causes of death for Americans under 35 years of age, while heart disease, cancer, cerebrovascular disease, cirrhosis, and pneumonia more frequently kill Americans over age 35. Increases in juvenile-onset and adult-onset obesity, smoking, and alcohol consumption; decreased exercise and manual labor; and changes in diet have probably all contributed to the increased incidence of and mortality from these diseases in adult life.

During the past 80 years a great deal has been learned in the field of nutrition. The early part of this century marked the discovery of various vital components, the vitamins. With the recent development of more sophisticated methods of investigation, the requirements for more and more trace elements are being defined. Research in nutrition has expanded greatly during the past 50 years, giving added support to the relationships between specific dietary components and various chronic diseases. Recently, scientists from the American Society for Clinical Nutrition, an organization composed of physicians and nutritionists involved in clinical nutrition research, undertook an extensive review of the literature and presented a symposium entitled "The Evidence Relating Six Dietary Factors to the Nation's Health" [2]. These six causative factors were *cholesterol* and *dietary fat* as factors in atherogenesis; *carbohydrate* and *sucrose* as

TABLE 21.1. Mortality for leading causes of death, United States, 1978

Rank	Cause of death	Number of deaths	Death rate* per 100,000 population	Percent of total deaths
	All causes	1,927,788	809.9	100.0
1	Heart disease	729,510	300.4	37.8
2	Cancer	396,992	169.9	20.6
3	Cerebrovascular disease	175,629	70.8	1.0
4	Accidents	105,561	45.8	5.5
5	Influenza and pneumonia	58,319	23.6	3.0
6	Chronic obstructive lung disease	50,488	21.1	2.6
7	Diabetes mellitus	33,841	14.2	1.8
8	Cirrhosis	30,066	13.4	1.6
9	Arteriosclerosis	28,940	11.1	1.5
10	Suicide	27,294	11.6	1.4
11	Diseases of infancy	22,033	12.1	1.1
12	Homicide	20,432	8.7	1.1
13	Aortic aneurysm	14,028	5.8	0.8
14	Congenital anomalies	12,968	6.8	0.7
15	Pulmonary infarction	10,941	4.6	0.6
	Other and ill-defined	210,606	89.9	10.8

*Age-adjusted to the 1970 U.S. census population.
Source: National Center for Health Statistics, 1978.

factors in atherosclerotic heart disease, diabetes mellitus, and dental caries; *calories* as a factor in disease; *alcohol* as a factor in liver disease and atherosclerosis; and *sodium* (dietary salt) as a factor in hypertension.

The National Cancer Institute has also recently issued a statement on diet, nutrition, and cancer [3]. The Institute reviewed a number of studies and observations, including those documenting a lower incidence of breast cancer in countries with a low fat diet and a lower incidence of colon cancer among populations with a high fiber diet. They concluded that the evidence suggests changes in dietary habits may benefit overall health.

Based upon these reviews and the opinions of the nation's foremost scientists, the Surgeon General has issued a report on health promotion and disease prevention, *Healthy People* [4]. This document called for a reordering of national health priorities, with a shift of direction and resources toward the prevention of disease and the promotion of good health. At about the same time, the U.S. Department of Agriculture (USDA), the U.S. Department of Health, Education and Welfare (USDHEW, now the U.S. Department of Health and Human Services), and the Food and Nutrition Board of the National Research Council issued similar guidelines [5, 6]. Although differing on some points, all the reports basically advocate the same dietary guidelines, aimed at reducing the morbidity and mortality from chronic diseases. The following section discusses the USDA and USDHEW guidelines in detail.

TABLE 21-2. Ten leading causes of death by age and sex, 1978

Rank	Age 1–14		Age 15–34		Age 35–54		Age 55–74		Age 75+	
	Male	Female	Male	Female	Male	Female	Male	Female	Male	Female
1	Accidents	Accidents	Accidents	Accidents	Heart disease	Cancer	Heart disease	Heart disease	Heart disease	Heart disease
2	Cancer	Cancer	Homicide	Cancer	Cancer	Heart disease	Cancer	Cancer	Cancer	Cerebrovascular disease
3	Congenital anomalies	Congenital anomalies	Suicide	Suicide	Accidents	Accidents	Cerebrovascular disease	Cerebrovascular disease	Cerebrovascular disease	Cancer
4	Homicide	Homicide	Cancer	Homicide	Cirrhosis	Cerebrovascular disease	Accidents	Diabetes	Pneumonia, influenza	Pneumonia, influenza
5	Pneumonia, influenza	Pneumonia, influenza	Heart disease	Heart disease	Suicide	Cirrhosis	Chronic obstructive lung disease	Accidents	Chronic obstructive lung disease	Arteriosclerosis
6	Heart disease	Heart disease	Cirrhosis	Cerebrovascular disease	Homicide	Suicide	Cirrhosis	Pneumonia, influenza	Arteriosclerosis	Diabetes
7	Meningitis	Cystic fibrosis	Pneumonia, influenza	Pneumonia, influenza	Cerebrovascular disease	Diabetes	Pneumonia, influenza	Cirrhosis	Accidents	Accidents
8	Cerebrovascular disease	Cerebrovascular disease	Cerebrovascular disease	Congenital anomalies	Pneumonia, influenza	Pneumonia, influenza	Diabetes	Chronic obstructive lung disease	Diabetes	Chronic obstructive lung disease
9	Cerebral palsy	Cirrhosis	Congenital anomalies	Cirrhosis	Diabetes	Homicide	Emphysema	Emphysema	Emphysema	Pulmonary infarction
10	Suicide	Meningitis	Diabetes	Diabetes	Chronic obstructive lung disease	Pulmonary infarction	Aortic aneurysm	Pulmonary infarction	Cirrhosis	Aortic aneurysm

Source: Vital Statistics of the United States, 1978.

Dietary Guidelines
EAT A VARIETY OF FOODS

All of the nutrients that are needed can be obtained by eating a variety of basic foods. Choices from all four food groups (milk, meat and poultry, fruits and vegetables, cereals and grains) should be included in the diet every day (Fig. 21-1). This goal has become even easier to achieve during the past few decades, with improved methods of packaging, preservation, and shipping, so that a wide variety of processed, frozen, and fresh foods are available all year.

MAINTAIN IDEAL WEIGHT

The daily caloric intake should be appropriate for the individual's sex, height, and state of health (see Table 21-3). The number of calories available for consumption per capita has been steadily rising since its lowest level around 1960. Although 3500 calories per person per day are available, the Nationwide Household Food Consumption Survey of 1977 showed that the actual caloric intake has declined, which may indicate that more food is being wasted [7]. An estimated 20 percent of edible food is discarded, lowering the per capita availability of calories to 2800 per day [8]. This level is above the recommended daily allowances for most age groups and, in the absence of regular exercise, may contribute to the development of obesity.

AVOID TOO MUCH FAT, SATURATED FAT, AND CHOLESTEROL

The consumption of fats has increased steadily since 1910. Dietary fats constituted 42 percent of the total calories in 1979, compared with 32 percent in 1910 [9]. The source of dietary fat has, however, changed dramatically during this century: In 1910, 17 percent of total fat came from vegetable sources (monounsaturated and polyunsaturated), whereas today 43 percent comes from these sources. Decreased demand for butter, lard, and some dairy products [10], increased demand for salad and cooking oils, and the increased availability and popularity of leaner cuts of meat have brought about this increase in the polyunsaturated content and decrease in the saturated fat content of the American diet. The cholesterol content of the American diet has remained the same as it was in 1910, about 500 mg per day, although more cholesterol is now derived from poultry and fish and less from eggs, lard, and butter [9]. Whether or not diet changes can change serum cholesterol levels and whether a change in serum levels can affect the incidence of and mortality from heart disease are highly controversial issues.

These changes in the American diet are partially consistent with changes that have been suggested as ways of complying with the U.S. dietary goals [5]: decreasing the consumption of meat and increasing the consumption of poultry and fish; decreasing the consumption of foods high in fat and partially substituting polyunsaturated fat for saturated fat; substituting nonfat milk for whole milk; and decreasing the consumption of butterfat, eggs, and other high cholesterol sources.

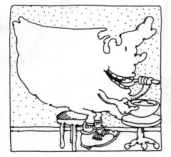

EAT FOODS WITH ADEQUATE STARCH AND FIBER

Foods containing starch or fiber have been shown to be more beneficial for gastrointestinal function and overall health than more processed foods. Foods with adequate starch include baked potatoes, rice, breads, and grains. Foods with fiber include fresh fruits and vegetables, grains, and cereals (Fig. 21-2).

FIG. 21-1. A diet consisting of foods from all four food groups is a requirement for good nutritional health.

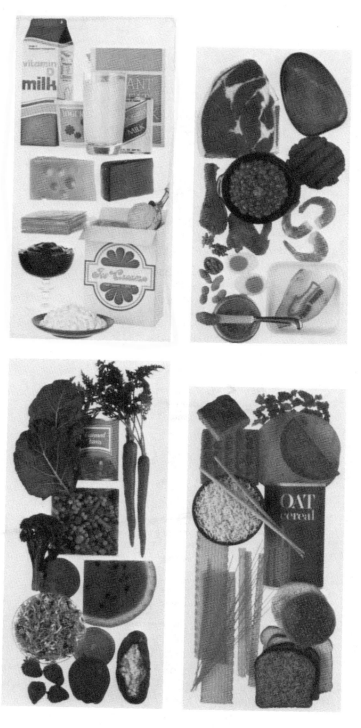

TABLE 21-3. Food servings recommended for different age groups

Food Group	Recommended number of servings				
	Child	Teenager	Adult	Pregnant woman	Lactating woman
Milk	3	4	2	4	4
1 cup milk, yogurt, *or*					
Calcium equivalent:					
1½ slices (1½ oz) cheddar cheese*					
1 cup pudding					
1¾ cups ice cream					
2 cups cottage cheese*					
Meat	2	2	2	3	2
2 ounces cooked, lean meat, fish, poultry, *or*					
Protein equivalent:					
2 eggs					
2 slices (2 oz) cheddar cheese*					
½ cup cottage cheese*					
1 cup cooked dried beans, peas					
4 tbsp peanut butter					
Fruit-vegetable	4	4	4	4	4
½ cup cooked or juice					
1 cup raw					
Portion commonly served such as medium-size apple or banana					
Grain, whole grain, fortified, enriched	4	4	4	4	4
1 slice bread					
1 cup ready-to-eat cereal					
½ cup cooked cereal pasta, grits					

*Count cheese as serving of milk *or* meat, not both simultaneously.
Note: Others complement but do not replace foods from the Four Food Groups. Amounts should be determined by individual caloric needs.
Source: National Dairy Council, 1978.

A decreased consumption of cereal and grain products and potatoes has resulted in a decrease in the crude fiber content of the American diet from 7 gm a day in 1910 to about 5 gm a day today [11]. These figures are difficult to interpret, since total dietary fiber may be much higher. A renewed interest in dietary fiber has recently led to the increased production of new whole-grain breads and high-fiber breakfast cereals. This new trend is in keeping with changes suggested in the U.S. dietary goals, including increasing the consumption of fruits, vegetables, and whole grains and decreasing the consumption of sugar and foods high in sugar content.

FIG. 21-2. "An apple a day . . ." is not just a silly saying. Apples contribute fiber and important vitamins, both necessary for good nutrition. (U.S. Department of Agriculture photo.)

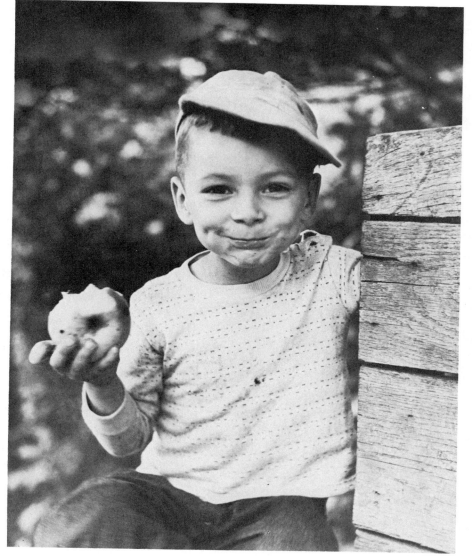

AVOID TOO MUCH SUGAR

Excesses of concentrated carbohydrates are thought to be one of the causes of dental caries and obesity in this country. There has been a steady decline in the amount of carbohydrate and the proportion of carbohydrate derived from starches in the American diet since 1910. In 1910, starches accounted for about 337 gm per day, compared with 185 gm today; this is due primarily to a decreased utilization of grain products and potatoes [9, 12]. Although the total amount of carbohydrate in the diet has declined, the proportion of sugars has increased. The amount of refined cane and beet sugar (sucrose), caloric sweeteners (corn syrup, honey, and molasses), and all other sources of sugar has in-

TABLE 21-4. Sodium content of selected foods

High (100–700 mg/100 gm)
  Seafood: tuna, clams, caviar, lobster, sardines, scallops, shrimp
  Meat/Organs: brains, eggs, beef kidneys, beef liver
  Vegetables: beet greens, celery, swiss chard, olives, peas
  Dairy products: butter, buttermilk, cheeses (cream, Parmesan, swiss, cheddar, cottage)
  Miscellaneous: pickles, table salt, kelp, brewer's yeast

Medium (50–100 mg/100 gm)
  Seafood: flounder, haddock, halibut, herring, lingcod, shad, perch, oysters, red snapper, salmon, sea bass, bluefish, carp, cod, croaker
  Meat/Organs: goose, beef heart, lamb, beef, chicken, duck, pork, turkey, liver, veal
  Nuts/Seeds: sesame
  Vegetables: beets, kale, spinach, turnips, watercress
  Dairy products: milk

Low (1–50 mg/100 gm)
  Nuts/Seeds: coconuts, filberts, peanuts, sunflower, walnuts, almonds, brazils, cashews
  Fruits: berries (blackberries, blueberries, boysenberries, cranberries, strawberries) apples, apricots, avocados, bananas, oranges, papaya, prunes, grapes, raisins
  Vegetables: green beans, broccoli, brussels sprouts, cabbage, carrots, bean sprouts, cucumbers, eggplant, lentils, potatoes, okra, onions, squash, green peppers
  Grains: barley, brown rice, rye, wheat
  Miscellaneous: chocolate, molasses, mushrooms

Source: R. J. Kutsky, *Handbook of Vitamins, Minerals and Hormones* (2nd ed.). New York: Van Nostrand Reinhold, 1981.

creased from 198 lb per person per year in 1969 to 213 lb in 1979 [13]. Foods high in refined sugar, which should be used sparingly, include jellies and jams, candies, sweetened prepared fruits, pies, cakes, soft drinks, chocolate, and cocoa.

AVOID TOO MUCH SODIUM

The average adult consumes about 10 to 12 gm of sodium per day. High sodium intakes have been linked with hypertension, heart disease, and kidney disease. The Senate Select Committee and the National Research Council both agree that limiting salt intake to 3 to 8 gm per day by decreasing consumption of salt and foods high in salt is advisable [5]. Some high sodium foods to avoid include pickles, foods prepared or packed in brine, and foods with salted tops (see Table 21-4).

DRINK ALCOHOL IN MODERATION

The rising incidence of alcoholism, mortality from cirrhosis, and birth defects are all directly related to the amount of alcohol consumed in America. Teenage alcoholism has become a severe problem in recent years and partially explains the high incidence of deaths from accidents in this age group. The amount of alcohol consumed has not changed much this past decade, although there is a trend toward use of white table wines, distilled white spirits (e.g., gin and vodka), and rum [14].

TABLE 21-5. Applying the United States dietary goals

Typical diet	Suggested revision
Breakfast	
Scrambled eggs	Cottage cheese[a]
Fried bacon	Sliced bananas[d]
White bread toast	Whole wheat toast[b]
Butter	Honey[a]
Whole milk	Skim milk[a]
Lunch	
Cheeseburger	Fish filet[a]
Dill pickles	Lettuce and tomatoes[d]
French fries	Baked potato[b,d]
Cola	Iced tea[c]
Apple pie	Fresh pear[b,c]
Dinner	
Grilled steak	Broiled chicken[a]
Baked potato and sour cream	Boiled rice[a,b]
Peas and carrots	Fresh salad[b]
Iced layer cake	Sherbet[c]
Vodka and tonic	Wine[e]

Dietary goals:
[a]Avoid too much fat, saturated fat, and cholesterol.
[b]Eat foods with adequate starch and fiber.
[c]Avoid too much sugar.
[d]Avoid too much sodium.
[e]Drink alcohol in moderation.

Conclusion

It is now known that much illness is preventable, and diet has been shown to be an important factor in prevention. Applying the principles of good nutrition, as illustrated in Table 21-5, is one of the best ways of ensuring a longer, healthier life.

References

1. McGinnis, J. M. Prevention: Today's dietary challenges. *J. Am. Diet. Assoc.* 77:129, 1980.
2. Symposium: Report of the Task Force on the Evidence Relating Six Dietary Factors to the Nation's Health. *Am. J. Clin. Nutr.* 32[suppl.]:12, 1979.
3. Upton, A. C. Status of the Diet, Nutrition, and Cancer Program. Testimony before the Subcommittee on Nutrition, Senate Committee on Agriculture, Nutrition, and Forestry. October 2, 1979.
4. U.S. Department of Health, Education and Welfare. *Healthy People: The Surgeon General's Report on Health Promotion and Disease Prevention* (DHEW Pub. No. [PHS] 79-55071). Washington, D.C.: Government Printing Office, 1979.
5. U.S. Department of Agriculture and U.S. Department of Health, Education and Welfare. *Nutrition and Your Health: Dietary Guidelines for Americans.* Washington, D.C.: Government Printing Office, 1980.
6. Food and Nutrition Board, National Research Council. *Toward Healthful Diets.* Washington, D.C.: National Academy Press, 1980.

7. Cronin, F. J.   Changes in nutrient levels and foods used by households in the United States, spring, 1965 and 1977. Presented to the 1980 Agricultural Outlook Conference, Session 11, Washington, D.C., 1979.

8. *A Status Report on the American Diet and Health, 1980.* Minneapolis: General Mills, 1980.

9. Marston, R., and Page, L.   Nutrient content of the national food supply. *Natl. Food Rev.* 5, 1978.

10. U.S. Department of Agriculture.   *Agricultural Statistics, 1979.* Washington, D.C.: Government Printing Office, 1979.

11. Heller, S. N., and Hackler, L. R.   Changes in the crude fiber content of the American diet. *Am. J. Clin. Nutr.* 31:510, 1978.

12. Gortner, W. A.   Nutrition in the United States, 1900–1974. *Cancer Res.* 35:3246, 1975.

13. U.S. Department of Agriculture.   *Sugar and Sweetener Report* 5(2):1, 1980.

14. Leinen, N. J.   1979 food industry outlook. *Food Process.* March 1979.

Suggested Readings

Celender, I. M., Shapero, M., and Sloan, A. E.   Dietary trends and nutritional status in the United States. *Food Technol.* 32:39, 1978.

Dosti, R., Kidushim, D., and Wolke, M.   *Light Style: The New American Cuisine.* San Francisco: Harper & Row, 1979.

Egan, M. C.   Public health nutrition services: Issues today and tomorrow. *J. Am. Diet. Assoc.* 77:423, 1980.

Guidelines for a national nutrition policy. *Nutr. Rev.* 38:96, 1980.

Harper, A. E.   Recommended dietary allowances—1980. Special report. *Nutr. Rev.* 38:290, 1980.

Harper, A. E.   Dietary guidelines for Americans. *Am. J. Clin. Nutr.* 34:121, 1981.

Jukes, T. H.   The predicament of food and nutrition. *Food Technol.* 33:42, 1979.

Lachance, P. A.   The role of cereal grain products in the U.S. diet. *Food Technol.* 35:49, 1981.

Leveille, G. A.   Recommendations for rational changes in the U.S. diet. *Food Technol.* 32:75, 1978.

McNutt, K. W.   An analysis of Dietary Goals for the United States, second edition. *J. Nutr. Educ.* 10:61, 1978.

McNutt, K. W.   The National Nutrition Consortium's programs and plans for the 1980's. *Food Technol.* 34:68, 1980.

Position paper on a national nutrition policy. *J. Am. Diet. Assoc.* 76:596, 1980.

Schafer, R. B., and Keith, P. M.   Influences on food decisions across the family life cycle. *J. Am. Dietet. Assoc.* 78:144, 1981.

Schmandt, J., Shorey, R. A., Kinch, L., and members of the Nutrition Policy Research Project.   *Nutrition Policy in Transition.* Lexington, Mass.: Lexington Books, 1980.

Tarrant, J. R.   *Food Policies.* New York: Wiley, 1980.

Toward a national nutrition policy. *Nutr. Policy Issues* (General Mills) No. 9, December 1980.

U.S. dietary goals: For and against. *J. Nutr. Educ.* 9:152, 1977.

Wheeler, E. F.   Food choice and the U.S. dietary goals. *J. Hum. Nutr.* 32:325, 1978.

Whitehead, R. G.   Dietary goals—past and present. *R. Soc. Health J.* 101:58, 1981.

Winikoff, B. (ed.).   *Nutrition and National Policy.* Cambridge, Mass.: The M.I.T. Press, 1978.

Chapter 22

ASSESSMENT OF NUTRITIONAL STATUS

Although advanced stages of malnutrition may be readily determined by observation, less obvious signs must be revealed in a systematic assessment of nutritional status. Nutritional assessment is particularly important in infants and children because early detection and intervention can prevent permanent disorders [1]. However, in providing an objective picture of nutritional status based on normal values, this procedure should become part of the routine examination of every patient/client in the hospital or primary care setting. Nutritional assessment permits determination of baseline nutritional status and serial assessment of nutritional support measures [1].

During nutritional assessment, several types of information are obtained and compared to standards representing normal nutriture (state of balance between tissue nutrient needs and actual nutrient supply). The information collected can be biochemical, anthropometric (scientific measurements of body size and structure), clinical, and dietary. Nutritional assessment allows the classification of individuals into three categories [2]:

1. Those who are already malnourished and in need of immediate nutritional rehabilitation
2. Those with limited nutrient stores or very high nutrient needs who are at risk of becoming frankly malnourished if not given special nutritional support
3. Those with adequate stores who do not require special nutritional therapy

Dietary Information

The easiest and most direct methods for determining the sources and amounts of nutrients consumed are observation and questioning. Although open to much interpretation (by the interviewer and the client), dietary studies of this sort do provide subjective data on the quality and quantity of the diet, indicating inadequacies or excesses.

Many methods have been devised to collect information on dietary intakes. When a family or group of persons is being studied, *food records* or *food lists* are often used to document food usage. Food records are an inventory of foods on hand, with daily accounts of foods brought into the home. Food lists estimate quantities of foods used over a specified period. These two methods are frequently used by the Food Consumption Branch of the Consumer and Food Economics Research Division, Agricultural Research Service, U.S. Department of Agriculture. The household record of food used and the household dietary questionnaire (in Appendix 22-1) are used for this purpose.

Dietary studies of individuals provide more precise information on nutrient intakes and allow for comparisons with clinical and laboratory findings from the same individual. The *24-hour recall*, which involves having the person, or parent of a child, recall the total food intake during the past 24 hours, is frequently used (in Appendix 22-1). The 24-hour recall is done more than once, if possible. The disadvantages of this method are that it relies on the individual's memory and that the previous day may not be representative of a typical day's food intake. Other methods may be more accurate and representative of typical intake but require more time and professional personnel and cost more. These methods include individual *food records* kept by weight, measures, or estimated quantities over a period of time (in Appendix 22-1); *questionnaires* (in Appendix 22-1); and *interviews*. When administered by a nutritionist, the *dietary history* or interview can provide valuable information on food habits, socioeconomic and cultural conditions, food tolerances and intolerances, appetite and taste changes, physical abilities (chewing, swallowing, motor skills, and mobility), shopping and cooking practices, and facilities for refrigeration and storage.

Kandzari and Howard have developed a tool to be used by nurses to assess nutritional health in the family [3]. With this record, the nurse indicates for each item whether the family or family member meets the criterion. Each section is scored and totals are compared to the ideal totals so that the nurse and family can see what areas should be addressed (in Appendix 22-2).

The information collected by these methods can be interpreted by comparing it with the recommended intakes of foods from the four basic food groups. Once the amounts of specific foods have been determined, they can then be compared with the U.S. recommended dietary allowances (RDAs) for specific age groups. The RDAs for individual nutrients by age group are discussed in Chaps. 23 to 27.

Clinical Assessment

The dietary information is based on information collected by history, recall, and interviewing. Data from clinical assessment is based on physical and biochemical findings.

PHYSICAL FINDINGS

Physical signs and symptoms can be valuable indicators of nutrient deficiencies. These signs appear fairly quickly in body systems with a rapid turnover of cells (e.g., mucous membranes of the mouth) and in those age groups with rapid skeletal and muscular growth (infants and children). The World Health Organization Expert Committee on Medical Assessment of Nutritional Status has proposed a classification of these physical findings [4]. This valuable guide helps in the diagnosis and interpretation of the clinical features of malnutrition by dividing the physical signs most frequently associated with malnutrition into three groups:

1. Signs that are most often associated with nutritional deficiencies (cheilosis, glossitis).
2. Signs that may be related to malnutrition but are often found where other health and environmental problems also exist (dehydration, weight loss).
3. Signs that do not have any relation to malnutrition; often these are difficult to

interpret and may require the expertise of a physician or other health professional specially trained in nutritional diagnosis.

The signs of malnutrition are usually multiple and may be compounded by environmental factors (e.g., wind or sun exposure), variations in personal hygiene, or cultural factors. Signs for the same deficiency may vary depending on the age of the person being examined. For example, scurvy (vitamin C deficiency) in a growing child may manifest as painful, swollen joints, whereas in an adult it may appear as bruises (ecchymoses). Physical findings are open to interpretation by the examiner and should be followed up by laboratory confirmation when possible. The physical signs indicative or suggestive of malnutrition (groups 1 and 2) are given in Table 22-1.

ANTHROPOMETRIC MEASUREMENTS

Anthropometry (from the Greek, *anthropos*, human being, plus *metron*, measure) is the scientific measurement of the human body. It is a quick, simple, and inexpensive method of assessing a person's nutritional status, particularly protein and calorie reserves. Some of the common measurements used are height, weight, head and chest circumferences (infants and young children only), arm muscle circumference, and skinfold thickness. The recommended anthropometric measurements for various ages are given in Table 22-2. It is important to remember that these measurements are nonspecific indicators of growth and development. Below-normal readings do not necessarily indicate poor nutritional status.

Height and *weight* should be obtained by direct measurement. Height should be measured without shoes, and weight should be recorded using a balance beam scale. Height and weight charts for infants and children are given in Figs. 22-1 and 22-2. Weight charts for adults are shown in Table 22-3. Because of osteoporotic changes, height and weight may not be accurate reflections of body composition and nutritional status in persons over age 60. *Weight loss*, calculated as a percentage of ideal weight, may be a helpful indicator of nutritional status. It is usually further defined as recent (within the last 6 to 12 months) and involuntary [1].

$$\text{Percentage weight loss} = \frac{\text{current weight} - \text{usual weight}}{\text{usual weight}} \times 100$$

Recent weight loss exceeding 10 percent of usual weight indicates a need for extensive nutritional assessment and possibly aggressive measures of nutritional support [1]. An evaluation of weight changes is given in Table 22-4.

In infants and young children measurements of head and chest circumference are useful parameters of growth. The *head circumference* is measured at the occipitofrontal circumference (over the temples); the *chest circumference* at the level of the nipples (Fig. 22-3). For newborn infants, the *ponderal index*, using

TABLE 22-1. Physical signs indicative or suggestive of malnutrition

Body area	Normal appearance	Signs associated with malnutrition
Hair	Shiny; firm; not easily plucked	Lack of natural shine; dull and dry; thin and sparse; fine, silky, and straight; color changes (flag sign); can be easily plucked
Face	Skin color uniform; smooth, healthy appearance; not swollen	Skin color loss (depigmentation); skin dark over cheeks and under eyes (malar and supraorbital pigmentation); lumpiness or flakiness of skin of nose and mouth; swollen face; enlarged parotid glands; scaling of skin around nostrils (nasolabial seborrhea)
Eyes	Bright, clear, shiny; no sores at corners of eyelids; membranes a healthy pink and moist; no prominent blood vessels or mound of tissue or sclera	Eye membranes pale (pale conjunctivae); redness of membranes (conjunctival injection); Bitot's spots; redness and fissuring of eyelid corners (angular palpebritis); dryness of eye membranes (conjunctival xerosis); cornea has dull appearance (corneal xerosis); cornea is soft (keratomalacia); scar on cornea; ring of fine blood vessels around corner (circumcorneal injection)
Lips	Smooth, not chapped or swollen	Redness and swelling of mouth or lips (cheilosis), especially at corners of mouth (angular fissures and scars)
Tongue	Deep red in appearance; not swollen or smooth	Swelling; scarlet and raw tongue; magenta (purplish color) tongue; smooth tongue; swollen sores; hyperemic and hypertrophic papillae; atrophic papillae
Teeth	No cavities; no pain; bright	May be missing or erupting abnormally; gray or black spots (fluorosis); cavities (caries)
Gums	Healthy; red; do not bleed; not swollen	"Spongy" and bleed easily; recession of gums
Glands	Face not swollen	Thyroid enlargement (front of neck); parotid enlargement (cheeks become swollen)
Skin	No signs of rashes, swellings, dark or light spots	Dryness (xerosis); sandpaper feel (follicular hyperkeratosis); flakiness; swollen and dark; red swollen pigmentation of exposed areas (pellagrous dermatosis); excessive lightness or darkness (dyspigmentation); black-and-blue marks caused by skin bleeding (petechiae); lack of fat under skin
Nails	Firm, pink	Spoon-shaped (koilonychia); brittle, ridged
Muscular and skeletal systems	Good muscle tone; some fat under skin; can walk or run without pain	Muscles have "wasted" appearance; baby's skull bones are thin and soft (craniotabes); round swelling of front and side of head (frontal and parietal bossing); swelling of ends of bones (epiphyseal enlargement); small bumps on both sides of chest wall on ribs (beading of ribs); baby's soft spot on head does not harden at proper time (persistently open anterior fontanelle); knock-knees or bowlegs; bleeding into muscle (musculoskeletal hemorrhages); person cannot get up or walk properly
Internal systems		
Cardiovascular	Normal heart rate and rhythm; no murmurs or abnormal rhythms; normal blood pressure for age	Rapid heart rate (above 100 = tachycardia); enlarged heart; abnormal rhythm; elevated blood pressure
Gastrointestinal	No palpable organs or masses (in children, however, liver edge may be palpable)	Liver enlargement; enlargement of spleen (usually indicates other associated diseases)
Nervous	Psychological stability; normal reflexes	Mental irritability and confusion; burning and tingling of hands and feet (paresthesia); loss of position and vibratory sense; weakness and tenderness of muscles (may result in inability to walk); decrease and loss of ankle and knee reflexes

Source: G. Christakis, Nutritional assessment in health programs. *American Journal of Public Health* 63:28, 1973.

TABLE 22-2. Recommended anthropometric measurements for various ages

Neonates and infants	School-aged children, adolescents
Weight	Weight
Recumbent length (crown–heel)	Standing height
Head circumference	Triceps skinfold
Chest circumference	Arm circumference
Triceps skinfold	Adults (including elderly)
Preschoolers	Weight
Weight	Standing height
Standing height	Triceps skinfold
Head circumference	Subscapular skinfold
Chest circumference	Arm circumference
Triceps skinfold	
Arm circumference	

Source: G. Christakis, Nutritional assessment in health programs. *American Journal of Public Health* 63:21, 1973.

both weight and length, gives an indication of the proportionality of intrauterine growth [5]:

$$\text{Ponderal index} = \frac{100 \times \text{weight in grams}}{(\text{length in centimeters})^3}$$

The *upper arm circumference* is measured by encircling the upper arm at the midpoint between the acromion (top of the shoulder) process and olecranon (the elbow) in the relaxed, nondominant hanging arm of a standing person (Fig. 22-4A) with a tape measure. This measurement includes both muscle and subcutaneous fat. The *triceps skinfold thickness* is an indirect measurement of adipose tissue stores (subcutaneous fat). It is considered to be a good index of overall body fatness. Because fat is the main storage form of energy in the body, this measurement is also considered to be an accurate index of the body's energy stores. At the same midpoint as for the upper arm circumference measurement, the skin and subcutaneous adipose tissue is grasped and lifted from underlying muscle tissue. The skinfold calipers are applied below the fingers to the fatfold (Fig. 22-4B). The measurement is read from the meter on the calipers. Several measurements of the triceps skinfold should be taken, and the average figure used as the final value. Measurements of subcutaneous adipose tissue may be taken from other areas, but the triceps is the most common site. (See Chap. 29 for further discussion of skinfold measurements.) The *arm muscle circumference* is derived from the upper arm circumference and triceps skinfold measurements. It is an indirect gross indicator of lean body or muscle mass:

$$\text{Arm muscle circumference} = \frac{\text{arm circumference} - (3.14 \times \text{triceps skinfold})}{(\text{all measurements in millimeters})}$$

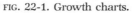

FIG. 22-1. Growth charts.
A. Infant girls.
B. Infant boys. (Data from Ross Laboratories, Columbus, Ohio, 1980.)

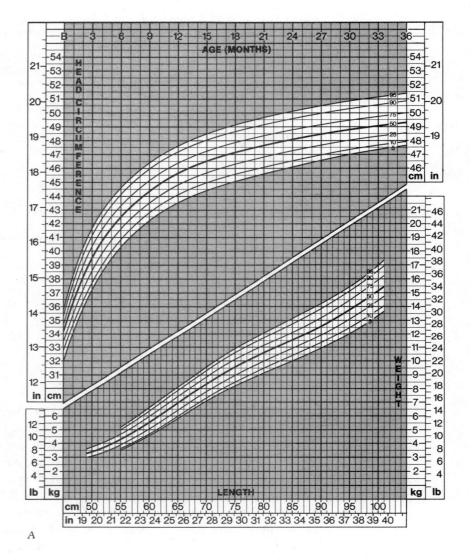

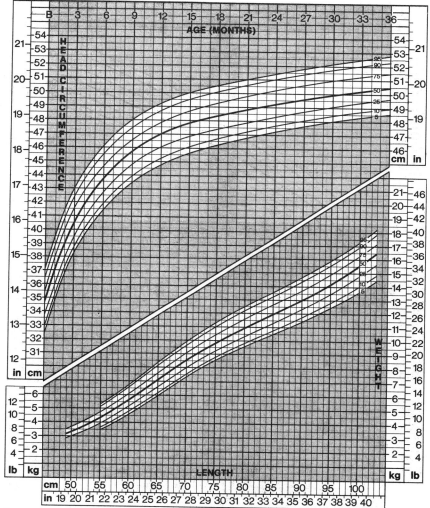

B

FIG. 22-2. Growth charts for children aged 2 to 18 years.
A. Girls.
B. Boys. (Adapted from P. V. V. Hamill, et al., *Physical growth: National Center for Health Statistics percentiles. American Journal of Clinical Nutrition* 32:607, 1979. Data from the National Center for Health Statistics [NCHS], Hyattsville, Md.)

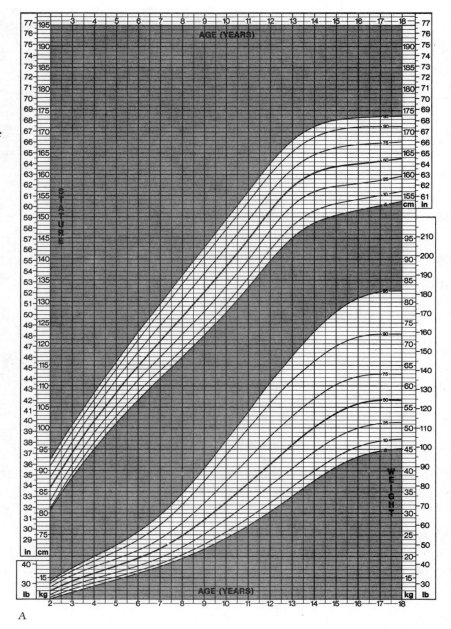

A

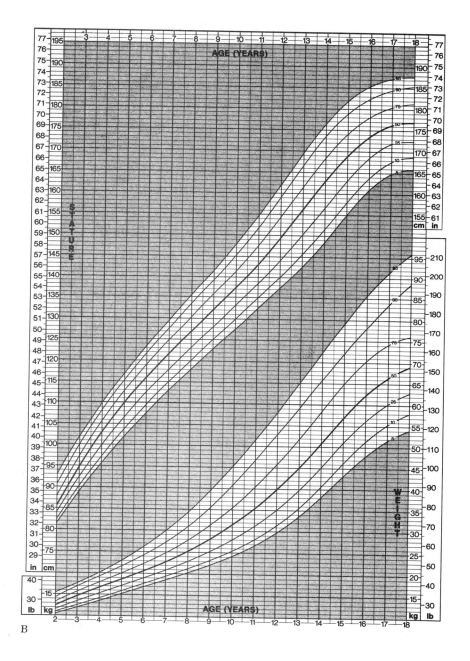

B

TABLE 22-3. Average weights for men and women

Height	Weight (lb)		
	Small frame	Medium frame	Large frame
Men			
5 ft 2 in.	128–134	131–141	138–150
5 ft 3 in.	130–136	133–143	140–153
5 ft 4 in.	132–138	135–145	142–156
5 ft 5 in.	134–140	137–148	144–160
5 ft 6 in.	136–142	139–151	146–164
5 ft 7 in.	138–145	142–154	149–168
5 ft 8 in.	140–148	145–157	152–172
5 ft 9 in.	142–151	148–160	155–176
5 ft 10 in.	144–154	151–163	158–180
5 ft 11 in.	146–157	154–166	161–184
6 ft 0 in.	149–160	157–170	164–188
6 ft 1 in.	152–164	160–174	168–192
6 ft 2 in.	155–168	164–178	172–197
6 ft 3 in.	158–172	167–182	176–202
6 ft 4 in.	162–176	171–187	181–207
Women			
4 ft 10 in.	102–111	109–121	118–131
4 ft 11 in.	103–113	111–123	120–134
5 ft 0 in.	104–115	113–126	122–137
5 ft 1 in.	106–118	115–129	125–140
5 ft 2 in.	108–121	118–132	128–143
5 ft 3 in.	111–124	121–135	131–147
5 ft 4 in.	114–127	124–138	134–151
5 ft 5 in.	117–130	127–141	137–155
5 ft 6 in.	120–133	130–144	140–159
5 ft 7 in.	123–136	133–147	143–163
5 ft 8 in.	126–139	136–150	146–167
5 ft 9 in.	129–142	139–153	149–170
5 ft 10 in.	132–145	142–156	152–173
5 ft 11 in.	135–148	145–159	155–176
6 ft 0 in.	138–151	148–162	158–179

Note: Figures include 5 lb of clothing for men, 3 lb for women; and shoes with 1-in. heels for both.
Source: Metropolitan Life Insurance Co., 1983.

TABLE 22-4. Evaluation of weight change

Time	Significant weight loss (% weight change*)	Severe weight loss (% weight change*)
1 week	1–2	> 2
1 month	5	> 5
3 months	7.5	> 7.5
6 months	10	>10

*See text for definition of percentage weight change.
Source: G. L. Blackburn, et al., Nutritional and metabolic assessment of the hospitalized patient. *Journal of Parenteral and Enteral Nutrition* 1:11, 1977.

FIG. 22-3. Anthropometric measurements in infants. A. Head circumference. B. Chest circumference. (Photos by Paul Wissel)

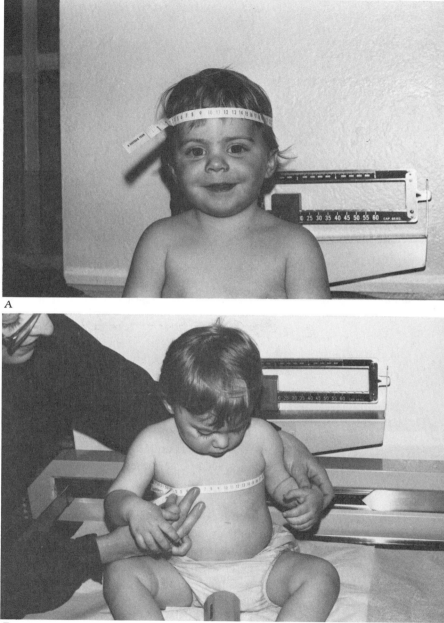

A

B

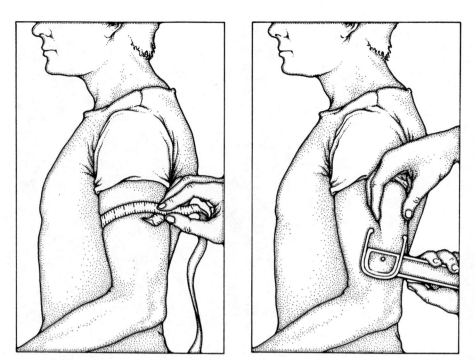

FIG. 22-4. Anthropometric measurements in adults.
A. Upper arm circumference.
B. Triceps skinfold thickness. (From M. Beyers and S. Dudas, *The Clinical Practice of Medical-Surgical Nursing* [2nd ed.]. Boston: Little, Brown, 1984.)

The arm muscle circumference has been shown to correlate well with other measures of total muscle mass. Since muscle is the major protein reserve of the body, this measurement is considered to be a good index of the body's protein reserves. Triceps skinfold and arm muscle circumference are useful because they are inexpensive, accurate, and objective methods of determining gross body composition.

There are some disadvantages associated with the techniques of anthropometric measurement. Specialized equipment is required, and one must be carefully trained in its use and limitations. Anthropometric measurements do not guarantee better diagnosis of nutritional problems, and they should be compared to reference standards derived from the patient's population group. When this is not possible, interpretation of data is necessary, and accuracy may be sacrificed.

Laboratory Assessment

Laboratory assessment provides more objective and precise measurements of nutritional status than dietary information and clinical assessments. The purpose of laboratory assessment is to detect marginal nutritional deficiencies and to supplement or enhance other assessment methods. Laboratory assessment utilizes biochemical tests to measure levels of nutrients or to evaluate biochemical functions of the body that depend on a certain level of essential nutrients.

Two types of tests are generally used: those indicating the *circulating level* of a nutrient in the blood or urine (identifying the presence of a nutritional problem), and *functional tests*, which measure the effect of the nutrient deficiency on the enzyme system utilizing it.

The following are usually assessed to determine nutritional status [6]:

1. Serum protein, particularly albumin level
2. The blood-forming nutrients: iron, folic acid, vitamins B_6 and B_{12}
3. Water-soluble vitamins: thiamin, riboflavin, niacin, and ascorbic acid (vitamin C)
4. Fat-soluble vitamins: A, D, E, and K
5. Minerals: iron, iodine, and other trace elements
6. Levels of blood lipids (cholesterol and triglycerides), glucose, and enzymes implicated in heart disease, diabetes, and other chronic diseases
7. Urinary levels of water-soluble vitamins, protein
8. Stool for guaiac (occult blood) and fat
9. Tests for immunologic function

The current criteria for laboratory evaluation of nutritional status are summarized in Table 22-5.

Several specific tests, most of which evaluate protein reserves and immune function, are discussed below.

CREATININE-HEIGHT INDEX

Creatinine is a normal product of muscle metabolism that is excreted in the urine. With normal renal function and an adequate fluid intake, the daily creatinine excretion is relatively constant. Creatinine is released from muscle in an amount proportional to the muscle mass. With a decrease in muscle mass, as in protein-calorie malnutrition, the amount of urinary creatinine decreases. The creatinine-height index (CHI) has been proposed as a measure of the percentage of body weight composed of muscle. The index is the 24-hour excretion of creatinine divided by the standard creatinine excretion for a person of the same height and sex:

$$CHI = \frac{\text{actual 24-hour urinary creatinine excretion}}{\text{ideal 24-hour urinary creatinine excretion}}.$$

The "ideal" creatinine excretion for men is 23 mg/kg body weight/24 hours; for women, it is 18 mg/kg body weight/24 hours [7]. Unfortunately, the need for a 24-hour urine collection and the assumption of normal kidney function (which is not always present) make this test somewhat impractical as a routine screening procedure.

SERUM ALBUMIN

With starvation, muscle releases amino acids, which are then used by the liver to synthesize albumin and other proteins. In severe protein-calorie malnutrition,

TABLE 22-5. Current criteria for laboratory evaluation of nutritional status

Nutrient (units)	Age of subject (years)	Deficient	Marginal	Acceptable
		Status		
Hemoglobin[a] (gm/100 ml)	6–23 mo	Up to 9.0	9.0–9.9	10.0+
	2–5	Up to 10.0	10.0–10.9	11.0+
	6–12	Up to 10.0	10.0–11.4	11.5+
	13–16M	Up to 12.0	12.0–12.9	13.0+
	13–16F	Up to 10.0	10.0–11.4	11.5+
	16+M	Up to 12.0	12.0–13.9	14.0+
	16+F	Up to 10.0	10.0–11.9	12.0+
	Pregnant (after 6+ mo)	Up to 9.5	9.5–10.9	11.0+
Hematocrit[a] (packed cell volume in percent)	Up to 2	Up to 28	28–30	31+
	2–5	Up to 30	30–33	34+
	6–12	Up to 30	30–35	36+
	13–16M	Up to 37	37–39	40+
	13–16F	Up to 31	31–35	36+
	16+M	Up to 37	37–43	44+
	16+F	Up to 31	31–37	38+
	Pregnant	Up to 30	30–32	33+
Serum albumin[a] (gm/100 ml)	Up to 1		Up to 2.5	2.5+
	1–5		Up to 3.0	3.0+
	6–16		Up to 3.5	3.5+
	16+	Up to 2.8	2.8–3.4	3.5+
	Pregnant	Up to 3.0	3.0–3.4	3.5+
Serum protein[a] (gm/100 ml)	Up to 1		Up to 5.0	5.0+
	1–5		Up to 5.5	5.5+
	6–16		Up to 6.0	6.0+
	16+	Up to 6.0	6.0–6.4	6.5+
	Pregnant	Up to 5.5	5.5–5.9	6.0+
Serum ascorbic acid[a] (mg/100 ml)	All ages	Up to 0.1	0.1–0.19	0.2+
Plasma vitamin A[a] (μg/100 ml)	All ages	Up to 10	10–19	20+
Plasma carotene[a] (μg/100 ml)	All ages	Up to 20	20–39	40+
	Pregnant		40–79	80+
Serum iron[a] (μg/100 ml)	Up to 2	Up to 30		30+
	2–5	Up to 40		40+
	6–12	Up to 50		50+
	12+M	Up to 60		60+
	12+F	Up to 40		40+
Transferrin saturation[a] (percent)	Up to 2	Up to 15.0		15.0+
	2–12	Up to 20.0		20.0+
	12+M	Up to 20.0		20.0+
	12+F	Up to 15.0		15.0+
Serum folacin[b] (ng/ml)	All ages	Up to 2.0	2.1–5.9	6.0+

TABLE 22-5 (CONTINUED)

Nutrient (units)	Age of subject (years)	Status		
		Deficient	Marginal	Acceptable
Serum vitamin B_{12}[b] (pg/ml)	All ages	Up to 100		100 +
Thiamin in urine[a] (µg/g creatinine)	1–3	Up to 120	120–175	175 +
	4–5	Up to 85	85–120	120 +
	6–9	Up to 70	70–180	180 +
	10–15	Up to 55	55–150	150 +
	16 +	Up to 27	27–65	65 +
	Pregnant	Up to 21	21–49	50 +
Riboflavin in urine[a] (µg/g creatinine)	1–3	Up to 150	150–499	500 +
	4–5	Up to 100	100–299	300 +
	6–9	Up to 85	85–269	270 +
	10–16	Up to 70	70–199	200 +
	16 +	Up to 27	27–79	80 +
	Pregnant	Up to 30	30–89	90 +
RBC transketolase-TPP-effect[b] (ratio)	All ages	25 +	15–25	Up to 15
RBC glutathione reductase-FAD-effect[b] (ratio)	All ages	1.2 +		Up to 1.2
Tryptophan load[b] (mg xanthurenic acid excreted)	Adults (dose: 100 mg/kg body weight)	25 + (6 hr) 75 + (24 hr)		Up to 25 Up to 75
Urinary pyridoxine[b] (µg/g creatinine)	1–3	Up to 90		90 +
	4–6	Up to 80		80 +
	7–9	Up to 60		60 +
	10–12	Up to 40		40 +
	13–15	Up to 30		30 +
	16 +	Up to 20		20 +
Urinary n'methyl nicotinamide[a] (mg/g creatinine)	All ages	Up to 0.2	0.2–5.59	0.6 +
	Pregnant	Up to 0.8	0.8–2.49	2.5 +
Urinary pantothenic acid[b] (mcg)	All ages	Up to 200		200 +
Plasma vitamin E[b] (mg/100 ml)	All ages	Up to 0.2	0.2–0.6	0.6 +
Transaminase index[b] (ratio)				
EGOT	Adult	2.0 +		Up to 2.0
EGPT	Adult	1.25 +		Up to 1.25

Key: M = male; F = female; RBC = red blood cell; TPP = thiamin pyrophosphate; FAD = flavin adenine dinucleotide; EGOT = erythrocyte glutamine oxalacetic transaminase; EGPT = erythrocyte glutamic pyruvic transaminase.
[a]Adapted from the Ten State Nutrition Survey.
[b]Criteria may vary with different methodology.
Source: G. Christakis, Nutritional assessment in health programs. *American Journal of Public Health* 63:28, 1973.

the release of amino acids is not sufficient to maintain serum albumin levels. Low levels are usually accompanied by a decrease in muscle mass. A correlation has been shown between arm muscle circumference and serum albumin levels in adults with protein-calorie malnutrition [8, 9]. Changes in serum albumin levels may not be reliable, though, since alterations can occur in liver disease, renal disease, inflammation, and congestive heart failure [10].

NITROGEN STUDIES

Nitrogen balance, the difference between nitrogen intake and output, is used to determine the severity of protein catabolism (tissue breakdown) and to monitor the adequacy of an individualized nutritional support regimen. *Positive* balance indicates nitrogen retention or tissue anabolism. *Negative* balance indicates nitrogen loss or tissue catabolism. *Zero* balance signifies nitrogen equilibrium. The determination of nitrogen balance requires meticulous evaluation of both intake (food) and output (urinary, fecal, dermal, and other losses) and is usually done only in specialized research units.

DELAYED HYPERSENSITIVITY SKIN TESTS

Intradermal injections of common recall antigens, such as dust, pollen, or hair, provide an inexpensive, safe, and reliable method of assessing cell-mediated immune function. Recall antigens stimulate the immune system to respond to substances to which the body has already formed antibodies. Normal immunity is defined as a certain number of positive skin test responses, depending on the set of skin tests used. An induration (a small, raised inflamed area) of the antigen site at 24 to 48 hours after injection is indicative of a positive test response. Absence of any positive skin test result indicates abnormal immune status or immunocompetence. This is associated with protein-calorie malnutrition and increased morbidity and mortality. Reestablishment of immunocompetence has been achieved with nutritional repletion [11, 12].

Levels of Assessment by Age Group

Many tests and measurements have been described on the previous pages. To do all of these assessments on every person would be costly, time-consuming, and very impractical. For this reason, the American Public Health Association has proposed guidelines for *minimal*, *midlevel*, and *in-depth* nutritional assessment of various age groups (Tables 22-6 through 22-9) [6].

The minimal level of assessment represents the simplest evaluation of nutritional status and general health and can be done with the least amount of time, cost, and personnel. Both the midlevel and in-depth assessments build on information in the previous level by using other resources to provide more sophisticated information. As the data collected become progressively more sophisticated, the interrelationships between nutritional states and biologic variables may become more evident.

TABLE 22-6. Levels of nutritional assessment for infants and children

Level of approach*	History: Dietary	Medical and socioeconomic	Clinical evaluation	Laboratory evaluation
Birth to 24 months				
Minimal	Source of iron; Vitamin supplement; Milk intake (type and amount)	Birth weight; Length of gestation; Serious or chronic illness; Use of medicines	Body weight and length; Gross defects	Hematocrit; Hemoglobin
Midlevel	Semiquantitative; Iron: cereal, meat egg yolks, supplement; Energy nutrients; Micronutrients: calcium, niacin, riboflavin, vitamin C; Protein; Food intolerances; Baby foods: processed commercially; home cooked	Family history: diabetes, tuberculosis; Maternal height, prenatal care; Infant immunizations, tuberculin test	Head circumference; Skin color, pallor, turgor; Subcutaneous tissue paucity, excess	RBC morphology; Serum iron; Total iron binding capacity; Sickle cell testing
In-depth	Quantitative 24-hour recall; Dietary history	Prenatal details; Complications of delivery; Regular health supervision	Cranial bossing; Epiphyseal enlargement; Costochondral beading; Ecchymoses	Same as above, plus vitamin and appropriate enzyme assays; protein and amino acids; hydroxyproline, etc., should be available
Age 2–5 years	Determine amount of intake	Probe about pica; medications	Add height at all levels; Add arm circumference at all levels; Add triceps skinfolds at in-depth level	Add serum lead at midlevel; Add serum micronutrients (vitamins A, C, folate, etc.) at in-depth level
Age 6–12 years	Probe about snack foods; Determine whether salt intake is excessive	Ask about medications taken, drug abuse	Add blood pressure at midlevel; Add description of changes in tongue, skin, eyes for in-depth level	All of above plus BUN

Key: RBC = red blood cell; BUN = blood urea nitrogen.
*It is understood that what is included at a minimal level would also be included or represented at successively more sophisticated levels of approach. However, it may be entirely appropriate to use a minimal level of approach to clinical evaluations and an in-depth approach to laboratory evaluations.
Source: G. Christakis, Nutritional assessment in health programs. *American Journal of Public Health* 63:28, 1973.

TABLE 22-7. Levels of nutritional assessment for adolescents

Level of approach	History — Dietary	History — Medical and socioeconomic	Clinical evaluation	Laboratory evaluation
Minimal	Frequency of use of food groups, Habits, patterns, Snacks, Socioeconomic status	Previous diseases and allergies, Abbreviated system review, Family history	Height, Weight	Urine, protein, sugar; Hemoglobin
Midlevel	Above, Qualitative estimate 24-hour recall	Above in more detail	Above, Arm circumference, Skinfold thickness, Skin appearance	Above, Blood taken by vein for albumin (serum), serum iron and TIBC, vitamins A and beta carotene, RBC indices, BUN, cholesterol, zinc
In-depth	Above, Quantitative estimate by recall (3–7 days)	Above	Above, X-ray of wrist, bone density	Above, Blood tests: folate and vitamin C, alkaline phosphatase, RBC transketolase, RBC glutathione, lipids; Urine: creatinine, nitrogen, zinc, thiamin, riboflavin, loading tests (xanthurenic acid/FIGLU); Hair root: DNA, protein, zinc, other metals

Key: RBC = red blood cell; BUN = blood urea nitrogen; FIGLU = formiminoglutamic acid.
Source: G. Christakis, Nutritional assessment in health programs. *American Journal of Public Health* 63:28, 1973.

TABLE 22-8. Levels of nutritional assessment for adults

Level of approach	History — Dietary	History — Medical and socioeconomic	Clinical evaluation	Laboratory evaluation
Minimal	Present food habits Meal patterns "Empty calories" Dietary supplements	Name, age, sex Address Socioeconomic level Number in family Brief medical history (including family)	Height, weight Blood pressure	Hemoglobin A simplified Dipstix evaluation, which would identify presence of protein and glucose in blood, urinary pH
Midlevel	Semiquantitative determination of food intake	Sequential history: present health, history, review of systems, family history, social history (e.g., Cornell Medical Index), smoking history	Anthropometric measurements (skinfold thickness, etc.), brief examination by physician or physician's assistant, chest x-ray as indicated	Evaluations for serum cholesterol, vitamin A, vitamin C, and folic acid; urine excretion of thiamin
In-depth	Household survey data Quantitative 24-hour recall Dietary history Diet patterns as they might influence lipogenic characteristics	All of the above Personal interview by physician Family history of cardiovascular disease	Comprehensive health status evaluation by an appropriate health team, by or under supervision of a physician	Serum triglyceride level, plus nutrients in midlevel Urine or serum evaluation of pyridoxine status (vitamin B_6 nutriture) Evaluation of protein nutriture by height, weight, and chronologic age indices Serum essential and nonessential amino acid ratios Evaluation of vitamin B_{12} nutriture by serum analysis Serum iron and serum iron binding capacity Adipose tissue aspiration and fatty acid analysis by gas-liquid chromatography

Source: G. Christakis, Nutritional assessment in health programs. *American Journal of Public Health* 63:28, 1973.

TABLE 22-9. Levels of nutritional assessment for the elderly

Level of approach	History		Clinical evaluation	Laboratory evaluation
	Dietary	Medical and socioeconomic		
Minimal	Meals eaten per day, week; regularity Frequency of ingestion of protective foods (four food groups) Supplemental vitamins, protein concentrates, mineral mixes General knowledge of nutrition, sources of information	Chronic illness and/or disability; occupational hazard exposure; use of tobacco, alcohol, drugs Symptoms such as bleeding, fainting, loss of memory, dyspnea, headache, pain, changed bowel and/or bladder habits, altered sight and/or hearing; condition of teeth and/or dentures Therapy (prescribed or self-administered) such as drugs, alcohol, vitamins, food fads, prescription items, eyeglasses, hearing aids Names, addresses, and phone numbers of persons providing medical or health care, close family, friends Lives alone, with spouse, or companion Sources of income	Height, weight; cachexia; obesity Blood pressure; pulse rate, rhythm Pallor, skin color and texture Condition of teeth and/or dentures, oral hygiene Affect during interview and examination Vision and hearing appraised subjectively and objectively by examiner Any gross evidence of neglect	Hemoglobin Blood and/or urine sugar Urinalysis (color, odor, bile, and sediment by gross inspection; pH, glucose, albumin blood, and ketones by stick test) Feces (color, texture, gross blood; occult blood by guaiac test)

Midlevel*			
Above data Food preferences and rejections Overt food fads Meal preparation facilities and knowledge Food budget Usual daily diet Protective foods (meats, dairy products, fruits and vegetables, cereals) Nutrients (protein, fat, carbohydrates, iron, vitamins, minerals, trace elements, and water) Empty calorie food (alcohol, candy, sucrose)	Above data Family history of spouse, parents, siblings, other relatives, persons living in same household Pain: location, frequency, character, duration Mental hygiene: attitudes, fears, prejudices, symptoms of psychoses, possible psychosomatic symptoms and signs Income: amount and adequacy for nutrition, housing, health, utilities, clothing, transportation, etc.	Above data Head and neck examinations (otoscopic, ophthalmoscopic, dental and oral cavity, nose, throat) Chest (inspection, palpation, auscultation and percussion, bimanual examination of breast tissue) Abdomen (inspection, auscultation, percussion, and palpation) Rectal and pelvic Inspection and palpation of extremities (evaluation for temperature, edema, pulse, discoloration, ulcers) Gross neurologic evaluation: motor and sensory If indicated, include Complete sensory and motor neurologic examination Sigmoidoscopy Ophthalmologic examination (ophthalmoscopic examination with pupils dilated, refraction, dark adaptation, color perception, visual field examination) Audiometry	Above data Serum lipids (including beta-lipoproteins) Serum iron and iron binding capacity Urinalysis Electrocardiogram Peripheral blood smear for differential white blood cell count and red cell morphology Chest film Postvoiding residual urine by catheterization (if indicated) If indicated, include Serum total protein and albumin; serum creatinine and/or blood urea nitrogen Roentgenographic evaluation of bones and joints suspected of being fractured, harboring infection, and affected by rheumatic and/or metabolic bone disease and/or metastatic or primary neoplastic disease Glucose tolerance tests
In-depth*			
Above data 24-hour dietary recall, preferably for each of several widely separated days; analysis of nutrient intake; evaluation of adequacy, e.g., relate to activity, body weight, laboratory data, affect Past and present food preparation and practices Dining practices and facilities, including companionship	Above data System review Social history Economic history including specifics on sources and amounts of income Mental evaluation (attitudes toward aging)		

TABLE 22-9 (CONTINUED)

| Level of approach | History | | Clinical evaluation | Laboratory evaluation |
	Dietary	Medical and socioeconomic		
				Blood and/or urine vitamin assays for water-soluble and fat-soluble vitamins
				Trace element assays of blood, urine, and/or tissue
				Kidney-ureter-bladder film for stones in urinary tract or gall bladder
				Bacteriologic cultures of any chronic infections
				Barium enema, upper gastrointestinal series, gall bladder series, intravenous pyelography
				Fluoroscopy of chest
				Angiography for coronary arteries, aorta, peripheral vessels
				Bone marrow for unexplained anemia
				Renal clearance studies
				Histologic evaluation of biopsies of tissue suspected of being neoplastic

*The aged, quite unlike children and youth, are the end result of lifetimes of physiologic aging, diseases, and disabilities and cannot be evaluated as if they belonged to younger cohorts. In the above table, it is assumed that midlevel evaluation procedures may be carried out in ambulatory care settings and that in-depth procedures may be conducted as hospital or research procedures. The placement of these in actual practice will depend on availability of facilities and personnel.
Source: G. Christakis, Nutritional assessment in health programs. *American Journal of Public Health* 63:28, 1973.

References

1. Hooley, R. A.   Clinical nutritional assessment: A perspective. *J. Am. Diet. Assoc.* 77:682, 1980.
2. Gray, G. E., and Gray, L. K.   Anthropometric measurements and their interpretation: Principles, practices, and problems. *J. Am. Diet. Assoc.* 77:534, 1980.
3. Kandzari, J., and Howard, J., with Rock, M.   *The Well Family: A Developmental Approach to Assessment.* Boston: Little, Brown, 1981.
4. Jelliffe, D. B.   The Assessment of the Nutritional Status of the Community (WHO Monograph No. 53). Geneva: World Health Organization, 1966.
5. Lubchenco, L. O., Hansman, C., and Boyd, E.   Intrauterine growth in length and head circumference as estimated from live births at gestational ages from 26 to 42 weeks. *Pediatrics* 37:403, 1966.
6. Christakis, G.   Nutritional assessment in health programs. *Am. J. Public Health* 63:28, 1973.
7. Bistrian, B. R., et al.   Therapeutic index of nutritional depletion in hospitalized patients. *Surg. Gynecol. Obstet.* 141:512, 1975.
8. Bistrian, B. R., et al.   Protein status of general surgical patients. *J.A.M.A.* 230:858, 1974.
9. Bistrian, B. R., et al.   Prevalence of malnutrition in general medical patients. *J.A.M.A.* 235:1567, 1976.
10. Blackburn, G. L., and Thornton, P. A.   Nutritional assessment of the hospitalized patient. *Med. Clin. North Am.* 63:1103, 1979.
11. Pietsch, J. B., Meakins, J. L., and MacLean, L. D.   The delayed hypersensitivity response: Application in clinical surgery. *Surgery* 82:349, 1977.
12. MacLean, L. D.   Host resistance in surgical patients. *J. Trauma* 19:297, 1979.

Suggested Readings

Arnold, J. C., et al.   Utilization of family characteristics in nutritional classification of preschool children. *Am. J. Clin. Nutr.* 34:2546, 1981.

Bishop, C. W., Bowen, P. E., and Ritchey, S. J.   Norms for nutritional assessment of American adults by upper arm anthropometry. *Am. J. Clin. Nutr.* 34:2530, 1981.

Blackburn, G. L., et al.   Nutritional and metabolic assessment of the hospitalized patient. *J. Parenter. Enter. Nutr.* 1:11, 1977.

Butterworth, C. E.   The skeleton in the hospital closet. *Nutr. Today* March/April 1974.

Chandra, R. K., and Scrimshaw, N. S.   Immunocompetence in nutritional assessment. *Am. J. Clin. Nutr.* 33:2694, 1980.

Daza, C. H., and Read, M. S.   Health-related components of a nutritional surveillance system. *Bull. Pan Am. Health Organ.* 14:327, 1981.

Driver, A. G., and McAlevy, M. T.   Creatinine height index as a function of age. *Am. J. Clin. Nutr.* 33:2057, 1980.

Durnin, J. V. G. A., and Womersley, J.   Body fat assessed from total body density and its estimation from skinfold thickness: Measurements on 481 men and women aged from 16 to 72 years. *Br. J. Nutr.* 32:77, 1974.

Frisancho, A. R.   Triceps skin fold and upper arm muscle size norms for assessment of nutritional status. *Am. J. Clin. Nutr.* 27:1052, 1974.

Frisancho, A. R.   New norms of upper limb fat and muscle areas for assessment of nutritional status. *Am. J. Clin. Nutr.* 34:2540, 1981.

Graystone, J. E., and Cheek, D. B.   The role of body composition in the assessment of growth and nutrition. *J. Hum. Nutr.* 32:258, 1978.

Hair: A diagnostic tool to complement blood serum and urine. *Science* 202:1271, 1978.

Improved nutrition can boost immune status. *J.A.M.A.* 239:1598, 1978.

Jensen, T. G., and Dudrick, S. J.   Implementation of a multidisciplinary nutritional assessment program. *J. Am. Dietet. Assoc.* 79:258, 1981.

Morgan, J.   The dietary survey and the assessment of food intake in the preschool child: A review. *J. Hum. Nutr.* 34:376, 1980.

Neumann, A. K., et al.   Evaluation of small-scale nutrition programs. *Am. J. Clin. Nutr.* 26:446, 1973.

Scherwin, H. S., et al.   Food eating patterns and health: A reexamination of the Ten-State and Hanes I Surveys. *Am. J. Clin. Nutr.* 34:568, 1981.

U.S. Department of Health, Education and Welfare, Centers for Disease Control.   *Nutrition Surveillance* (Pub. No. [CDC] 75-8295). Atlanta: CDC, 1975.

U.S. Department of Health, Education and Welfare.   *Preliminary Findings of the First Health and Nutrition Examination Survey, United States, 1971–72* (Pub. No. [HRA] 74-1219-1), 1972.

U.S. Department of Health, Education and Welfare.   *Ten-State Nutrition Survey, 1968–1970* (Pub. No. [HSM] 72-8130-8134), 1972.

Winborn, A. L., et al.   A protocol for nutritional assessment in a community hospital. *J. Am. Dietet. Assoc.* 78:129, 1981.

Appendix 22-1

DIETARY QUESTIONNAIRES

Household Record of Food Used for One Week

Record no.:   Date record started:

Meals eaten this week

Person	Sex	Age	Number of meals eaten at home or lunches carried	Number of meals eaten out, not using home food supply

On the following pages, we would like a record of the foods and drinks used in your home for one week.

1. When you start the record, write down the amount of food on hand which you may use during the week.
2. As food is brought into the house from store, farm, or elsewhere during the week, write down the amount.
3. At the end of the week, write down the amount of food left.

HOW TO KEEP THE RECORD:

Under Amount put down the numbers, weights, measure, or sizes.

Under Kind of Food write the exact name of the food, for example, "cornflakes," not cereal. Write whether foods are fresh, canned, dried, or frozen.

Under Price for Amount Bought, put down price.

Under Source, write whether foods are from store, own farm, bought from farm, dairy, bakery, gift, etc. If food is home-canned or home-frozen, record this, and tell the original source of the fresh food.

Amount	Kind of food	Price for amount bought	Source

End of week:

AMOUNT OF FOOD LEFT OVER:

Amount	Kind of food

Household Dietary Questionnaire

Name: Address: Date:

1. Persons fed: (give sex and age for each)

2. Grade of school completed by homemaker:
3. Occupation of head of household:
4. Yearly income: $
   Sources of income:
5. Where do you usually get your food supplies?
   If purchased:

   Kind of store?
   Distance to store?
   How often shop for food?
   Cash or credit?
   Transportation?
   Why?

   If home-produced, what?

   Do you home-preserve?   What? How much?

   Other sources?

   Are food stamps available?   Do you purchase?
   How much do you pay? $ What value do you get?

   Are donated or surplus foods available?   Do you use?
6. How much did you spend for food last week?
   Is this the usual amount?
7. Do you feel you have adequate storage facilities for food?
8. Do you feel you have adequate cooking facilities?
   What kind?   Working oven?
9. Do you feel you have adequate refrigeration?
   What kind?

24-Hour Recall

Name:
Date and time of interview:
Length of interview:
Date of recall:
Day of the week of recall: 1-M   2-T   3-W   4-Th   5-F   6-Sat   7-Sun

I would like you to tell me everything you (your child) ate and drank from the time you (he) got up in the morning until you (he) went to bed at night and what you (he) ate during the night. Be sure to mention everything you (he) ate or drank at home, at work (school), and away from home. Include snacks and drinks of all kinds and everything else you (he) put in your (his) mouth and swallowed. I also need to know where you (he) ate the food. Now let us begin.

What time did you (he) get up yesterday?

Was it the usual time?

When was the first time you (he) ate or had anything to drink yesterday morning?
    (List on the form that follows.)

Where did you (he) eat? (List on form that follows.)

Now tell me what you (he) had to eat and how much?

(Occasionally the interviewer will need to ask):
When did you (he) eat again? or, Is there anything else?
Did you (he) have anything to eat or drink during the night?

Was intake unusual in any way?   Yes   No
(If answer is yes)   Why?
                     In what way?

What time did you (he) go to bed last night?

Do(es) you (he) take vitamin or mineral supplements?
            Yes   No
(If answer is yes)   How many per day?
                     Per week?

What kind? (Insert brand name if known.)
Multivitamins
Ascorbic acid
Vitamins A and D
Iron
Other

Suggested Form for Recording Food Intake

Time	Where eaten	Food	Type and/or preparation	Amount	Food code*	Amount code*

Code

 H = Home
 R = Restaurant, drug store, or lunch counter
 CL = Carried lunch from home
 CC = Child-care center
 OH = Other home (friend, relative, baby-sitter, etc.)
 S = School, office, plant, or work
 FD = Food dispenser
 SS = Social center, eligible senior citizen, etc.

*Do not write in these spaces.

Dietary Questionnaire for Children

Name:

Date:

1. Does the child eat at regular times each day?

2. How many days a week does he eat—
    A morning meal?
    A lunch or mid-day meal?
    An evening meal?
    During the night?*

3. How many days a week does he have snacks—
    In mid-morning?
    In mid-afternoon?
    In the evening?
    During the night?*

4. Which meals does he usually eat with your family?
    None   Breakfast   Noon meal   Evening meal

5. How many times per week does he eat at school, child-care center, or day camp?
    Breakfast   Lunch   Between meals

6. Would you describe his appetite as good?   fair?   poor?

7. At what time of day is he most hungry?
    Morning   Noon   Evening

8. What foods does he dislike?

9. Is he on a special diet now? Yes   No
    If Yes, why is he on a diet? (Check)
        For weight reduction (own prescription)
        For weight reduction (doctor's prescription)
        For gaining weight
        For allergy, specify
        For other reason, specify
    If No, has he been on a special diet within the past year? Yes   No
        If Yes, for what reason

10. Does he eat anything which is not usually considered food? Yes   No
    If Yes, what?   How often?

11. Can he feed himself? Yes   No
    If Yes, with his fingers?   with a spoon?

12. Can he use a cup or glass by himself? Yes   No

13. Does he drink from a bottle with a nipple? Yes   No
    If Yes, how often?   At what time of day or night?

14. How many times per week does he eat the following foods (at any meal or between meals)? Circle the appropriate number:

Bacon	0 1 2 3 4 5 6 7 >7, specify:
Tongue	0 1 2 3 4 5 6 7 >7, specify:
Sausage	0 1 2 3 4 5 6 7 >7, specify:
Luncheon meat	0 1 2 3 4 5 6 7 >7, specify:
Hot dogs	0 1 2 3 4 5 6 7 >7, specify:

*Include formula feeding for young children

Dietary Questionnaire for Children (continued)

Liver—chicken	0 1 2 3 4 5 6 7 >7, specify:
Liver—other	0 1 2 3 4 5 6 7 >7, specify:
Poultry	0 1 2 3 4 5 6 7 >7, specify:
Salt pork	0 1 2 3 4 5 6 7 >7, specify:
Pork or ham	0 1 2 3 4 5 6 7 >7, specify:
Bones (neck or other)	0 1 2 3 4 5 6 7 >7, specify:
Meat in mixtures (stew, tamales, casseroles, etc.)	0 1 2 3 4 5 6 7 >7, specify:
Beef or veal	0 1 2 3 4 5 6 7 >7, specify:
Other meat	0 1 2 3 4 5 6 7 >7, specify:
Fish	0 1 2 3 4 5 6 7 >7, specify:

15. How many times per week does he eat the following foods (at any meal or between meals)? Circle the appropriate number:

Fruit juice	0 1 2 3 4 5 6 7 >7, specify:
Fruit	0 1 2 3 4 5 6 7 >7, specify:
Cereal—dry	0 1 2 3 4 5 6 7 >7, specify:
Cereal—cooked or instant	0 1 2 3 4 5 6 7 >7, specify:
Cereal—infant	0 1 2 3 4 5 6 7 >7, specify:
Eggs	0 1 2 3 4 5 6 7 >7, specify:
Pancakes or waffles	0 1 2 3 4 5 6 7 >7, specify:
Cheese	0 1 2 3 4 5 6 7 >7, specify:
Potato	0 1 2 3 4 5 6 7 >7, specify:
Other cooked vegetables	0 1 2 3 4 5 6 7 >7, specify:
Raw vegetables	0 1 2 3 4 5 6 7 >7, specify:
Dried beans or peas	0 1 2 3 4 5 6 7 >7, specify:
Macaroni, spaghetti, rice, or noodles	0 1 2 3 4 5 6 7 >7, specify:
Ice cream, milk pudding, custard, or cream soup	0 1 2 3 4 5 6 7 >7, specify:
Peanut butter or nuts	0 1 2 3 4 5 6 7 >7, specify:
Sweet rolls or doughnuts	0 1 2 3 4 5 6 7 >7, specify:
Crackers or pretzels	0 1 2 3 4 5 6 7 >7, specify:
Cookies	0 1 2 3 4 5 6 7 >7, specify:
Pie, cake, or brownies	0 1 2 3 4 5 6 7 >7, specify:
Potato chips or corn chips	0 1 2 3 4 5 6 7 >7, specify:
Candy	0 1 2 3 4 5 6 7 >7, specify:
Soft drinks, Popsicles, or Koolaid	0 1 2 3 4 5 6 7 >7, specify:
Instant Breakfast	0 1 2 3 4 5 6 7 >7, specify:

16. How many servings per day does he eat of the following foods? Circle the appropriate number:

Bread (including sandwich), toast, rolls, muffins (1 slice or 1 piece is 1 serving)	0 1 2 3 4 5 6 7 >7, specify:
Milk (including on cereal or other foods) (8 ounces is 1 serving)	0 1 2 3 4 5 6 7 >7, specify:
Sugar, jam, jelly, syrup (1 tsp is 1 serving)	0 1 2 3 4 5 6 7 >7, specify:

17. What specific kinds of the following foods does he eat most often?
    Fruit juices
    Fruit
    Vegetables
    Cheese
    Cooked or instant cereal
    Dry cereal
    Milk

Dietary Questionnaire for Adults and Adolescents

Name: Sex   Date of birth

Address: Marital status   Date

1. Grade of school completed?

2. Still in school?

3. Occupation

4. Are you employed?   Full time?   Part time?

5. Income level $ Sources of income
    Where appropriate:

6. Are you pregnant?   Stage?   Lactating?
    If pregnant have you changed the way you eat or drink? How?
       On whose advice?

7. Where do you usually get your food supplies?
       If home-produced, what?
       Do you home-preserve? What? How much?
       If purchased:
          Kind of store?   Cash or credit?
          Distance to store?   Transportation?
          How often shop for food?   Why?
       Are food stamps available?   Do you purchase?
          How much do you pay? $ What value do you get? $
       Are donated or surplus foods available?   Do you use?

8. Do you feel you have adequate storage facilities for food in your home?

9. Do you feel you have adequate cooking facilities?
       What kind?   Working oven?

10. Do you feel you have adequate refrigeration?   What kind?

11. Do you eat at regular times each day?

12. How many days a week do you eat
       A morning meal?
       A lunch or midday meal?
       An evening meal?
       During the evening or night?

13. How many days a week do you have snacks, and what do you have then?
       In midmorning
       In midafternoon
       In the evening
       During the night

Dietary Questionnaire for Adults and Adolescents (continued)

14. Where do you usually eat your meal?
    Morning   Midday   Evening

15. With whom do you usually eat?
    Morning   Midday   Evening

16. How many times a week do you usually eat away from home?

17. Would you say your appetite is good?   fair?   poor?

18. What foods do you particularly dislike?

19. Are you on a special diet?   If yes, what kind?   Who prescribed?

20. Are there foods you don't eat for other reasons?

21. Do you eat anything not usually considered food (e.g., clay, dirt, starch, other)?
    If yes, what?   When?   How much?

22. Do you add salt to your food at the table?

23. Do you have any difficulty chewing?

24. How many times per week do you eat the following foods (at any meal or between meals)? Circle the appropriate number:

Bacon	0 1 2 3 4 5 6 7 >7, specify:
Tongue	0 1 2 3 4 5 6 7 >7, specify:
Sausage	0 1 2 3 4 5 6 7 >7, specify:
Luncheon meat	0 1 2 3 4 5 6 7 >7, specify:
Hot dogs	0 1 2 3 4 5 6 7 >7, specify:
Liver—chicken	0 1 2 3 4 5 6 7 >7, specify:
Liver—other	0 1 2 3 4 5 6 7 >7, specify:
Poultry	0 1 2 3 4 5 6 7 >7, specify:
Salt pork	0 1 2 3 4 5 6 7 >7, specify:
Pork or ham	0 1 2 3 4 5 6 7 >7, specify:
Bones (neck or other)	0 1 2 3 4 5 6 7 >7, specify:
Meat in mixtures (stew, tamales, casseroles, etc.)	0 1 2 3 4 5 6 7 >7, specify:
Beef or veal	0 1 2 3 4 5 6 7 >7, specify:
Other meat	0 1 2 3 4 5 6 7 >7, specify:
Fish	0 1 2 3 4 5 6 7 >7, specify:
Cheese and cheese dishes	0 1 2 3 4 5 6 7 >7, specify:
Eggs	0 1 2 3 4 5 6 7 >7, specify:
Dried beans or pea dishes	0 1 2 3 4 5 6 7 >7, specify:
Peanut butter or nuts	0 1 2 3 4 5 6 7 >7, specify:

25. How many servings per day do you eat of the following foods? Circle the appropriate number:

Bread (including sandwich), toast, rolls, muffins (1 slice or 1 piece is 1 serving)	0 1 2 3 4 5 6 7 >7, specify:
Milk (including on cereal or other foods) (8 ounces is 1 serving)	0 1 2 3 4 5 6 7 >7, specify:
Sugar, jam, jelly, syrup (1 tsp is 1 serving)	0 1 2 3 4 5 6 7 >7, specify:
Butter or margarine (1 tsp is 1 serving)	0 1 2 3 4 5 6 7 >7, specify:

26. How many times per week do you eat the following foods (at any meal or between meals)? Circle the appropriate number:

Fruit juice	0 1 2 3 4 5 6 7 >7, specify:
Fruit	0 1 2 3 4 5 6 7 >7, specify:
Cereal—dry	0 1 2 3 4 5 6 7 >7, specify:
Cereal—cooked or instant	0 1 2 3 4 5 6 7 >7, specify:
Pancakes or waffles	0 1 2 3 4 5 6 7 >7, specify:
Potato	0 1 2 3 4 5 6 7 >7, specify:
Other cooked vegetables	0 1 2 3 4 5 6 7 >7, specify:
Raw vegetables	0 1 2 3 4 5 6 7 >7, specify:
Macaroni, spaghetti, rice, or noodles	0 1 2 3 4 5 6 7 >7, specify:
Ice cream, milk pudding, custard, or cream soup	0 1 2 3 4 5 6 7 >7, specify:
Sweet rolls or doughnuts	0 1 2 3 4 5 6 7 >7, specify:
Crackers or pretzels	0 1 2 3 4 5 6 7 >7, specify:
Cookies	0 1 2 3 4 5 6 7 >7, specify:
Pie, cake, or brownies	0 1 2 3 4 5 6 7 >7, specify:
Potato chips or corn chips	0 1 2 3 4 5 6 7 >7, specify:
Candy	0 1 2 3 4 5 6 7 >7, specify:
Soft drinks, Popsicles, or Koolaid; sherbets	0 1 2 3 4 5 6 7 >7, specify:
Instant Breakfast	0 1 2 3 4 5 6 7 >7, specify:
Artificially sweetened beverage	0 1 2 3 4 5 6 7 >7, specify:
Coffee or tea	0 1 2 3 4 5 6 7 >7, specify:
Beer	0 1 2 3 4 5 6 7 >7, specify:
Wine	0 1 2 3 4 5 6 7 >7, specify:
Whiskey, vodka, rum, scotch, gin	0 1 2 3 4 5 6 7 >7, specify:

27. What specific kinds of the following foods do you eat most often?
Fruit juices
Fruit
Vegetables
Cheese
Cooked or instant cereal
Dry cereal
Milk
Cream or cream substitute
Butter or margarine
Salad dressings

Appendix 22-2   NURSING ASSESSMENT TOOL FOR EVALUATING NUTRITIONAL HEALTH*

	Usually (2 pts)	Some-times (1 pt)	Never (0 pt)	Not appli-cable
I. Family promotes nutritional wellness by				
A. Formulating a daily mealtime plan	——	——	——	——
B. Identifying six food-exchange categories	——	——	——	——
C. Identifying three examples from each of the six food exchanges	——	——	——	——
D. Encouraging each family member to eat three meals a day or the number appropriate for age†				
1. Mother	——	——	——	——
2. Father	——	——	——	——
3. Child	——	——	——	——
4. Child	——	——	——	——
5. Other	——	——	——	——
E. Serving meals at approximately the same time each day	——	——	——	——
F. Drinking water or fluid with each meal	——	——	——	——
G. Drinking water or fluid between meals	——	——	——	——
H. Sharing one meal a day	——	——	——	——
I. Providing a relaxed mealtime	——	——	——	——
J. Providing an unhurried mealtime atmosphere	——	——	——	——
K. Providing a bright, well-lighted, ventilated room	——	——	——	——
L. Valuing mealtime as an event, not just a habit	——	——	——	——
M. Providing fresh fruits and vegetables whenever available	——	——	——	——
N. Establishing guidelines about mealtime atmosphere	——	——	——	——
O. Identifying cultural influences on eating habits	——	——	——	——
P. Understanding meaning and significance of food to life-style	——	——	——	——
Q. Obtaining sufficient financial resources for nutritional wellness	——	——	——	——
R. Participating in daily exercise†				
1. Mother	——	——	——	——
2. Father	——	——	——	——
3. Child	——	——	——	——
4. Child	——	——	——	——
5. Other	——	——	——	——

*Source: J. H. Kandzari and J. R. Howard with M. S. Rock, *The Well Family*. Boston: Little, Brown, 1981.
†If there are greater or fewer than five members in the family, add or subtract them for this item and adjust the "total points possible" accordingly in the summary.

	Usually (2 pts)	Some-times (1 pt)	Never (0 pt)	Not appli-cable
S. Planning family exercise activities	——	——	——	——
T. Feeling good about self*				
1. Mother	——	——	——	——
2. Father	——	——	——	——
3. Child	——	——	——	——
4. Child	——	——	——	——
5. Other	——	——	——	——
U. Describing self using positive terms*				
1. Mother	——	——	——	——
2. Father	——	——	——	——
3. Child	——	——	——	——
4. Child	——	——	——	——
5. Other	——	——	——	——
V. Remaining within 10 percent of desired weight*				
1. Mother	——	——	——	——
2. Father	——	——	——	——
3. Child	——	——	——	——
4. Child	——	——	——	——
5. Other	——	——	——	——
W. Valuing nutritional wellness	——	——	——	——

Total points possible   86
Total not applicable   ——
Total applicable   ——
Total points attained   ——

II. Practicing nutritional wellness during developmental stages

  A. Infancy

	Usually (2 pts)	Some-times (1 pt)	Never (0 pt)	Not appli-cable
1. Feeding breast milk or formula	——	——	——	——
2. Holding baby close during feedings	——	——	——	——
3. Feeding promptly	——	——	——	——
4. Following recommended feeding intervals	——	——	——	——
5. Adding iron supplements by age 4 to 5 months	——	——	——	——
6. Feeding appropriate sources of iron	——	——	——	——
7. Introducing solid foods in conjunction with developmental cues	——	——	——	——
8. Offering a variety of food textures and colors	——	——	——	——

*If there are greater or fewer than five members in the family, add or subtract them for this item and adjust the "total points possible" accordingly in the summary.

	Usually (2 pts)	Some-times (1 pt)	Never (0 pt)	Not appli-cable
9. Allowing tactile experiences with food	___	___	___	___
10. Avoiding possible allergens	___	___	___	___
11. Introducing new foods one at a time	___	___	___	___
12. Allowing child to determine quantities of food	___	___	___	___
13. Allowing child to self-feed according to developmental cues	___	___	___	___
14. Providing foods according to recommended food exchange	___	___	___	___

Total points possible   28
Total not applicable   ___
Total applicable   ___
Total points attained   ___

B. Toddler stage

	Usually	Some-times	Never	Not applicable
1. Gauging food intake expectations according to child's growth rate	___	___	___	___
2. Encouraging use of child's favorite dishes and utensils	___	___	___	___
3. Offering easily chewed foods	___	___	___	___
4. Allowing food choices within recommended food exchange	___	___	___	___
5. Allowing child mobility during mealtime	___	___	___	___
6. Encouraging self-feeding	___	___	___	___
7. Allowing child to explore food with hands and eyes	___	___	___	___
8. Supervising all mealtimes	___	___	___	___
9. Avoiding extremely hot or cold foods	___	___	___	___
10. Keeping hazardous or poisonous substances out of reach	___	___	___	___
11. Meeting nutritional needs of child in a relaxed manner	___	___	___	___
12. Providing foods according to recommended food exchanges	___	___	___	___

Total points possible   24
Total not applicable   ___
Total applicable   ___
Total points attained   ___

C. Preschool stage

	Usually	Some-times	Never	Not applicable
1. Recognizing child's eagerness to learn	___	___	___	___
2. Teaching food practices by a. Eating wholesome foods	___	___	___	___

	Usually (2 pts)	Some-times (1 pt)	Never (0 pt)	Not appli-cable
b. Avoiding eating in front of television set	——	——	——	——
c. Avoiding use of foods as bribes	——	——	——	——
d. Encouraging a relaxed attitude at mealtime	——	——	——	——
3. Teaching child about nutrition				
a. Pointing out nutritious foods in books and magazines	——	——	——	——
b. Role playing appropriate eating behaviors	——	——	——	——
c. Playing games that teach about nutrition	——	——	——	——
d. Screening food advertisements on TV	——	——	——	——
e. Allowing child to help select nutritious foods at the store	——	——	——	——
4. Inquiring about food attitudes and practices in the school programs	——	——	——	——
5. Encouraging nutritional education in the school	——	——	——	——
6. Recognizing changes in growth rate and corresponding changes in food intake	——	——	——	——
7. Recognizing normal decrease in milk intake	——	——	——	——
8. Offering foods that have been periodically refused	——	——	——	——
9. Offering easily chewed meals and meat substitutes	——	——	——	——
10. Offering finger foods	——	——	——	——
11. Offering simple, mild-tasting foods at room temperature	——	——	——	——
12. Offering complementary foods	——	——	——	——
13. Offering foods according to recommended food exchanges	——	——	——	——
14. Encouraging self-feeding	——	——	——	——
15. Ignoring negative mealtime behaviors	——	——	——	——
16. Praising positive mealtime behaviors	——	——	——	——
17. Allowing choice in choosing reward system	——	——	——	——
18. Encouraging physical activity and exercise	——	——	——	——

	Usually (2 pts)	Some-times (1 pt)	Never (0 pt)	Not appli-cable
19. Providing toys that provide physical exercise	___	___	___	___
20. Encouraging participation in family exercise activities	___	___	___	___

Total points possible   54
Total not applicable   ___
Total applicable   ___
Total points attained   ___

D. School age

	Usually	Some-times	Never	Not appli-cable
1. Recognizing the impact of teacher, peers, and parents in the development of self-concept	___	___	___	___
2. Recognizing slower pattern of growth and changes in food intake	___	___	___	___
3. Providing foods according to the recommended food ex-changes	___	___	___	___
4. Recognizing influences on the development of values by				
a. Eating with friends	___	___	___	___
b. Eating outside the home	___	___	___	___
c. Exposure to junk foods	___	___	___	___
d. Reemphasizing importance of nutritious foods	___	___	___	___
e. Encouraging child to select foods for family meals and school lunches	___	___	___	___
f. Screening food advertise-ments on TV	___	___	___	___
g. Helping the child develop a consumer awareness in re-lation to TV advertising	___	___	___	___
5. Assuring some time for family members to get meals together	___	___	___	___
6. Encouraging physical activity at home and school	___	___	___	___
7. Providing and encouraging nutritious snacks	___	___	___	___
8. Avoiding concentrated sugar in food and drink	___	___	___	___
9. Praising child when he selects nutritious snacks	___	___	___	___
10. Serving nutritious snacks to visitors	___	___	___	___
11. Encouraging nutrition educa-tion in school health cur-riculum	___	___	___	___

	Usually (2 pts)	Some-times (1 pt)	Never (0 pt)	Not appli-cable
12. Encouraging activities in school that teach nutrition	___	___	___	___
13. Working through school organizations to assure nutritious school lunches	___	___	___	___
14. Monitoring whether child eats lunches at school	___	___	___	___
15. Involving child in preparation and planning of brown bag lunch utilizing the food exchange list	___	___	___	___

Total points possible   42
Total not applicable   ___
Total applicable   ___
Total points attained   ___

E. Adolescence

	Usually	Some-times	Never	Not applicable
1. Adapting nutritional patterns to changing growth rate	___	___	___	___
2. Providing foods according to the recommended food exchanges	___	___	___	___
3. Understanding the nutritional implications of the growth spurt	___	___	___	___
4. Understanding the social importance of friends and food	___	___	___	___
5. Supplementing fast food meals with nutrients at home	___	___	___	___
6. Providing family mealtimes	___	___	___	___
7. Participating in sports and physical activities daily	___	___	___	___
8. Assisting in meal planning, meal preparation, and budgeting	___	___	___	___

Total points possible   16
Total not applicable   ___
Total applicable   ___
Total points attained   ___

F. Young adulthood

	Usually	Some-times	Never	Not applicable
1. Adapting food intake to maintenance levels	___	___	___	___
2. Eating foods according to the recommended food exchanges	___	___	___	___
3. Adapting food patterns to changing life events by a. Menu planning	___	___	___	___

	Usually (2 pts)	Some-times (1 pt)	Never (0 pt)	Not appli-cable
b. Food preparation	___	___	___	___
c. Budgeting	___	___	___	___
d. Shopping	___	___	___	___
4. Exercising regularly	___	___	___	___

Total points possible   14
Total not applicable   ___
Total applicable   ___
Total points attained   ___

G. Pregnancy and lactation
1. Assessing food patterns in terms of future role modeling   ___ ___ ___ ___
2. Modifying food practices as necessary to achieve desired model   ___ ___ ___ ___
3. Eating foods during pregnancy according to the recommended food exchanges   ___ ___ ___ ___
4. Increasing intake by 300 cal per day during pregnancy   ___ ___ ___ ___
5. Eating three meals a day plus bedtime snack during pregnancy   ___ ___ ___ ___
6. Increasing fluid intake during pregnancy   ___ ___ ___ ___
7. Avoiding alcohol and caffeine   ___ ___ ___ ___
8. Eating foods during lactation according to the recommended food exchanges   ___ ___ ___ ___
9. Increasing intake by 500 cal per day during lactation   ___ ___ ___ ___
10. Drinking liquid before nursing   ___ ___ ___ ___

Total points possible   20
Total not applicable   ___
Total applicable   ___
Total points attained   ___

H. Middle age
1. Realizing impact of decreasing metabolic rate on nutritional wellness   ___ ___ ___ ___
2. Following a meal plan based on the recommended food exchanges   ___ ___ ___ ___
3. Balancing nutrients and calories to prevent obesity   ___ ___ ___ ___
4. Eating nourishing foods at social events   ___ ___ ___ ___

	Usually (2 pts)	Sometimes (1 pt)	Never (0 pt)	Not applicable
5. Adapting eating patterns to life-style	___	___	___	___
6. Obtaining exercise profile	___	___	___	___
7. Exercising a minimum of 30 minutes per day, 4 days a week at the exercise heart rate	___	___	___	___
8. Realizing benefits of a planned exercise program	___	___	___	___
9. Supporting community-wide sports activities	___	___	___	___
10. Understanding impact of psychosocial crises on nutritional wellness	___	___	___	___
11. Modifying life-style to achieve or maintain optimal weight	___	___	___	___
12. Meeting nutritional needs in the workplace through				
a. Nutritious snacks	___	___	___	___
b. Lunch breaks	___	___	___	___
c. Nutritious lunch foods	___	___	___	___
d. Changing activity levels during breaks	___	___	___	___
e. Promotion of availability of nutritious foods	___	___	___	___
f. Promotion of safe storage of bag lunches	___	___	___	___
g. Promotion of pleasant eating spaces	___	___	___	___

Total points possible   36
Total not applicable   ___
Total applicable   ___
Total points attained   ___

I. Old age

	Usually (2 pts)	Sometimes (1 pt)	Never (0 pt)	Not applicable
1. Realizing physiologic changes that affect nutrition	___	___	___	___
2. Adapting caloric intake to compensate for changes in metabolic rate and physical activity	___	___	___	___
3. Eating foods according to recommended food exchanges	___	___	___	___
4. Understanding how values influence food choices	___	___	___	___
5. Planning nutritious meals consistent with income levels	___	___	___	___
6. Using community resources as necessary or desired to improve nutrition	___	___	___	___

	Usually (2 pts)	Some-times (1 pt)	Never (0 pt)	Not appli-cable
7. Participating in planned and regular exercise programs	___	___	___	___
Total points possible				14
Total not applicable				___
Total applicable				___
Total points attained				___

	Yes (2 pts)	No (1 pt)	Not appli-cable
III. Nutritional issues, agencies, and resources			
A. Family expresses knowledge about the following issues:			
1. Food labeling	___	___	___
2. Food dating	___	___	___
3. Natural versus synthetic vitamins	___	___	___
4. Excess vitamin intake	___	___	___
5. Vitamin C as a cure for colds	___	___	___
6. Vitamin E as a cure-all	___	___	___
7. Processed baby foods	___	___	___
8. Use of skim milk for infants	___	___	___
9. Prevention of specific diseases	___	___	___
10. Relationship between colon cancer and high fat diet	___	___	___
11. Use of fiber in the diet	___	___	___
12. Use of sugar	___	___	___
13. Use of presweetened cereals	___	___	___
14. Use and safety of saccharin	___	___	___
15. Role of salt intake in hypertension	___	___	___
16. Effects of food faddism	___	___	___
17. Safety of vegetarian diets	___	___	___
18. Safety of food additives	___	___	___
Total points possible			36
Total not applicable			___
Total applicable			___
Total points attained			___

	Yes	No	Not appli-cable
B. Family is aware of function and purposes of agencies and resources involved in nutrition research, financial support, and education			
1. International			
a. Food and Agricultural Organization	___	___	___
b. World Health Organization	___	___	___
c. UN Children's Fund	___	___	___
d. Agency for International Development	___	___	___
2. Federal			
a. Department of Health and Human Services	___	___	___

	Yes (2 pts)	No (1 pt)	Not applicable
b. Department of Agriculture	——	——	——
c. Food and Drug Administration	——	——	——
d. National Institutes of Health	——	——	——
e. Public Health Service	——	——	——
f. Consumer Information Center	——	——	——
g. Nutrition Foundation	——	——	——
h. Administration on Aging	——	——	——
3. Private and local			
a. American Dietetic Association	——	——	——
b. Society for Nutrition Education	——	——	——
c. Local community groups and agencies	——	——	——

Total points possible 30
Total not applicable ——
Total applicable ——
Total points attained ——

Assessment Tool Summary

	Subtotal points possible	Subtotal not applicable	Subtotal applicable	Subtotal points attained
I. Promotion of nutritional wellness	86	——	——	——
II. Practicing nutritional wellness during developmental stages				
A. Infancy	28	——	——	——
B. Toddler stage	24	——	——	——
C. Preschool stage	54	——	——	——
D. School age	42	——	——	——
E. Adolescence	16	——	——	——
F. Young adulthood	14	——	——	——
G. Pregnancy and lactation	20	——	——	——
H. Middle age	36	——	——	——
I. Old age	14	——	——	——
III. Nutritional issues, agencies, and resources				
A. Nutritional issues	36	——	——	——
B. Agencies and resources	30	——	——	——

Total points possible 400
Total not applicable ——
Total applicable ——
Total points attained ——

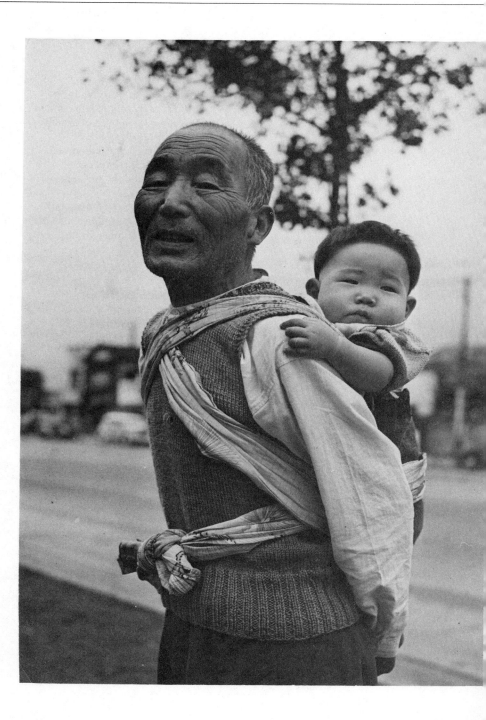

NUTRITIONAL NEEDS THROUGH THE LIFE CYCLE

The human body is an amazing machine, constantly renewing itself. At different stages of life, nutritional needs vary, depending on the body's requirements. The most rapid period of growth is before birth, when individual cells are differentiating into separate organs; for this reason, maternal nutrition is of vital importance. During infancy, growth of bones, muscles, and other systems is rapid, making proper nutrition at this time so important. During childhood growth slows down somewhat, but body systems continue to develop at a steady rate. Another growth spurt occurs again at adolescence, until adult height and weight are finally reached. In adulthood and in old age, proper nutrition is needed for maintenance and repair of the body, resistance to infection, and cell renewal. At each stage of life good nutrition provides a sound basis for health and well-being. In this section, also, nutrition is discussed in terms of its impact on dental health and the development of obesity and leanness.

Chapter 23

NUTRITION IN INFANCY

Infancy is one of the most critical nutritional periods of the life cycle. Growth during the first year of life is more rapid than at any other period beyond intrauterine life. Because of this rapid growth, a constant and adequate supply of essential nutrients is vital. In the absence of adequate essential nutrients, clinical signs of nutritional deficiencies appear much sooner in infants than in other age groups and have graver consequences. For example, protein deficiency in early life may result in permanent deficiencies in cell growth that manifest themselves as physical and mental retardation and learning defects [1]. Nutrition during this stage can affect health throughout life.

Nutrition Requirements
ENERGY

The reserves of fat and water with which full-term infants are born are adequate for only a few days. Calories from food are needed by the second or third day of life. Per unit of body weight, the energy requirements of infants exceed those of all other age groups. From birth to 6 months of age, the recommended dietary allowance (RDA) is 115 calories per kilogram, and from 6 months to 1 year it is 105 calories per kilogram. This is 1¼–1⅓ times the requirement for young schoolchildren, and almost three times that for men. During the first 4 months of life about one-third of the caloric intake is used exclusively for growth. During this period infants usually double their birth weight and spend most of their time sleeping.

Contributing to infants' high caloric needs is their greater surface area in proportion to their weight and the consequent greater heat loss; calories are also needed for activity. Between the ages of 4 and 12 months, the infant becomes more physically active, and only about 10 percent or less of the caloric intake is used for growth (Fig. 23-1) [2]. By 1 year of age the birth weight has usually tripled.

Since each ounce of breast milk or infant formula at proper dilution contains about 20 calories, about 23 oz per day would be required to supply the average 4 kg (8.8 lb) infant with its caloric needs (20 calories per oz × 23 oz = 460 calories; 4 kg × 115 calories per kg = 460 calories). Intakes less than 80 calories/kg/day are usually inadequate, and those above 120 calories/kg/day are usually associated with the development of obesity. The caloric needs of low-birth-weight (LBW) or premature infants and those recovering from illness or malnutrition are greater (see Special Needs of the Premature or Low-Birth-Weight Infant, below).

FLUIDS

The average infant requires about 150 ml (5 oz) of fluid/kg body weight/day. This is usually taken as breast milk or infant formula, but under conditions in which extra fluid is lost from the skin, lungs, or gastrointestinal tract, such as fever, hot weather, or diarrhea, additional water should be given. Extra fluids may also be necessary when solid foods are introduced into the diet, replacing

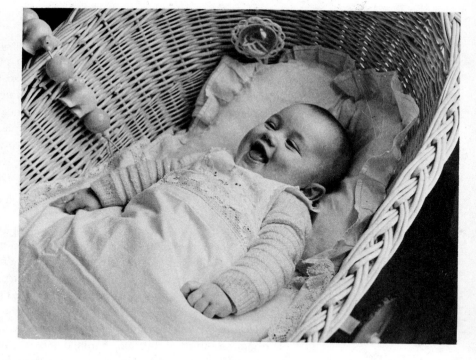

FIG. 23-1. Until now about one-third of this healthy 5-month-old baby's caloric intake has been used exclusively for growth. Now, because she is growing less rapidly and becoming more physically active, less energy will be expended on actual growth (about 10 percent or less) and more on maintaining heat and activity. (World Health Organization photo by R. Doisneau.)

some of the breast milk or formula. This is especially true if the solid food is high in protein, sodium, or potassium.

PROTEIN

As with the energy requirement, the need for protein per unit of body weight is greater during infancy than at any other period. From birth to age 6 months, the RDA is 2.2 gm/kg/day; for infants 6 months to 1 year of age it is 2.0 gm/kg/day. During the first 4 months of life the average increase in body protein is about 3.5 gm per day; during the next 8 months, about 3.1 gm per day [3]. This results in a weight gain of about 7 kg by the end of the first year and an increase of 14.6 percent in the protein content of the body. For infants over 6 months of age, the liberal protein requirements allow for about a 75 percent efficiency of utilization of proteins from a mixed diet.

FAT

Although there is no specific requirement for fat in the diet of infants, it does contribute calories and essential fatty acids and is a carrier of fat-soluble vitamins. Commercial formulas contain about 35 to 50 percent of calories as fat, cow's milk formula about 46 percent, and human milk about 48 percent.

The infant must be supplied with the essential fatty acid linoleic acid. Studies in animals have shown that prenatal and postnatal essential fatty acid deficiency results in a retardation of brain development and a reduction in some of the myelin (nerve sheath) components [4]. To prevent essential fatty acid deficiency, the recommended intake of linoleic acid is 300 mg per 100 calories or 3 percent of the total calories [2]. Commercial formulas supply about 3 percent, cow's milk formula, 1 to 2 percent, and human milk about 6 to 9 percent of the total calories as linoleate.

CARBOHYDRATE

Lactose, the naturally occurring carbohydrate found exclusively in milk, has many nutritional advantages. It is slowly metabolized and aids in the intestinal absorption of calcium. It also promotes the growth of *Lactobacillus bifidus* in the intestines, which provides some protection against gastrointestinal infections.

MINERALS

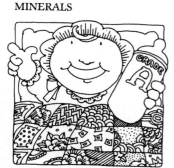

CALCIUM

Breast milk provides about 60 mg of calcium/kg body weight/day (300 mg per liter of milk), of which the infant retains about two-thirds. The calcium content of cow's milk formula is about twice as great (600 to 700 mg per liter), providing about 170 mg/kg/day, but the infant only retains about 25 to 30 percent [5]. In view of these findings, the Food and Nutrition Board of the National Research Council has recommended 60 mg per kilogram body weight as the daily calcium allowance.

IRON

The risk of developing iron-deficiency anemia is greatest when the iron stores established in utero have been depleted: after 2 months in LBW and premature infants and after 4 to 6 months in full-term infants. Although clear-cut evidence in human infants is lacking, animal studies indicate that iron-deficiency anemia early in postnatal life results in biochemical abnormalities in some organs, including the brain, that persist long after the anemia has been corrected [6]. The infant will be born with inadequate stores of iron if the mother is severely iron deficient, if the infant is born prematurely, if the placenta separates prematurely, if there are injuries during the birth process, if there are illnesses requiring maternal transfusions, or if the umbilical cord is clamped too early.

The RDA for iron is 10 mg per day during the first 6 months of life and 15 mg per day during the second 6 months. Normal infants can maintain optimal hemoglobin levels with a supplementation of iron of 1 mg/kg/day starting at about the third month [5]. LBW infants (less than 2500 gm at birth) may require 2 mg/kg/day starting at birth. The recommended allowance of 1.5 mg/kg/day is based on the average need during the first year of life.

The iron present in breast milk is absorbed more efficiently than the iron in prepared formulas or cow's milk [7], and breast-fed infants rarely develop iron-deficiency anemia. Iron-fortified dry cereal is a good supplemental iron source for the breast-fed infant and should be introduced no later than 4 to 6 months of age. For formula-fed infants, iron-fortified formula and dry cereals are the best iron sources.

Full-term infants should be screened for iron-deficiency anemia (hemoglobin less than 11 gm per 100 ml, or hematocrit less than 33 percent) between the ages of 9 and 12 months, and LBW or premature infants between 6 and 9 months [8].

FLUORIDE

The inclusion of this essential dental nutrient in the diet from birth has been shown to have dramatic beneficial effects on later dental health. It has been estimated that the infant receives as little as 0.1 mg per day from breast milk or cow's milk formula and as much as 1.2 mg per day from certain commercial formulas [9]. The Food and Nutrition Board suggests a daily intake of 0.1 to 1.0 mg per day during the first year of life, and 0.5 to 1.5 mg per day during the subsequent 2 years, as being safe and adequate.

VITAMINS

VITAMIN A

Human milk contains about 49 µg per 100 ml of retinol, and a daily intake of about 860 ml would supply 420 µg of retinol, the recommended allowance for infants up to 6 months of age. With the addition of solid foods plus milk, the recommendation for infants aged 6 months to 1 year is 400 retinol equivalents (300 as retinol and 100 as beta carotene) (1 µg retinol = 10 IU vitamin A).

VITAMIN D

The vitamin D content of human milk is far below the needs of the growing infant. Although a level of 2.5 µg (100 IU) of vitamin D per day will prevent rickets and will ensure normal mineralization of bone in infants, 10 µg (400 IU) has been shown to promote better calcium absorption and increased growth. It is therefore recommended by the Food and Nutrition Board that infants receive this higher level. It should be ensured that the infant receive this vitamin D allowance in the diet or by supplements, since exposure to sunlight may be inadequate to meet these needs.

VITAMIN E

The concentration of vitamin E in the plasma of newborn infants is about one-third that in adults, and in LBW infants the level is even lower. These levels begin to rise within a few days after birth and reach normal childhood concentrations by 1 month of age. In infants fed breast milk, this level rises more rapidly than in those fed cow's milk formula. Some studies have linked vitamin E deficiency in LBW infants to their eating of commercial formulas made with polyunsaturated fat and a low vitamin E content [10]. Signs of vitamin E deficiency include an increased susceptibility of erythrocytes (red blood cells) to hemolysis (breakdown). This may appear clinically as anemia. In all infant formulas, and especially those fed to LBW infants, the level of vitamin E, as well as iron and polyunsaturated lipids, should be carefully monitored.

The vitamin E content of human milk, 2 to 5 IU per liter, is assumed to be sufficient for nursing infants. The American Academy of Pediatrics [11] suggests that for the special needs of the LBW infant, commercial formulas should provide

0.7 IU of vitamin E per 100 calories, at least 1.0 IU of linoleic acid per gram, and a supplement of 5 IU of water-soluble alpha tocopherol.

VITAMIN K

A deficiency of this vitamin has been reported in some newborn infants before the establishment of intestinal flora. Newborn infants are often administered vitamin K at birth to prevent hemorrhage, since vitamin K–dependent clotting factors are low for approximately 1 week after birth. The American Academy of Pediatrics recommends that all formulas contain a minimum of 4 μg of vitamin K per 100 calories [10]. This amount is sufficient to prevent deficiency, and the bacterial flora engendered by milk feeding contribute to an adequate vitamin K supply. Breast milk contains about 12 μg per day (15 μg per liter). Since after infancy the bacterial flora synthesize vitamin K, there are no specific recommended allowances made for this vitamin.

VITAMIN C

The precise requirement for vitamin C in infancy is not known, but it has been shown that the amount in human milk from a well-nourished mother (30 to 55 mg per liter) and prepared formulas (50 mg per quart) provides an adequate margin of safety against the signs of scurvy. All newborn infants, but especially if they are premature, may have an increased requirement for vitamin C for the metabolism of tyrosine, an amino acid [12]. To protect against the possible adverse effects of tyrosinemia (high levels of tyrosine in the blood), an intake of 100 mg per day is recommended for infants.

FOLIC ACID

The recommended daily allowance of folic acid has been estimated to be 5 μg/kg/day. Human and cow's milk both contain about 2 to 3 μg per 100 mg, and most of this is present in an absorbable form. Since folic acid is destroyed by heat processing, formulas made from pasteurized, sterilized, or powdered cow's milk may be lacking this essential vitamin, and infants fed these formulas should receive additional folic acid to ensure an adequate intake [13].

THIAMIN

The thiamin content of human milk is sufficient to supply the minimum daily requirement of about 0.03 mg/kg/day or about 0.27 mg per 1000 calories. To provide a margin of safety in milk formulas, the allowance recommended is 0.5 mg per 1000 calories. From birth to 6 months, the RDA is 0.3 mg; from 6 months to 1 year, it is 0.5 mg. This higher allowance is easily met after the introduction of enriched cereals.

When the mother's diet is low or lacking in thiamin, such as in areas where the diet consists mainly of unenriched white rice or white flour, this lack is reflected in the breast milk. Clinical signs of deficiency in infants appear suddenly and are severe, often involving cardiac failure.

TABLE 23-1. Recommended daily dietary allowances for infants

Feature or nutrient	0.0–0.5 years	0.5–1.0
Weight (kg, lb)	6, 13	9, 20
Length (cm, in.)	61, 24	71, 28
Energy (cal)	Weight (kg) × 115	Weight (kg) × 105
Protein (gm)	Weight (kg) × 2.2	Weight (kg) × 2.0
Fat-soluble vitamins		
Vitamin A (IU)	4200	4000
Vitamin D (IU)	400	400
Vitamin E (IU)	4.6	6.2
Water-soluble vitamins		
Vitamin C (mg)	35	35
Thiamin (mg)	0.3	0.5
Riboflavin (mg)	0.4	0.6
Niacin (mg)	6	8
Pyridoxine (mg)	0.3	0.6
Folacin (µg)	30	45
Vitamin B_{12} (µg)	0.5	1.5
Minerals		
Calcium (mg)	360	540
Phosphorus (mg)	240	360
Magnesium (mg)	50	70
Iron (mg)	10	15
Zinc (mg)	3	5
Iodine (µg)	40	50

Source: Food and Nutrition Board, National Research Council, *Recommended Dietary Allowances* (9th ed.). Washington, D.C.: National Academy Press, 1980. Pp. 130, 138.

NIACIN

The amino acid tryptophan is converted into niacin by the human body. Human milk contains about 0.17 mg of niacin and 22 mg of tryptophan per 100 ml. With an adequate maternal intake, breast milk meets the niacin requirements of the infant. The RDA for infants up to 6 months of age is 6 mg of niacin, with two-thirds being supplied by tryptophan. For infants aged 6 months to 1 year, the RDA is 8 mg of niacin.

A summary of the RDAs for infants is given in Table 23-1.

Breast-feeding

Breast milk is the ideal food for the newborn infant and is nutritionally unique. Because it provides the infant with maximal immunologic defenses and minimizes the risk of allergic reactions and overfeeding, breast milk should be the baby's only food source for 4 to 6 months.

The main advantages of breast-feeding, as expressed by a joint statement by the American Academy of Pediatrics and the Canadian Paediatric Society, are the transmission of maternal immunity in the colostrum, or early milk, and the reinforcement of "bonding," which is considered necessary for the emotional nurturing of the newborn [14].

The mother transmits certain elements of her own resistance to the infant while its own immune system is developing. Human milk contains a number of antibodies to certain intestinal microorganisms, protecting the infant from gastrointestinal infections. Lactoferrin lowers the iron concentration of milk by chelation (binding iron) and thereby inhibits bacterial proliferation. This protein, lactoferrin, is the protection given by breast milk against diarrheal diseases. Other factors in breast milk are active against streptococci and staphylococci. High levels of secretory immunoglobulin A (IgA) are also transmitted in colostrum at delivery and even 1 year later in breast milk. Several other components, including the "bifidus factor," complement, and lysozyme, together with the high concentration of lactose found in breast milk, are responsible for the proliferation of *L. bifidus* bacteria in the ileum and large intestine of breast-fed infants. Because of the metabolic by-products of these bacteria, such infants are very resistant to invasive enteric bacteria and protozoa. Infant formulas that have been heat treated do not supply such immunologic protection.

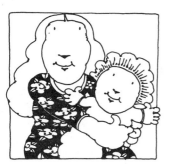

The lipids in human milk are better absorbed by infants than those in cow's milk. This is especially important in LBW or premature infants, who have poor fat absorption. Although the caloric content of breast milk and cow's milk formulas are similar, the amount taken at each feeding may differ widely. With bottle-feeding, the mother or caretaker controls the intake; with breast-feeding, the infant does.

About 60 percent of the protein in human milk is lactalbumin, whereas the protein in cow's milk is mostly casein. Lactalbumin is rich in sulfur-containing amino acids, of which cysteine is thought to be vital for proper brain development during this period.

The iron in breast milk is well absorbed, making breast-fed infants less prone to iron-deficiency anemia. The low iron concentration found in human milk is also important because transferrin and lactoferrin (found in higher concentrations in human milk) lose their bacteria-fighting qualities with iron saturation.

One year is the optimum period of breast-feeding for the infant, but any time period is better than none at all. For the working mother, the breast milk can be expressed by hand, refrigerated (for a period not to exceed 24 hours), and bottle-fed as an ideal alternate method.

Breast milk, when available in adequate amounts, produces optimal growth and health in the newborn. Although there may be trace amounts of insecticides and chemicals in human milk, reflecting their presence in the maternal diet and environment, human milk is still the preferred food for the newborn.

A comparison of the composition of human milk, cow's milk, and evaporated milk is given in Table 23-2.

TABLE 23-2. Human milk and cow's milk[a]

Nutrient	Human	Cow's	Evaporated
Percent water (ml/100 ml)	87.6	87.2	73
Percent total solids (gm/100 ml)	12.4	12.7	27
Energy			
(cal/100 ml)	71	69	152
(cal per oz)	20	20	44
Protein (gm/100 ml)[b]	1.2	3.3	7.3
Fat (gm/100 ml)	3.8	3.7	8.2
Carbohydrate (gm/100 ml)[c]	7.0	4.8	10.6
Ash (gm/100 ml)	0.2	0.7	1.6
Minerals (per liter)			
Sodium (mEq)	7	22	55
Potassium (mEq)	13	35	77
Chloride (mEq)	11	29	46
Calcium (mg)	340	1170	2750
Phosphorus (mg)	140	920	2112
Magnesium (mg)	40	120	264
Iron (mg)	1.5	1.0	2.2
Zinc (mg)	3–5	3–5	8.4
Iodine (μg)	30	10–200	460
Copper (mg)	400	300	660
Vitamins (per liter)[d]			
A (IU)	1898	1025	1850
D (IU)	21	13[e]	420
E (IU)	6.6	1	1.3
K (μg)	15	60	0–160
C (mg)	43	11	5.5
Thiamin (μg)	160	440	280
Riboflavin (mg)	0.36	1.75	1.9
Niacin (mg)	1.47	0.94	1.0
B_6 (pyridoxine) (μg)	100	640	370
Folacin (μg)	52	55	55
B_{12} (μg)	0.3	4	1.0–1.9
Pantothenic acid (mg)	1.84	3.46	3.5

[a] Average, undiluted composition.
[b] Human milk: 60% whey protein, 40% casein; cow's milk: 18% whey protein, 82% casein.
[c] As lactose.
[d] Evaporated milk values based on 1:1 dilution.
[e] Marketed cow's milk usually fortified to 400 IU.
Source: D. Reina, Infant nutrition. *Clinics in Perinatology* 2:373, 1975.

Prepared Formulas

Before the turn of the century, if a woman died in childbirth, her newborn would also soon die unless a wet nurse could be found to feed it as well as her own. At that time very little was known about the nutritional requirements of infants, and there were no infant formulas. When cow's milk or milk from other animals was given, the infant usually died within the first 2 weeks of life. Because human milk has a very low protein content, these deaths were probably the result of protein or electrolyte intoxication.

Infant mortality in the United States during the late nineteenth and early

TABLE 23-3. Commonly used formulas

Contents	Enfamil	Similac	SMA	Soy isolates[a]
Components				
Protein	Nonfat milk	Nonfat milk	Whey and nonfat milk	Soy isolate
Fat	Vegetable oils	Vegetable oils	Vegetable and oleo oils	Vegetable oils
Carbohydrate	Lactose	Lactose	Lactose	Corn syrup and/or sucrose
Major constituents (gm/100 ml)				
Protein	1.5	1.55	1.5	1.8–2.5
Fat	3.7	3.6	3.6	3.0–3.6
Carbohydrates	7.0	7.1	7.2	6.4–6.8
Ash (minerals)	0.36	0.37	0.3	0.4–0.5
Cal/oz[b]	20	20	20	20
Percent of calories				
Protein	9	9	9	12–15
Fat	50	48	48	45–48
Carbohydrate	41	43	43	39–40
Minerals/liter				
Sodium (mEq)	11	11	6.5	9–24
Potassium (mEq)	19	19	14.3	15–28
Chloride (mEq)	12	17	10	7–15
Calcium (mg)	536	600	445	700–950
Phosphorus (mg)	454	440	300	500–690
Magnesium (mg)	46	40	53	50–80
Copper (mg)	0.6	0.4	0.4	0.4–0.6
Zinc (mg)	1.1	5	3.2	2.0–5.3
Iodine (µg)	67	40	69	70–160
Iron (mg)[c]	1.5	Trace	12.7	8.5–12.7
Vitamins/liter				
A (IU)	1650	2500	2650	2100–2500
D (IU)	413	400	423	400–423
E (IU)	12.4	15	9.5	9–11
K (mg)	—[d]	—[d]	—[d]	0.9–0.15
C (mg)	52	55	58	50–55
Thiamin (µg)	510	650	710	400–700
Riboflavin (µg)	620	1000	1060	600–1060
Niacin (mg)	8.25	7	7	5.0–8.4
Pyridoxine (µg)	410	400	423	400–530
Folacin (µg)	100	50	32	50–100
B_{12} (µg)	2.0	1.5	1.1	2.0–3.0
Pantothenate (mg)	3.1	3	2.1	2.6–5.0

[a] Prosobee, Isomil, Nursoy, Neo-mulsoy, i-soyalac (contains tapioca starch).
[b] Diluted per manufacturer's specifications.
[c] Enfamil with iron contains 12.7 mg/liter; Similac with iron, 12 mg/liter.
[d] Vitamin K not added because milk base supplies ample amounts.
Source: D. Reina, Infant nutrition. *Clinics in Perinatology* 2:373, 1975.

TABLE 23-4. Special formulas

Formula	Recommended dilution (milk:water)	Calories/ounce	Protein (gm/100 ml)	Fat (gm/100 ml)	Carbohydrates (gm/100 ml)	Minerals (gm/100 ml)	Sodium (mEq/liter)	Potassium (mEq/liter)	Chloride (mEq/liter)	Calcium (mg/liter)	Phosphorus (mg/liter)	Iron (mg/liter)	Vitamins
Nutramigen	1:2	20	2.2	2.6	8.6 (sucrose)	0.56	17	26	23	50	52	12.7	Added
Meat base[a]	13:19.5	17.4	2.7	3.1	4.0 (sucrose, starch)	0.33	12	12	17	52	40	9.7	Added
Lambase	1:1	20	2.4	2.4	7.9 (maltose, dextrose, starch)	0.3	24	28	7	46	45	7.9	Added
Cho-Free	1:1	20	1.8	3.5	6.4[b]	0.5	17	25	6		47	8.4	Added
Probana	1:2	20	4.2	2.2	7.9 (dextrose, lactose)	0.6	26	31	28	58	58	1.5	Added
Portogen	1:3	20	2.7	3.2[c]	7.7 (sucrose, maltodextrins)	0.7	17	33	23	48	46	12.7	Added
Pregestimil	1:2	20	2.2	2.8[c]	8.8 (glucose)	0.6	14	24	23	48	47	12.7	Added
Lofenelac	1:2	20	2.2[d]	2.7	8.7 (tapioca starch)	0.6	21	27	23	47	47	12.7	Added
Lonalac	1:3.5	20	3.4	3.5	4.8 (lactose)	0.6	1.1	27	14	56	57	1	Added[e]
Similac 60/40	1:2	20	1.5	3.5	7.5 (lactose)	0.2	7	15	13	20	12	12	Added

[a]Low in carbohydrate. Ordinarily add carbohydrate before feeding.
[b]12.5% dextrose added. Because of hypoglycemia, ketosis, avoid use without carbohydrates.
[c]Medium-chain triglycerides.
[d]Casein hydrolysate specially processed to remove most of the phenylalanine.
[e]Vitamins C and D not added.
Source: D. Reina, Infant nutrition. *Clinics in Perinatology* 2:373, 1975.

twentieth centuries was high, ranging from 288.9 per 1000 infants under 1 year of age in 1880 to 133.9 per 1000 infants in 1910 [15]. At that time, the causes of infant death were grouped into four classes: (1) contagious disease, (2) respiratory disease, (3) diarrheal disease, and (4) congenital disease (including marasmus, a form of protein-caloric malnutrition). With control of infectious diseases and improvements in refrigeration and water supplies, infant morbidity and mortality decreased. Jeremiah Milbank made his fortune by perfecting canned condensed milk, creating the Borden Milk Company, and provisioning the Northern armies during the Civil War. His fortune, as the Milbank Fund, would become one of the leading philanthropic sources in maternal and child health in this country. The process developed by Milbank modified the casein curds of unpasteurized cow's milk, which had previously been indigestible for infants. Evaporated milk, as a result of this process, became the most widely accepted ingredient for home-prepared infant formulas and as recently as 1960 was being given to 80 percent of bottle-fed infants [16].

In 1915 the modern infant formulas began with the introduction of a skim cow's milk formula to which had been added various fats and oils to simulate the fatty acid content of human milk. Manufacturers attempted to include each new nutrient discovered in human milk in formula.

Today most infant formulas are based on cow's milk, although there are special formulas based on soybean isolate given to infants who are allergic to cow's milk. There are also special formulas for infants who are underweight or have medical problems or inborn errors of metabolism. The contents of commonly used formulas are summarized in Table 23-3; special formulas, in Table 23-4.

Special Needs of the Premature or Low-Birth-Weight Infant
NEUROPHYSIOLOGIC DEFICIENCIES

Premature or LBW infants (less than 2500 gm at birth) have unique problems associated with feeding (Fig. 23-2). Unlike normal, full-term infants, they may have a poor sucking reflex, an uncoordinated swallowing mechanism, delayed gastric emptying, or a combination of these. The immature neurologic development of these infants predisposes them to vomiting and aspiration.

Adequate nutrition during this time is vital, especially in these infants, because they are born with poor nutritional reserves. Iron and vitamin supplementation is very important in the premature infant. Since iron stores are not deposited until the last months of gestation, premature infants frequently become iron deficient. This is during a critical period (from conception through first year) of brain growth, and nutritional deficiency can result in irreversibly altered brain growth and development [17]. Methods of feeding currently in practice include total intravenous alimentation (total parenteral nutrition), intravenous supplementation of oral feedings, and nasojejunal feedings [17]. Human milk appears to be the best food, even for the premature infant.

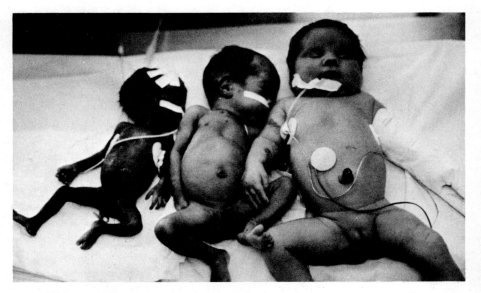

FIG. 23-2. Three babies of the same gestational age. Weights are 600, 1400, and 2750 gm, respectively. (From S. Korones, *High-Risk Newborn Infants* (3rd ed.). St. Louis: Mosby, 1981. By permission.)

CALORIES

The LBW infant may require as many as 110 to 200 calories/kg/day. Exposure to cold may increase this need as much as 2½ times; therefore protection from heat losses may increase the rate of gain in these infants [18].

PROTEIN

The protein requirement of 2.2 gm/kg/day for the normal, full-term infant is inadequate for the LBW infant. Although the precise requirement for the LBW or premature infant is not known, the distribution of amino acids found in human milk seems to approximate closely the needs of these infants. If the respiratory distress syndrome is present at birth, the rate of protein catabolism is doubled, which also increases both the protein and caloric requirements.

FAT

Because of a decreased secretion of bile acids and the immaturity of the gastrointestinal tract, fat absorption in these infants is poor. The fat content should be between 40 and 50 percent of the total calories. The fat present in human milk is absorbed better by the LBW infant than is the fat in cow's milk.

CARBOHYDRATE

LBW infants can metabolize carbohydrates almost as well as full-term infants. Lactose is the carbohydrate of choice, since it promotes the proliferation of *L. bifidus* in the gut, providing some protection against infections.

ORAL FEEDING

When the weight exceeds 1500 gm and the infant has a well-developed sucking reflex, nipple feedings should be started. If the sucking reflex has not yet fully developed, or if the infant tires easily, nasogastric tube feedings may be necessary. The infants should be carefully monitored for signs of intolerance to the feedings, such as abdominal distention, diarrhea, or vomiting.

BREAST-FEEDING

Immunoglobulins and white cells of the colostrum confer immunity against bacterial infections, especially gastroenteritis. The amount of iron and protein present in breast milk may also inhibit bacterial growth. Lactoferrin, an iron-binding protein present in human milk, competes with microorganisms for the iron that is present, inhibiting their growth.

Introduction of Solid Foods

Human milk or prepared formula meets the nutritional requirements of the infant for the first 4–6 months of life. The introduction of solid food before this time period has no nutritional advantage and may even expose the infant's gastrointestinal tract to food antigens. It also carries the risk of overfeeding.

At birth and for some months thereafter, the neuromuscular development of the infant is appropriate for swallowing liquids and sucking. The ability of the tongue and swallowing mechanism to deal with nonliquid food indicates the developmental readiness for semisolid food. For most infants, this developmental stage occurs between 3 and 6 months of age.

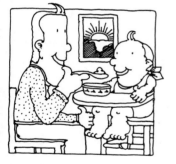

Another factor important in the timing and nature of solid food use is the influence of early feeding practices on lifelong dietary habits. The caloric intake during this period should be adequate for normal growth and activity. The use of food as a form of gratification for either the infant or the caretaker may lay the foundation for lifetime obesity, the most common type of malnutrition in this country (see Chap. 29). If solid foods are introduced too early, before 4 to 6 months of age, they will cause the infant to drink less milk and thereby lose essential nutrients. If the milk intake remains constant, a trend to overfeeding is established.

The introduction of solid foods into the diet at age 4 to 6 months supports the normal infant's psychological, psychomotor, and educational development. New foods should be chosen to meet the nutritional needs of the infant. They should be introduced at weekly intervals so that food sensitivity can be identified. An appropriate first supplemental food is iron-fortified infant cereal, mixed with breast milk or formula. By the age of 9 to 10 months, the infant usually shows signs of wanting to feed himself. The foods chosen should complement both his nutritional and developmental needs. The introduction of a variety of foods, ranging in consistency, taste, color, and temperature, is important. By 9 months of age, foods from the family table can be introduced. It is important to remember that dietary habits established in infancy and childhood influence lifelong health and well-being.

The following is a suggested sequence for introducing solid foods [19]:

AGE	FOODS TO BE INTRODUCED
Birth to 12 months	Breast milk, iron-fortified formula, or evaporated milk formula
4 to 6 months	Infant cereal (dry type)
5 to 7 months	Vegetables, fruits, and their juices
6 to 8 months	Protein foods (cheese, yogurt, cooked beans, meat, fish, chicken, egg yolk)
10 to 12 months	Whole egg, regular milk

References

1. Goldman, H. I., et al. Effects of early dietary protein intake on low birth weight infants: Evaluation at 3 years of age. *J. Pediatr.* 78:126, 1971.
2. Woodruff, C. The science of infant nutrition and the art of infant feeding. *J.A.M.A.* 240:657, 1978.
3. Fomon, S. J. *Infant Nutrition* (2nd ed.). Philadelphia: Saunders, 1974. P. 575.
4. McKenna, M. C., and Campagnoni, A. T. Effect of pre- and postnatal essential fatty acid deficiency on brain development and myelination. *J. Nutr.* 109:1195, 1979.
5. Food and Nutrition Board, National Research Council. *Recommended Dietary Allowances* (9th ed.). Washington, D.C.: National Academy Press, 1980. Pp. 130, 138.
6. Dallman, P. R., et al. Brain iron: Persistent deficiency following short-term iron deprivation in the young rat. *Br. J. Haematol.* 31:209, 1975.
7. Saarinen, U. M., Siimes, M. A., and Dallman, P. R. Iron absorption in infants: High bioavailability of breast milk iron as indicated by the extrinsic tag method of iron absorption and the concentration of serum ferritin. *J. Pediatr.* 91:36, 1977.
8. American Academy of Pediatrics, Committee on Standards of Child Health Care. *Standards of Child Health Care* (2nd ed.). Evanston, Ill.: American Academy of Pediatrics, 1972. P. 10.
9. Wiatrowski, E., et al. Dietary fluoride intake of infants. *Pediatrics* 55:517, 1975.
10. Food and Nutrition Board, National Research Council. *Recommended Dietary Allowances* (9th ed.). Washington, D.C.: National Academy Press, 1980. Pp. 63, 70.
11. American Academy of Pediatrics, Committee on Nutrition. Nutritional needs of low birth weight infants. *Pediatrics* 60:519, 1977.
12. Irwin, M. I., and Hutchins, B. K. A conspectus of research on vitamin C requirements of man. *J. Nutr.* 106:823, 1976.
13. Ghitis, J. The labile folate of milk. *Am. J. Clin. Nutr.* 18:452, 1966.
14. Breast-feeding lauded by pediatricians. *J.A.M.A.* 240:2612, 1978.
15. Baker, S. J. The reduction of infant mortality in New York City. *Am. J. Dis. Child.* 5:151, 1913.
16. Hopkins, H. Next to mother's milk, there's infant formula. *FDA Consum.* 14:11, 1980.
17. Heird, W. C., and Driscoll, J. M. Newer methods for feeding low birth weight infants. *Clin. Perinatol.* 2:309, 1975.
18. Sinclair, J. C., et al. Supportive management of the sick neonate. *Pediatr. Clin. North Am.* 17:863, 1970.
19. Current infant feeding practices. *Nutr. & the MD* January 1980.

Suggested Readings

American Academy of Pediatrics, Committee on Nutrition. Iron supplementation for infants. *Pediatrics* 58:765, 1976.

Barness, L. A.   Nutrition for the low birth weight infant. *Clin. Perinatol.* 2:345, 1975.

Barness, L. A.   Infant feeding: Benefits of formulas. *Professional Nutritionist* 12:4, 1980.

Cravioto, J.   Nutrition, stimulation, mental development, and learning. *Nutr. Today* 16:4, 1981.

Ferris, A. G., et al.   The effect of diet on weight gain in infancy. *Am. J. Clin. Nutr.* 33:2635, 1980.

Fomon, S. J., et al.   Recommendations for feeding normal infants. *Pediatrics* 63:52, 1979.

Gastrointestinal Development and Neonatal Nutrition: Report of the seventy-second Ross Conference on Pediatric Research. Columbus, Ohio, 1977.

Gurney, J. M.   The problems of feeding the weaning age group: An overview of available solutions. *Cajanus* 12:43, 1979.

Iron Nutrition in Infancy: Report of the sixty-second Ross Conference of Pediatric Research. Columbus, Ohio, 1970.

Jefferson, D. L.   Child feeding in the United States in the nineteenth century. *J. Am. Diet. Assoc.* 30:335, 1954.

Jensen, R. G., Hagerty, M. M., and McMahon, K. E.   Lipids of human milk and infant formulas: A review. *Am. J. Clin. Nutr.* 31:990, 1978.

MacKeith, R., and Wood, C.   *Infant Feeding and Feeding Difficulties* (5th ed.). New York: Churchill Livingstone, 1977.

Mata, L.   Breast-feeding: Main promoter of infant health. *Am. J. Clin. Nutr.* 31:2058, 1978.

Pelto, G. H.   Perspectives on infant feeding: Decision-making and ecology. *Food Nutr. Bull.* 3:16, 1981.

Pipes, P. L.   *Nutrition in Infancy and Childhood.* St. Louis: Mosby, 1981.

Recommendations for Infant Feeding Practices. Sacramento: California Department of Health Services, Maternal and Child Health, 1979.

Richard, K., and Gresham, E.   Nutritional considerations for the newborn requiring intensive care. *J. Am. Diet. Assoc.* 66:592, 1975.

Rothermel, P. C., and Faber, M. M.   Drugs in breast milk: A consumer's guide. *Birth Fam. J.* 33:276, 1979.

Schwab, M. G.   The rise and fall of the baby's bottle. *J. Hum. Nutr.* 33:276, 1979.

Scrimshaw, N. S., and Underwood, B. A.   Timely and appropriate complementary feeding of the breast-fed infant: An overview. *Food Nutr. Bull.* 2:19, 1980.

Sinatra, F. R.   Chronic diarrhea in infancy: A nutritional disorder. *Nutr. & the MD* 7, 1981.

Sinha, D. P.   Definitions and overview of the problems of feeding the weaning age group. *Cajanus* 12:25, 1979.

Therapeutic trials in mild iron deficiency in infants. *Nutr. Rev.* 40:139, 1982.

Walker, B.   Lead content of milk and infant formulas. *J. Food Protect.* 43:178, 1980.

Winick, M.   Infant nutrition: Formula or breast feeding? *Professional Nutritionist* 12:1, 1980.

Wood, A. L.   The history of artificial feeding of infants. *J. Am. Diet. Assoc.* 31:474, 1955.

Woodruff, C. W.   Supplementary foods for infants. *Contemp. Nutr.* 6, 1981.

Year One: Nutrition, Growth, Health. Columbus, Ohio: Ross Laboratories, 1975.

Yeung, D. L., et al.   Infant fatness and feeding practices: A longitudinal assessment. *J. Am. Dietet. Assoc.* 79:531, 1981.

Yeung, D. L., et al.   Sodium intakes of infants from 1 to 18 months of age. *J. Am. Dietet. Assoc.* 80:242, 1982.

Chapter 24

NUTRITION IN CHILDHOOD AND ADOLESCENCE

Today's children are taller and heavier than those of even a generation ago. Although stature is genetically determined, environmental factors such as disease and nutrition influence genetic expression. The eradication of many diseases, including those of nutritional origin, and improvements in the quality and quantity of the available diets have permitted growth to reach maximal levels of the genetic potential of the individual.

The development of protective vaccines for plague, cholera, typhoid, tuberculosis, and yellow fever in the late 1800s and more recently for poliomyelitis and measles has greatly improved childhood health. Bovine tuberculosis was linked to childhood tuberculosis, and the incidence of both decreased dramatically with the introduction of pasteurized milk. The spread of epidemic diseases such as typhoid fever, scarlet fever, and diphtheria by milk was recognized around the turn of the century. Infantile diarrhea (cholera infantum), which increased dramatically during the summer, was mainly caused by impure milk and was responsible for most of the infant mortality at that time. The provision of pure milk was a very important factor in the reduction of infant mortality.

The introduction of antibiotics during the 1940s and 1950s greatly reduced childhood diseases and mortality. Fortification of foods with vitamins and minerals has also greatly improved childhood health. The fortification of milk with vitamin D has probably done more to eradicate rickets and bone deformities than any other public health measure. This treatment of milk has also greatly reduced the incidence of pelvic deformities, a major cause of maternal mortality during childbirth.

The nutritional requirements for childhood and adolescence are primarily for the building and maintenance of new tissues and for increased physical activity. Proper nutrition during this period is often judged by the adequacy of growth in both height and weight. Figures indicating the normal ranges of height and weight at different ages are presented in Chap. 22.

Physiologic Considerations

Growth from age 1 until about age 12 proceeds at a gradual, steady rate. After the first year, the rate of growth slows and dramatic changes in body structure begin to occur. Bone and muscle accumulate a larger mass and greater density. Much of the fat present during infancy is lost, muscles become stronger, and bones lengthen and increase in density. Until adolescence, the trend of lengthening of long bones and increasing musculature continues; then growth continues in spurts.

The fat depot increases steadily for the first 9 months after birth, then it plateaus; there are two more fat growth spurts before the adult fat cell number becomes fixed: at about age 7 and at puberty [1]. If the child is overfed during any of these critical periods, the number of fat cells may increase beyond the normal number [1]. The number of fat cells acquired during this time may be related to adult obesity and a lifelong battle against fatness. This excess weight acquired in childhood is often difficult to lose as an adult.

Appetites decrease around 1 year of age, paralleling a decrease in the growth rate. After 1 year of age the appetite fluctuates, demanding more food during periods of rapid growth and less during periods of quiescence. During the preadolescent period, nutrient stores are being built up. During adolescence growth may be so rapid that nutrient intake is insufficient, and nutrient stores may be drawn upon.

The growth rate accelerates during adolescence as the child physically enters adulthood. Adolescence is a time not only of increased physical growth, development of secondary sexual characteristics, and sexual maturation, but also of changes in interests and emotional and mental attitudes. Adolescence is a period of increased need for all nutrients; in addition, it is a time when there is a change from childhood to adult food choices and habits.

Nutritional Requirements

The dietary allowances recommended by the Food and Nutrition Board, National Research Council, are summarized in Tables 24-1 (childhood) and 24-2 (adolescence).

TABLE 24-1. Recommended daily dietary allowances for children

Feature or nutrient	1–3 years	4–6 years	7–10 years
Weight (kg, lb)	13, 29	20, 44	28, 62
Height (cm, in.)	90, 35	112, 44	132, 52
Energy (cal)	1300	1700	2400
Protein (gm)	23	30	34
Fat-soluble vitamins			
Vitamin A (IU)	4000	5000	7000
Vitamin D (IU)	400	400	400
Vitamin E (IU)	7.75	9.30	10.85
Water-soluble vitamins			
Vitamin C (mg)	45	45	45
Thiamin (mg)	0.7	0.9	1.2
Riboflavin (mg)	0.8	1.0	1.4
Niacin (mg)	9	11	16
Pyridoxine (mg)	0.9	1.3	1.6
Folacin (μg)	100	200	300
Vitamin B_{12} (μg)	2.0	2.5	3.0
Minerals			
Calcium (mg)	800	800	800
Phosphorus (mg)	800	800	800
Magnesium (mg)	150	200	250
Iron (mg)	15	10	10
Zinc (mg)	10	10	10
Iodine (μg)	70	90	120

Source: Adapted from Food and Nutrition Board, National Research Council, *Recommended Dietary Allowances* (9th ed.). Washington, D.C.: National Academy Press, 1980.

TABLE 24-2. Recommended daily dietary allowances for adolescents

Feature or nutrient	Males 11–14 years	Males 15–18 years	Males 19–22 years	Females 11–14 years	Females 15–18 years	Females 19–22 years
Weight (kg, lb)	45, 99	66, 145	70, 154	46, 101	55, 121	55, 121
Height (cm, in.)	157, 62	175, 69	178, 70	157, 62	163, 64	163, 64
Energy (cal)	2700	2800	2900	2200	2100	2100
Protein (gm)	45	56	56	46	46	44
Fat-soluble vitamins						
Vitamin A (IU)	10,000	10,000	10,000	8000	8000	8000
Vitamin D (IU)	400	400	300	400	400	300
Vitamin E (IU)	12.4	15.5	15.5	12.4	12.4	12.4
Water-soluble vitamins						
Vitamin C (mg)	50	60	60	50	60	60
Thiamin (mg)	1.4	1.4	1.5	1.1	1.1	1.1
Riboflavin (mg)	1.6	1.7	1.7	1.3	1.3	1.3
Niacin (mg)	18	18	19	15	14	14
Pyridoxine (mg)	1.8	2.0	2.2	1.8	2.0	2.0
Folacin (μg)	400	400	400	400	400	400
Vitamin B_{12} (μg)	3.0	3.0	3.0	3.0	3.0	3.0
Minerals						
Calcium (mg)	1200	1200	800	1200	1200	800
Phosphorus (mg)	1200	1200	800	1200	1200	800
Magnesium (mg)	350	400	350	300	300	300
Iron (mg)	18	18	10	18	18	18
Zinc (mg)	15	15	15	15	15	15
Iodine (μg)	150	150	150	150	150	150

Source: Adapted from Food and Nutrition Board, National Research Council, *Recommended Dietary Allowances* (9th ed.). Washington, D.C.: National Academy Press, 1980.

CALORIES

The average caloric requirement for boys and girls ranges from 1300 calories at 1 to 3 years to 2400 calories at 7 to 10 years. For boys aged 11 to 14, the average requirement is 2700 calories; it increases to 2900 calories for those aged 19 to 22. Since adolescence occurs earlier in girls, the caloric requirement drops from 2200 calories at 11 to 14 to 2100 calories at 15 to 22. The caloric requirement for boys is greater than for girls because boys are usually more physically active and grow to a larger stature.

PROTEIN AND MINERALS

Skeletal growth continues throughout childhood and adolescence. Even after linear growth has ceased, the skeleton continues to mineralize and becomes heavier. The main components of mature bone, calcium and phosphorus, must be supplied in adequate amounts in the diet for normal skeletal development. The recommended daily allowance (RDA) for calcium and phosphorus is 800 mg of each for both boys and girls during all of childhood, increasing to 1200 mg for both sexes during adolescence (11 to 18 years).

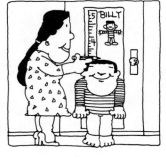

Muscle growth parallels skeletal growth and involves a positive nitrogen balance, an increase in muscle tissue, and an increase in the blood volume and its components. Adequate calories are necessary to spare the dietary protein for such tissue expansion. While some growth may continue with less than optimal food intakes, it is likely to result in poorly mineralized bones, nitrogen-poor soft tissues, a decrease in physical activity and metabolism, borderline or frank anemia, and a decreased resistance to infection.

The daily protein requirement increases steadily from childhood through adolescence (see Tables 24-1 and 24-2).

IRON

Iron-deficiency anemia is among the most common nutritional problems of young children in the United States. Children with low iron stores have been shown to be less attentive, more easily distracted, more apathetic, and more irritable than children with sufficient stores [2].

The daily iron requirement increases from 10 mg at birth to 15 mg by 6 months of age and remains at this level until age 4. Between ages 4 and 10 it drops to 10 mg. Paralleling the adolescent growth spurt, the requirement increases to 18 mg for boys between 11 and 18 and then drops back down to 10 mg for ages 19 to 22. For females, the requirement increases to 18 mg at age 11 and remains at that level until age 50, dropping back down to 10 mg only at age 51. This reflects not only the increased iron demands of the adolescent growth spurt in girls, but also the additional iron needs for menstruation. For childbearing women, the RDAs are even higher.

FLUORIDE

Fluoridated water, especially if consumed from birth, has been shown to reduce tooth decay in growing children. The Surgeon General states that tooth decay can be reduced by two-thirds by fluoridation [3]. Fluoride works by being incorporated into the hard structure of the tooth, making it more resistant to decay, and by inhibiting plaque formation. In communities where the water is not fluoridated, fluoride supplements and topical fluoride treatments should be used. Brushing after each meal, particularly after eating sweet foods, and after the last meal or snack of the day is important, as are regular dental checkups.

VITAMINS

Vitamin D is essential for the absorption and deposition of calcium and phosphorus into bone. Although exposure to sunshine during the summer may supply an adequate amount for endogenous vitamin D synthesis (by the body), few children receive sufficient exposure in the winter.

Vitamin D supplementation is usually initiated during infancy and should be continued during childhood if the requirement is not met through dietary sources. The daily requirement is 400 IU throughout childhood and adolescence to age 18 for both sexes. The requirement for both vitamin D and calcium can be met by the daily consumption of one quart of vitamin D–fortified milk.

The daily requirements for the B vitamins and vitamin C reflect the gradually increasing caloric need throughout childhood. The requirement for vitamin A reflects body weight, increasing also throughout childhood and attaining adult levels by adolescence.

The Preschool Child

Children are born without distinct food likes or dislikes. The food habits a child develops are learned.

The atmosphere of dining greatly influences eating behavior. Since children can be sensitive imitators, eating habits, table manners, and general mealtime atmosphere are quickly picked up from other family members.

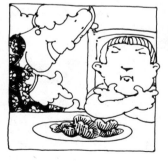

Children should enjoy a wide variety of foods, and new foods should be introduced only one at a time. Like adults, children develop food preferences, which, if reasonable, should be respected. Variety in tastes, textures, and colors can stimulate food acceptance and make mealtime more pleasant. Because children's senses of taste and smell are very keen, foods should be lightly seasoned and mildly flavored. Crunchy foods are often well accepted and may easily be combined with other textures: apple slices with cheese, celery with peanut butter, shredded carrots with raisins.

Portions should be small to moderate, appropriate for a child's needs and appetite. Children are more likely to finish if the serving is small, and they can be reassured that second helpings are available.

Until coordination is sufficiently developed, toddlers and preschoolers prefer to use their fingers rather than utensils (Fig. 24-2). The transition from fingers to forks and spoons may occur earlier when children are allowed to feed themselves (Fig. 24-3). Table 24-3 outlines the normal development of self-feeding.

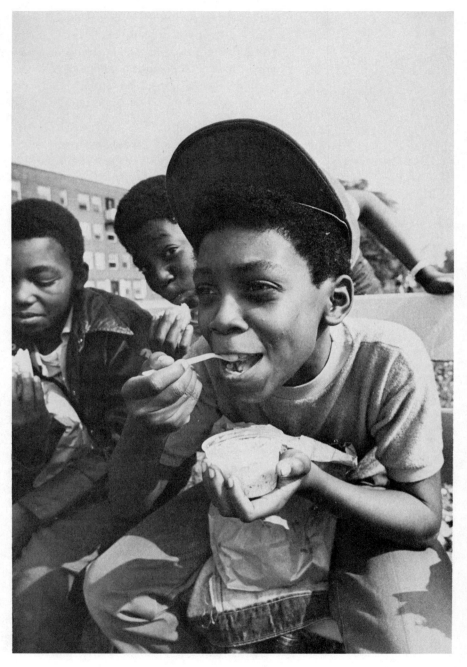

FIG. 24-1. Between-meal snacks often supply essential nutrients for children on the go. (U.S. Department of Agriculture photo by Larry Raza.)

5. Expenditure of school lunch money on candy and soft drinks, which constitute a substitution of "empty" calories for what might have been a well-balanced diet
6. Occasional self-imposed dieting by girls to achieve a standard of slimness
7. Self-imposed dieting by boys in an effort to improve unsightly acne

FEDERAL NUTRITION
PROGRAMS

The National School Lunch Act was passed by Congress in 1946 to channel surplus agricultural products into the improvement of the health and nutrition of the nation's children. This act stipulates that every public school make lunches available to its children and that the federal government reimburse the school for all or part of the cost when the families cannot pay. The secretary of the U.S. Department of Agriculture established nutrition standards to ensure nutritionally adequate meals. The school lunches must include specified servings of milk, protein-rich foods (meat, eggs, legumes, cheese, or peanut butter), fruits and vegetables, bread or other grain foods, and butter or margarine. The lunches are designed to provide at least one-third of the RDAs. In 1975 this program was available to 90 percent of all schoolchildren in the United States and cost almost $3 billion per year in federal money, with nearly 25 million lunches served every day [5].

Since the purpose of the school lunch program is defeated if the child will not eat what is served, an effort has been made to serve both what the children want to eat and what is good for them. This has been done by increasing the variety of what is served, varying portion sizes, involving students in menu planning, and offering longer serving hours so that students can eat when they are hungry. In view of the changing ideas of what is healthful, the requirement for butter or margarine has been dropped, and the whole milk has been changed to skim or low-fat milk.

In 1954, the Special Milk Program was established with the purpose of increasing milk consumption. The program provides extra nutrition for those children who were unable to have lunch at school.

The Child Nutrition Act of 1966 provided for a pilot breakfast program as well as additional lunch funds for especially needy children. Amendments in 1975 made the breakfast program permanent. This program serves over 2 million children daily, the majority of whom pay little or nothing.

All of these programs grew from and were patterned after the School Lunch Act. From a budget of $100 million in 1946, these programs have expanded to $2.7 billion in 1980 [6].

SPECIAL PROBLEMS OF
ADOLESCENT GIRLS

Many girls who are chubby throughout childhood become conscious of their appearance during adolescence and attempt to restrict their food intake. When dieting becomes compulsive, resulting in severe malnutrition and an aversion to food, it is considered to be the syndrome termed *anorexia nervosa*. This nutritional problem is discussed in greater detail in Chap. 34. Those for whom dieting fails may withdraw from sports and social activities and overindulge in food.

This may also occur in males but is less common. More about obesity is presented in Chap. 29.

With the age of first pregnancy decreasing progressively in recent years, adequate nutrition among female adolescents is extremely important. Inadequate nutrient stores can severely limit the normal growth of both the female adolescent and her future infant. See Chap. 26, Nutrition in Pregnancy and Lactation, for further details.

Dietary Recommendations

Calories and essential nutrients must be provided if the growing child is to reach his or her maximum growth potential. These requirements are best met by three meals per day and afternoon and bedtime snacks that include milk.

An adequate breakfast has been shown to be vital for a number of reasons. With adequate amounts of protein, fat, and carbohydrate, the blood sugar level increases, sustaining mental alertness and physical activity until lunchtime. An inadequate breakfast or no breakfast at all may lead to a decreased attention span and inefficiency at school during the late morning hours. This may result in a poor attitude and difficulty with academic work. Breakfast should include about one-third of the daily caloric requirement and one-third or more of the protein allowance.

Because of the high protein requirement during adolescence, poultry, fish, meat, and eggs are important. At least one quart of milk should be taken daily as the major source of calcium, protein, and riboflavin. It may be made into puddings or custards; cheese in sandwiches or main dishes as a substitute.

Desserts should be eaten only after meals so that they do not interfere with appetite before the more essential food items are eaten.

Exercise, rest, recreation, and good nutrition are all components of a healthful environment for a growing child.

References

1. Knittle, J. L.   Obesity in childhood: A problem in adipose tissue cellular development. *J. Pediatr.* 81:1048, 1972.
2. U.S. Department of Health, Education and Welfare.   *Malnutrition, Learning and Behavior.* Washington, D.C.: Government Printing Office, 1976.
3. U.S. Surgeon General.   *Statement on Fluoridation.* Washington, D.C.: Government Printing Office, 1978.
4. Burton, B. T.   *Human Nutrition* (3rd ed.). New York: McGraw-Hill, 1976. P. 209.
5. A Tuesday in the White House (White House Conference on Nutrition, April 13, 1975). *Nutr. Today* Sept/Oct-Nov/Dec: 20, 53, 1975.
6. Martin, J.   Child nutrition programs: 1946 to 1980. *School Foodservice J.* January, 1980.

Suggested Readings

ADA's views on school lunch presented to Congress. *J. Am. Diet. Assoc.* 70:630, 1977.
Béhar, M.   Nutrition and child health. *WHO Chron.* 33:125, 1979.
Birch, L. L., et al.   Mother-child interaction and the degree of fatness in children. *J. Nutr. Educ.* 13:17, 1981.

Caghan, S. B. The adolescent process and the problem of nutrition. *Am. J. Nurs.* 75:1728, 1975.

Damrau, F., and Damrau, A. M. Use of soft drinks by children and adolescents. *Rocky Mountain Med. J.* 60:37, 1963.

Daniels, W. J. Nutrition and adolescence. *Diet. Curr.* 3:(4), 1976.

Dietary practices in adolescence. *Nutr. & the MD* 7, 1981.

Fisk, D. A successful program for changing children's eating habits. *Nutr. Today* May/June 1979.

Kadushin, A. Child welfare services: Past and present. *Child. Today* May-June 1976.

Martin, E. A., and Beal, V. A. *Robert's Nutrition Work With Children.* Chicago: University of Chicago Press, 1978.

McKigney, J. I., and Munro, H. N. *Nutrient Requirements in Adolescence.* Cambridge, Mass.: M.I.T. Press, 1976.

McWilliams, M. *Nutrition for the Growing Years* (3rd ed.). New York: Wiley, 1980.

Nourish your neurons. The National School Lunch Week Menu. *School Food Serv. J.* 35:31, 1981.

Nutrition in adolescence. Eighth Annual Marabou Symposium. *Nutr. Rev.* 39:37, 1981.

Peavy, L. S., and Pagenkopf, A. L. *Grow Healthy Kids.* New York: Grosset & Dunlap, 1980.

Thomas, J. A., and Call, D. L. Eating between meals: A nutrition problem among teenagers? *Nutr. Rev.* 31:137, 1973.

Tsang, R. C., and Nichols, B. L. (eds.). *Nutrition and Child Health: Perspectives for the 1980's.* New York: Alan R. Liss, 1981.

Vaden, A. G. Child nutrition school programs. *Prof. Nutr.* 13:7, 1981.

Vonde, D. A. S., and Beck, J. *Food Adventures for Children.* Redondo Beach, Calif.: Plycon Press, 1980.

Waserman, M. An overview of child health care in America. *Child. Today* 1976.

Wills, B. B. Food becomes fun for children. *Am. J. Nurs.* 78:2082, 1978.

Zigler, E. F. The unmet needs of America's children. *Child. Today* May-June 1976.

Chapter 25

THE ADULT DIET:
REQUIREMENTS AND TRENDS

Changes in the traditional family unit and life-style during recent years, including increased numbers of wives and mothers working part-time or full-time outside the home, more single parents, later marriages, and the decline of the extended family, have altered the traditional family eating patterns, including the adult diet. A wider variety of foods, the availability of completely new foods, the increased accessibility of cultural and ethnic food items, and a faster-paced life-style demanding speed and uniformity have resulted in some distinct changes in food choices during the past 30 years or so. Also at a higher level than ever before are the incidences of heart disease, cancer, cerebrovascular disease, diabetes, arteriosclerosis, and cirrhosis. These six of the ten leading causes of death have been directly related to changes in the American diet [1].

This chapter will first explore the nutritional requirements of the normal adult. These requirements are low compared with those for other age groups, since rapid growth has ceased and needs are for maintenance only. Nutritional deficiencies are slower to develop in adults, and nutritional status is more likely to be influenced by life-style factors (e.g., caffeine and alcohol consumption) than by daily diet. For this reason, the remainder of the chapter will discuss caffeine, fiber, alcohol, and "fast foods"—all probable components of the modern-day adult diet.

Nutritional Requirements

By the end of adolescence, adult heights and weights have normally been achieved. In the absence of chronic or acute illnesses, nutrient requirements remain essentially the same from early adulthood through middle age. Table 25-1 summarizes the Food and Nutrition Board's recommended dietary allowances (RDAs) for adults.

CALORIES

For both sexes, the caloric requirement decreases from that for the 19 to 22 age group. For men, it drops from 2900 to 2700 calories; for women, from 2100 to 2000 calories. This reflects a slow decline in basal metabolic rate and a decrease in physical activity. Dietary habits should decrease and daily exercise regimens should increase to fit this reduced need. Whereas during adolescence calories are needed for both growth and maintenance, during the adult years they are only needed for maintenance. With the adolescent growth spurt completed, continued caloric intake at adolescent levels will soon result in adult obesity and its accompanying health problems.

PROTEIN

The daily protein requirement remains the same as for the 19 to 22 age group: 56 gm for men and 44 gm for women. This daily intake replenishes tissue proteins and components of blood and antibodies and allows for wound healing. The

TABLE 25-1. Recommended daily dietary allowances for adults aged 23–50

Feature or nutrient	Men	Women
Weight (kg, lb)	70, 154	55, 121
Height (cm, in.)	178, 70	163, 64
Energy (cal)	2700	2000
Protein (gm)	56	44
Fat-soluble vitamins		
Vitamin A (IU)	10,000	8000
Vitamin D (IU)	200	200
Vitamin E (IU)	14	12
Water-soluble vitamins		
Vitamin C (mg)	60	60
Thiamin (mg)	1.4	1.0
Riboflavin (mg)	1.6	1.2
Niacin (mg)	18	13
Pyridoxine (mg)	2.2	2.0
Folacin (μg)	400	400
Vitamin B_{12} (μg)	3.0	3.0
Minerals		
Calcium (mg)	800	800
Phosphorus (mg)	800	800
Magnesium (mg)	350	300
Iron (mg)	10	18
Zinc (mg)	15	15
Iodine (μg)	150	150

Source: Adapted from Food and Nutrition Board, National Research Council, *Recommended Dietary Allowances* (9th ed.). Washington, D.C.: National Academy Press, 1980.

protein requirement rises for women during pregnancy and lactation (see Chap. 26).

MINERALS AND VITAMINS

Although the bones continue to turn over their mineral content, after about age 20–24 there is no longer a net gain in bone mass or length. For this reason the vitamin D allowance drops from 300 IU at ages 19 to 22 to 200 IU for adults of both sexes, and the calcium and phosphorus requirements for both sexes drop from 1200 mg at ages 15 to 18 to 800 mg for ages 19 to 50. The decreased requirement for the B vitamins reflects a lower caloric intake. The higher iron allowance for women (18 mg versus 10 mg for men) stems from monthly losses during menstruation.

Caffeine

Caffeine acts as a true stimulant, producing a variety of effects within the body, including increased heart and respiration rates, increased blood pressure, and the release of various hormones. Its wake-up effect is greatest within about 1 hour [2]. In moderate daily amounts (50 to 200 mg) it seems to be a relatively harmless drug.

The world consumption of coffee has been estimated at 4 million tons per year [3]. This figure does not represent all caffeine consumed, however, since substantial amounts of caffeine are also ingested in cola beverages, tea, and chocolate. Coffee beans were originally found in Arabia, tea leaves in China, the kola nut in West Africa, and the cocoa bean in Mexico, although they are all now widely used around the world (Fig. 25-1).

PHARMACOLOGY

Caffeine, theophylline, and theobromine are all methylated xanthines, and their structural similarity to purine and uric acid facilitates their use in the body (Fig. 25-2). They have several common pharmacologic actions, including stimulation of cardiac muscle and the central nervous system, action on the kidney to produce diuresis (fluid loss), and relaxation of smooth muscle. Caffeine is the principal xanthine in coffee, theophylline in tea, and theobromine in chocolate and cocoa. Caffeine has the strongest influence on the central nervous system; theophylline, the second strongest. Theobromine has almost no central nervous system effect. Theophylline exerts its greatest effect on the musculoskeletal and cardiovascular systems.

Caffeine-containing beverages may contain substantial amounts of potassium while contributing little sodium, making them helpful for patients who must restrict their sodium intake but require potassium supplementation [4, 5].

BEVERAGE (6 oz)	SODIUM (mg)	POTASSIUM (mEq)
Coffee		
Brewed	0.6	2.6
Instant	1.4	1.7
Sanka		
Instant	0.2	2.2
Freeze-dried	0.3	2.3
Ground roast	2.0	4.0
Tea	0	2.5
Coca-Cola	2.0	2.3

The caffeine content of some common dietary sources is given in Table 25-2.

METABOLISM

Caffeine is quickly and completely absorbed from the gastrointestinal tract and reaches peak blood levels about 1 hour after ingestion. It passes rapidly into the central nervous system and various other tissues. It is demethylated and excreted in the urine as xanthine and uric acid (see Fig. 25-2). There is no day-to-day accumulation of caffeine, but doses as high as 3000 to 10,000 mg, if taken over a brief period, can be fatal [6]. Metabolic effects of high tissue concentrations of caffeine include increased muscle lactic acid; increased oxygen consumption; muscle twitches; increased levels of such hormones as plasma renin, norepinephrine, and epinephrine; and increased blood pressure and respiratory rate [3].

FIG. 25-1. Cocoa beans being sun dried in Cameroon, a country that exports large quantities of cocoa. (United Nations photo by Carolyn Redenius.)

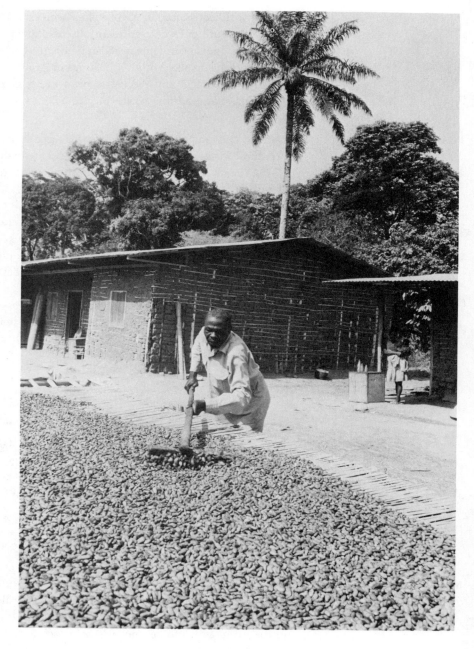

FIG. 25-2. The chemical structures of purine, xanthine, and derivatives.

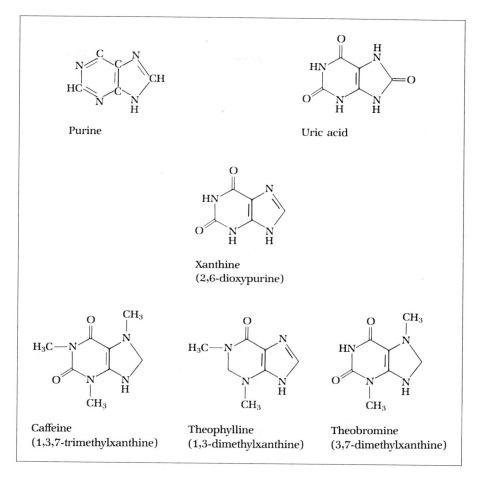

Purine

Uric acid

Xanthine
(2,6-dioxypurine)

Caffeine
(1,3,7-trimethylxanthine)

Theophylline
(1,3-dimethylxanthine)

Theobromine
(3,7-dimethylxanthine)

Caffeine increases the metabolic rate, and this stimulation is dose dependent. To evaluate caffeine's effectiveness in weight reduction regimens, various levels were used in normal and obese persons. The metabolic rate increased in both groups, but increases in fat oxidation were observed only in the normal group [7]. Therefore, caffeine does not aid weight reduction in the obese individual.

CENTRAL NERVOUS
SYSTEM EFFECTS

Although all the methylated xanthines stimulate the central nervous system when present in high concentrations, caffeine is the most potent. Doses in the range of 50 to 200 mg result in increased alertness and decreased drowsiness and fatigue. Intakes of 200 to 500 mg may produce nervousness, irritability, headaches, tremors, and gastrointestinal upsets.

Caffeine can be habit-forming. A sudden abstinence may cause a characteristic withdrawal reaction, whose most frequent symptom is an acute headache, sometimes accompanied by nausea and vomiting. Excessive use of caffeine may also result in headaches.

TABLE 25-2. Some common sources of caffeine

Source	Approximate amount of caffeine
Beverages	
Brewed coffee	85 mg/150 ml
Instant coffee	60 mg/150 ml
Brewed black tea	50 mg/150 ml
Brewed green tea	30 mg/150 ml
Instant tea	30 mg/150 ml
Decaffeinated coffee	3 mg/150 ml
Coca-Cola	40–72 mg/12 oz
Cocoa	50 mg/6 oz
Milk chocolate	3 mg/oz
Prescription medications	
APC (aspirin, phenacetin, and caffeine	32 mg/tablet
Cafergot (ergotamine tartrate and caffeine)	100 mg/tablet
Darvon Compound (propoxyphene hydrochloride and APC)	32 mg/tablet
Fiorinal (butabital and APC)	40 mg/tablet
Migral (ergotamine tartrate, cyclizine hydrochloride, and caffeine)	50 mg/tablet
Over-the-counter preparations	
Anacin, aspirin compound, Bromo-Seltzer	32 mg/tablet
Cope, Easy-Mens, Empirin Compound, Midol	32 mg/tablet
Vanquish	32 mg/tablet
Excedrin	60 mg/tablet
Pre-Mens	66 mg/tablet
Many cold preparations	30 mg/tablet
No Doz tablets	100 mg/tablet
Many stimulants	100 mg/tablet

Sources: P. E. Stephenson, Physiologic and psychotropic affects of caffeine on man. *Journal of the American Dietetic Association* 71:240, 1977; and D. S. Groisser, A study of caffeine in tea. *American Journal of Clinical Nutrition* 31:1727, 1978.

An overdose of caffeine can mimic the symptoms of an anxiety attack. In persons consuming a dozen or more cups of coffee per day, complaints of restlessness, agitation, dizziness, sleep difficulties, and recurring headaches may be more the result of excessive caffeine than any psychiatric problem. Children and adolescents may complain of rapid heartbeats (tachycardia) or insomnia related to the excessive consumption of cola beverages [8]. Elderly persons may be particularly sensitive to the stimulating effect of caffeine. Studies have shown that a decreased amount of deep sleep and a decrease in total sleep time resulted when coffee was taken before bedtime [9].

GASTROINTESTINAL EFFECTS

It has been well documented that caffeine stimulates gastric secretions. In normal persons there is only a transitory rise with high doses, but in ulcer patients there is a sustained elevation of acid secretion. Decaffeinated coffee has also been shown to stimulate acid secretion and decrease the effectiveness of the lower esophageal sphincter, which indicates that some other compounds in coffee may be responsible for these effects or may potentiate the action of caffeine.

CARDIOVASCULAR EFFECTS

Caffeine stimulates cardiac muscle, increasing the force of contraction, heart rate, and output. It also dilates blood vessels by relaxing the smooth muscle lining the vessel walls. In the brain, caffeine causes a constriction of blood vessels and a decreased cerebral blood flow. Caffeine can also cause extra heartbeats. It is not considered to be a risk factor for the development of arteriosclerosis. No correlation between coffee consumption and the risk of heart attack has been shown [10, 11].

SPECIAL PRECAUTIONS

Caffeine has recently been implicated as a cause of some birth defects, and all pregnant women should curtail their consumption of caffeine-containing products [12, 13]. Caffeine readily crosses the human placenta and enters the fetal circulation. During development and for the first few days after birth, the neonate lacks the appropriate enzymes necessary to dementhylate (metabolize) caffeine and may appear jittery, nervous, and have difficulty feeding or sleeping.

A daily consumption of 600 mg or more of caffeine may predispose a woman to reproductive difficulty. This level of intake has been related to increased incidences of spontaneous abortion, stillbirth, and premature birth [14].

RECOMMENDATIONS

It appears that, during pregnancy, caffeine intake in moderation is harmless. In excessive amounts it may cause headaches, tremors, and gastrointestinal upsets. Caution should be taken in the use of caffeine-containing foods and beverages with children, adolescents, and the elderly, since they seem to be especially sensitive to its stimulating effects. The use of caffeine-containing foods and beverages before bedtime may result in insomnia or a decrease in deep sleep.

Fiber

The positive influence of food fiber on health has been known since biblical times. Hippocrates advocated eating unbolted wheatmeal bread (made with flour still containing the bran). Roman wrestlers would eat only coarse wheaten bread because they believed it would preserve their strength.

In the late 1800s Sylvester Graham, a pioneer of food reform in the United States, advocated the use of bran for the relief of indigestion. He also advocated the use of graham (whole wheat) flour, which is still used today in the manufacture of graham crackers.

Another believer in the benefits of food fiber was J. H. Kellogg, who made ready-to-eat cereals available across the nation. He stimulated some research during the early twentieth century, but not until the 1970s and D. P. Burkitt's observations in rural Africa did current interest really bloom. Dr. Burkitt reported that the rural Africans, whose diets are high in fiber-rich foods, have a lower incidence of cardiovascular disease, cancer of the colon, appendicitis, and hemorrhoids than the population in the United States and other countries where diets are low in fiber [15].

DEFINITIONS

Dietary fiber is defined as the sum of all components of food (mostly polysaccharides and lignin) that are not digested by the gastrointestinal tract [16]. This mixture includes hemicelluloses, pectic substances, gums, and certain other carbohydrates as well as lignin and cellulose (see Chaps. 4 and 13 for definitions). In the large bowel many of the polysaccharides, but not lignin, or cellulose, are degraded and metabolized by the intestinal microflora. This final stage of breakdown and the products produced may be an important part of the physiologic role of dietary fiber.

Traditionally the *crude fiber* content of food was used in analyzing foods. The crude fiber is the residue remaining after a food sample has been treated in the laboratory with a solvent, hot acid, and hot alkali. Dietary fiber, defined as all the food components not broken down by enzymes in the human digestive tract, is a more valuable, applicable definition and may represent as much as seven times the crude fiber content [16]. Table 25-3 gives the total dietary fiber content of some selected foods.

Different types of dietary fiber are digested differently, resulting in a range of physiologic effects. The digestion of hemicellulose (present in high amounts in white flour) involves attracting water from surrounding tissues by osmosis, and the result may be a cathartic (laxative) effect [31]. The dietary fibers found in sugar cane are very abrasive to the gastrointestinal tract, and others, such as lignin, may actually be constipating [31].

Excessive intakes of dietary fiber, especially pectin, may cause a decrease in vitamin B_{12} absorption. Substantial losses of such minerals as zinc, iron, calcium, copper, and magnesium owing to their binding by phytic acid, present in many dietary fibers, have been reported [31]. By its sheer bulk, dietary fiber may reduce the total amount of food consumed and may result in a deficiency of certain nutrients or even of calories. In areas where malnutrition is prevalent this may be a very real problem. Large amounts of dietary fiber can aggravate ulcerative colitis and could even cause an enlargement and twisting of the sigmoid colon.

GASTROINTESTINAL EFFECTS

LAXATIVE

Dietary fiber has been shown to be of value by its ability to increase the water content of the feces, producing bulkier but softer stools. It has also been shown to prevent hemorrhoids.

DIET THERAPY

Diverticulosis, characterized by the development of outpouchings in weak areas in the bowel wall that become inflamed, has traditionally been treated with a low-residue (low-fiber) diet. Recently, successful treatment with a high-fiber diet

TABLE 25-3. Total dietary fiber content of selected foods

Food	Fiber (gm/100 gm)	Food	Fiber (gm/100 gm)
Flours		Chips	11.90
White	3.15	Canned (drained)	2.51
Brown	7.87	Legumes	
Whole meal	9.51	Beans, baked (canned)	7.27
Bran	44.00	Beans, runner (boiled)	3.35
Breads		Peas (frozen)	7.75
White	2.72	Peas, garden (canned)	6.28
Brown	5.11	Peas, processed (canned)	7.85
Whole meal	8.50	Peppers (cooked)	0.93
Breakfast cereals		Tomatoes (fresh)	1.40
All-bran	26.70	Tomatoes (canned)	0.85
Cornflakes	11.00	Sweet corn (cooked)	4.74
Grapenuts	7.00	Sweet corn (canned)	5.69
Rice Krispies	4.47	Fruits	
Puffed Wheat	15.41	Apples (flesh only)	1.42
Sugar Puffs	6.08	Apples (peel only)	3.71
Shredded Wheat	12.26	Bananas	1.75
Special K	5.45	Cherries (flesh and skin)	1.24
Vegetables		Grapefruit (canned)*	0.44
Leafy vegetables		Guavas (canned)*	3.64
Broccoli tops (boiled)	4.10	Mandarin oranges (canned)*	0.29
Brussels sprouts (boiled)	2.86	Mangoes (canned)*	1.00
Cabbage (boiled)	2.83	Peaches (flesh and skin)	2.28
Cauliflower (boiled)	1.80	Pears (flesh only)	2.44
Lettuce (raw)	1.53	Pears (peel only)	8.59
Onions (raw)	2.10	Plums (flesh and skin)	1.52
Root vegetables		Rhubarb (raw)	1.78
Carrots, young (boiled)	3.70	Strawberries (raw)	2.12
Parsnips (raw)	4.90	Strawberries (canned)*	1.00
Rutabaga (raw)	2.40	Sultanas	4.40
Turnips (raw)	2.20	Nuts	
Potatoes		Brazils	7.73
Main crop (raw)	3.51	Peanuts	9.30
French fried	3.20		

*Fruit and syrup.
Source: Adapted from D. A. T. Southgate, et al., A guide to calculating intakes of dietary fibre. *Journal of Human Nutrition* 30:303, 1976.

has lent support to the theory that the disease results from a deficiency of dietary fiber [32]. The incidence of diverticulosis has increased steadily in industrialized countries, paralleling a decrease in the amount of fiber in the diet. In areas where the diet has remained high in fiber, such as Africa and China, the incidence of the disease has changed little [31].

CANCER PREVENTION

It has been theorized that dietary fiber may provide protection from cancer of the colon and rectum. This hypothesis presumes that the slow movement of the feces that occurs with a low-fiber diet allows more time for carcinogens (cancer-causing compounds) present in the colon to initiate cancer [17]. According to this theory, the extra bile salts, fat, and water bound by added fiber act as solvents to remove chemical factors that may be carcinogenic. A high-fiber diet may also alter the number and type of microorganisms in the colon and inhibit their production of potential carcinogens.

Currently, there is no proof linking transit time in the bowel to colon cancer, nor is there evidence that constipation causes cancer. Furthermore, it has not been demonstrated that dietary fiber itself has an effect on the intestinal flora of humans.

CARDIOVASCULAR EFFECTS

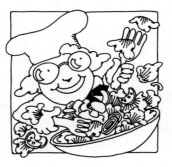

Dietary fiber may reduce serum cholesterol levels by decreasing the time it takes for food to travel through the gastrointestinal tract, resulting in a decreased absorption of dietary cholesterol [31]. Dietary fiber may also reduce the absorption of bile salts, essential for the digestion and absorption of fats. Dietary fiber may bind bile acids, preventing the absorption of cholesterol, fat, and the reabsorption of bile acids derived from the body's cholesterol. This would cause the body's stores of cholesterol to be drawn upon to synthesize more bile acids, lowering serum cholesterol levels.

Although high serum cholesterol levels have been recognized as one of the risk factors in arteriosclerosis, it is not known whether the risk can be reduced by lowering cholesterol levels. In addition, different dietary fibers produce different effects. For example, adding barley or rolled oats to the diet decreases serum cholesterol levels in rats [31]; rolled oats have a similar effect in humans [33]. The influence of whole wheat is variable, whereas bran does not appear to alter serum levels at all.

METABOLIC EFFECTS

IN DIABETES

Recently it was shown that blood sugar levels of patients taking insulin were higher with a low-fiber diet than with a high-fiber diet [34]. The cause of this mechanism has not yet been determined, but this may prove to be an area in which dietary fiber may be very useful.

IN WEIGHT LOSS

High-fiber diets may also aid in weight reduction regimens. There is a decrease in the caloric density with increasing fiber content and an increased feeling of satiety. Dietary fiber would also decrease the transit time through the intestine, reducing the amount of nutrients absorbed.

RECOMMENDATIONS

At present, the evidence on high-fiber diets is inconclusive. Persons consuming a low-fiber diet are also likely to be eating increased amounts of refined carbohydrates, fats, and animal products. The beneficial effect of a high-fiber diet may result from an increased amount of trace elements or other nutrients present with the fiber. The beneficial effects of dietary fiber probably originate from more than one of its components. Therefore, by adding only one type of fiber to the diet, little will be gained. Until more research is completed, it seems best to include a variety of foods in the diet, emphasizing fresh or frozen foods and avoiding overuse of processed foods, which, in addition to fiber, are also often lacking in essential nutrients.

Alcohol

Alcohol (ethanol or ethyl alcohol) is used by humans for several purposes, including as a preservative, a disinfectant, a drug, and a food. As a source of energy it differs from protein, fat, and carbohydrate in that it cannot be utilized by muscle and is metabolized at a fixed rate unaffected by the serum concentration. One gram of ethyl alcohol contains 7 kcal.

Alcohol is produced by the fermentation of sugars by yeasts. Beer and ale are made from fermenting malted (sprouted) barley; wine from grapes; liquor from grains. The alcoholic content of distilled beverages is expressed as proof, which is the percent of alcohol multiplied by 2: 100 proof means 50% alcohol. Table 25-4 summarizes the composition of some common alcoholic beverages.

An estimated 100 million adults in the United States use alcohol. Of these, about 9 million overconsume alcohol to the extent that it interferes with family, work, and social interaction; they are alcoholics. Because it is so socially acceptable, alcohol abuse is the most prevalent drug addiction in Western society.

Chronic alcohol use has both short-term and long-term effects on many body systems. Altered functioning results in gastrointestinal, nutritional, hematologic, and even psychological systems; some of the effects are reversible, others are not. A summary is given in Table 25-5.

METABOLISM

Alcohol is quickly and completely absorbed by the gastrointestinal tract and appears in the bloodstream soon after ingestion. Because it is soluble in both water and lipid, alcohol diffuses through cell membranes and into all cells. Gastric absorption is increased by the presence of carbonated liquids (the carbon dioxide component) and is delayed by a high concentration of alcohol, high sugar content, coldness, and the presence of food, especially food rich in protein and fat. When alcohol passes into the duodenum and intestines, the intestinal mucosa absorbs it rapidly and completely, regardless of the presence of food.

More than 90 percent of ingested alcohol is metabolized by the liver; about 10 percent passes through the lungs and kidneys. The amount in expired air and urine is directly proportional to blood concentrations. This is the principle used by police departments in determining if a person is legally drunk. The breath analyzer test indicates the person's blood level of alcohol; levels 0.10 percent or higher are grounds for arrest in most states.

The rate at which the liver metabolizes (oxidizes) alcohol appears fairly constant in almost everyone. In the chronic alcoholic, though, the metabolic rate seems to increase. Prolonged intake of more alcohol than the liver can metabolize leads to the development of a supplemental system for alcohol metabolism in

TABLE 25-4. Nutritional value of some common alcoholic beverages

Type	Amount (oz)	Calories	Protein (gm)	Carbohydrate (gm)	Alcohol (gm)	Calcium (mg)	Magnesium (mg)	Phosphorus (mg)	Iron (mg)	Thiamin (µg)	Riboflavin (µg)	Niacin (mg)	Vitamin C (mg)	Vitamin A (IU)	Vitamin D (IU)
Ale, mild	8	98	1.1	8.0	8.9	30	—	41	0.2	Tr	69	0.5	0	0	0
Beer, average	8	114	1.4	10.6	8.9	10	—	62	0	Tr	72	0.5	0	0	0
Brandy															
California	1	73	—	—	10.5	—	—	—	—	—	—	—	—	—	—
Cognac	1	73	—	—	10.5	—	—	—	—	—	—	—	—	—	—
Cider, fermented	6	71	—	1.8	9.4	—	—	—	—	—	—	—	—	—	—
Cordial															
Anisette	⅔	74	—	7.0	7.0	—	—	—	—	—	—	—	—	—	—
Apricot brandy	⅔	64	—	6.0	6.0	—	—	—	—	—	—	—	—	—	—
Benedictine	⅔	69	—	6.6	6.6	—	—	—	—	—	—	—	—	—	—
Crème de menthe	⅔	67	—	6.0	7.0	—	—	—	—	—	—	—	—	—	—
Curaçao	⅔	54	—	6.0	6.0	—	—	—	—	—	—	—	—	—	—
Daiquiri	3½	122	0.1	5.2	15.1	4	—	3	0.1	14	1	Tr	8	0	0
Eggnog	4	335	3.9	18.0	15.0	44	—	74	0.7	35	113	Tr	Tr	84	21
Gin, dry	1½	105	—	—	15.1	—	—	—	—	—	—	—	—	—	—
Gin rickey	4	150	Tr	1.3	21.0	2	—	1	Tr	7	Tr	Tr	4	—	0
Highball	8	166	—	—	24.0	—	—	—	—	—	—	—	—	—	0
Manhattan	3½	164	Tr	7.9	19.2	1	—	1	Tr	3	2	Tr	0	35	—
Martini	3½	140	0.1	0.3	18.5	5	—	1	0.1	Tr	Tr	Tr	0	4	—
Mint julep	10	212	—	2.7	29.2	—	—	—	—	—	—	—	—	—	—
Old-fashioned	4	179	—	3.5	24.0	—	—	—	—	—	—	—	—	—	—
Planter's punch	3½	175	0.1	7.9	21.5	4	—	3	0.1	14	1	Tr	8	0	0
Rum	1½	105	—	—	15.1	—	—	—	—	—	—	—	—	—	—
Tom Collins	10	180	0.3	9.0	21.5	6	—	6	Tr	30	Tr	Tr	21	0	0
Whiskey															
Rye	1½	119	—	—	17.2	—	—	—	—	—	—	—	—	—	—
Scotch	1½	105	—	—	15.1	—	—	—	—	—	—	—	—	—	—
Wine															
Champagne	4	84	0.2	3.0	11.0	—	—	—	—	—	—	—	—	—	—
Muscatel or port	3½	158	0.2	14.0	15.0	—	—	—	—	—	—	—	—	—	—
Sauterne, California	3½	84	0.2	4.0	10.5	—	—	—	—	—	—	—	—	—	—
Sherry	2	84	0.2	4.8	9.0	—	—	—	—	—	—	—	—	—	—
Vermouth, French	3½	105	—	1.0	15.0	—	—	—	—	—	—	—	—	—	—
Vermouth, Italian	3½	167	—	12.0	18.0	—	—	—	—	—	—	—	—	—	—

Key: Tr = trace; — indicates no significant data available.
Source: C. F. Church and H. N. Church, Food Values of Portions Commonly Used (12th ed.). Philadelphia: Lippincott, 1975. P. 6.

TABLE 25-5. Effects of alcohol on body systems

Gastrointestinal
    Suppresses appetite
    Irritates gastric mucosa (gastritis)
    Irritates esophagus, stomach, intestines, and liver
    Decreases pancreatic enzymes
    Impairs absorption of proteins, fat, thiamin, folic acid, and fat-soluble vitamins
Renal
    Increases urinary losses of amino acids, magnesium, potassium, zinc, and water
Hematologic
    Alters red blood cell formation (anemia)
    Increases levels of fat in the blood
Psychological
    Impairs learning (requires protein synthesis)
    Loss of memory, with cover-up lies (confabulation)

the liver. Under these circumstances, the ability of the liver to metabolize alcohol may double. The ability of the liver to remove other substances it normally metabolizes, such as drugs, also increases. This is important to physicians prescribing medication for chronic alcohol users; the blood levels of these drugs are about half those in the nonalcoholic person.

The liver metabolizes alcohol at a constant rate, regardless of the blood concentration. Usually the greater the concentration of the substance to be oxidized, the more rapidly the liver does the job—not so with alcohol. It averages about 10 ml per hour, or 5 to 6 hours to fully oxidize the alcohol in 4 oz of whiskey or 2½ pints of beer [18]. This relatively slow and constant rate of metabolism places a definite limit on the amount of alcohol that can be consumed over a given period of time before the accumulation of unmetabolized alcohol in the body becomes intoxicating. Unmetabolized alcohol in the bloodstream affects all organs, including the brain. It acts as a depressant and anesthetic. Its first effect is on the brain area that controls judgment and thought, releasing the drinker's inhibitions. If more alcohol builds up, speech and vision will be affected, then voluntary muscles (a staggering walk will result). The last to be affected are the areas of the brain controlling heartbeat and respiration, although the drinker has usually passed out by this time, while the liver gradually reduces the level of circulating alcohol.

The breakdown of alcohol requires a constant supply of the B vitamins niacin and thiamin. Since the liver preferentially metabolizes alcohol over other substances, it uses up the available supply of these B vitamins in the process. The lack of thiamin and niacin impairs the metabolism of glucose; the heavy drinker, therefore, is prone to episodes of hypoglycemia (low blood sugar). Adequate amounts of glucose are also needed for the metabolism of alcohol, specifically to free up niacin for continued alcohol breakdown. During heavy drinking, when all available glucose is being shuttled to metabolize alcohol, the absence of glucose may be severe enough to produce coma and death because the brain is being deprived of glucose.

DEVELOPMENT OF
LIVER DAMAGE

After handling excessive amounts of alcohol over a period of time, the liver may accumulate fat. Alcohol slows down and interferes with protein synthesis. The accumulation of fat results partly from the liver's failure to synthesize proteins to package fat for transport in the bloodstream. Liver cells surrounded by fat are deprived of an adequate blood supply and often die, leaving scar tissue. With continued heavy drinking and fatty infiltration, the liver tissue hardens, resulting in *cirrhosis*. This is the seventh leading cause of death in the United States and is overwhelmingly caused by alcohol abuse [19]. Fewer than one in seven alcoholics develop liver damage, however. The severe and irreversible clinical picture of liver impairment appears to be caused by malnutrition in addition to the primary insult to the liver by alcohol. Recently, however, cirrhosis has been experimentally produced with alcohol and a diet considered adequate [20].

SPECIAL PRECAUTIONS

Because alcohol crosses all cell membranes and interferes with protein synthesis, its use during pregnancy can be especially hazardous. The rate of protein synthesis is more rapid in the prenatal period than at any other time during life. Heavy alcohol consumption during the first 13 weeks after conception, the embryonic period, is extremely dangerous because this is the time when organogenesis, the differentiation of cells into various organs, is occurring. Heavy alcohol use at any time during pregnancy can result in altered protein synthesis and growth retardation but during the first half of pregnancy is more likely to cause permanent damage in the baby, including postnatal growth deficiency; facial, joint, and cardiac malformations; and later speech and learning disabilities [21].

The Food and Drug Administration (FDA) estimates that a risk is established by drinking 3 oz of absolute alcohol or six drinks per day. The International Conference on Birth Defects warns that even moderate drinking (less than two cocktails or glasses of wine or beer per day) may have dangerous effects, especially during the first month or two. Since peak blood alcohol concentration is probably the most critical factor in causing malformations, most women should not have more than two drinks per day. The National Council on Alcoholism advises pregnant women that it is a safe and responsible decision to abstain from drinking during gestation [22].

RECOMMENDATIONS

1. Eat before and during drinking; the presence of food, especially protein and fat, will slow the gastric absorption of alcohol.
2. Drink slowly; it takes about 1½ hours to metabolize 12 oz of beer, 5 oz of wine, or 1½ oz of whiskey.
3. Drink other fluids with alcoholic beverages. Because alcohol causes water to be lost from the body, resulting in thirst and dehydration, fluids need to be replaced.
4. Remember, alcohol impairs judgment and thought first. Never drive or allow

others to drive while under the influence of alcohol. Coffee will make the driver more alert, but he or she is still as intoxicated.

Fast Foods

The percentage of the food industry's share in the American food dollar has risen steadily from about 38 percent in the late 1960s to almost 50 percent by 1980 [23–25]. This growth is mostly accounted for by the increase in franchised food outlets and their response to the public's desire for fast food of uniform quality.

As stated earlier, the traditional family unit and life-style are changing, with more adults working full-time or part-time. In exchange for the convenience of the foods provided, the American public is willing to spend more on food. Cost comparison studies done by the U.S. Department of Agriculture indicate that restaurant fast foods cost about twice as much as similar foods prepared at home [26]. Part of the popularity of fast foods may be the result of advertising: In 1976, the food industry spent $370 million on advertising, with McDonald's spending almost a third of that amount ($111 million) [27]. The advertising must be working, because sales for the top fast-food chains have been overwhelming [27]:

McDonald's	$2730 million
Kentucky Fried Chicken	$1165 million
Burger King	$ 742 million
Dairy Queen	$ 684 million
Pizza Hut	$ 374 million

The menus of fast-food chains are by necessity very limited. With more meals being eaten in these establishments, the daily diet tends to be composed of relatively few foods. The increased consumption of ice cream, beef, fish, and potatoes over the past decade has probably been the result of the thriving fast-food industry. Generally, the foods tend to be high in calories, although recently low-calorie beverages are being offered at more chains. The selections are generally adequate in protein (beef, fish, shakes with milk solids) but may be lacking in other nutrients such as vitamins A and C. A meal of a hamburger, French fries, and a shake would supply about one-third of the RDA for thiamin, niacin, riboflavin, and vitamins B_{12} and D, but also about half the recommended daily calories.

Two other nutritional problems with the typical fast-food meal are fiber and sodium. The fiber content of most fast foods tends to be very low, the sodium content very high. These may be important considerations if a person is on a special dietary regimen. Table 25-6 summarizes the nutritional content of selected fast foods.

RECOMMENDATIONS

1. It is important for the consumer to realize that he is paying more for the convenience of fast foods.
2. Although generally adequate in protein and calories, most fast-food meals are

TABLE 25-6. Nutritional content of selected fast foods

	Calories	Protein (gm)	Carbohydrate (gm)	Fat (gm)	Vitamin A (IU)	Thiamin (mg)	Riboflavin (mg)	Niacin (mg)	Vitamin C (mg)	Vitamin D (IU)	Calcium (mg)	Iron (mg)	Sodium (mg)
Burger King													
Cheeseburger	305	17	29	13	195	0.01	0.02	2.20	0.5	—	141	2.0	562
Hamburger	252	14	29	9	21	0.01	0.01	2.20	0.5	—	45	2.0	401
Whopper	606	29	51	32	641	0.02	0.03	5.20	13.0	—	37	6.0	909
French fries	214	3	28	10	0	0.01	0.01	2.42	16.0	—	12	1.0	5
Vanilla shake	332	11	50	11	9	0.01	0.05	0.27	tr	—	390	0.2	159
Whaler	486	18	64	46	141	0.01	0.01	1.04	1.3	—	70	1.0	735
Hot dog	291	11	23	17	0	0.04	0.02	2.00	0	—	40	2.0	841
Kentucky Fried Chicken													
Original Recipe Dinner[a]	830	52	56	46	750[b]	0.38[b]	0.56[b]	15.0[b]	27.0[b]	—	150[b]	4.5[b]	2285
Extra Crispy Dinner[a]	950	52	63	54	750[b]	0.38[b]	0.56[b]	14.0[b]	27.0[b]	—	150[b]	3.6[b]	1915
Individual Pieces[c]													
Drumstick	136	14	2	8	30	0.04	0.12	2.7	0.6	—	20	0.0	—
Keel	283	25	6	13	50	0.07	0.13	—	1.2	—	—	0.9	—
Rib	241	19	8	15	58	0.06	0.14	5.8	1.0	—	55	1.0	—
Thigh	276	20	12	19	74	0.08	0.24	4.9	1.0	—	39	1.4	—
Wing	151	11	4	10	—	0.03	0.07	—	1.0	—	—	0.6	—
9 pieces[c]	1892	152	59	116	—	0.49	1.27	—	—	—	—	8.8	—
McDonald's													
Egg McMuffin	352	18	26	20	361	0.36	0.60	4.3	1.6	40	187	3.2	914
Big Mac	541	26	39	31	327	0.35	0.37	8.2	2.4	37	175	4.3	962
Cheeseburger	306	16	31	13	372	0.24	0.30	5.5	1.6	14	158	2.9	725
Filet-O-Fish	402	15	34	23	152	0.28	0.28	3.9	4.2	37	105	1.8	709
French fries	211	3	26	11	52	0.15	0.03	2.9	11.0	3	10	0.5	113
Hamburger	257	13	30	9	231	0.23	0.23	5.1	1.8	11	63	3.0	526
Quarter Pounder	418	26	33	21	164	0.31	0.41	9.8	2.3	23	79	5.1	711
Quarter Pounder with Cheese	518	31	34	29	683	0.35	0.59	15.1	2.9	36	251	4.6	1209
Apple pie	300	2	31	19	69	0.02	0.03	1.3	2.7	5	12	0.6	414
Cherry pie	298	2	33	18	213	0.02	0.03	0.4	1.3	5	12	0.4	456
McDonaldland Cookies	294	4	45	11	48	0.28	0.23	0.8	1.4	10	10	1.4	330
Vanilla shake	323	10	52	8	346	0.12	0.66	0.6	2.9	354	346	0.2	250

Key: tr = trace; — indicates no significant data available.

[a]Dinner comprises mashed potatoes and gravy, cole slaw, roll, and three pieces of chicken: (1) wing, rib, and thigh; (2) wing, drumstick, and thigh; or (3) wing, drumstick, and keel.

[b]Calculated from percentage of the U.S. Recommended Daily Allowance.

[c]Edible portion of chicken.

Sources: For Burger King: Chart House, Oak Brook, Ill., 1978; for Kentucky Fried Chicken: Nutritional Content of Average Serving, Heublein Food Service and Franchising Group, 1976; for McDonald's: Nutritional Analysis of Food Served at McDonald's Restaurants, WARF Institute, Madison, Wisc., 1977.

TABLE 25-7. Exchanges for fast foods

	Bread	Meat	Fat	Other	Calories
Arby's					
Regular	2	3			355
Junior	2	2			282
Super	3	3	1	1v	468
Ham 'N Cheese	2	4			428
Turkey Deluxe	2	3	1		400
Beef & Cheese	2	4			428
Potato Cake	1		1		113
Coleslaw				1v	70
Diet Dr. Pepper				f	0
Barbecue Sauce: 1 pkg				f	10
Horsey Sauce			1		45
Arthur Treacher's					
Treacher's Basket	2	3	4		531
Treacher's Boat	2	5	6		771
Krunch Pups	1½	1	3		312
Shrimp	2	2	3		421
Original Dinner	2	5	5		726
Mate	2	7	6		921
Coleslaw, 4 oz			2	1v	115
Milk				1m	160
Braum's					
Hamburger	2	3	1		420
Cheeseburger	2	4	2		540
Corndog	1½	1	3		312
French Fries					
Small order	1½		2		192
Large order	3		5		339
Steak Sandwich	3	4	3		639
Burger Chef					
Hamburger	2	1	2		321
Double Hamburger	2	2½	1		368
Super Chef	3	3½	2		556
Big Chef	3	3	3		564
French Fries	2		2		226
Fish Sandwich	2	2	3		421
Mariner Dinner	2	4	5		651
Rancher Dinner	1	5	3		578
Casa Bonita					
Dinner #1: 2 beef enchiladas, 1 cheese	6	2	8		908
Dinner #2: 3 tacos	6	3	5		848
Dinner #3: 1 tamale, 1 beef enchilada, 1 taco	6	3	8		983
Dinner #4: 1 beef enchilada, 1 cheese enchilada, 1 taco	6	2	7		863
Deluxe	8	4½	6		1141
American	5	6	12		1330
Dairy Queen Stores, Inc.					
King Burger	4	4			572
Beef Burger	4	2			422

TABLE 25-7 (CONTINUED)

	Bread	Meat	Fat	Other	Calories
Dairy Queen Stores, Inc. (continued)					
Jiffy Burger	2	1			211
Steak Sandwich	4	2	2		512
Fish Sandwich	4	3	3		632
Grilled Cheese	2	2	2		376
Hot Dog	2	1			211
Tacos	1	1½			182
Steak Finger Basket	4	4	6		832
French Fries	1½		2		192
Onion Rings	2		4		306
Burrito	2	2	2		376
Sugar Free Dr. Pepper				f	0
Der Wienerschnitzel					
Hot Dog	2	1	1		256
Chili Dog	2	1½	1		293
Kraut Dog	2	1	1		256
Cheese Dog	2	2	1		331
Mustard Dog	2	1	1		256
French Fries					
Large order	2		4		306
Small order	1		2		158
Polish Sandwich	2	3	4		531
Dickies Fish and Chips					
Fish, French Fries, and Coleslaw	3	4	8		854
Shrimp, French Fries, and Coleslaw	3	2	6		614
El Chico					
Nooner 1: enchilada, chili, fried rice, taco	4½	3	8		881
Nooner 2: enchilada, cheese taco, chili, chili con queso, beans	3	3	3		564
Nooner 3: chalupa, chili con queso, meat taco, rice	4½	3	3		666
Nooner 4: chalupa, refried beans, taco salad, enchilada, chili, rice	6	2	4		728
Burrito Lunch: 1 burrito and refried beans	3	4	5		719
Burrito Dinner: 2 burritos and refried beans	4	8	9		1267
Poblano Chili Relleno Dinner	3	3	3		564
Quesdaillas	5	4	5		855
Chalupas Jalisco Style	3½	4	5		753
Chicken Enchiladas	4½	3	3		666
Kentucky Fried Chicken					
Fried Chicken, mashed potato, coleslaw, roll					
3-Piece Dinner					
Original	4	5	4		817
Crispy	4	5	6		907

TABLE 25-7 (CONTINUED)

	Bread	Meat	Fat	Other	Calories
Kentucky Fried Chicken (continued)					
2-Piece Dinner					
Original	3	3	3		564
Crispy	3	3	5		664
McDonald's					
Hamburger	2	1			260
Cheeseburger	2	1½			306
Quarter Pounder	2	3			420
Filet-O-Fish	2½	1½	3½		400
Egg McMuffin	1½	2	1		350
Pork Sausage		1	1½		185
Scrambled Eggs		1½	1		160
100% Orange Juice: 6 oz				1½ fr	60
Sirloin Stockade					
Dinners served with baked potatoes					
with butter and Texas toast					
Club Steak	4	4	3		707
Sizzling Sirloin Steak	4	6	3		857
Stockade Strip Steak	4	7	3		932
Rancher Steak	4	9	3		1082
Filet Steak: Tenderloin	4	6	4		892
Chicken Fried Steak	5	4	4		810
Kabob	4	4	3		707
Ground Sirloin Steak	4	6	3		857
Hamburger	2	3			361
Fish Platter	4	5	4		817
Shrimp	4	2	3		557
German Sausage	4	4	7		877
Taco Bell					
Taco	½	1	1		154
Bell Burger	2	1½	1		283
Bell Burger with cheese	2	2	2		376
Beef Burrito	2	3	3		496
Bean Burrito	3		3		339
Enchirito	2	2	3		421
Burrito Supreme	2½	2	3		480
Tostado	1½	1	2	1v	267
Combination Burrito	2½	2	2		410
Frijoles	1½	½	4		309
Taco Bueno					
Taco	1	1	1		188
Bean Burrito	2	1	1		256
Combination Burrito	2	3	2		451
Meat Burrito	1	4	2		458
Deluxe Burrito	1	2	1		263
Chili Burger	2	2½			323
Frijoles	1½		3		237
Frito Pie	2½	½	3		362
Chalupa	2	1	1		256
Deluxe Chalupa	1	3	1		338
Taco Tico					
Taco	½	1	1		154

TABLE 25-7 (CONTINUED)

	Bread	Meat	Fat	Other	Calories
Taco Tico (continued)					
Burrito	3	2	2		444
Taco Burger	2	2	1		331
Sancho	2	3	2		451
Soft Taco	½	1	1		154
Refried Beans	2		2		226
Tostado	2½		3		305
Enchilada	½	2	2		274
Tamale	1½	1	1		222
Chili	1½	2	1		297
Tamale Pie	2	1½	2		338
Taco Dinner Plate	3½	4	5		756
Nacho	1½		1		150
Salad with dressing			2	1v	115
Wendy's					
Hamburger	3	3	1		474
Double Hamburger	3	6	1		699
Cheeseburger	3	4	1		549
French Fries	2		4		306
Frostie	4		3		407
Diet Pepsi				f	0

Key: v = vegetable, m = milk, f = free, fr = fruit.
Note: The food groups listed are based on the exchange system developed by the American Diabetes Association and The American Dietetic Association.
Source: Adapted from St. Francis Hospital, Diabetes Center, Tulsa, Oklahoma, *Eating Out Made Simple*, 1979.

very low in fiber and vitamins A and C. The diet should include alternative food sources of these nutrients, such as fresh fruits and vegetables.

The fast-food industry may provide a valuable service as a more accepted form of school lunch [28–30]. As the food industry responds to the needs and desires of the American public, more nutrition information, a wider variety of foods, and a more complete balance of nutrients may be provided. See Table 25-7 for an exchange chart for fast foods.

References

1. Select Committee on Nutrition and Human Needs, U.S. Senate. *Eating in America: Dietary Goals for the United States.* Cambridge, Mass.: M.I.T. Press, 1977. P. 1.
2. Robertson, D., et al. Effects of caffeine on plasma renin activity, catecholamines and blood pressure. *N. Engl. J. Med.* 298:181, 1978.
3. Robertson, D., et al. Effects of caffeine on plasma renin activity, catecholamines and blood pressure. *N. Engl. J. Med.* 298:181, 1978.
4. Coffee and cardiovascular disease. *Med. Lett. Drugs Ther.* 19:65, 1977.
5. Church, C. F., and Church, H. N. *Food Values of Portions Commonly Used* (12th ed.). Philadelphia: Lippincott, 1975. P. 6.
6. Dimaio, V. J. M., and Garriott, J. C. Lethal caffeine poisoning in a child. *Forensic Sci.* 3:275, 1974.

7. Acheson, K. J., et al.   Caffeine and coffee: Their influence on metabolic rate and substrate utilization in normal weight and obese individuals. *Am. J. Clin. Nutr.* 33:989, 1980.

8. Third International Caffeine Workshop. *Nutr. Rev.* 39:183, 1981.

9. Brezinova, V.   Effect of caffeine on sleep: EEG study in late middle age people. *Br. J. Clin. Pharm.* 1:203, 1974.

10. Yano, K., Rhoads, G. G., and Kagan, A.   Coffee, alcohol and risk of coronary heart disease among Japanese men living in Hawaii. *N. Engl. J. Med.* 297:405, 1977.

11. Coffee drinking and acute myocardial infarction: Report from the Boston Collaborative Drug Surveillance Program. *Lancet* 2:1278, 1972.

12. Weathersbee, P. S., and Lodge, J. R.   Caffeine: Its direct and indirect influence on reproduction. *J. Reprod. Med.* 19:55, 1977.

13. Luke, B.   Does caffeine influence reproduction? *Am. J. Maternal Child Nurs.* 7:240, 1982.

14. Weathersbee, P. S., Olsen, L. K., and Lodge, J. R.   Caffeine in pregnancy. *Postgrad. Med.* 62:64, 1977.

15. Burkitt, D. P.   Some diseases characteristic of modern Western civilization. *Br. Med. J.* 1:274, 1973.

16. Southgate, D. A. T., et al.   A guide to calculating intakes of dietary fibre. *J. Hum. Nutr.* 30:303, 1976.

17. Institute of Food Technologists' Expert Panel on Food Safety and Nutrition and the Committee on Public Information.   Dietary fiber: A scientific status summary. *Food Technol.* 33:35, 1979.

18. Iber, F. L.   In alcoholism, the liver sets the pace. *Nutr. Today* January/February 1971.

19. National Center for Health Statistics.   Mortality for leading causes of death. 1977.

20. Patek, A. J.   Alcohol, malnutrition and alcoholic cirrhosis. *Am. J. Clin. Nutr.* 32:1304, 1979.

21. Luke, B.   Maternal alcoholism and fetal alcohol syndrome. *Am. J. Nurs.* 77:1924, 1977.

22. Luke, B.   *Maternal Nutrition.* Boston: Little, Brown, 1979. Pp. 137–148.

23. Safeway: Selling nongrocery items to cure the supermarket blahs. *Business Week*, p. 52, Mar. 7, 1977.

24. Sherk, C. K.   Changes in food consumption patterns. *Food Technol.* 25:914, 1971.

25. LeBovit, C.   The changing pattern of eating out. *Nat. Food Situation* (U.S. Department of Agriculture), No. 144, May 1973, p. 30.

26. Isom, P.   Nutrition value and cost of fast-food meals. *Family Economics Review*, p. 10, Fall 1976.

27. Fast-food stars: Three strategies for growth. *Business Week*, p. 56, July 11, 1971.

28. Does fast food get an "A" in school lunch? *CNI Weekly Report*, p. 4, Nov. 3, 1977.

29. New York to try fast-food lunches. *CNI Weekly Report*, p. 4, Dec. 1, 1977.

30. Satchell, M.   McDonald's operates school's cafeteria, kids love it. *San Antonio News*, p. 9-A, Aug. 10, 1976.

31. Dietary fiber: A scientific status summary by the Institute of Food Technologists' Expert Panel on Food Safety and Nutrition and the Committee on Public Information. *Food Technology* 33:35, 1979.

32. Dietary fiber: Institute of Food Technologists' Expert Panel on Food Safety and Nutrition and the Committee on Public Information. *Contemp. Nutr.* Sept., 1979.

33. De Groat, A. P., Lugken, R., and Pikaar, N. A. Cholesterol-lowering effects of rolled oats. *Lancet* 2:303, 1963.

34. Anderson, J. W., Midgley, W. R., and Wedman, B. Fiber and diabetes. *Diabetes Care* 2:369, 1979.

Suggested Reading

Alcohol-induced brain damage and its reversibility. *Nutr. Rev.* 38:11, 1980.

Alfin-Slater, R. B., and Kritchevsky, D. (eds.). *Nutrition and the Adult: Macronutrients.* New York: Plenum Press, 1980.

Appledorf, H. How good are "fast foods"? *Prof. Nutr.* 14:1, 1982.

Baker, D., and Holden, J. M. Fiber in breakfast cereals. *J. Food Sci.* 46:396, 1981.

Boeker, E. A. Metabolism of alcohol. *J. Am. Diet. Assoc.* 76:550, 1980.

Burg, A. N. How much caffeine in a cup of tea and coffee. *Tea Coffee Trade J.* 1:40, 1975.

Burkitt, D. P., and Trowell, H. C. (eds.). *Refined Carbohydrate Foods and Disease: Some Implications of Dietary Fiber.* New York: Academic, 1975.

Caffeine update. *Nutr. MD* September 1981.

Cavaiani, M. *The High-Fiber Cookbook.* Chicago: Contemporary Books, 1980.

'Coffee, cola, or cocoa': And fibrocystic breast disease. *Nutr. MD* May, 1982.

Eastwood, M. A., and Robertson, J. A. The place of dietary fibre in our diet. *J. Hum. Nutr.* 32:53, 1978.

Food and fibre: Fifth Annual Marabou Symposium. *Nutr. Rev.* March 1977.

Harland, B., and Hecht, A. Grandma called it roughage. *FDA Consum.* July/August 1977.

Holloway, W. D., Tasman-Jones, C., and Lee, S. P. Digestion of certain fractions of dietary fiber in humans. *Am. J. Clin. Nutr.* 31:927, 1978.

Irwin, M. I. *Nutritional Requirements of Man: A Conspectus of Research.* New York: The Nutrition Foundation, 1980.

Kelsy, J. L. Effect of diet fiber level on bowel function and trace mineral balances on human subjects. *Cereal Chem.* 58:2, 1981.

Kies, C. Edible fiber: Practical problems. *Contemp. Nutr.* February 1982.

Lecos, C. Caution light on caffeine. *FDA Consum.* 14:6, 1980.

Lecos, C. More cups lifted sans caffeine. *FDA Consum.* 14:23, 1980.

Lieber, C. S. Liver adaptation and injury in alcoholism. *N. Engl. J. Med.* 288:356, 1973.

Luke, B. The nutritional implications of alcohol abuse. *RN* 39:32, 1976.

Luke, B. Maternal alcoholism and the fetal alcohol syndrome. *Am. J. Nurs.* 77:1924, 1977.

Rezabek, K. (ed.). *Nutritive Value of Convenience Foods* (2nd ed.). Hines, Ill.: West Suburban Dietetic Association, 1979.

Roe, D. A. Nutritional concerns in the alcoholic. *J. Am. Diet. Assoc.* 78:17, 1981.

Second International Caffeine Workshop. *Nutr. Rev.* 38:196, 1980.

Slover, H. T., Lanza, E., and Thompson, R. H. Lipids in fast foods. *J. Food Sci.* 45:1583, 1980.

Starbird, E. A. The bonanza bean, coffee. *Nat. Geogr.* 159:388, 1981.

U.S. Department of Agriculture. *Nutrition: Food at Work for You.* Washington, D.C.: Government Printing Office, 1978.

Winick, M. Nutritional disorders of American women. *Nutr. Today* 10:26, 1975.

Winick, M. The relationship of diet, nutrition, and health during various stages of life. *Food Technol.* 32:42, 1978.

Chapter 26

NUTRITION IN PREGNANCY AND LACTATION

A person's nutritional state can profoundly affect ultimate height, age of sexual maturation, ability to conceive, and, for women, the success of childbearing, the length of time between conceptions, and the age of menopause. Many studies have been done comparing these events in different populations all over the world. Almost all evidence points to nutrition as the deciding factor in health and reproductive capacity [1, 2].

By comparing the attainment of adult height by social class in Europe in the nineteenth century (the upper classes being better nourished than the lower classes), the influence of nutrition can be seen: Most men of the lower class did not complete height growth until age 23 to 25, compared with age 21 to 23 for those of the upper classes and age 18 to 20 for present day well-nourished men [3]. During the nineteenth century, most women did not complete their growth in height until age 20 to 21, compared with age 16 to 18 today.

Nature has timed the ability to reproduce with physical growth and development. The onset and maintenance of menstrual cycles are associated with the attainment of a minimum weight for height, representing a critical fat store [3]. The average age of menarche (age of onset of menstruation) is given in Table 26-1. Undernourished females are more likely to have menarche later, menopause earlier, and a higher frequency of irregular cycles. They are also more likely to have miscarriages and stillbirths than well-nourished women. If the undernourished woman delivers her infant successfully, she will have a longer period of lactational amenorrhea (time interval without menses during breast-feeding) after childbirth, resulting in a longer interval until the next conception. In males, malnutrition will also delay the onset of sexual maturation, reduce libido (sexual drive), and decrease sperm number and motility. In severe malnutrition, sperm production ceases completely.

Undernourished populations are less fecund (able to reproduce) than are well-nourished humans. This can be viewed as an ecologic adaptation to reduced availability of food in the environment. Although Charles Darwin described this relationship between nutrition and fertility in other animals, all of his observations also apply to humans [4]:

1. Domestic animals which have regular, plentiful food without working to get it are more fertile than the corresponding wild animals.
2. "Hard living retards the period at which animals conceive."
3. An individual's fertility is affected by variation in the amount of food.
4. It is difficult to fatten a cow that is lactating.

The effects of maternal malnutrition may be both immediate and long-term. In the most severe cases, maternal starvation or acute undernutrition can cause a cessation of menstruation (amenorrhea), and conception cannot occur. This was

TABLE 26-1. Average age at menarche

Nation or group	Age (years)
United States	12.5–12.8
Cuba	12.4
India	13–14
Sri Lanka	13.4
South African Bantus	15.0
Bangladesh	15.7
19th century Britain	15.5–16.5
Bundi of New Guinea	18.8

Sources: R. E. Frisch, Population, food intake, and fertility. *Science* 199:22, 1978; and J. Bongaarts, Does malnutrition affect fecundity? A summary of evidence. *Science* 208:564, 1980.

seen in the decline in birthrates during the food crises in seventeenth and eighteenth century Europe, the 1974–1975 famine in Bangladesh, and the famines during recent world wars. If severe malnutrition is imposed upon a previously well-nourished woman, a reduction in infant birth weight will result. When the woman has been chronically malnourished for some time before the period of starvation, the results will be an increase in spontaneous abortions, stillbirths, prematurity, and low-birth-weight (LBW) infants, and increased maternal and infant morbidity and mortality. These situations occurred in Holland and Russia during World War II [5, 6]. The long-term effects of maternal malnutrition on the offspring have been more difficult to document since it is not ethical to withhold food from a pregnant woman. In the many studies done in animals, it has been shown that nutritional deprivation, especially of protein and calories, during pregnancy, adversely affects cognitive, emotional, and neurologic development of the offspring. Generally, the earlier and more prolonged the period of deprivation, the more profound and irreversible are the abnormalities [7].

A woman beginning pregnancy brings with her a lifetime of nutritional experiences. It is this "bank" that determines her nutritional status and, indirectly, the health of her child. This chapter will discuss the nutritional demands of pregnancy and lactation, the factors placing a woman at nutritional risk, and historic and cultural food practices during this period in the life cycle.

Nutritional Requirements
HISTORY

Throughout recorded history, the dietary habits of the pregnant woman have received careful scrutiny and consideration. Nutritional and medical advice given during pregnancy reflects the religious, scientific, and social beliefs of the times; such advice has been intended to aid the miracle of creation.

In ancient China, during the Chou dynasty (1155 B.C.), the type of meat in the pregnant woman's diet received special attention. She was warned against eating goat's meat because it would produce a sickly child; donkey meat would result in a lengthy pregnancy and difficult labor; and turtle meat would produce a short-necked offspring. Pig's feet were considered a delicacy, boiled in dilute acid until soft, and eaten bones and all (an excellent source of calcium!) [8].

In ancient Rome the consumption of wolves' flesh by the pregnant woman was felt to cause premature birth. A diet of young stork, however, would make the eyes of the mother and child clear. Mouse meat would produce black eyes in the child [9]. A belief first recorded during this period and surviving to this day was that the fetus would be marked, or even die, as the result of denial of the mother's desire for a specific food.

The nutritional advice from biblical times through the sixteenth and seventeenth centuries was basically liberal and nutritionally sound. During this time obstetrics was dominated by female midwives, and pregnancy was considered a normal life function that should be aided rather than manipulated. This philosophy changed, however, during the late eighteenth century when more male physicians assumed the responsibility for the care and delivery of the unborn child. Death of the mother and child during childbirth was not uncommon during this period, because of contracted pelvis in the mother. Purging, bleeding, and underfeeding were the rules of the day in an effort to limit the size of the infant [10]. Since surgical delivery was not yet routine, this seemed to be the only other way of delivering the infant. Although these practices led to equivocal results and were criticized by many, they were used for a number of years.

This trend of starving the mother to diminish the size of the child continued through the nineteenth century and into the early twentieth century. A refinement of this regimen was introduced in 1889 by a Russian doctor, Ludwig Prochownick. He claimed that by giving a diet restricted in carbohydrates and fluids, but rich in proteins, the infant would be born of average length, but deficient in fat tissue, thus facilitating delivery [11, 12]. Since the philosophy of the times and for decades later was that the nutrition of the mother was not related to that of the infant, and that the fetus was actually an effective parasite, the Prochownick diet was widely accepted and practiced for over half a century.

Although many held to the Prochownick diet or other restrictions, the voices of opponents began to be heard. In 1935 Strauss blamed protein-restricted diets for causing toxemia [13]; Toverud, in 1938, showed that maternal vitamin and mineral deficiencies had far-reaching effects on developing teeth [14]; and Dieckmann observed in 1932 that frequent pregnancies coupled with a poor diet had a cumulative effect [15]. During the second half of the twentieth century more scientific research has been done, and evidence has been acquired clearly linking deficient maternal diets with poor reproductive outcomes.

In the 1940s the first edition of *Recommended Dietary Allowances* of the Food and Nutrition Board, National Research Council, was published. Revised eight times since, it uses the latest scientific knowledge to set dietary standards by age and sex and for pregnancy and lactation. The publishing of accepted standards for levels of various nutrients was a big advancement toward better maternal nutrition. Up to this time, physicians were prescribing diets according to their own theories, not usually based on scientific data.

In the late 1960s Eastman and Jackson published their historic study of nearly 12,000 deliveries at the Johns Hopkins Hospital in Baltimore [16]. They showed that two factors—increased weight gain and higher pregravid (prepregnancy) weight—each paralleled independently of the other increased mean birth weight. They stressed that weight gains of less than 14 pounds depleted maternal tissues and were unwise. In 1968 the Collaborative Study of Cerebral Palsy also concluded that greater weight gain was related not only to higher birth weight but also to improved infant growth and performance during the first postnatal year [17].

As more is learned, ideas about maternal nutrition will probably change again. It is important to realize, however, that because the prenatal period is the most rapid growth period during the entire life cycle, both quantity and quality are essential components of a varied diet. Good nutrition is probably the most important insurance for a healthy mother and baby.

NUTRIENTS

The metabolic and hormonal changes of pregnancy are designed to create an environment most favorable for the developing fetus. Requirements for all nutrients are increased. If the mother is under age 22, a higher increase is indicated, partially for her own continued growth. Table 26-2 summarizes the Food and Nutrition Board's recommended dietary allowances (RDAs) for pregnancy and lactation. A daily food plan incorporating the RDAs for pregnancy and lactation is given in Table 26-3.

CALORIES

The additional caloric needs imposed by pregnancy are related to increased maternal metabolism, added maternal tissues, and the growth of the fetus and placenta. The total energy cost of a full-term pregnancy, based on these factors, is estimated to be about 80,000 calories [18]. Energy needs increase little during the first trimester (13 weeks), and then remain constant until term (the fortieth week) (Fig. 26-1). During the second trimester (weeks 14 to 26) the extra energy cost is due primarily to maternal factors, such as an increase in blood volume, accumulation of fat, and growth of the uterus and breasts; during the third trimester (weeks 27 to 40), additional calories are mostly needed for growth of the placenta and fetus [18]. During pregnancy, the additional needs translate into about 300 calories per day added to the allowance for nonpregnant women. For women ages 15 to 22, the caloric requirement is 2400 calories per day; for those ages 23 to 50, it is 2300 calories per day.

The caloric requirements during lactation are proportional to the quantity of breast milk produced. A maternal caloric intake of 80 to 95 calories per 100 ml of milk produced is needed [19]; an average daily production of 850 ml requires

TABLE 26-2. Recommended daily dietary allowances

Feature or nutrient	Pregnancy			Lactation		
	15–18 years	19–22 years	23–50 years	15–18 years	19–22 years	23–50 years
Weight (kg, lb)	55, 121	55, 121	55, 121	55, 121	55, 121	55, 121
Height (cm, in.)	163, 64	163, 64	163, 64	163, 64	163, 64	163, 64
Energy (cal)	2400	2400	2300	2600	2600	2500
Protein (gm)	76	74	74	66	64	64
Fat-soluble vitamins						
Vitamin A (IU)	5000	5000	5000	6000	6000	6000
Vitamin D (IU)	600	500	400	600	500	400
Vitamin E (IU)	14	14	14	15.4	15.4	15.4
Water-soluble vitamins						
Vitamin C (mg)	80	80	80	100	100	100
Thiamin (mg)	1.5	1.5	1.4	1.6	1.6	1.5
Riboflavin (mg)	1.6	1.6	1.5	1.8	1.8	1.7
Niacin (mg)	16	16	15	19	19	18
Pyridoxine (mg)	2.6	2.6	2.6	2.5	2.5	2.5
Folacin (μg)	800	800	800	500	500	500
Vitamin B_{12} (μg)	4.0	4.0	4.0	4.0	4.0	4.0
Minerals						
Calcium (mg)	1600	1200	1200	1600	1200	1200
Phosphorus (mg)	1600	1200	1200	1600	1200	1200
Magnesium (mg)	450	450	450	450	450	450
Iron (mg)	30–60*	30–60*	30–60*	18	18	18
Zinc (mg)	20	20	20	25	25	25
Iodine (μg)	175	175	175	200	200	200

*This high requirement cannot be met by diet; supplemental iron is required.
Source: Adapted from Food and Nutrition Board, National Research Council, Washington, D.C.: National Academy of Sciences, 1980.

approximately an additional 750 calories per day. With a normal weight gain of 11 to 12.5 kg (24.2 to 27.5 lb) during pregnancy, about 2 to 4 kg (4.4 to 8.8 lb.) is stored as maternal body fat. During lactation, these fat stores are mobilized to provide 200 to 300 calories per day for the first 3 months. Therefore, only an additional 500 calories are needed above nonpregnancy allowances. If maternal weight gain was inadequate, or if lactation continues beyond 3 months, or if more than one infant is being nursed, additional calories are needed. The allowance for women ages 15 to 22 is 2600 calories per day; for ages 23 to 50, 2500 calories per day.

PROTEIN

The normal breakdown of tissue proteins (catabolism) ceases during pregnancy, and nitrogen balance becomes positive. This hormonally controlled mechanism provides a continuous supply of extra protein to the fetus for tissue synthesis. The mother may also utilize some of this extra protein by deposition in maternal tissues for later use by the fetus in case of protein deprivation before delivery and

TABLE 26-3. Daily food plan for pregnancy and lactation

Food	Serving	Number of servings		
		First half of pregnancy	Second half of pregnancy	Lactation
Dairy products				
Whole milk, skim milk, or butter-milk	8 oz	2–4	4	4–5
Yogurt	8 oz			
Cottage cheese	12 oz			
Ice cream	6 oz			
Processed cheese	1½ oz			
Hard (aged) cheese	1 oz			
Meat group (lean meat, fish, poultry, cheese, beans)	1 oz	3–4	6–8	8
Eggs	1	1	1–2	1–2
Vegetables (dark green or deep yellow)	½ cup	1	1	1–2
Vitamin C foods (citrus fruits, tomatoes, cabbage, greens)	½ cup	1–2	2	2
Other fruits and vegetables	½ cup	1	2	2
Breads and cereals (whole-grain or enriched)	1 oz (1 slice)	3	4–5	5
Butter or margarine		As needed for calories		

Source: B. Luke, Lactose intolerance during pregnancy: Significance and solutions. *American Journal of Maternal and Child Nursing* 2:92, 1977. Copyright © 1977, American Journal of Nursing Company. Reproduced, with permission, from *MCN*, March/April, Vol. 2, No. 2.

for needs during lactation. A liberal protein intake during lactation is also important to satisfy the extra requirements needed for the production of the protein-rich breast milk. For women ages 15 to 18, the daily protein requirement during pregnancy is 76 gm and 66 gm during lactation. For women ages 19 to 50, the requirements are 74 gm and 64 gm, respectively, during pregnancy and lactation.

CARBOHYDRATES

The minimum levels of dietary carbohydrate necessary to prevent ketosis (the result of utilizing fat stores for energy) doubles during pregnancy. For the average nonpregnant woman, about 100 gm per day is adequate; during pregnancy 200 gm or more is needed. This increased requirement is hormonally induced

FIG. 26-1. Normal weight gain during pregnancy. (From A. Pillitteri, *Maternal-Newborn Nursing* [2nd ed.]. Boston: Little, Brown, 1981.)

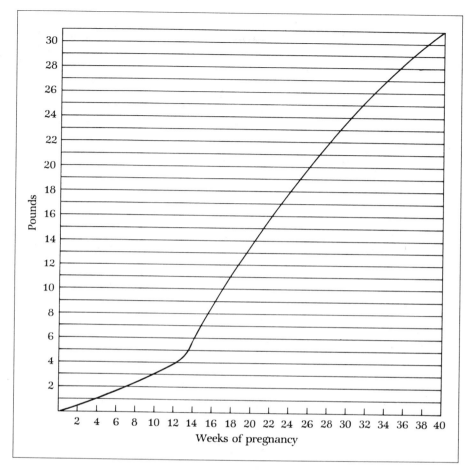

and helps ensure a continuous supply of glucose to the developing fetus, who cannot utilize the products of fat breakdown for energy.

VITAMINS

The increase in the allowance for *vitamin A* to 5000 IU per day for all age groups during pregnancy allows for its storage in the fetus. During lactation, requirements are increased even higher, to 6000 IU per day for all age groups, to provide for the vitamin A secreted in breast milk.

During gestation and lactation, calcium and *vitamin D* requirements increase. The allowance for vitamin D is increased 200 IU per day above the nonpregnant state: 600, 500, and 400 IU per day, respectively, for ages 15 to 18, 19 to 22, and 23 to 50. Because increased calcium needs continue through lactation, these same allowances are also recommended during that period.

The requirement for *folic acid* doubles during gestation (800 μg per day for all age groups) and increases by 25 percent over nonpregnancy levels during lactation (500 μg). The increase is due to the accelerated protein anabolism during pregnancy and lactation. A deficiency of this vitamin leads to impaired cell division and alterations in protein synthesis. *Megaloblastic anemia,* a type of anemia seen in pregnancy, is caused by a deficiency of this vitamin. Folic acid is present in a variety of foods, especially liver, leafy vegetables, and fruits. Requirements of the other water-soluble vitamins also increase and can be met by additional amounts of milk, fruits and vegetables, protein, and calories (see Table 26-3).

MINERALS

The intestinal absorption of *iron* occurs with greater efficiency during pregnancy. This protective mechanism allows for both fetal and maternal storage of the additional iron. The maternal stores are mobilized during pregnancy for the expansion of the blood volume and during lactation for the iron present in the breast milk. A deficiency of iron results in microcytic, hypochromic anemia called *iron-deficiency anemia,* which is especially common in women who had low iron stores before pregnancy and in whom the increased demands of gestation have aggravated the deficiency. The RDA of 18 mg for women in all age groups is difficult to meet by diet alone, and therefore a supplement of 30 to 60 mg per day of iron is often given during the second and third trimesters.

The increase in metabolic rate during pregnancy is paralleled by an increased activity of the thyroid gland and secretion of thyroid hormone. Since *iodine* is a vital component of thyroid hormone, requirements for this element are increased during pregnancy and lactation. The two most common sources of iodine are iodized salt and seafood. The requirement during pregnancy for all age groups is 175 μg per day, during lactation 200 μg per day. Diets deficient in iodine result in the development of goiter.

As an additional mechanism to ensure optimal fetal nutrition, maternal absorption of *calcium* increases and its excretion decreases during pregnancy. About 30 gm of calcium is accumulated during pregnancy, mostly as the calcification of the fetal skeleton during the last third of pregnancy. To cover the increased needs, an additional 400 mg per day above nonpregnant levels is recommended, or 1600 mg per day for ages 15 to 18, and 1200 mg per day for ages 19 to 50. Poor calcium intakes during pregnancy may result in decreased bone density in the newborn [20]. During lactation, approximately 250 mg of calcium is lost per day as breast milk. To meet this demand, calcium intakes at pregnancy levels are recommended.

Nutritional Risk Factors
BEFORE PREGNANCY

A woman enters pregnancy with the sum of a lifetime of nutritional and health habits. Her emotional, psychological, and educational maturity also reflects her past growth and experience. All of these factors can and do influence the course and outcome of her pregnancy as well as her ability to handle the physical and emotional demands of motherhood.

ADOLESCENCE

A pregnant woman 18 years of age or younger is often termed a *juvenile gravida;* she is at nutritional risk by virtue of her age. Her chronologic age is not as important as her *reproductive biologic age* (chronologic age minus age of menarche). Females with a reproductive biologic age less than 3 years are at particular risk for reproductive problems. The risk of infant death is twice as high for teenage mothers as for those in their twenties. Mothers age 15 and younger are twice as likely to have low-birth-weight babies [21]. During this time, the woman is still growing herself, and pregnancy imposes additional nutritional demands. Recent research has shown, however, that if the nutritional requirements of both adolescence and pregnancy are met, the risks can be reduced and the complication rates can approach those of the general population [22, 23]. Women who are 5 or more years past menarche are not considered to be at additional risk, since their own growth has been completed.

DEVIATIONS IN PREGRAVID WEIGHT

Next to the length of gestation, the two best predictors of infant birth weight are the maternal pregravid weight and the amount of weight gained during gestation. Both *underweight* (10 percent or more below ideal weight for height) and *overweight* (20 percent or more above ideal weight for height) women are at special risk during pregnancy (Table 26-4). Despite normal weight gains, some

TABLE 26-4. Ideal and deviations of pregravid weight for height (lb)

Height	Underweight[a]	Ideal weight	Normal range[b]	Moderate obesity[c]	Massive obesity[d]
4'9"	≤94	104	95–124	125–155	≥156
4'10"	≤96	107	97–127	128–159	≥161
4'11"	≤99	110	100–131	132–164	≥165
5'0"	≤102	113	103–134	136–168	≥170
5'1"	≤104	116	105–138	139–173	≥174
5'2"	≤106	118	107–140	142–176	≥177
5'3"	≤111	123	112–146	148–183	≥185
5'4"	≤115	128	116–152	154–191	≥192
5'5"	≤119	132	120–157	158–197	≥198
5'6"	≤122	136	124–162	163–203	≥204
5'7"	≤126	140	127–167	168–209	≥210
5'8"	≤130	144	131–171	173–215	≥216
5'9"	≤133	148	135–176	178–221	≥222
5'10"	≤137	152	138–181	182–226	≥228

[a] Ideal weight minus 10% or more.
[b] Ideal weight minus 9% to ideal weight plus 19%.
[c] Ideal weight plus 20% to ideal weight plus 49%.
[d] Ideal weight plus 50% or more.
Source: Adapted from B. Luke, *Maternal Nutrition.* Boston: Little, Brown, 1979. P. 5.

degree of intrauterine growth retardation is often seen in the infants of these women. For the underweight woman, a larger proportion of the weight gained during gestation is diverted to correct her own weight deficit. The obese woman requires a larger provision of calories just for her own metabolic maintenance. In both instances, less nutrients are available for the developing fetus, resulting in less than optimal intrauterine growth [24]. It is best to begin pregnancy within the normal weight range.

OBSTETRIC AND MEDICAL HISTORY

The *total number of pregnancies* is important, since high parity (number of pregnancies) carries the risk of depletion of maternal stores, especially with interconceptional intervals of less than 1 year. The *outcome of previous pregnancies* and *complications in the infants* are also important, because many problems related to maternal nutrition will manifest themselves in the condition of the infant. Withdrawal symptoms may result from maternal drug use; fetal alcohol syndrome from maternal alcoholism. Stillbirths or infants greater than 9 lb may be related to undiagnosed or uncontrolled maternal diabetes. Prematurity or intrauterine growth retardation can result from poor maternal nutrition or anemia. A history of such complications in previous pregnancies indicates the need for preventive measures during the present pregnancy.

The *maternal course and complications* may be caused or influenced by inadequate maternal nutrition. Some of these complications include premature labor and birth, preeclampsia (hypertensive disease of pregnancy), anemia, hemorrhage, postpartum infections, and poor wound healing.

Family history of disease, as well as medical, surgical, and psychiatric experiences, should be evaluated in relation to maternal nutritional status. Some diseases and the medications used to treat them may interfere with the ingestion, absorption, and utilization of nutrients.

LIFE-STYLE AND HABITS

The excessive use of alcohol, cigarettes, and even coffee (and other caffeine-containing foods) has been shown to have an adverse effect on the growth and development of the unborn child. *Alcohol,* as discussed in Chap. 25, interferes with protein synthesis and can cause a syndrome of malformations in the infant. The influence of smoking is dose-related during pregnancy, with the number of cigarettes smoked per day being inversely proportional to birth weight. Infants of smokers tend to be 150 to 325 gm lighter at birth than those born to nonsmokers and twice as likely to weigh less than 2500 gm (LBW). Smoking has also been associated with increased stillbirth, neonatal mortality, and prematurity rates, and an increase in placental complications. Another alarming result of cigarette smoking is a retardation of skeletal and brain growth; the latter may manifest years later as learning disabilities [25–27]. These results may stem from the effects of cigarette smoke and its components on the infant or the placenta, from maternal or infant nutrition, or from a combination of these factors. *Drug use* during pregnancy, whether self-administered or prescribed, may have a deleterious effect on the developing infant. *Caffeine* may act as a drug when taken in excessive amounts, and all caffeine-containing foods should be used with moderation in pregnancy (see Chap. 25 for more details on caffeine). All medications should be used with caution and only under the supervision of a health professional during pregnancy and lactation.

Self-prescribed diets during pregnancy may also be detrimental to the unborn child by possibly excluding vital nutrients. Strict vegetarians may develop a deficiency of vitamin B_{12}, a nutrient found exclusively in animal sources. *Pica*, the craving for nonfood substances or foods in excessive quantities, has been associated with pregnancy for hundreds of years. Current theories speculate that it may be the cause or the effect of iron deficiency precipitated by the additional demands of gestation [28]. Pica may exclude nutritionally balanced foods from the diet. *Ethnic or cultural customs* may pose special dietary restrictions. Such practices should be respected but appropriate supplements made available.

Poor nutrition may also result from an *inadequate income*. U.S. Department of Agriculture food stamps and the supplemental food program for women, infants, and children (WIC) are available to eligible women and their families, providing a variety of foods. Eligibility for the WIC program is based on economic need and nutritional risk factors as discussed here.

DURING PREGNANCY

As stated earlier in the discussion of nutritional requirements, a poor diet during pregnancy may cause a variety of problems. Inadequate nutrient stores before conception quickly appear as frank deficiencies during gestation, precipitated by the additional demands. Two types of anemia, as discussed in relation to iron and folic acid requirements, result from deficiencies of these vital nutrients. A deficiency of protein or protein and calories can cause intrauterine growth retardation in the unborn child and possible adverse long-term effects (Fig. 26-1).

Inadequate weight gain (less than 20 to 25 lb) and excessive weight gain (more than 35 lb) have both been associated with increased fetal and maternal complications, including preeclampsia and toxemia, which are hypertensive diseases of pregnancy. Weight reduction should never be attempted during pregnancy because of potential adverse effects on fetal growth and development. "Morning sickness," excessive vomiting, usually seen during early pregnancy but may continue until delivery, is thought to be related to rising hormone levels and may cause weight loss. If the vomiting is severe enough to cause ketosis, intravenous feedings may be necessary.

Lactation

The advantages of breast-feeding are many and the contraindications few. The main advantages of breast-feeding over bottle-feeding are that breast-feeding provides a nutritionally superior food in a safe, convenient form; it helps eliminate the additional fat acquired during pregnancy; and it is of great psychologi-

FIG. 26-2. Mother's milk is the most important source of nutrients at least during the first months of an infant's life. (World Health Organization photo by J. Abcede.)

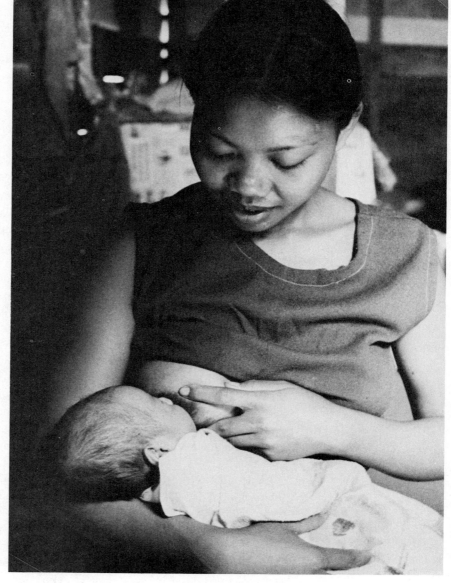

cal value to the mother and infant (Fig. 26-2). For a discussion of the unique immunologic properties and nutrient composition of breast milk, see Breast-feeding in Chap. 23.

The contraindications to breast-feeding include active maternal tuberculosis (breast-feeding exposes the infant to infection), serious chronic disease or marked undernutrition, and mastitis (inflammation of the breast). The ability to

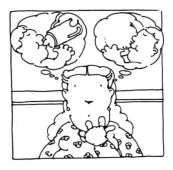

nurse is adversely affected by maternal obesity, infection of the nipple or breast, pregnancy, and adverse psychological factors. It has been stated that [29]

the effects of emotional stresses on the secretion of milk are very striking. Usually worry, anxiety, fatigue, or any prolonged emotional stress tends to reduce secretion of milk and may arrest it entirely. The psychological state of the mother, more than any other single factor, appears to determine success or failure in nursing the infant.

A woman should not be forced to breast-feed her infant or be made to feel guilty if she doesn't. It is a personal choice that should be respected. Breast-feeding may be inconvenient or embarrassing for her, and alternate methods of feeding her child should be supported.

DIET AND SUPPLEMENTATION

The maternal diet affects only the fat composition and the water-soluble vitamin content of breast milk. The fat composition of breast milk reflects that of the fat taken in the diet; when insufficient calories are derived from the diet, fat from the maternal tissues is mobilized and its composition is reflected in the breast milk. The levels of protein and calcium remain constant even if these nutrients are low or lacking in the maternal diet. The long-term effects of such deficiencies on the lactating women include protein malnutrition and skeletal calcium depletion. The trace elements (iron, copper, and fluoride) and fat-soluble vitamins also remain at a constant level in breast milk, but the content of water-soluble vitamins reflects maternal dietary intake. Because breast milk is low in iron, fluoride, and vitamin D, breast-fed infants should receive supplements of these nutrients. The mother should not need to take any supplements, except for iron, to replenish stores depleted by pregnancy, if her diet is adequate. Nutritional supplements are necessary when there is a deficient intake of one or more nutrients. For example, if a lactating woman is intolerant to lactose, the sugar found exclusively in milk, calcium supplements or alternate low lactose sources of calcium should be found.

SPECIAL PRECAUTIONS

Almost every drug taken by the nursing mother appears in the breast milk. Among those that could reach high enough levels to have an effect on the baby are antibiotics, laxatives, narcotics, sedatives, tranquilizers, analgesics, and stimulants. Included in this list are caffeine, nicotine, and alcohol, all of which are known to have an adverse effect on the growing infant if taken in sufficient amounts. Pesticides have also been found in breast milk, and although the long-term effects are unknown, more stringent monitoring of environmental pollutants is warranted. Table 26-5 indicates which drugs are excreted in breast milk and how the infant may be affected.

Folklore and Food Practices During the Reproductive Cycle

In most cultures food is equated with health, and dietary patterns may change in response to illness and to normal physiologic states associated with the female reproductive cycle. Certain foods may be seen as preventing illness, too much or

TABLE 26-5. Drug excretion in breast milk and effect on the infant

Drug	Excreted	Implications
Analgesics		
Acetaminophen (Datril, Tylenol)	Yes	No significant effect on infant from therapeutic doses
Acetylsalicylic acid (aspirin)[a]	Yes	Tendency toward bleeding noted; if given to nursing mother, should be given after nursing; check infant for adequate sources of vitamin K
Codeine	Yes	No significant effect on infant reported from therapeutic doses
Heroin[b]	Yes	Controversial reports as to the long-term effect on infant; usually goes through withdrawal depending on maternal dose
Meperidine hydrochloride (Demerol)	Yes	No significant effect on infant from therapeutic doses
Methadone hydrochloride[a]	Yes	Controversial as to whether user should breast-feed; if she does, the daily dose should be given after the feeding, and the next feeding should be by bottle
Morphine	Yes	No significant effects on infant from therapeutic doses
Pentazocine (Talwin)	No	
Phenylbutazone[a] (Azolid, Butazolidin)	Yes	Drug should be used judiciously; manufacturer states that it is excreted in cord blood and breast milk; infant should be monitored; may increase kernicterus—highly protein-bound
Propoxyphene hydrochloride (Darvon)	Yes	No significant effect on infant from therapeutic doses
Anticoagulants		Differing opinions as to whether mother on anticoagulants should nurse; all agree that if she does, infant should be monitored with the mother
Bishydroxycoumarin[a] (Dicumarol)	Yes	May cause hypoprothrombinemia in infant; monitor infant
Heparin sodium	No	
Phenindione[b] (Dindeyan, Hedulin)	Yes	May cause hypoprothrombinemia; one incident of massive hematoma in infant whose mother received it
Warfarin sodium[a] (Coumadin)	Yes	May cause hypoprothrombinemia; monitor infant
Anticonvulsants		
Phenytoin[a] (Dilantin)	Yes	Methemoglobulinemia in breast-fed infant; enzyme induction may occur
Primidone[b] (Mysoline)	Yes	Manufacturer recommends breast-feeding be avoided, since substantial amounts found in breast milk; drowsiness may occur in newborn
Antidiabetics		
Chlorpropamide (Diabinese)	Yes	No significant effect on infant from therapeutic doses
Insulin	Yes	Destroyed in the infant's GI tract
Tolbutamide (Dolipol, Mobenol, Orinase, Tolbutol)	Yes	No significant effects on infant from therapeutic doses
Tolazamide (Tolinase)	?	Has not been completely evaluated; 6.7 times more potent than tolbutamide
Antihistamines		
Chlorpheniramine maleate (Chlor-Trimeton)	Yes	May cause drowsiness in the infant
Diphenhydramine (Benadryl, Benhydril)	Yes	No adverse effects on infant from therapeutic doses
Promethazine hydrochloride (Phenergan)	Yes	No significant effects on infant from therapeutic doses
Trimeprazine tartrate (Temaril)	Yes	No significant effects on infant from therapeutic doses

TABLE 26-5 (CONTINUED)

Drug	Excreted	Implications
Anticholinergics		
Atropine sulfate[b]	Yes	May inhibit lactation and may cause atropine intoxication in infant; although documentation scarce, best avoided until further research available
Scopolamine	Yes	No significant effects on infant from therapeutic doses
Antihypertensives, diuretics		
Acetazolamide[a] (Diamox)	Yes	Infant may develop idiosyncratic reaction to this sulfonamide diuretic
Furosemide (Lasix)	No	Women ill enough to receive Lasix should not breastfeed
Hexamethonium	Yes	Rarely used drug; very toxic
Reserpine[b] (Serpasil)	Yes	May cause nasal stuffiness, drowsiness, and diarrhea in infant, galactorrhea in mother
Spironolactone (Aldactone)	No	Watch for potassium deficiency and dehydration in mother
Thiazides[b]	Yes	Manufacturer suggests avoiding; watch fluid, electrolyte balance
Anti-infectives		With all anti-infectives that cross into breast milk, the possibility of sensitization of the infant must be considered
Amantadine hydrochloride[b] (Symmetrel)	Yes	May cause skin rash and vomiting; manufacturer suggests avoiding
Aminoglycosides[a]	Yes	Should be reserved for severe infection; avoid in high G-6-PD–deficient populations, as hemolysis may occur
Ampicillin	Yes	No significant effects on infant from therapeutic doses
Chloramphenicol[a] (Chloromycetin)	Yes	May affect infant's bone marrow; avoid use, particularly during the first 2 weeks of life
Erythromycin[a] (E-Mycin, Erythrocin, Ilosone, Ilotycin)	Yes	Appears in breast milk in concentrations higher than that of maternal plasma; sensitization possible; estolate form (Ilosone) may cause jaundice
Isoniazid[b]	Yes	If possible, avoid use during lactation; if given, infant must be monitored for toxicity
Mandelic acid[b]	Yes	Probably best avoided during lactation; for this urinary antiseptic to be effective, urine must be strongly acid and fluids must be limited
Metronidazole[b] (Flagyl)	Yes	No adverse oral or GI effects noted in infants, but some authors feel that because of possible carcinogenicity it would be best to avoid, as long-term effects are not known
Nalidixic acid[b] (NegGram)	Yes	Hemolytic anemia, especially in G-6-PD–deficient populations
Penicillin	Yes	Possibility of sensitization; may alter intestinal flora of infant
Quinine	Not in clinically significant amounts	In very high maternal doses, thrombocytopenia in infants
Sulfonamides[a]	Yes	Avoid in high G-6-PD populations; high doses for long-term use are questionable; may cause kernicterus; avoid in the first 2 weeks of life
Tetracyclines[b]	Yes	Slows bone growth and deposits in bones and teeth
Cancer chemotherapeutic agents[b]		Breast-feeding is generally considered ill-advised in patients receiving chemotherapy

TABLE 26-5 (CONTINUED)

Drug	Excreted	Implications
Hormones		
Estrogen, progestogen, androgens[b]	Yes	Breast-feeding not indicated if mother is on oral contraceptives; may alter the composition of breast milk (decreasing the amounts of protein, fats, and minerals); long-term effects on infants have not been adequately determined
Corticosteroids[b]	Yes	Should be avoided by the nursing mother, as they may interfere with normal function and cause growth suppression
Laxatives		
Aloe[a]	Yes	Conflicting evidence regarding catharsis in infants; avoid in high doses
Cascara sagrada[b]	Yes	Thought to cause diarrhea in infants
Danthron[b] (Dorbane, Dorbantyl, Doxan, Doxidan)	Yes	Conflicting reports regarding the cathartic effect of these drugs; probably best avoided
Dioctyl sodium sulfosuccinate (Colace)		No reports of having caused any problems in the infant
Milk of magnesia	No	No adverse reactions noted
Phenolphthalein (Evac-U-Lax, Ex-Lax, other nonprescription drugs)	Yes	No significant effects noted in usual doses
Psyllium hydrophilic mucilloid (Metamucil)	Yes	No adverse reactions noted
Senna compounds[a]	Yes	Controversial reports with moderate doses; high doses may cause diarrhea in infants
Muscle relaxants		
Carisoprodol[b] (Rela, Soma)	Yes	According to manufacturer, 2 to 4 times more concentrated in breast milk than in maternal blood plasma; infant may experience CNS depression and GI upset
Methocarbamol (Robaxin)	Yes	No significant effects on infant from therapeutic doses
Oxytocics		
Ergot preparations[b]	Yes	May suppress lactation by blocking the release of prolactin; symptoms in the infant may include vomiting, diarrhea, cardiovascular changes
Oxytocin	Yes	Oxytocin nasal spray used prior to breast-feeding appears to increase the volume of milk produced; may be used for hemorrhaging mother; very short half-life
Psychotropics, psychotherapeutics		
Butyrophenones, haloperidol[a] (Haldol)		Manufacturer recommends that benefits must outweigh risks in the use of these drugs, since their safe use in pregnancy and lactation has not been established
Chlordiazepoxide[a] (Librium)	Yes	No significant effects on infant from therapeutic doses; some authors suggest using caution
Diazepam[a] (Valium)	Yes	May cause weight loss, lethargy, jaundice in the infant; some authors feel that breast-feeding should be discontinued if high doses are given to mother
Imipramine[a] (Tofranil)	Yes	Safe use during lactation has not been established
Lithium carbonate[b] (Lithonate, Lithane)	Yes	May alter electrolyte balance; most authors state that indications for its use should be unequivocal; long-term effect on infant unknown; best avoided until further evidence available
Phenothiazines[a] (Compazine, Thorazine, etc.)	Yes	All phenothiazines are excreted in breast milk, and except for reported jaundice in the infant and galactorrhea, no other effects are known at this time

TABLE 26-5 (CONTINUED)

Drug	Excreted	Implications
Sedatives, hypnotics		
Barbiturates[b]	Yes	May increase the activity of hepatic drug-metabolizing enzymes; high single dose may cause more drowsiness than small, multiple doses
Bromides[b] (ingredient in many nonprescription sleeping medications)	Yes	May cause rash and drowsiness in infant; difficulty in feeding, lethargy, hypotonia or hypertonia
Chloral hydrate (Noctec, Somnos)	Yes	Drowsiness in infant
Chloroform[b]	Yes	Anesthetic effect in infant
Glutethimide[a] (Doriden)	Yes	May cause drowsiness in infant; one author suggests avoiding during lactation; manufacturer suggests caution during lactation
Meprobamate[b] (Equanil, Miltown)	Yes	Very high level in milk (2–4 times maternal plasma); alternate drug advised; if given, infant should be monitored for signs of meprobamate toxication
Thyroid and antithyroid preparations		
Carbimazole[b] (Neo-Mercazole)	Yes	May cause goiter in infant
Methimazole[b] (Tapazole)	Yes	Manufacturer recommends that user not breast-feed
Thiouracil[b] (+ derivatives)	Yes	Excreted in high levels (3–12 times maternal plasma levels); may cause goiter or agranulocytosis
Thyroid	Yes	No significant effects on infant with therapeutic doses
Thyroxine sodium[b] (Choloxin)	Yes	Manufacturer states that use in pregnancy and lactation is contraindicated
Iodides		
^{131}I[b] (radioactive)	Yes	All radioactive agents should be avoided in the breast-feeding mother
Iodides[b] (contained in many nonprescription cough preparations)	Yes	Infant's thyroid functioning may be affected; avoid taking large or frequent doses of iodide-containing cough preparations; may have thyrotropic effect on infant or cause rash
Vitamins, minerals, food products		
Vitamins		
B$_1$ (thiamin)	Yes	Mothers with severe deficiency (beriberi) should not nurse because of excretion of toxic substances, sodium pyruvate and methylglyoxal, which have caused infant death
B$_6$ (pyridoxine)	Yes	Some authors report that it successfully suppressed lactation in doses of 150–200 mg by mouth 3 times per day
B$_{12}$ (cyanocobalamin)	Yes	No effect with therapeutic doses
D (calciferol)	Yes	High doses may cause hypercalcemia in infant
K	Yes	No significant effects on infant with therapeutic doses
Caffeine[a] (many nonprescription drugs contain caffeine: Awake, 100 mg; No Doz, 100 mg; Sta-Alert, 100 mg; Vivarin, 200 mg; coffee and tea, 100–150 mg per cup)	Yes	Unless large amount ingested, no significant effect on infant; ingestion of large quantities of tea or coffee can cause irritability and poor sleeping patterns in infants
Carrots	Yes	In large quantity, may cause yellow discoloration of skin
Egg protein	Yes	Allergic sensitization possible
Fava beans	Yes	In G-6-PD–deficient infants, hemolysis has occurred
Fluoride (toothpaste, water supply, tablets)	Yes	Not significant in usual quantities; excess may affect tooth enamel; La Leche League advises either *not* breast-feeding or to stop taking fluoride tablets; may cause GI upsets, rash in infants

TABLE 26-5 (CONTINUED)

Drug	Excreted	Implications
Vaccines, immunosuppressives		
DPT	Yes	Probably no immunity transfer to baby
Poliovirus	Yes	If infant is immunized after 6 weeks, probably negligible effect on antibody titer
Rh₀ (D) immune globulin (human) (Gamulin Rh, RhoGAM)	No	
Rubella	No	Probably no transfer of live virus to infant
Other		
Alcohol (ethyl alcohol)	Yes	No significant effect in moderate amount; prolonged ingestion of large amounts may intoxicate infant; large doses may also inhibit the milk ejection reflex, whereas small amount of alcohol prior to nursing may enhance the milk "let-down"
Clomiphene citrate (Clomid)		May suppress lactation
Dihydrotachysterol[a] (DHT)	Yes	May cause hypercalcemia in infant (osteoporosis, bone dysgenesis)
L-dopa		May suppress lactation by inhibiting prolactin secretion
Lead[b]		Caution against the use of lead acetate ointment in breast creams, as it may lead to encephalitis
Marijuana[b]	Yes	May interfere with DNA and RNA formation
Mercury[b]	Yes	In cases of mercury contamination in the environment, watch infant for CNS symptoms and mercury intoxication
Nicotine[a]	Yes	Probably very little effect on infant with moderate use (20 cigarettes per day or less); may decrease milk production; one recorded case of nicotine intoxication in infant (restlessness, vomiting, diarrhea, insomnia, circulatory disruptions)—mother smoked 20 cigarettes per day; infants of smoking mothers absorb smoke through GI tract, respiratory tract, and skin as well

Key: GI = gastrointestinal; G-6-PD = glucose 6-phosphate dehydrogenase; CNS = central nervous system.
[a] Use with caution in nursing mother.
[b] Avoid drug whenever possible.
Source: E. J. Dickason, et al., *Maternal and Infant Drugs and Nursing Intervention.* New York: McGraw-Hill, 1978. Copyright © 1978 McGraw-Hill Book Company. Used with the permission of McGraw-Hill Book Company.

too little of others as causing illness, and still others as having curative properties. In many parts of the world, menstruation, pregnancy, and the postpartum period are all thought to be potentially troublesome for women if the diet is not carefully monitored and manipulated.

MENSTRUATION

In a study of folklore surrounding food, it was found that foods to be avoided during menstruation included sweets, chocolate, carbonated beverages, lemons, grapefruit, bananas, lettuce, tomatoes, cabbage, sauerkraut, spices, sausage, pickles, vinegar, and pork [30]. Sweets were thought to keep the menstrual flow "going longer," while all the other foods were capable of causing the flow to stop because they were "cold" or "too acid." The belief that some foods have intrinsic properties of hotness and coldness irrespective of actual temperature is part of the hot-cold theory of disease. It stems from the Hippocratic theory of illness and health in which the body is seen as composed of four humors: blood, phlegm, black bile, and yellow bile. Each humor is associated with properties of hot or cold and wetness or dryness, and good health results from keeping the humors in balance. An excess of any one humor would cause disease. Although beliefs based on this theory are found in many parts of the world, it is most prominent in the Latin American cultures. Menstruation, postabortion, and postpartum states are viewed as cold intervals, since the body is losing a hot substance, blood. Cold foods are avoided during these periods. Cold foods include fresh fruits (especially citrus), tomatoes, and green vegetables. Avoidance of such foods eliminates from the diet vitamins (A, C, folic acid) needed in greater amounts when blood is lost during these states.

PREGNANCY

Pregnancy is considered to be a hot state, since there is an accumulation rather than a loss of blood. Foods to be avoided were usually "very hot" or "very cold": chili, chocolate, pork, beans, ice, tomatoes, citrus fruits, melons, ice cream, gelatin, and coffee [30]. The doctrine of *maternal impressions*, another widely held belief in many areas of the world, states that any strong emotional state of the mother, including the craving for a specific food, is somehow directly imprinted on the child. Infants born with a "strawberry" or "chocolate" birthmark were so inflicted because the mother craved that substance and touched her own body while desiring the food. Since food cravings are more commonly associated with pregnancy than with any other bodily state, the desire for a particular food is most often attributed to the developing fetus. An extension of this thinking is that the fetus desires the particular food and will be harmed (marked) if he or she does not receive it.

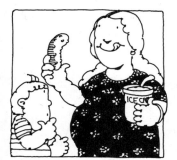

The craving or aversion for certain foods during pregnancy may have a true physiologic basis. In a recent study it was found that the most pronounced cravings were for dairy products and sweets such as chocolate and fruits [31]. It was suggested that the craving for these foods was related to the increased need for calcium and calories during pregnancy and a preferential desire for foods rich in sugars and calcium. The craving for pickles and other salty items may be related to sodium balance during pregnancy. Changes in the kidney may result in sodium depletion during a normal pregnancy [32], and the desire for sodium-rich foods may be a physiologic response to restore sodium balance. In the cravings study, many women reported an aversion to coffee, alcohol, and cigarette smoke. It was hypothesized that the nausea and vomiting evoked by these substances was a protective mechanism for the fetus, since components of all three can have adverse effects on the unborn child [31].

Also common during pregnancy is *pica*, the craving for clay, starch, dirt, or ice cubes. As discussed earlier, this habit may be the cause or the effect of iron-deficiency anemia. For some women the practice of pica represents a tradition. It may also be used to aid heartburn or as a source of minerals (especially if clay and dirt are eaten). Pica may not only displace more nutritionally rich foods from the diet but may also cause severe medical problems, including intestinal obstruction and parasites.

POSTPARTUM PERIOD AND LACTATION

As with menstruation, certain foods in the hot-cold theory are thought to impede the postpartum blood flow. Tonics containing hot foods and chocolate, garlic, cinnamon, and cheese were advised to be included during this period [33].

Because babies are believed by some to be hot from the womb, they are thought to reject breast milk, which is cold to them. They must be rid of the phlegm in their stomachs before they can tolerate breast milk, and castor oil or olive oil is administered to help achieve this [30]. Acid foods and cabbage are thought to sour the breast milk; red raspberry tea, to increase the milk supply. Because hot foods are often thought to cause rashes, many Latin American mothers prefer to feed their infants cold foods or to add something cool to the formula: barley water, magnesium carbonate, or chamomile tea (laxatives) or mannitol (a diuretic).

While many folk and cultural practices during the female reproductive cycle are harmless, others may potentiate poor nutrition for mother and child. Individual practices should be evaluated as to their impact on the health and nutrition of the woman and her infant, and alternatives given if the tradition is harmful.

Dietary Recommendations

1. A variety of foods based on the four food groups is always best but especially during pregnancy and lactation.
2. Choose foods rich in protein, calcium, iron, vitamins, and minerals.
3. As pregnancy advances and the growing fetus allows less room for a full stomach, frequent small meals may be better than several large ones.
4. Avoid drugs, medications, smoking, and the excessive use of alcohol and coffee.
5. Avoid excesses of any one food, which may displace other nutrients from the diet.
6. Seek prenatal care early, for your own health and your baby's.

References

1. *Assessment of Maternal Nutrition.* Chicago: American College of Obstetricians and Gynecologists, and American Dietetic Association, 1978.
2. *Nutrition in Maternal Health Care.* Chicago: American College of Obstetricians and Gynecologists, 1974.
3. Frisch, R. E.   Population, food intake, and fertility. *Science* 199:22, 1978.
4. Darwin, C., quoted in Frisch [3].
5. Smith, C. A.   The effect of wartime starvation in Holland upon pregnancy and its product. *Am. J. Obstet. Gynecol.* 53:599, 1947.
6. Antonov, A. N.   Children born during the siege of Leningrad in 1942. *J. Pediatr.* 30:250, 1947.

7. Osofsky, H. J.   Relationships between nutrition during pregnancy and subsequent infant and child development. *Obstet. Gynecol. Surv.* 30:227, 1975.

8. Nixon, W. C. W.   Diet in pregnancy. *J. Obstet. Gynaec. Br. Emp.* 49:614, 1942.

9. Mussey, R. D.   Nutrition and human reproduction: An historical review. *Am. J. Obstet. Gynecol.* 57:1037, 1949.

10. Lucas (1788), in Spencer, H. R.   An address on some changes in obstetric practice since the foundation of the Medical Society of London. *Br. Med. J.* 2:639, 1923.

11. Prochownick, L.   Ein Versuch zum Ersatz der Kinsflichen fruhgeburt. *Ehl. Gynak.* 13:577, 1889.

12. Prochownick, L.   Ernahruengscuren in der Schwangershaft. *Ther. Mn.,* 15:387, 446, 1901.

13. Strauss, M. B.   Observations on the etiology of the toxemias of pregnancy: The relationship of nutritional deficiency, hypoproteinuria, and elevated venous pressure to water retention in pregnancy. *Am. J. Med.* 190:811, 1935.

14. Toverud, G.   Preventive dentistry in the preschool period and particularly during foetal life. *Dental Mag. Oral Topics* 55:299, 1938.

15. Dieckmann, W. J.   Osteomalacia in pregnancy. *Am. J. Obstet. Gynecol.* 23:478, 1932.

16. Eastman, N. J., and Jackson, E.   Weight relationships in pregnancy. *Obstet. Gynecol. Surv.* 23:1003, 1968.

17. Singer, J. E., Westphal, M., and Niswander, K.   Relationship of weight gain during pregnancy to birthweight and infant growth and development in the first year of life: A report from the Collaborative Study of Cerebral Palsy. *Obstet. Gynecol.* 31:417, 1968.

18. Hytten, R. E., and Leitch, I.   *The Physiology of Human Pregnancy* (2nd ed.). Oxford: Blackwell, 1971.

19. Food and Nutrition Board, National Research Council.   *Recommended Dietary Allowances* (9th ed.). Washington, D.C.: National Academy Press, 1980. P. 27.

20. Krishnamachari, K. A. V. P., and Iyengar, L.   Effect of maternal malnutrition on the bone density of the neonate. *Am. J. Clin. Nutr.* 28:482, 1975.

21. *Teenage Pregnancy: The Problem That Hasn't Gone Away.* New York: Alan Guttmacher Institute, 1981. P. 29.

22. Dwyer, J. F.   Managing the teenage pregnancy. *Obstet. Gynecol. Observ.* 12:2, 1975.

23. Prenatal clinic for teenagers provides a comprehensive program. *Contemp. Obstet. Gynecol.* 3:79, 1972.

24. Luke, B., and Petrie, R. H.   Intrauterine growth: Correlation of infant birth weight and maternal postpartum weight. *Am. J. Clin. Nutr.* 33:2311, 1980.

25. Luke, B., Hawkins, M. M., and Petrie, R. H.   Influence of smoking, weight gain, and pregravid weight for height on intrauterine growth. *Am. J. Clin. Nutr.* 34:1410, 1981.

26. Goldstein, H.   Factors influencing the height of seven-year-old children: Results from the National Child Development Study. *Hum. Biol.* 43:92, 1971.

27. Davie, R., Butler, N. R., and Goldstein, H.   *From Birth to Seven: The Second Report of the National Child Development Study.* London: Longman and National Children's Bureau, 1972.

28. Luke, B.   Understanding pica in pregnant women. *Am. J. Matern. Child Nurs.* 2:97, 1977.

29. Rudolph, A. M.   *Pediatrics* (16th ed.). New York: Appleton-Century-Crofts, 1977. P. 204.

30. Snow, L. F., and Johnson, S. M.   Folklore, food, female reproductive cycle. *Ecology Food Nutr.* 7:41, 1978.

31. Hook, E. B.   Dietary cravings and aversions during pregnancy. *Am. J. Clin. Nutr.* 31:1355, 1978.

32. Ehrlich, E. N., and Lindheimer, M. D.   Sodium metabolism and the hypertensive disorders of pregnancy. *J. Reprod. Med.* 8:106, 1972.

33. Harwood, A.   The hot-cold theory of disease: Implications for treatment of Puerto Rican patients. *J.A.M.A.* 216:1153, 1971.

Suggested Readings

Adequacy of lactation in well-nourished mothers. *Nutr. Rev.* 40:136, 1982.

Aftergood, L., and Alfin-Slater, R. B.   Women and nutrition. *Contemp. Nutr.* March, 1980.

Alcohol use during pregnancy: A report by the American Council on Science and Health. *Nutr. Today* 17:29, 1982.

Arena, J. M.   Contamination of the ideal food. *Nutr. Today* 5:2, 1970.

Assessment of Maternal Nutrition. Chicago: American College of Obstetricians and Gynecologists, 1978.

Beerens, H., Romand, C., and Neut, C.   Influence of breast-feeding on the bifid flora of the newborn intestine. *Am. J. Clin. Nutr.* 33:2434, 1980.

Breast-feeding and avoidance of food antigens in the prevention and management of allergic disease. *Nutr. Rev.* 36:181, 1978.

Carruth, B. R.   Adolescent pregnancy and nutrition. *Contemp. Nutr.* October 1980.

Chandra, R. K.   Immunological aspects of human milk. *Nutr. Rev.* 36:265, 1978.

Chapman, N.   Incorporating nutrition into family planning services. *J. Nutr. Educ.* 10:129, 1978.

Eating Right for Your Baby. Sacramento: California Department of Health Services, 1978.

Evans, R. W., et al.   Maternal diet and infantile colic in breast-fed infants. *Lancet* 1:1340, 1981.

Falkner, F.   Maternal nutrition and fetal growth. *Am. J. Clin. Nutr.* 34:769, 1981.

Ferguson, B. B., Wilson, D. J., and Schaffner, W.   Determination of nicotine concentrations in human milk. *Am. J. Dis. Child.* 130:837, 1976.

Filer, L. J.   Maternal nutrition in lactation. *Clin. Perinatol.* 2:353, 1975.

Foman, S. J., and Strauss, R. G.   Nutrient deficiencies in breast-fed infants. *N. Engl. J. Med.* 299:355, 1978.

Food and Nutrition Board.   *Nutrition Services in Perinatal Care.* Washington, D.C.: National Academy Press, 1981.

Gibson, R. A., and Kneebone, G. M.   Fatty acid composition of human colostrum and mature breast milk. *Am. J. Clin. Nutr.* 34:252, 1981.

Goldfarb, J., and Tibbetts, E.   *Breast-feeding Handbook: A Practical Reference for Physicians, Nurses, and Other Health Professionals.* Hillside, N.J.: Enslow Publishers, 1980.

Henley, E. C., and Bahl, S.   Nutrition across the woman's life cycle: Special emphasis on pregnancy. *Nurs. Clin. North Am.* 17:99, 1982.

Hughes, M.   Healthy mothers, healthy babies. *J. Am. Dietet. Assoc.* 80:215, 1982.

Impact of maternal alcohol intake on birth weight. *Nutr. Rev.* 40:48, 1982.

Iron absorption from breast milk or cow's milk. *Nutr. Rev.* 35:203, 1977.

Jacobson, H. N.   Maternal nutrition in the 1980's. *J. Am. Dietet. Assoc.* 80:216, 1982.

Kabara, J. J.   Lipids as host-resistance factors of human milk. *Nutr. Rev.* 38:65, 1980.

Kennedy, E. T., and Gershoff, S.   Effect of W.I.C. supplemental feeding on hemoglobin and hematocrit of prenatal patients. *J. Am. Dietet. Assoc.* 80:227, 1982.

Kennedy, E. T., et al.   Evaluation of the effect of W.I.C. supplemental feeding on birth weight. *J. Am. Dietet. Assoc.* 80:220, 1982.

Luke, B., Dickinson, C., and Petrie, R. H.   Intrauterine growth: Correlations of maternal nutritional status and rate of gestational weight gain. *Europ. J. Obstet. Gynecol. Reprod. Biol.* 12:113, 1981.

Luke, B. *Maternal Nutrition*. Boston: Little, Brown, 1979.

McMillan, J. A., Landaw, S. A., and Oski, F. A. Iron sufficiency in breast-fed infants and the availability of iron from human milk. *Pediatrics* 58:686, 1976.

Meal Planning During Pregnancy. Minneapolis: General Mills Nutrition Department, 1978.

Morbidity in breast fed and artificially fed infants. *Nutr. Rev.* 38:114, 1980.

Myres, A. W. Breast-feeding: A national priority for infant health. *J. Can. Dietet. Assoc.* 42:130, 1981.

Naeye, R. L. Nutritional/nonnutritional interactions that affect the outcome of pregnancy. *Am. J. Clin. Nutr.* 34:727, 1981.

Nutritional demands of lactating women. *Nutr. & the MD* February, 1982.

Nutrition During Pregnancy and Lactation. Sacramento: California Department of Health Services, 1975.

Oral contraceptives and nutrition. *J. Am. Dietet. Assoc.* 68:419, 1976.

Overbach, A. M., and Rodman, M. J. *Drugs Used With Neonates and During Pregnancy*. Oradell, N.J.: Medical Economics, 1975.

Pittard, W. B. Breast milk immunology: A frontier in infant nutrition. *Am. J. Dis. Child.* 133:83, 1979.

Raman, L. Influence of maternal nutritional factors affecting birthweight. *Am. J. Clin. Nutr.* 34:775, 1981.

Report of the third meeting of the ACC/SCN consultative group on maternal and young child nutrition. *Food Nutr. Bull.* 3:20, 1981.

Rogan, W. J., Bagniewska, A., and Damstra, T. Pollutants in breast milk. *N. Engl. J. Med.* 302:1450, 1980.

Rothermel, P. C., and Faber, M. M. Drugs, in breastmilk: A consumer's guide. *Birth Fam. J.* 2:76, 1975.

Rowland, M. G. M., Paul, A. A., and Whitehead, R. G. Lactation and infant nutrition. *Br. Med. Bull.* 37:77, 1981.

Shahani, K. M., Kwan, A. J. M., and Friend, B. A. Role and significance of enzymes in human milk. *Am. J. Clin. Nutr.* 33:1861, 1980.

Sulik, K. K., Johnston, M. C., and Webb, M. A. Fetal alcohol syndrome: Embryogenesis in a mouse model. *Science* 214:936, 1981.

Thenen, S. W. Folacin content of supplemental foods for pregnancy. *J. Am. Dietet. Assoc.* 80:237, 1982.

Thorp, V. J. Effect of oral contraceptive agents on vitamin and mineral requirements. *J. Am. Dietet. Assoc.* 76:581, 1980.

Toxemia of pregnancy: The dietary calcium hypothesis. *Nutr. Rev.* 39:124, 1981.

Update: Drugs in breast milk. *Med. Lett.* 21:21, 1979.

U.S. Department of Health and Human Services, Public Health Service. *Caffeine and Pregnancy*. Washington, D.C.: Government Printing Office, 1981.

Van den Berg, B. J. Maternal variables affecting fetal growth. *Am. J. Clin. Nutr.* 34:772, 1981.

Chapter 27

GERIATRIC NUTRITION

Senior citizen, older American, geriatric individual: the elderly have many labels and definitions. The Social Security system has selected 65 years as the retirement age. The Older American Act of 1973 defined persons 60 years and older as eligible for programs for older Americans. The "young old" are defined as those in the transition stage from middle age such as those in their sixties, seventies, and eighties, and the "very old" as those in their late nineties or older.

Growing older is not necessarily synonymous with growing ill and weak. Only about 5 percent of those over age 65 are in nursing homes or other institutions, whereas about 95 percent continue to live independently [1]. In 1970 there were an estimated 20 million elderly in this country, increasing by about half a million per year. The increase in this segment of the American population has been attributed to improvements in health care, diagnostic techniques, treatment, and preventive medicine, all of which increase survival rates and decrease the disabling effects of disease. Federal assistance in the form of special insurance and health care programs has brought more elderly into the health care system and made them active participants in preventive programs. Special needs of the elderly, especially the nutritional needs for health maintenance and for improving the effects of treatment, are important to recognize if treatment and care are to be effective.

Physiologic Changes with Aging

The process of aging includes a physiologic decline. This process is not uniform, however; various organs and systems lose their functional capacity at different rates. The greatest change that occurs with aging is in the ability of an organ or system to respond to challenge; this response is neither as rapid nor as effective as in the younger adult.

BASAL METABOLIC RATE

The basal metabolic rate (the rate of energy expenditure at complete rest) decreases by a little over 2 percent per decade in adults [2], or by about 20 percent between the ages of 20 and 90. When combined with the decrease in activity levels of most elderly adults, this results in a reduced daily caloric requirement [3].

PULMONARY FUNCTION

Pulmonary capacity declines by about 40 percent with advancing age. These changes may limit the capacity for exercise but do not normally impose restrictions on normal daily activities. This decline is compounded and accelerated by such variables as smoking and smog.

CARDIOVASCULAR SYSTEM

Decreased functioning of the cardiovascular system occurs with advancing age. Hardening of the vessels occurs, with calcium being deposited and a loss of elasticity resulting. The changes responsible for this reduced efficiency include increased rigidity of the arterial walls, reduced contractility of the heart muscle, and reduced cardiac output. Changes in the pulmonary and cardiovascular systems with age manifest as a longer time period for the rate of respiration and pulse to return to normal after exercise or exertion. Many of these changes may be related to life-long dietary habits.

RENAL FUNCTION

From age 25 to 80, the glomerular filtration rate decreases by about 50 percent, paralleling a decrease in the renal plasma flow. After about age 40, the body's ability to regenerate nephrons (the functional unit of the kidney) ceases, and the total number of functioning nephrons gradually declines. Because there are fewer nephrons in the elderly than in the young person, the solute load per nephron is higher. This results in a decreased ability of the aging kidney to form either a dilute or a concentrated urine [4]. This becomes important during periods of excessive fluid loss (e.g., humid, hot weather) when dehydration may result, and in congestive heart failure when fluid overload may result.

SKELETAL STRUCTURE

Although human bones are remolded throughout life by the processes of absorption (loss of minerals from bone) and deposition (addition of minerals to bone), by about the third or fourth decade of life the former process becomes more rapid than the latter, resulting in a net loss of bone, or negative calcium balance. An overall decrease in skeletal mass occurs as a result of a progressive loss from the inner core of the bones and a thinning of the walls. When the loss of skeletal mass is severe, it is termed *osteoporosis*.

The loss of bone mass occurs with advancing age in all persons but progresses more rapidly in postmenopausal women and Caucasians [5]. As a result, bones become increasingly vulnerable to fracture. In older persons, fractures of the wrist and femoral neck are common. The vertebrae may collapse, causing a shortening and bowing of the spine with resultant reduced height and stooped posture.

Several factors can lead to more rapid bone loss and negative calcium balance [6]:

I. Unavailability of calcium for mineralization
   A. Inadequate dietary intake of calcium
   B. Imbalance of calcium-phosphorus ratio
   C. Presence of calcium binders inhibiting the absorption of dietary calcium
II. Reduced physical activity or immobilization
III. Alteration in endocrine controls influencing calcium metabolism [7]
IV. Reduced renal function

Advanced osteoporosis is irreversible. Adequate intake of dietary calcium and sufficient physical activity are prudent preventive measures.

GASTROINTESTINAL FUNCTION

It has been shown that digestive enzymes and hydrochloric acid are reduced in the elderly. The motility of the colon is also decreased, which, when combined with a decline in physical activity, results in constipation. Although life-long dietary and bowel habits are the primary determinants of bowel function, changes in the gastrointestinal tract are contributing factors to decreased bowel motility.

DENTITION

The American Dental Association estimates that about three-fourths of all individuals 70 years of age and older have lost all their teeth, and about 80 percent of those who have lost their teeth either do not replace them or replace them with poorly fitting dentures. Part of the problem may be lack of funds or availability of services. Tooth loss may result from the loss of supporting bone in the jaw because of periodontal disease, which can be the result of life-long poor dietary or dental habits. This loss of bone is seen in other parts of the skeleton as osteoporosis.

The loss of teeth, or the use of painful, ill-fitting dentures, may severely limit the food choices and nutritional intake of the elderly person. Problems with dentition can result in modifications in eating habits and even overt malnutrition. Chewing becomes difficult, and inadequately masticated food is difficult to swallow. Therefore foods high in fiber such as fruits and vegetables may be eliminated from the diet, thus reducing the intake of fiber with a resultant decrease in gastrointestinal motility and consequent problems with elimination. Fruits and vegetables also provide a rich source of vitamin C, which is necessary for wound healing, tissue repair, and maintenance of cellular walls. The avoidance of meat, another food difficult to eat with poor dentition, greatly decreases the intake of protein of high biologic value, a readily absorbed form of iron, and an abundant source of the B vitamins. Lethargy, anemia, and susceptibility to infection may be signs of these modifications in diet, and their link to poor dental health may not at first seem obvious.

SENSORY FUNCTION

With advancing age, the ability to adapt to dim light decreases, as does the ability of the eye's lens to focus at different distances. This latter condition is termed *presbyopia* and occurs in nearly all elderly persons. Cataracts, the clouding of the lens as a result of changes in the metabolism of the lens material, also is a frequent condition among the elderly.

The loss of hearing acuity also may be part of aging. This slow, progressive decline in hearing acuity, termed *presbycusis*, often manifests itself as an inability to distinguish speech patterns from background noise and tones of high frequency.

The number of taste buds present at age 30 declines by about one-third by age 70. In addition, the ability to discriminate flavors at low concentrations is lost. There is a loss in the number of taste buds, particularly those that detect sweet and salt [8]. The reduction in olfactory sensitivity may compound this reduced ability to enjoy food. Unless a person is following a medical dietary regimen, the eating of bland foods is not necessary; actually, seasonings may need to be increased to enhance eating enjoyment.

When combined, impaired vision, hearing, taste, and smell may lead to a general apathy of older persons toward meals. The elderly may experience problems in food preparation and, when eating with others, difficulty in communicating in a group.

NEUROMUSCULAR
COORDINATION

Fine neuromuscular coordination declines with age; this decline may manifest itself as difficulty in adequately manipulating eating utensils. This may have two results. First, to avoid embarrassment in the company of others from spilling food or the inability to cut meat, the elderly person may avoid eating with others. Secondly, the person may realize that the lack of coordination is hazardous when working with boiling water, sharp kitchen utensils, and open gas flames. To avoid this danger, the person may choose foods that do not require preparation. This limiting of food choices for physical reasons has other implications. Ready-made foods that do not require much preparation are much more expensive, and because most elderly persons are on a severely limited budget, this may result in an overall compromised nutritional intake. Pastries, cookies, candies, and breads, often the prepared foods chosen, do not offer a balance of nutrients.

Table 27-1 provides a summary of common physiologic changes, their effects on nutrition, and some suggested therapies to compensate for them.

**Life-Long Dietary
Habits**

Life-long inadequate dietary habits may leave the elderly adult in a state of marginal deficiency for a number of nutrients. Acute or chronic diseases in this age group can place demands on low or deficient nutrient reserves, precipitating frank (overt) deficiencies.

Because most of the elderly were forming their food habits 60 or 70 years ago when the types and varieties of foods were very different than they are today, many in this age group may choose foods familiar to them from a time when selection was more limited. For example, fresh citrus fruits were available only seasonally during the first half of this century, whereas now a wider variety of better quality citrus is accessible year round. Similarly, many new types and forms of cereals and cereal products have become available during the past 20 to 30 years. Still, many of the elderly cling to a way of eating engrained in their youth and are resistant to new types of foods, familiar foods in different forms (whole-grain oats as granola), or foods thought to be out of season (strawberries in December).

Although it is difficult to change life-long habits, new foods can be introduced one at a time in an unpressured, nonjudgmental manner.

Economic Factors

Because income from Social Security and most pension plans has remained static while inflation has soared, the real income of most elderly is low. In 1974, about half of all persons over age 65 had an income of less than $1480, and 25 percent

TABLE 27-1. Summary of age-related changes and suggested therapy

Physiologic change	Effect	Suggested therapy
Decreased basal metabolic rate	Reduced caloric requirement	Choose less calorically dense foods
Decreased pulmonary function	Reduced exercise capacity	Avoid excessive exertion Avoid smoking, smog
Decreased cardiovascular function	Reduced exercise capacity	Avoid excessive exertion
Decreased renal function	Reduced ability to concentrate or dilute urine	Avoid dehydration and overhydration
Loss of mineral from bone	Fractures of wrist and femoral neck common	Ensure adequate dietary calcium intake Get sufficient physical activity
Slowed gastrointestinal function	Reduced bowel motility; constipation, hemorrhoids	Ensure adequate dietary fiber, fluid intake Get sufficient physical activity
Impaired dentition	Difficulty in eating; possible malnutrition	Get proper dental care and/or dentures Eat a balanced variety of soft, easily chewed foods
Impaired hearing	Avoidance of social interaction; isolation, loneliness	Have hearing tested and appliance made
Impaired sight	Difficulty reading and remaining independent	Have sight tested and eyeglasses made Get help with shopping, cooking
Impaired taste	Poor appetite; apathy toward eating and meals	Use additional spices

had an income of less than $1000 [9]. It is simple to see that food budgets for the elderly are often severely restricted. Most frequently, retirement income is much less than that earned during the working years. Maintaining a previous life-style is often difficult, and, reluctant to accept charity, many elderly persons will try to maintain a former standard of living at the expense of such basics as food. In an attempt to choose foods that are inexpensive yet will satisfy hunger and provide energy, many of the elderly will substitute high carbohydrate foods such as breads, pastries, and cereals for more expensive foods such as fresh produce, meats, and milk, which provide essential protein, minerals, and vitamins. The lower priced, high carbohydrate foods are usually lacking in these vital nutrients.

Psychosocial Factors

In addition to the many physiologic changes that accompany aging, those in this age group face numerous social and psychological adjustments as well. A number of these changes involve loss—of friends, neighbors, relatives, income, mobility, and even self-esteem and independence.

Most families today are widely dispersed geographically, decreasing the social contacts and support that family relationships can provide. One of the most difficult adjustments for the elderly person to make is to the loss of a spouse. Women outnumber men in the older age categories, since women have a longer

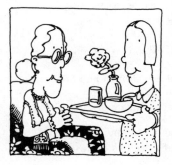

life span than men. Living alone preserves independence, but such isolation may lead to changes in the eating habits of the elderly. Loneliness, lack of motivation, and inadequate cooking or refrigeration facilities may lead to snacking at irregular intervals rather than eating regular, balanced meals and result in poor dietary intake. Persons often eat more, more slowly, and with more pleasure in the company of others. Church groups, senior citizens' groups, and other social clubs may provide environments conducive to both social interaction and better eating habits.

The physiologic changes such as decreased joint mobility and impaired vision and hearing, as well as social and economic changes, may alter the elderly person's ability to move within his or her own environment. The physical changes may make the rigors of driving a car or using public transportation too demanding. Fear for personal safety may also restrict mobility. Shopping may become increasingly difficult. The replacement of corner grocery stores with large supermarkets may offer a wider variety of foods at lower cost, but a supermarket may be more difficult for the elderly adult to get to using public or private transportation. The supermarket may seem overwhelming when the person does arrive; it may be especially confusing for those with impaired vision or physical disabilities.

Nutritional Requirements

Such factors as heredity, environment, nutritional status, illness, stress, and dietary intake during the early years of life have been shown to be important in overall health in later years. When compounded by an acute or chronic illness and single or multiple medications nutritional status and requirements are also affected. The influence of disease and medications is discussed separately in other chapters. General nutritional requirements for the elderly are discussed below.

CALORIES

As stated earlier, the basal metabolic rate decreases with advancing age. This decrease, combined with reduced physical activity, results in a decreased caloric need. For women between ages 23 and 50, the Food and Nutrition Board of the National Research Council recommends about 2000 calories daily; for those between 51 and 75, 1800 calories (a reduction by 10 percent); and for women 76 years of age and older, 1600 calories (a reduction from mature adult recommendations by 20 percent) [10]. For men between the ages of 23 and 50, the recommended energy intake is 2700 calories daily; 2400 calories for ages 51 to 75; and 2050 calories for men age 76 and older [10].

Although obesity is a common problem in late middle age, increasing susceptibility to the degenerative diseases arthritis, hypertension, diabetes, and atherosclerosis, extreme underweight is more prevalent among those over age 70. The lack of sufficient calories required for the biochemical reactions vital to life processes causes a breakdown in cellular metabolism. The clinical signs of such calorie malnutrition include a lack of vigor and interest in surroundings and an increased susceptibility to disease. The malnutrition-underweight syndrome in the elderly is probably the result of age-related changes and their effect on nutritional status plus the economic restrictions on buying power.

PROTEIN

Lean body mass decreases with age [11], with a greater decrease observed in women than in men. This is partially due to a decreased rate of protein anabolism (tissue formation) and a reduction in physical exercise. For most elderly, total essential amino acid needs are greater. The recommended daily dietary allowance (RDA) for protein for those over 50 is 56 gm for men and 44 gm for women [10]. Since the energy intake is reduced in this age group while the protein recommendations are similar to those for other age groups, a greater proportion of the dietary intake should be in the form of protein. The Food and Nutrition Board recommends that 12 percent or more of the caloric intake be in the form of protein, since the elderly are more prone to recurring episodes of chronic diseases requiring repletion of protein reserves during convalescence [10]. Some examples of foods providing low-cost, high-quality protein are eggs, canned or powdered milk, and peanut butter.

FAT AND CARBOHYDRATE

The Council on Foods and Nutrition of the American Medical Association and the Food and Nutrition Board recommend a reduction in the consumption of saturated fats and carbohydrates to reduce overall caloric intake and to maintain ideal body weight [12]. They also advise reductions in sodium and cholesterol intake.

Abnormal glucose tolerance is fairly common among the elderly, being more frequent among women than men [13]. This is often due to delayed insulin response and can be controlled by spacing and restricting the intake of carbohydrate and calories.

MINERALS

Osteoporosis is prevalent among the elderly and is related to changes in hormone balance, physical activity, and protein and calcium intake. Some studies indicate that the calcium needs of women are greater than those of men, although the Food and Nutrition Board recommends a daily dietary allowance of 800 mg for each.

The use of fluoride by the elderly is encouraged. The incidence of osteoporosis, collapsed vertebrae, and reduced bone density is higher among elderly populations residing in areas where the fluoride content of the water is low [14].

Iron-deficiency anemia may be seen in the elderly because of the decreased secretion of hydrochloric acid or as a manifestation of a chronic underlying disease [15]. The RDA for iron for both men and women over the age of 50 is 10 mg.

VITAMINS

The vitamin requirements for the elderly are essentially the same as for the younger adult. Vitamin D may be especially important in the diet of the elderly, in its relationship with bone mineralization and the development of osteoporosis.

TABLE 27-2. Recommended daily dietary allowances for adults 51 years old or older

Feature or nutrient	Men	Women
Weight (kg, lb)	70, 154	55, 121
Height (cm, in.)	178, 70	163, 64
Energy (cal)	2400*	1800*
Protein (gm)	56	44
Fat-soluble vitamins		
Vitamin A (IU)	10,000	8000
Vitamin D (IU)	200	200
Vitamin E (IU)	14	12
Water-soluble vitamins		
Vitamin C (mg)	60	60
Thiamin (mg)	1.2	1.0
Riboflavin (mg)	1.4	1.2
Niacin (mg)	16	13
Pyridoxine (mg)	2.2	2.0
Folacin (μg)	400	400
Vitamin B_{12} (μg)	3.0	3.0
Minerals		
Calcium (mg)	800	800
Phosphorus (mg)	800	800
Magnesium (mg)	350	300
Iron (mg)	10	10
Zinc (mg)	15	15
Iodine (μg)	150	150

*The energy allowance for men over 75 is 2050 cal; for women over 75, 1600 cal.
Source: Food and Nutrition Board, National Research Council, *Recommended Daily Dietary Allowances*. Washington, D.C.: National Academy of Sciences, 1980.

FLUIDS

As stated earlier, the number of functioning nephrons per kidney decreases with age, and therefore the solute load per nephron is greater. To facilitate the excretion of this solute load, adequate fluid intake is essential. In conditions in which additional water is lost, such as excessive perspiration, diarrhea, vomiting, or the prescribed use of diuretics, the need for ample fluid intake is even greater.

Table 27-2 summarizes the RDAs for this age group.

Intervention Programs

A number of special programs for the elderly have been started to help alleviate malnutrition and isolation in this age group. Such services as Meals on Wheels provide nutritional assistance to the elderly. The National Nutrition Program (Title VII of the Older American Act), enacted in 1973, is operated through state agencies on aging. Through this act, the federal government has allocated $250 million to meet up to 90 percent of the cost of providing at least one hot meal daily that provides one-third of the RDAs 5 days per week. The purpose of this program is to provide nutritious meals to persons 60 years of age and older who

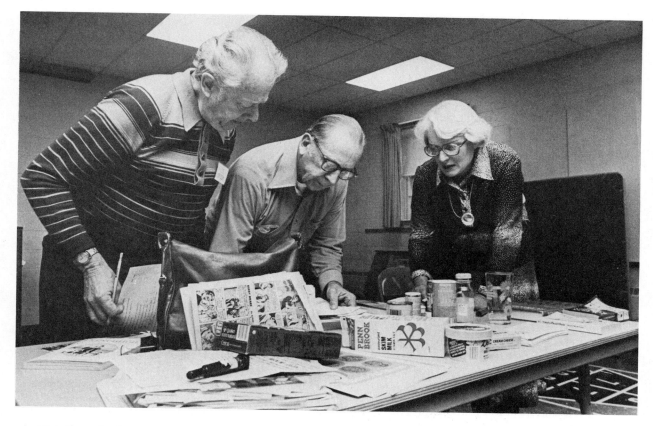

FIG. 27-1. Extension home economists from the U.S. Department of Agriculture (USDA) sponsor workshops on food shopping. Their emphasis is on how to prepare nutritious meals economically. (USDA photo by Fred Witte.)

do not eat adequately because of lack of funds, knowledge, mobility, or incentive [16].

Congregate Meals, another federally funded nutrition program for the elderly, is designed to meet both nutritional and social needs. Transportation is provided to centrally located meeting places where a nutritious meal is served in an atmosphere also providing recreational, educational, and social experiences.

The Food Stamp Program, federally funded and administered through local welfare departments, is available to those of all age groups with low incomes. Food stamps are issued according to income and number of persons in the household and are redeemable for food items at most grocery stores.

Home health services available through private and public agencies by physician referral provide nursing and homemaker care. Home health aides and homemakers can assist with food shopping and preparation, and visiting public health nurses can provide nursing services and education.

Many local communities and churches offer unique services for the elderly adult in their area. These and other possibilities should be explored to provide help to the aged and to keep them active and included as a vital and needed part of the community (Fig. 27-1). It is critical for the health professional to be aware of the services available within the community. They can serve as a link to the elderly, helping to educate them regarding nutrition and serving as advocates of preventive health care.

References

1. Weiner, W. B., Brok, A. J., and Snadowsky, A. M. *Working with the Aged.* Englewood Cliffs, N.J.: Prentice-Hall, 1978.
2. Durnin, J. V. G. A. *Energy, Work and Leisure.* London: Heineman, 1967.
3. Busse, E. W. How mind, body, and environment influence nutrition in the elderly. *Postgrad. Med.* 63:118, 1978.
4. Lindeman, R. D. Age Changes in Renal Function. In R. Goldman and M. Rockstein (eds.), *The Physiology and Pathology of Human Aging.* New York: Academic, 1975.
5. Albanese, A. A. *Bone Loss: Causes, Detection and Therapy.* New York: Alan R. Liss, 1977.
6. *Dietary Modifications in Disease: Aging and Nutrition.* Columbus, Ohio: Ross Laboratories, 1979.
7. Estrogens given after menopause protect against fractures. *Nutr. Rev.* 38:80, 1980.
8. Schiffman, S. C. Changes in Taste and Smell in Old Persons. In *Advances in Research.* Durham, N.C.: Duke University Center for the Study of Aging and Human Development, 1978. Pp. 1–6.
9. Guthrie, H. A. *Introductory Nutrition* (4th ed.). St. Louis: Mosby, 1979. P. 493.
10. Food and Nutrition Board, National Research Council. *Recommended Dietary Allowances* (9th ed.). Washington, D.C.: National Academy Press, 1980.
11. Forbes, G. B., et al. Adult lean body mass declines with age: Some longitudinal observations. *Metabolism* 19:653, 1970.
12. American Medical Association. Diet and Coronary Heart Disease: A joint statement of the AMA Council on Food and Nutrition and the Food and Nutrition Board, National Academy of Sciences–National Research Council. *J.A.M.A.* 222:1647, 1972.
13. Zeytinoglu, I. Y., et al. The process of aging: Serum glucose and immunoreactive insulin levels during the oral glucose tolerance test. *J. Am. Geriatr. Soc.* 17:1, 1969.
14. Bernstein, D. G., et al. Prevalence of osteoporosis in high- and low-fluoride areas in North Dakota. *J.A.M.A.* 198:499, 1966.
15. Matzner, Y., et al. Prevalence and causes of anemia in the elderly. *Isr. J. Med. Sci.* 14:1165, 1978.
16. Administration on Aging, Office of Human Development Services, National Clearinghouse on Aging. *National Nutrition Program for Older Americans* (HEW fact sheet). 1978.

Suggested Readings

Behnke, J. A., Finch, C. E., and Moment, G. B. (eds.). *The Biology of Aging.* New York: Plenum Press, 1978.

Cheung, L. Y.-S., et al. The Chinese elderly and family structure: Implications for health care. *Pub. Health Rep.* 95:491, 1980.

Elwood, T. W. Nutritional concerns of the elderly. *J. Nutr. Educ.* 7:50, 1975.

For the elderly, cool can be too cold. *FDA Consum.* 14:20, 1980.

Greger, J. L., and Geissler, A. H. Effect of zinc supplementation on taste acuity of the aged. *Am. J. Clin. Nutr.* 31:633, 1978.

Harrill, I., and Cervone, N. Vitamin status of older women. *Am. J. Clin. Nutr.* 30:431, 1977.

Heavey, R. P. Premenopausal prophylactic calcium supplementation. *J.A.M.A.* 245:1362, 1981.

Hormones, nutrients and postmenopausal bone loss. *Nutr. Rev.* 40:13, 1982.

Kirkendall, W. M., and Hammond, J. J. Hypertension in the elderly. *Arch. Intern. Med.* 140:1155, 1980.

Leaf, A. Getting old. *Sci. Am.* 229:44, 1973.

Leeming, J. T. Skeletal disease in the elderly. *Br. Med. J.* 4:472, 1973.

Masoro, E. J., et al. Nutritional probe of the aging process. *Fed. Proc.* 39:3178, 1980.

Mayer, J. Aging and nutrition. *Geriatrics* 29:57, 1974.

Meal Planning for the Golden Years. Minneapolis: General Mills Nutrition Department, Betty Crocker Food and Nutrition Center, 1979.

Montgomery, R. D., et al. The aging gut: A study of intestinal absorption in relation to nutrition in the elderly. *Q. J. Med.* 47:197, 1978.

Natow, A. B., Heslin, J. A., and Natow, A. Geriatric Nutrition. Boston: CBI Publishing, 1980.

Rockstein, M., and Sussman, M. L. (eds.). *Nutrition, Longevity, and Aging*. New York: Academic, 1976.

Shock, N. W. Physiological aspects of aging. *J. Am. Diet. Assoc.* 54:491, 1970.

Stiedman, M., Jansen, C., and Harrill, I. Nutritional status of elderly men and women. *J. Am. Diet. Assoc.* 73:132, 1978.

Taggart, H. McA., et al. Deficient calcitonin response to calcium stimulation in post-menopausal osteoporosis? *Lancet* 1:475, 1982.

Tomaiolo, P. P., Enman, S., and Kraus, V. Preventing and treating malnutrition in the elderly. *J. Parent. Ent. Nutr.* 5:46, 1981.

Watkin, D. Aging: Symposium. *Am. J. Clin. Nutr.* 26:1095, 1973.

Watkin, D. Logical bases for action in nutrition and aging. *J. Am. Geriatr. Soc.* 26:193, 1978.

Weg, R. B. *Nutrition and the Later Years*. Los Angeles, Calif.: University of Southern California Press, 1978.

Wheeler, M. Osteoporosis. *Med. Clin. North Am.* 60:1213, 1976.

Young, R. C., and Blass, J. P. Nutrition in the aged. *Nutr. & the MD* January, 1981.

Chapter 28

NUTRITION AND DENTAL HEALTH

The health of the teeth and oral cavity can have a profound influence on the rest of the body. During infancy the types of foods that can be eaten are limited not only by the physiologic maturity of the gastrointestinal system but also by the lack of teeth. Any disease that causes pain or lesions (sores) in the mouth or loss of teeth compromises nutritional status by limiting food intake. This chapter will discuss tooth development, oral signs of dietary deficiencies, the current theories on the development of dental caries (tooth decay), and preventive dental practices.

Unlike other tissues of the body, the oral cavity is not sterile and is actually the site of the growth and multiplication of many types of microorganisms. Because of its structure and function, the oral cavity is subject to a greater variety of environmental stresses and trauma than other, more protected body tissues. The teeth and gums are exposed to recurrent physical and chemical wear by the diversity of foods in the daily diet, which vary in temperature, acidity, and texture.

Nutrition influences not only the development of the oral tissues but also their maintenance and ability to resist disease. Most susceptible to diseases of nutritional origin are the soft tissues of the mouth, including the gums, oral and labial mucosa, and tongue. Because most of these frank nutritional deficiencies have been substantially reduced over the past few decades, attention has shifted to the health and development of the teeth proper: dietary influences during development and the daily dietary effect on dental caries (tooth decay).

Tooth Development

The teeth, the hardest of all body materials, are composed of three calcified tissues: *dentin, enamel* (outer coating of the dentin), and the *cementum* (the dentin coating below the gums). The pulp of the tooth is located in the center, contains blood vessels and nerve tissue, and extends from the tooth into the jaw (Fig. 28-1). Both the enamel and the dentin are composed of a protein framework, or matrix, which becomes mineralized before the tooth erupts. This protein matrix is filled in with calcium phosphate in the form of apatite crystals. Tiny channels penetrate the bony dentin from the pulp to furnish nutrients to the outer surface of the tooth. Unfortunately, neither dentin nor enamel can regenerate or repair itself after decay or mechanical injury.

The life of a tooth can be divided into three stages: the period when the crown of the tooth is being formed and calcified in the jaw; the period when the tooth erupts and the roots grow; and the period when the mature tooth functions in the mouth [1]. Table 28-1 outlines the approximate ages corresponding to these stages. The period when the tooth is being formed and calcified in the jaw ranges from 14 weeks after conception for the first primary ("baby") teeth to age 8 to 10 years for the last permanent teeth.

FIG. 28-1. A longitudinal section through an incisor with dentin and enamel in cross section. (From M. Borysenko, et al., *Functional Histology* [2nd ed.]. Boston: Little, Brown, 1984.)

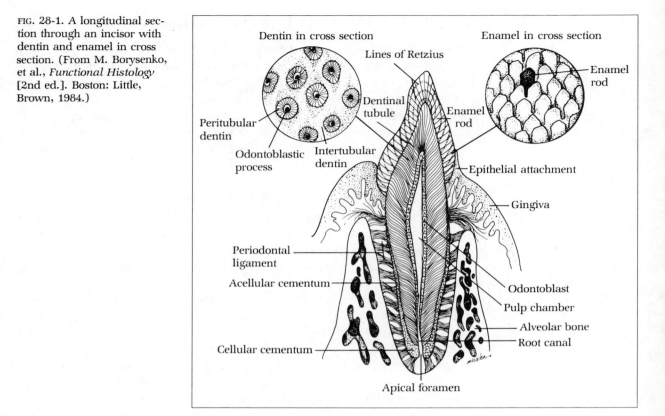

INFLUENCE OF VITAMIN DEFICIENCIES ON TOOTH DEVELOPMENT

During development, genetic factors largely determine the structure and composition of the teeth, although nutritional factors can influence and modify the process. In *vitamin A deficiency*, the enamel is hypoplastic (underdeveloped, with a decreased number of cells) and malformed, the dentin is poorly calcified, and the pulp may be infiltrated with small calcified growths. In *vitamin C deficiency*, the dentin may be irregular or missing, and weakness develops in the supporting jawbone, resulting in looseness of the teeth. *Vitamin D deficiency* leads to improper calcification of the dentin and hypoplasia of the enamel. Unlike deficiencies of vitamins A and C, there is a definite correlation between vitamin D deficiency during development and a later incidence of tooth decay.

DIETARY INFLUENCES ON TOOTH DEVELOPMENT

Although genetic and nutritional factors during development determine the structure and composition of the teeth, the oral environment and dietary conditions are powerful influences during the long period after development and maturation are complete.

A diet rich in sticky carbohydrates, especially when eaten between meals, creates conditions on the tooth surface favorable to microbial growth, which may lead to tooth decay. In addition, a deficiency of the trace element fluoride in the

TABLE 28-1. Chronology of human dentition

Tooth	Calcification begins	Crown completed	Eruption	Root completed	Root resorption begins
Primary					
I	14 wk*	4 mo	6–8 mo	1½–2 yr	5–6 yr
II	16 wk*	5 mo	8–10 mo	1½–2 yr	5–6 yr
III	17 wk*	9 mo	16–20 mo	2½–3 yr	6–7 yr
IV	15½ wk*	6 mo	12–16 mo	2–2½ yr	4–5 yr
V	18–19 wk*	10–12 mo	20–30 mo	3 yr	4–5 yr
Upper permanent					
1	3–4 mo	4–5 yr	7–8 yr	10 yr	
2	1 yr	4–5 yr	8–9 yr	11 yr	
3	4–5 yr	6–7 yr	11–12 yr	13–15 yr	
4	1½–1¾ yr	5–6 yr	10–11 yr	12–13 yr	
5	2–2½ yr	6–7 yr	10–12 yr	12–14 yr	
6	8 mo*	2½–3 yr	6–7 yr	9–10 yr	
7	2½–3 yr	7–8 yr	12–14 yr	14–16 yr	
8	7–9 yr	12–16 yr	17–30 yr	18–25 yr	
Lower permanent					
1	3–4 mo	4–5 yr	6–7 yr	9 yr	
2	3–4 mo	4–5 yr	7–8 yr	10 yr	
3	4–5 mo	6–7 yr	10–11 yr	12–14 yr	
4	1¾–2 yr	5–6 yr	10–12 yr	12–13 yr	
5	2¼–2½ yr	6–7 yr	11–12 yr	13–14 yr	
6	8 mo	2½–3 yr	6–7 yr	9–10 yr	
7	2½–3 yr	7–8 yr	12–13 yr	14–15 yr	
8	8–10 yr	12–16 yr	17–30 yr	18–25 yr	

*In utero (average).
Source: A. M. Rudolph, *Pediatrics* (16th ed.). New York: Appleton-Century-Crofts, 1977. P. 934.

diet may result in increased tooth decay. Fluoride is probably the most important dietary factor influencing dental health today.

Oral Signs of Dietary Deficiencies

Because the cells of the oral tissues undergo such rapid turnover, they require a continuous supply of essential nutrients. Oral signs can therefore give an early indication of dietary insufficiencies. (See Chaps. 11 and 34 for more detail.) The following oral signs are most commonly seen, although they are often present in conjunction with other clinical (physical) signs.

MUCOSAL SIGNS

Inflammation of the mucosa of the lips (cheilitis) or at the corners of the mouth (angular stomatitis) are signs of deficiencies of riboflavin, niacin, pyridoxine, folic acid, iron, vitamin B_{12}, or protein. Deficiencies of niacin or tryptophan may manifest as severely inflamed oral mucosa, occasionally with grayish-green patches. White ulcers with red borders are seen in folic acid or vitamin B_{12} deficiency.

GLOSSAL (TONGUE) SIGNS

A reddened, swollen tongue and increased salivation is indicative of niacin deficiency. Riboflavin deficiency results in a deep red coloring of the tongue. When only the tip and edges are reddened, sprue or a deficiency of one of the B vitamins should be suspected. A shiny, smooth tongue, indicative of papillary atrophy, is a sign of protein, iron, or vitamin B–complex deficiency. An early sign of vitamin B_{12} deficiency is a burning sensation, which is probably due to nerve irritation.

GINGIVAL (GUM) SIGNS

A deficiency of niacin makes the gingivae more susceptible to bacterial infection. Gingivitis (inflammation of the gums) is an inflammatory response to plaque (a film produced by carbohydrates and bacteria). Gingivitis leads to destruction of the connective tissue and bone that support the teeth and eventual loss of teeth. A lack of vitamin C, vital to collagen formation, leads to defects in the capillary walls, with resultant bleeding and loose teeth.

Dental Caries
DEVELOPMENT OF TOOTH DECAY

It has been estimated that the average 15-year-old has 10 decayed, filled, or missing teeth and that $6 billion is spent annually in the United States to repair the damage caused by dental caries [2]. The susceptibility of a tooth to decay is influenced by genetic and nutritional factors active during its development and beyond. Poor diet and dental hygiene will weaken the teeth, lowering their ability to resist decay.

The mouth contains more than 60 different varieties of bacteria, some of which are vital for the maintenance of general health by virtue of their ability to produce protective antibodies. Some bacteria adhere to the surface of the tooth enamel, producing a sticky polysaccharide by-product. In combination with carbohydrates such as sucrose, these bacteria and their products form *dental plaque* over a period of days. This film on the tooth surface creates an ideal environment for the development of dental caries by attracting carbohydrates and promoting their breakdown. The fermentation of sugars by bacteria present in dental plaque produces organic acids (e.g., lactic acid). These end products of glycolysis (carbohydrate breakdown) cause the surface enamel of the tooth to dissolve, creating a cavity. Other bacterial products, especially proteases (enzymes that break down proteins) carry the cavity deeper through the enamel and dentin. Carbohydrates in the form of starch (e.g., in rice and potatoes) are much less likely than sucrose to promote tooth decay because they are cleared from the mouth before being broken down to simple sugars.

STREPTOCOCCUS MUTANS

One type of organism found predominantly in developing plaque is *Streptococcus mutans*, a bacterium stimulated to multiply by the ingestion of sucrose and implicated in the development of dental caries. Recent research has suggested treating tooth decay as an infectious disease caused by the specific antigen *S. mutans* [3]. The human oral cavity, specifically dental plaque, is the only natural habitat for this organism. *S. mutans* is not found in children's mouths before teeth erupt, nor is it present after the complete loss of teeth [4]. *S. mutans* can metabolize many different types of carbohydrates, which explains its capacity to respond to a variety of foods. Plaque from carious (decayed) sites has been shown to contain a much higher concentration of these bacteria than does plaque from other sites, and *S. mutans* from carious sites is able to metabolize sucrose to lactic acid faster [5]. Such research suggests that *S. mutans* has a key role in caries formation.

Several treatments designed to suppress or modify *S. mutans* infections have been suggested. The topical application of an iodine solution to the teeth has been shown to reduce levels of these bacteria in plaque [6]. It has also been suggested that by allowing the host to be colonized by nonvirulent (non-caries-producing) strains of *S. mutans*, which have a reduced ability to produce acid from carbohydrates, bacterial infections could be controlled [7]. In another study the production of salivary antibodies was induced by the ingestion of capsules containing nonviable (nonliving) *S. mutans* [8]. Although still in the experimental stages, these treatments may be used in the future to suppress cariogenic bacteria.

NURSING-BOTTLE CARIES SYNDROME

Also known as baby-bottle caries, nursing-bottle caries syndrome is the name for rampant caries in children aged 1 to 4 years. When the child is pacified at bedtime with a bottle of sweet liquid (milk, fruit juice, sugar water, soda, sweetened tea), the teeth are continuously bathed by carbohydrates. The combination of a decreased salivary flow during sleep and the presence of carbohydrate results in decay of the erupted teeth. The tongue may or may not protect the lower front teeth. If the parents consider it necessary to put the baby to sleep with a bottle, water or just a safe pacifier (one with an adequate mouth guard to prevent it from accidentally being swallowed) could be used.

Preventive Dental Practices

Fluoride is a trace element recognized as an essential dietary nutrient by the Food and Nutrition Board of the National Research Council and as an essential mineral by the U.S. Food and Drug Administration (FDA).

Fluoride is found in almost all foods, the individual levels proportionate to the level of fluoride in the available water. Although water is the major dietary source, fluoride is also found in considerable amounts in seafoods (particularly fish with small, edible bones) and tea.

Fluoride's main action as a dental nutrient is to make teeth more caries resistant. Fluoride displaces some of the calcium phosphate crystals of apatite during tooth formation to form fluoroapatite, which is less soluble in acid and is more resistant to cariogenic factors. The acid destruction of the tooth enamel is also much slower when it contains fluoride. Fluoride is concentrated in dental plaque and interferes with the attachment of plaque to the teeth. Fluoride may also act by inhibiting certain enzymes that promote caries formation and the growth of oral bacteria that act on carbohydrates.

FLUORIDATION OF WATER

Currently, fluoridation of public drinking water is the simplest, most effective, and least expensive preventive health measure for dental caries. Fluoride is naturally present in drinking water, particularly deep artesian well water, but this varies by geographic location. In the Southwest it is present in very high levels, whereas in the Northeast it is detected only in trace amounts. *Fluoridation* redistributes this natural trace element according to medical and scientific guidelines. Epidemiologic studies comparing a number of cities have shown that the incidence of tooth decay varies inversely with the fluoride content of the drinking water. A level of 1 part per million (ppm) of fluoride (1 mg per liter = 1 ppm) has been agreed upon as the optimal concentration to prevent dental caries without risk of excessive fluoride intake. This level of fluoridation has been estimated to prevent dental caries by up to 65 percent [9]. Research has shown that fluoridation of water can reduce the professional time needed for children's dental care by 50 percent [10].

The World Health Organization, the National Cancer Institute, the Centers for Disease Control, and the National Heart, Lung and Blood Institute have each concluded that there is no evidence linking fluoride to cancer or to any other ill effects or symptoms.

FLUORIDE TREATMENTS

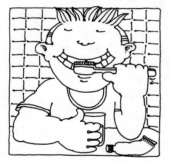

Only about 60 percent of Americans using public water supplies consume fluoridated water. In areas where fluoridation has not been adopted, alternative fluoride sources are available.

Since adult teeth are developing in the newborn infant, fluoride intake should begin as soon as possible. Studies have shown that daily fluoride supplements, starting from birth, are even more effective than fluoridated water or topical fluoride treatments in the reduction of dental caries [11]. Exposure of developing teeth to high concentrations of fluoride (greater than 2.5 ppm, or 2.5 mg per day) may result in *fluorosis* of the enamel [12]. This adverse effect, characterized by mottled, roughened, or stained enamel, is not seen when overexposure occurs after the teeth have erupted. At recommended levels, fluoridation does not cause mottling. If supplements are to be given, however, investigators suggest that a low dose (1 mg/day) of fluoride be given from birth to age 3 and that after age 5 or 6 the dose be increased beyond 1 mg per day [13].

Up to 10 times more fluoride is absorbed by enamel that has been partially demineralized by decay than by healthy enamel; this helps to retard the growth of the cavity. Therefore continued use of fluoride remains beneficial even in adulthood. Topical application may help teeth fight bacteria and make the enamel more resistant to acid.

An expert panel of the FDA states that dentifrices (toothpastes) containing sodium fluoride, sodium monofluorophosphate, or stannous fluoride are safe and effective cavity fighters [14]. They also recommend rinses and gels containing fluoride, provided they do not contain more than 120 mg total fluorine and have child-resistant caps.

Recommendations for Promoting Dental Health

1. The prenatal diet should be adequate in all respects, with special attention to vitamins A, C, and D; calcium; and phosphorus.
2. The available drinking water should contain 1.0 to 1.2 ppm fluoride; if more than 2 ppm is present, alternate sources of drinking water should be sought.
3. Sticky, high-sucrose foods and between-meal snacks should be avoided.
4. Foods that have a cleansing action on dental plaque, such as raw fruit and vegetables, should be encouraged.
5. Brushing and flossing after meals to remove dental plaque and regular dental checkups are healthful habits.
6. Overall optimal nutritional status is important for continued dental health and for general health.

References

1. Burton, B. T. *Human Nutrition* (3rd ed.). New York: McGraw-Hill, 1976. P. 226.
2. Sanders, H. J. Tooth decay. *Chemical Engineering News*, pp. 30–42, Feb. 25, 1980.
3. Loesche, W. J. Chemotherapy of dental plaque infections. *Oral Sci. Rev.* 9:65, 1976.
4. Schachtele, C. F. Bacteria, diet and the prevention of dental caries: I. *Contemp. Nutr.* 5:7, 1980.
5. Maryanski, J. H., and Wittenberger, C. L. Mannitol transport in *Streptococcus mutans. J. Bacteriol.* 124:1475, 1975.
6. Caufield, P. W., and Gibbons, R. J. Suppression of *Streptococcus mutans* in the mouths of humans by a dental prophylaxis and topically applied iodine. *J. Dent. Res.* 58:1317, 1979.
7. Hillman, J. D. Lactate dehydrogenase mutants of *Streptococcus mutans*: Isolation and preliminary characterization. *Infect. Immun.* 21:206, 1978.
8. McGhee, J. R., et al. Induction of secretory antibodies in humans following ingestion of *Streptococcus mutans. Adv. Exp. Biol. Med.* 107:177, 1978.
9. U.S. Department of Health, Education and Welfare, Public Health Service, Center for Disease Control. *Preventing Diseases, Promoting Health, Objectives for the Nation: Fluoridation.* Atlanta: Centers for Disease Control, 1979. P. 17.
10. Ast, D. B., et al. Time and cost factors to provide regular, periodic dental care for children in a fluoridated and nonfluoridated area: Final report. *J. Am. Dent. Assoc.* 80:770, 1970.
11. Aasenden, R., and Peebles, T. C. Effects of fluoride supplementation from birth on human deciduous and permanent teeth. *Arch. Oral Biol.* 19:321, 1974.
12. Toxic effects of fluoride in enamel formation. *Nutr. Rev.* 34:311, 1976.
13. Aasenden, R., and Peebles, T. C. Effects of fluoride supplementation from birth on dental caries and fluorosis in teenaged children. *Arch. Oral Biol.* 23:111, 1978.
14. Hecht, A. Brushing and rinsing to prevent cavities. *FDA Consum.* 14:22, 1980.

Suggested Readings

Alfono, M. C. Dental caries: The nature of the problem. *Cereal Foods World* 26:5, 1981.
Collier, D. R. Fluorine: An essential element for good dental health. *Contemp. Nutr.* 4:10, 1979.
Eklund, S. A., and Striffler, D. F. Anticaries effect of various concentrations of fluoride in drinking water: Evaluation of empirical evidence. *Pub. Health Rep.* 95:486, 1980.
Evaluation of the caries-producing ability of human foods. *Nutr. Rev.* 36:249, 1978.

Hefferen, J. J., and Volpe, T.   Foods, nutrition, and dental health program. *Cereal Foods World* 26:26, 1981.

Hewetson, J. M.   Diet and the control of dental disease in normal children: Practical applications. *J. Hum. Nutr.* 33:111, 1979.

Hume, W. R., and Sognnaes, R. F.   Diet and dental health. *Nutr. & MD* June, 1980.

Isman, R.   Fluoridation: Strategies for success. *Am. J. Pub. Health* 71:717, 1981.

Johnson, N. W.   Aetiology of dental disease and theoretical aspects of dietary control. *J. Hum. Nutr.* 33:98, 1979.

Mandel, I. D.   Dental caries. *Am. Sci.* 67:680, 1979.

Nizel, A. E.   *Nutrition in Preventive Dentistry: Science and Practice.* Philadelphia: Saunders, 1981.

Seventh Annual Marabou Symposium: Prevention of major dental disorders. *Nutr. Rev.* 38:134, 1980.

Stookey, G. K.   Reducing the caries potential of cereal products. *Cereal Foods World* 26:10, 1981.

Chapter 29

OBESITY AND LEANNESS

Although sleek and trim have traditionally been the ideal in American society, obesity is present in epidemic proportions. An estimated 20 percent of all adults in the United States are overweight to the extent that it interferes with health and longevity. This figure jumps to about 35 percent after age 40 [1]. Americans spend too much time eating and not enough time being physically active.

In addition to the discomfort and inconvenience, many diseases are caused or aggravated by obesity. These diseases include high blood pressure (hypertension), heart disease, gallbladder and liver disease, osteoarthritis, and diabetes, some of which may shorten the life span.

Overweight *may not* necessarily be synonymous with unhealthy. An athlete who is very muscular may be above his ideal weight for his height without being overweight or obese. Conversely, a person who is within his ideal weight range may have an excess accumulation of fat.

Obesity is a public health problem affecting 10 to 40 percent of school-aged children. An estimated 80 percent of obese children become obese adults [2]. Children of obese parents may themselves become obese because they eat the same foods and practice the same eating habits as their parents.

Definitions and Assessment

Obesity is a condition in which there is excessive deposition of body fat. A person who is 20 percent above his or her ideal weight for height and sex is *overweight*; a deviation of 50 percent is indicative of *obesity*. A person who is 100 pounds or more overweight is considered to be *morbidly obese*.

The degree of obesity can be evaluated by assessing the proportion of fat in the total body weight. For a normal male, about 12 percent of the total body weight is fat, and levels above 20 percent indicate obesity. For normal females, about 26 percent is normally fat, and more than 30 percent represents obesity [3]. Total body fat can be determined indirectly by measuring body density, total body water, or total potassium; however, these techniques are costly and not readily available. A practical, although less accurate, assessment of body fat can be made from measurements of skinfold thickness. Skinfold calipers (see Fig. 29-1) actually measure the amount of fat present below the skin (subcutaneous adipose tissue). It is recommended that measurements be made at four sites [3]:

1. Triceps, at a point equidistant from the tip of the acromion (tip of shoulder) and the olecranon (tip of elbow)
2. Subscapular, just below the tip of the inferior angle of the scapula (shoulder blades)
3. Biceps, at the midpoint of the muscle with the arm hanging vertically
4. Suprailiac, over the iliac crest (the hip bones) in line with the nipples

FIG. 29-1. Skinfold calipers.

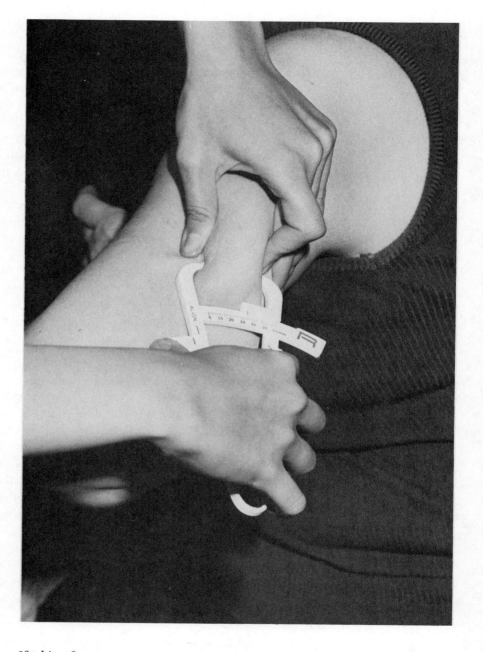

If taking four measurements is impractical, the measurement over the triceps is most useful. Obesity standards using the triceps skinfold thickness are given in Table 29-1. Other methods for assessing degree of obesity include the body weight for height and sex and weight charts defining obesity as those who exceed mean values by more than two standard deviations (see Chap. 22).

The obese state may be caused by a variety of factors. *Simple* or *developmental*

TABLE 29-1. Minimum triceps skinfold thickness indicating obesity in Caucasian Americans

Age (years)	Thickness (mm)	
	Males	Females
5	12	14
6	12	15
7	13	16
8	14	17
9	15	18
10	16	20
11	17	21
12	18	22
13	18	23
14	17	23
15	16	24
16	15	25
17	14	26
18	15	27
19	15	27
20	16	28
21	17	28
22	18	28
23	18	28
24	19	28
25	20	29
26	20	29
27	21	29
28	22	29
29	22	29
30–50	23	30

Source: C. C. Selzer and J. Mayer, *Postgrad. Med.* 38:A101, 1965.

obesity is the cumulative result of positive energy balance: the intake of more calories than are expended. The factors regulating energy balance are varied and complex, as discussed in Control of Appetite and Hunger, below. Psychogenic (psychological) factors are being recognized as more important in evaluating overweight and obese persons and planning appropriate therapy. *Emotional* or *reactive obesity* may be caused by overeating in response to tension, life situations, or an underlying emotional illness (e.g., depression or addiction to food). For a child in a home situation that offers little emotional security, food may be used as a substitute for the needed love. Heredity has also been considered in the development of obesity. A familial tendency to gain weight may be related to familial eating habits; its result is *acquired obesity*.

Society in general places a negative connotation on fatness, giving a high degree of importance to physical attractiveness. Overeating is often judged as poor impulse control, and gluttony is one of the seven deadly sins [4]. The medical profession also frequently exhibits this prejudice against the obese. In an article discussing the hazards of obesity in surgery, Bendezu and coworkers stated that ". . . the alternative (to surgical treatment for obesity) is to declare morbid obesity a just punishment for those who cannot control their eating and allow them to develop the complications that all recognize as diseases and to pay for the care of these complications" [5].

Control of Appetite and Hunger
PHYSIOLOGIC

The feeling of *hunger* consists of a series of brief cramping sensations in the area of the stomach, often accompanied by a gradual feeling of weakness and even irritability. The regulation of food intake is controlled by a mechanism beyond the stomach and hunger pains, since the desire to eat remains even after partial or total gastrectomy (removal of the stomach) or the severing of all nerves to the stomach. The gastric hunger sensation is a powerful stimulus for the initiation of eating, but it does not regulate the amount eaten at one time, since hunger pains cease soon after eating begins.

Experiments have shown that the intake of food is controlled by an area of the brain at the base of the brain stem, the *hypothalamus*. Two parts of the hypothalamus seem to be particularly important: the ventromedial hypothalamus (VMH) and the lateral hypothalamus (LH). Pathologic lesions in humans in the VMH may cause extreme overeating (hyperphagia) and abnormal obesity. This condition has been duplicated in laboratory animals by destroying the VMH. In contrast, lesions in the LH, in both humans and animals, cause a lowering of the desire to eat (anorexia) and eventual starvation. From such studies the VMH has been termed the *satiety center* and the LH the *appetite center*. It has been postulated that receptor cells in the VMH and LH are sensitive to blood levels of various nutrients, including carbohydrates, fats, and proteins. When the blood levels of these nutrients, particularly glucose, are low, the receptor cells of the LH are stimulated, triggering the appetite; when the levels are high, the VMH is signaled, indicating satiety. Many other factors, such as social customs, conscious or unconscious emotional drives, habits, and even environment (external signals), may override these involuntary regulatory mechanisms (internal signals).

PSYCHOLOGICAL

Many factors related to appetite are psychological, based on past memories and experiences that may date back to early childhood. Memories of early food experiences often determine likes and dislikes and food patterns that are not necessarily based on any logic. Food habits established in childhood, including quantity and quality of food, are often carried over into adulthood.

When adequate emotional gratification in the form of love and affection is received along with satisfaction of the physical needs for food, the growing child is likely to develop a positive attitude toward food and food intake. Disorders of appetite may stem from unconscious inner conflicts. For example, the adolescent who feels rejected by the peer group may seek solace in oral gratification and establish a pattern of overeating. An adult seeking acceptance and recognition may channel his frustration into overeating. Such oral gratification can decrease tension, anxiety, frustration, and dissatisfaction. Any weight reduction regimen should take these psychological factors into account. For long-term, lasting success at weight reduction, the overweight person must recognize the true reasons for his or her overindulgence in food.

Psychological problems may also manifest themselves as a desire not to eat, *psychogenic hypophagia*. A person who fails to attain love and recognition may feel isolated and depressed and lose the desire to eat (anorexia). *Anorexia nervosa*, self-induced starvation, is an extreme example of this condition, and is thought to be the physical manifestation of unresolved psychological conflicts (see Chap. 34).

Other factors in childhood may also leave their mark. A child raised in an atmosphere in which food is scarce and fought over is more likely to grow up with attitudes of suspicion and doubt, even when food supplies are plentiful. Food habits are formed during childhood, with children most often imitating the adults. Among the factors that ultimately mold adult habits are social and family traditions; ethnic, cultural, and religious patterns; and economic necessity. Agricultural factors also play a part in determining the availability, and therefore choice, of foods. Although modern agricultural technology and methods of transportation have made a wide variety of foods available throughout the world, many traditions are still followed: wheat remains the food staple of the United States, corn of Mexico, and rice of China.

Development of Obesity in Childhood

Many studies have shown that early nutrition has an important role in determining whether or not an infant or child will develop obesity later in life. Some investigators have found a strong correlation between adult obesity and obesity during childhood [6, 7]. Overnutrition during infancy, with its resultant obesity in childhood and adulthood, may be the direct product of bottle-feeding, early introduction of solid foods, and early weaning. Conversely, breast-feeding, delayed introduction of solid foods, and demand feeding (allowing the infant to set the amount of food consumed) are possible ways to prevent overfeeding and consequent obesity. Other researchers have suggested that significant correlations between childhood and adult weights do not occur until about age 5 [8].

PATHOGENESIS

One of the effects of overfeeding during infancy is an increase in the number (hyperplasia) of fat cells. The total number of fat cells is greater in children who were obese by age 1 year and in adults who were obese from childhood than in adults who became obese after puberty. Eighty percent of obese children become obese adults [9]. There appears to be a critical period of development between birth and age 5 when childhood weight shows a strong correlation with adult

FIG. 29-2. This baby looks healthy enough, but a health practitioner might recognize as an undesirable traditional practice this mother's determination to overfeed her baby. (World Health Organization photo by E. Schwab.)

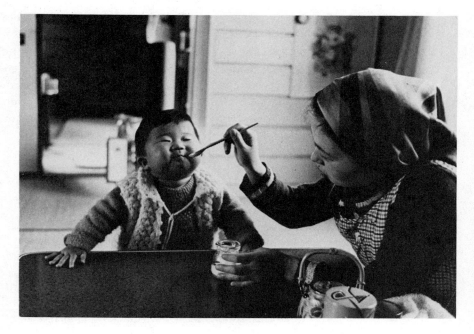

weight; peaks for the onset of juvenile obesity occur at age 4 and between ages 7 and 11 (Fig. 29-2) [9].

The number of fat cells increases steadily during the first 9 months of life. After this time there is a plateau with only slight increases until about age 7 when the number of fat cells increases again. The final increase occurs during adolescence. By adulthood, the number of fat cells appears to be relatively fixed, and alterations are mediated by changes in the lipid content of individual fat cells. Studies have shown that nutritional experiences during infancy and childhood can permanently change the number of fat cells, but once the adult number of fat cells is attained, it cannot be altered by nutritional means. Thus, the prevention of adult obesity, with its myriad health problems, is best achieved by preventing juvenile obesity.

RECOMMENDATIONS

The following recommendations are part of the nutrition education program of Weight Watchers International, Inc., designed to foster good eating habits for all segments of the population [10]:

For the first year of life

1. Do not insist that baby finish every bottle.
2. Do not worry if your baby refuses or sleeps through a feeding.
3. Do not use formula to quiet baby every time he cries.
4. Do not mistake thirst for hunger.
5. Do not start your baby on solid foods before your doctor suggests it.
6. Do not compare your baby with neighbors' babies.

For the overweight baby

1. Remember that for fat babies, unlike fat adults, the goal is not weight reduction.
2. Read baby food labels carefully and become generally familiar with caloric content.
3. Offer water between feedings to satisfy sucking and thirst needs.
4. Try to increase baby's activity.

For the toddler and young child

1. Remember how much less children eat than adults.
2. Do not insist your child eat everything on the plate.
3. Do not worry if your child's appetite falls off.
4. Do not offer dessert as a reward for finishing the main course.
5. Keep junk food out of the house. No one needs it.
6. Remember that children have a more acute sense of taste than adults.

For the overweight child or adolescent

1. Prepare meals that can be eaten by the overweight child and the rest of the family too.
2. Learn to prepare attractive yet calorie-controlled foods.
3. Serve meals in measured out portions rather than family style.
4. See that high calorie foods are not accessible.
5. Accentuate the positive.

Consequences of Obesity

The adult human body is designed by nature to function best within a narrow range of weight. The heart, skeleton, and even the amount of hormones produced by the various endocrine glands are geared to support the adult frame with deviations of only a few percent [11]. When burdened with excessive weight, adaptive changes occur in almost every body system, resulting in decreased efficiency or accelerated wear. Eventually, the cumulative effect of all these changes is a shortened life span.

RESPIRATORY PROBLEMS

Excess fat accumulates on the chest wall, actually making it difficult to breathe. Without adequate passage of air through the lungs, the blood does not receive sufficient oxygen. As a result of this, the body's tissues become deprived of oxygen, causing the obese person to tire easily. The lack of oxygen and buildup of carbon dioxide also cause lethargy and sleepiness. In an attempt to compensate for low oxygen in the blood, more red blood cells are produced, making the blood thicker and more likely to clot (that is, thrombosis may develop).

CARDIOVASCULAR PROBLEMS

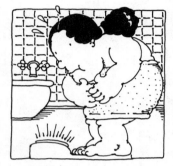

Although the two main conditions underlying the development of heart disease, hardening of the arteries (atherosclerosis) and high blood pressure (hypertension), are not limited to overweight persons, they are aggravated by obesity and usually improve with weight loss. Overweight persons tend to have elevated levels of fatty substances in their blood (see Chap. 40 for more detail). These substances are deposited in the inner lining of arteries, causing the walls to thicken, harden, weaken, and become narrow. Every artery in the body is susceptible to these changes, but the most important ones are the coronary arteries, which supply blood to the heart tissue itself, and those supplying the brain and kidneys. As the coronary arteries become more and more constricted, supplying less than the needed amount of blood to the heart tissue, pain (angina pectoris) results. If the coronary arteries become completely occluded (blocked), a heart attack (myocardial infarction) may result. Occlusions in arteries supplying the brain may result in stroke and paralysis; occlusions in those to the kidney may produce kidney damage.

Blood pressure tends to become elevated with an increase in body weight, although the exact mechanism is not known. Each pound of fat tissue is supplied with about two miles of extra blood vessels. Therefore, for each pound of fat, the heart must pump blood additional miles. Besides having a greater distance over which to pump blood, overweight persons have a greater volume of blood than do persons of normal weight. Both of these factors cause the heart to work harder with every beat. When atherosclerosis and hypertension are both present, the risk of myocardial infarction, stroke, and kidney damage is greatly increased. With a reduction in weight, the level of the fatty substances (and their accompanying risks) are lowered.

In addition to hypertension, the burden of obesity can have other effects on the heart. It enlarges and weakens, and its pumping becomes less effective. Because it cannot correctly circulate the body fluids, some collect in the lungs and other parts of the body (edema). When the heart becomes very weak and ineffective, it eventually fails (congestive heart failure).

DIABETES

The hormone insulin, which is produced by the pancreas, acts as a carrier of carbohydrate into cells all over the body. The carbohydrate is then used as energy by the cells or stored for use later. Diabetes results when there is an insufficient supply of insulin. With obesity, there is not enough insulin produced to supply all the extra cells, and glucose builds up in the blood. Eventually the glucose is lost by excretion (glycosuria). This condition is four times as prevalent in overweight persons as in those of normal weight. With weight loss and proper diet, diabetes can often be brought under control without the use of medication.

GYNECOLOGIC PROBLEMS

As with diabetes, obesity causes other hormonal imbalances in the body. These may manifest as irregular menstrual cycles, problems with fertility, and even excessive growth of facial and body hair. If an obese woman does become pregnant, she is at greater risk of developing complications, including preeclampsia (a hypertensive condition of pregnancy) and of requiring surgical (cesarean) delivery. The infant of an overweight mother runs a greater risk of being low birth weight, since a larger proportion of the mother's prenatal diet is used to maintain her own body tissues. All of these problems improve with weight loss, although it should only be attempted *before* conception.

OSTEOARTHRITIS

As stated earlier, the skeletal system is designed to support the muscles and organs of the human body within a narrow weight range. Although osteoarthritis, the degeneration of joint cartilage by wear, is considered to be part of the normal aging process, it is accelerated and aggravated by the physical burden of obesity. As the cartilage is worn down, the bones enlarge and do not fit together properly, which causes pain with movement. In overweight persons the most commonly affected joints are those that bear weight: the ankles, knees, and hips. Again, with weight reduction, this condition usually improves.

SKIN CONDITIONS

Because of the additional body weight, certain areas on the obese person's body undergo excessive friction and perspire excessively. This often results in painful skin irritation and inflammation. *Striae*, stretch marks or streaks, are often seen on the upper thigh and abdomen, the result of stretching and rupture of the elastic fibers in the skin. In addition, some hormonally induced skin problems are more prevalent in the obese.

SURGICAL RISKS

Most physicians recommend that the obese lose weight before any nonemergency surgical procedure. As discussed earlier, fat tissue has a rich blood supply, and the more that must be cut through, the more bleeding occurs and the more complex the operation becomes. In addition, the overweight person requires more anesthetic, adding to the possibility of respiratory and cardiac problems that can occur during surgery. Because fatty tissue does not heal well, there is a greater risk of wound infection and poor healing.

Treatment of Obesity

The treatment of obesity is at once the simplest and yet most complex of all disorders: simple in that, in the adult, all that is required is caloric restriction, and complex in that cellular, metabolic, socioeconomic, cultural, and psychological factors all militate against the maintenance of the reduced state. Unfortunately, in our society only the weight reduction period is emphasized and the obese subject is exposed to an endless variety of weight reduction programs, which include diets, drugs, hormones, hypnosis, psychotherapy, and surgical intervention . . . . This preoccupation of both the lay and medical community with weight loss alone has fostered the neglect of the post-reduction period, which is in fact the more difficult problem. Thus most obese subjects live in a vicious cycle of weight loss followed by weight gain, ad infinitum, going from one "cure" to another in search of a magic formula [9].

No one program will be effective for everyone, and the overweight individual should work with a nutritionist or physician in finding an appropriate regimen.

Meal patterns should be balanced and promote wise food choices. A program that provides protein, minerals, vitamins, and fiber without promoting excessive ketosis (accumulation of the products of fat breakdown) or undue hunger is acceptable. The planned diet should also take into account the degree of obesity: A balanced diet deficient only in calories is best for the person 30 percent or less overweight; a medically supervised protein-sparing fast may produce better results for the person 30 to 60 percent overweight; surgical therapy may be needed for the person 100 lb or more overweight. Just as it took time to acquire the additional weight, it takes time to shed it. Successful weight reduction regimens should include plans for immediate weight loss and the long-term maintenance of desired weight. Any weight reduction program will be short-lived if not followed by supportive therapy tailored to the tastes and life-style of the individual.

BEHAVIOR MODIFICATION

Everyone's food choices at one time or another are influenced more by external signals (surroundings, psychological state, social situation, the sight or smell of food nearby) than by internal signals (the normal appetite and hunger mechanisms). For the obese, the external signals may be operating most of the time, resulting in chronic overeating. Programs based on behavior modification try to determine why, when, where, and how much is eaten each day, in an attempt to educate the dieter to the external signals to which he or she is listening. Part of behavior modification may be to keep a food diary for a period of time, with the date, time, place, type of food, and amount eaten recorded, as well as the reason and emotional state. In this way dieters can learn what causes them to eat when—for example, perhaps a dieter eats sweets while watching television late at night, or has an ice cream sundae every afternoon on the way home from work. In combination with a balanced dieting regimen, behavior modification can be of great value in both immediate weight reduction and long-term maintenance.

LOW CALORIE DIETS

When based on a balanced variety of food, low calorie diets are the best method of weight reduction for most people. They have been used with success to lose a few or scores of pounds when part of a program of nutritional guidance, education, and supportive therapy. Many weight-reduction diets have been devised, some based on the inclusion or exclusion of specific foods or nutrients to "turn on" "fat-burning" mechanisms in the body. While some weight reduction may be achieved through water loss, the dietary imbalances produced by long-term dieting on such regimens can be very hazardous to your health. A comparison of some popular reducing diets is given in Table 29-2.

SEMISTARVATION KETOGENIC (FAT-MOBILIZING) REGIMENS

Although total fasting reduces hunger and induces rapid weight loss, lean body tissue accounts for one-third to one-half of the weight lost [12]. The loss of protein can be controlled by supplementation with dietary protein. Weight loss in excess of 40 pounds has been achieved with this method under close medical

TABLE 29-2. Some popular reducing diets

Type	Rationale	Deficiencies	Evaluation
High protein, high fat, low carbohydrate (Dr. Atkins)	To induce ketosis (burning of fat) to promote weight loss	Calories, carbohydrate, calcium, iron, vitamins A and C, thiamin, niacin, riboflavin	Unwise diet plan that may be hazardous to health
High roughage, no refined carbohydrates (Dr. Reuben)	To normalize the functioning of the gastrointestinal system	Calories, calcium, iron, niacin	Basically sound food choices; needs iron and vitamin supplementation
Weight Watchers	To assist and educate the dieter in new and sound eating habits	Calories	Wise food choices; plans for maintenance; excellent diet
Protein and water (Dr. Stillman)	To burn body fat rapidly and wash away the waste products with water	Calories, carbohydrate, calcium, vitamins A and C, thiamin	Unwise diet plan that may be hazardous to health
Grapefruit diet (Dr. Stillman)	More efficient burning of fat	Calories, carbohydrate, calcium, iron, vitamin A, thiamin, riboflavin	Unwise diet plan that may be hazardous to health

Source: Summarized from E. B. Spannhake, *Eye It Before You Diet.* Washington, D.C.: Sugar Association, 1977.

supervision [13]. This method of weight reduction does not educate the dieter to better eating habits, but it may induce enough weight loss in the moderately obese person to break the vicious cycle of dieting failure–weight gain–dieting failure. Medical supervision is essential with this regimen.

SURGERY

Surgery entails the greatest risks and the most serious complications of all the treatments for obesity. It is recommended for those 200 percent or more above their ideal weight for height and sex. Although the mortality can be as high as 11.5 percent and major complications about 50 percent, the surgical treatment of obesity provides a substantial weight loss (usually of about 30 percent of initial weight), with accompanying improvement in cardiovascular and respiratory function [14]. The surgical procedures now commonly in use include the jejunoileal (or intestinal) bypass and the gastric bypass. The principle behind the procedures is to bypass or shorten the absorptive surface of the gastrointestinal tract so that it utilizes less of what is eaten. In the first procedure, the jejunum and ileum are totally or partially bypassed; in the second, the stomach is. Both procedures have complications and risks, and the choice is mainly up to the surgeon's judgment. Some dietary restrictions and supplementations may be necessary. The advantages and disadvantages of the gastric and intestinal bypasses are outlined in Table 29-3.

Leanness

It may seem surprising at first thought, but many of the causes of *underweight* (10 percent or more below ideal weight for height and sex) are the same as those

TABLE 29-3. Advantages and disadvantages of surgical treatments for obesity

Treatment	Disadvantages (complications)	Advantages
Gastric bypass	Concentrated sweets may cause diarrhea Possible vitamin deficiencies Ulceration Bile reflux gastritis Reflux esophagitis	Average weight loss of 20–80 kg (44–176 lb) by end of first year Improvement of orthopedic conditions Lowered cholesterol levels Improved fertility and menstrual cycles for women Improved quality of life Improved psychological status
Intestinal bypass or shunt	Diarrhea (can be controlled with diet and medication) Possible liver failure Renal stones and gallstones Vitamin deficiencies (particularly B_{12} and D) Hypokalemia Hypomagnesemia	All of the above; average weight loss is greater than with gastric bypass Simpler operation than gastric bypass

Source: M. M. Cegielski and J. A. Saporta, Surgical treatment of massive obesity: Current status of the art. *Obesity/Bariatric Medicine* 7:156, 1978.

for obesity. Abnormalities of the appetite and satiety centers (internal signals) may exist, and metabolic and psychological factors may be involved. Childhood experiences, as discussed earlier, may also play a role. Habits, life-style, and social activities may all reinforce the underweight state. Moderate underweight carries no severe health risks, except these persons are more prone to infections than those of normal weight, and it may even prolong the life span.

Recommendations for weight gain are the direct opposite, in some respects, of those for weight loss. Although both regimens are based on a balanced variety of foods, the regimen for weight gain is planned around the highest calorie nutritious foods with the least amount of volume. Included are liberal servings of meat, starchy vegetables, bread, desserts, and milk shakes. Between-meal snacking is sometimes encouraged to include more calories in the daily menu.

Anorexia nervosa, an extreme example of underweight, has deep psychological roots and requires special medical and diet therapy. An in-depth discussion of this condition is given in Chap. 34.

References

1. National Institutes of Health, National Institute of Arthritis, Metabolism, and Digestive Diseases. *Facts About Obesity* (HEW fact sheet). 1979.
2. Burton, B. T. *Human Nutrition* (3rd ed.). New York: McGraw-Hill, 1976. P. 234.
3. Davidson, S., et al. *Human Nutrition and Dietetics* (6th ed.). London: Churchill Livingstone, 1975. P. 288.
4. Kalisch, B. J. The stigma of obesity. *Am. J. Nurs.* 72:1124, 1972.
5. Bendezu, R., et al. Certain metabolic consequences of jejunoileal bypass. *Am. J. Clin. Nutr.* 29:366, 1976.

6. Rose, H. E., and Mayer, J.   Activity calorie intake and the energy balance of infants. *Pediatrics* 41:18, 1968.

7. Lloyd, J. K., Wolff, O. H., and Whelen, W. S.   Childhood obesity: Long term study of height and weight. *Br. Med. J. [Clin. Res.]* 2:45, 1961.

8. Wolff, O. H.   Obesity in childhood. *Q. J. Med.* 24:109, 1955.

9. Knittle, J. L.   Obesity in childhood: A problem in adipose tissue cellular development. *J. Pediatr.* 81:1048, 1972.

10. *The Fat Child—Born or Made? Thoughts on Feeding from Infancy to Adolescence.* Manhasset, N.Y.: Weight Watchers International, 1978.

11. *Overweight and Your Health—The Vital Connection.* Manhasset, N.Y.: Weight Watchers International, 1978.

12. Runcie, J., and Hilditch, T. E.   Energy provision, tissue utilization, and weight loss in prolonged starvation. *Br. Med. J.* 2:352, 1974.

13. Bistrian, B. R.   Recent developments in the treatment of obesity with particular reference to semistarvation ketogenic regimens. *Diabetes Care* 1:379, 1978.

14. Bray, G. A., et al.   Surgical treatment of obesity: A review of our experience and an analysis of published reports. *Int. J. Obes.* 1:331, 1977.

Suggested Readings

Antal, S. C., and Kovacs, Z. G.   Gastric bypass operation in morbid obesity. *Israel J. Med. Sci.* 16:672, 1980.

Birch, L. L., et al.   Mother-child interaction and the degree of fatness in children. *J. Nutr. Educ.* 13:17, 1981.

Bray, G. A. (ed.).   *Obesity: Comparative Methods of Weight Control.* Westport, Conn.: Technomic Publishing, 1980.

Bray, G. A.   "Brown" tissue and metabolic obesity. *Nutr. Today* 17:23, 1982.

Brown, E. K., Settle, E. A., and Van Rij, A. M.   Food intake patterns of gastric bypass patients. *J. Am. Dietet. Assoc.* 80:437, 1982.

Brownell, K. D., and Stunkard, A. J.   Behavioral treatment of obesity in children. *Am. J. Dis. Child.* 132:403, 1978.

Cegielski, M. M., and Saporta, J. A.   Surgical treatment of morbid obesity: An update. *Obesity Bariatr. Med.* 10:44, 1981.

Chan, J. C. M., and Bartter, F. C.   Weight reduction: Renal, mineral, and hormonal excretion during semistarvation in obese patients. *J.A.M.A.* 245:371, 1981.

Cherfas, J. J.   Signals for food: Reinforcers or informants? *Science* 209:1552, 1980.

Davis, J. D., et al.   Sustained intracerebroventricular infusion of brain fuels reduces body weight and food intake in rats. *Science* 212:81, 1981.

The development of adipose tissue in infancy. *Nutr. Rev.* 37:194, 1979.

DeWind, L. T., and Payne, J. H.   Intestinal bypass surgery for morbid obesity: Long-term results. *J.A.M.A.* 236:2298, 1976.

Effects of preweaning and postweaning nutrition on adiposity in mice. *Nutr. Rev.* 38:253, 1980.

Feig, B. K.   *Parent's Guide to Weight Control for Children Ages 5 to 13 Years.* Springfield, Ill.: Charles C Thomas, 1980.

Felig, P.   Four questions about protein diets. *N. Engl. J. Med.* 298:1025, 1978.

Fenner, L.   Cellulite: Hard-to-budge pudge. *FDA Consum.* 14:4, 1980.

Fetal and infant nutrition and susceptibility to obesity. *Am. J. Clin. Nutr.* 31:2026, 1978.

Forbes, G. B.   Is obesity a genetic disease? *Contemp. Nutr.* August, 1981.

Gardner, F. S.   Patient education for weight loss: Comparing strategies. *J. Am. Dietet. Assoc.* 80:432, 1982.

Garn, S. M.   Socioeconomic aspects of obesity. *Contemp. Nutr.* July, 1981.

Holsted, C. H., and Stern, J. S.   ASCN workshop on obesity and its treatments. Sacramento, California, October 5, 1979. *Am. J. Clin. Nutr.* 33:1326, 1980.

Jordan, H. A., et al.   Role of food characteristics in behavioral change and weight loss. *J. Am. Dietet. Assoc.* 79:24, 1981.

Langford, R. W.   Teenagers and obesity. *Am. J. Nurs.* 81:556, 1981.

Lecos, C.   Fructose: Questionable diet aid. *FDA Consum.* 14:21, 1980.

Miller, B. K.   Jejunoileal bypass: A drastic weight control measure. *Am. J. Nurs.* 81:564, 1981.

Mojzisik, C. M., and Martin, E. W.   Gastric partitioning: The latest surgical means to control morbid obesity. *Am. J. Nurs.* 81:569, 1981.

Overfeeding in the first year of life. *Nutr. Rev.* 31:116, 1973.

Reeves, J.   Estimating fatness. *Science* 204:881, 1979.

Reisin, E., and Frohlich, E. D.   Obesity: Cardiovascular and respiratory pathophysiological alterations. *Arch. Intern. Med.* 141:431, 1981.

Roundtable: Maintenance after weight loss. *Obesity Bariatr. Med.* 9:168, 1980.

Schemmel, R. (ed.).   *Nutrition, Physiology, and Obesity.* Boca Raton, Fla.: CRC Press, 1980.

Sours, H. E., et al.   Sudden death associated with very low calorie weight reduction regimens. *Am. J. Clin. Nutr.* 34:453, 1981.

Strauss, E., and Yalow, R. S.   Cholecystokinin in the brains of obese and nonobese mice. *Science* 203:68, 1979.

Stuart, R. B., and Davis, B.   *Slim Chance in a Fat World: Behavioral Control of Obesity.* Champaign, Ill.: Research Press, 1978.

Updegraff, T. A., and Neufeld, N. J.   Protein, iron, and folate status of patients prior to and following gastric bypass surgery for morbid obesity. *J. Am. Dietet. Assoc.* 78:135, 1981.

Van Itallie, T. B.   Liquid protein mayhem (editorial). *J.A.M.A.* 240:144, 1978.

Volkman, F. R., et al.   High attrition rates in commercial weight reduction programs. *Arch. Intern. Med.* 141:426, 1981.

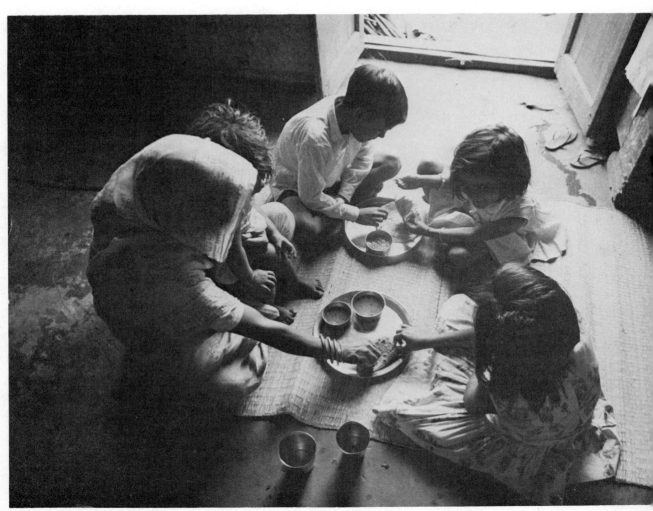

(WHO photo by P. Almasy.)

LIFE-STYLE CONSIDERATIONS

The daily diet can be viewed as a combination of nutrients needed to meet the metabolic demands of the individual. But for most of us, the food we eat represents a far wider range of values and meanings than mere nutrients. Food reflects our ethnic heritage, cultural past, economics and education, life-style factors, and even, for some, self-medication. This section deals with some of those special influences that transform the "daily diet" into a food plan unique to each individual. When planning a special diet, or modifying an existing one, the health professional must take these factors into consideration.

Chapter 30

GEOGRAPHIC AND CULTURAL VARIATION IN DIET

Beyond its nutritive, life-sustaining qualities, food has other, deeper meanings. It is a symbol of home, comfort, love, hospitality, pleasure, and security. It has religious, social, and ritual significance. Each group or culture defines what it considers to be edible and what is not. This varies greatly all over the world; for example, the Islams of Egypt would never eat the blood of an animal, yet the people of Finland bottle it and sell it as an ingredient in soup. Ants, grasshoppers, and caterpillars are considered inedible pests in the United States, but in Africa, they are delicacies. Even how one eats is culturally defined—in the Islamic countries it is proper to eat barefoot and with the right hand; such table manners would shock the British!

Cultural traditions help to unify people through a common sense of purpose, pride, dignity, and stability. It also serves as a unifying factor when separated from the homeland, such as the immigrants who came to America in the 1800s and 1900s. An understanding of the many aspects of cultural groups, including food customs, is essential for members of the health profession or any other profession that deals with a variety of people.

This chapter presents background, food groups, meal patterns, and special occasions of selected countries as well as the traditions of the major religions as they affect the diet. The countries and foods selected are only meant to be representative and not comprehensive; to cover each country would require volumes. The reference and selected readings at the end of this chapter will help direct the interested student to sources of more information.

Much of the material presented here was adapted from the book, *You Eat What You Are: A Study of Ethnic Food Traditions*, by Thelma Barer-Stein, Toronto: McClelland and Stewart, Ltd., 1979.

Africa

Africa, the second largest continent of the world, is a blend of more than 30 countries, 800 languages, and over 270 million persons. This continent has been the crossroads for travelers, explorers, and armies for thousands of years; the traditions and customs of the African people reflect this influence. Such exploring countries as France, the Netherlands, England, Spain, and Portugal have all left their mark on this subtropical territory. The urban population of Africa may still be more affected by European customs, while rural Africa has generally retained its own traditions. Africa suffers from many agricultural and technologic problems, including poor transportation methods, inadequate preservation and storage processes, poor soil, limited equipment, and shortage of trained personnel.

Fresh milk, usually from cows, goats, or sheep, is used, either plain or soured. Milk is used as part of soups or puddings, and may even be mixed with blood as a beverage.

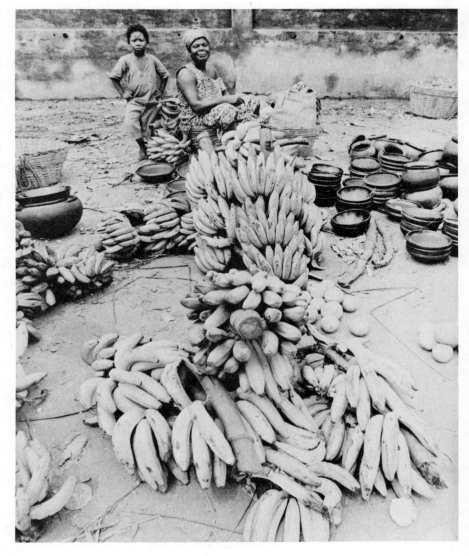

Fruits and vegetables are eaten in season. Mangoes and bananas are particularly popular (Fig. 30-1). Other tropical fruits and melons, such as figs, dates, oranges, papayas, avocados, and pineapples, are also available. Wild or cultivated vegetables in the African diet include okra, yams, corn, greens, pumpkin, plantain, cucumbers, onion, garlic, cabbage, and potatoes.

The use of meat in the daily diet is infrequent for the average rural African. Most of the meat and fowl that is available is tough and requires slow cooking with moisture, as in stews or soups. Preservation is a problem in some areas of Africa; smoking, salting, and drying are common. Cattle are frequently viewed as a sign of wealth, and therefore may not be used for food. Alternate sources of protein in the diet include black or red ants, grasshoppers, caterpillars, and mice. Along the coastal regions and near rivers and lakes, fish and seafood are eaten. A variety of legumes, nuts, and seeds are also used to supplement the protein intake.

The main starch food in the African diet is a paste made from starchy vegetables or roots and mixed with water to form a cereal. It may be made from wheat, rice, corn, millet, sorghum, or manioc, and is usually eaten with side dishes of spicy sauces. A type of yeast is made by adding sugar, water, and wheat flour to mashed ripe plantain and allowing the mixture to ferment. It acts as a leavening agent and adds a sour taste to the baked goods.

Hot and spicy seasonings and the liberal use of salt are common in African cooking. Seeds are often dried and ground into a paste and used for flavoring. Beer and wine are made locally; juices from tropical fruits are also popular.

MEAL PATTERNS

For much of rural Africa, the main meal of the day is dinner. Breakfast may consist of coffee or tea with milk or curds. Throughout the day, snacking on nuts, seeds, and fruits is common. Children are breast-fed for two years or longer, and are given a thin type of cereal after weaning. This, combined with the practice of giving the men in the family the best of the food first, results in a special type of malnutrition, kwashiorkor, among many African children (see Chap. 34, Malnutrition, for more details).

SPECIAL OCCASIONS

Although many Africans may adhere to Islam or Christianity, other, more deeply rooted traditions unique to their region may also be important. Besides the usual special occasions of birth, death, and marriage, the arrival of visitors may also be cause for celebration.

China

The Chinese culture is one of the oldest and largest on earth, dating back more than 4000 years and presently accounting for nearly one-fourth of the world's population—800 million people. China is actually a blend of many races and peoples and their foods reflect this rich cultural heritage. It is from China that we owe the development of gunpowder, porcelain, techniques of slope-terracing, the wheelbarrow, and paper money, among other things.

Many of the foods that are part of the Chinese culture were developed or brought to China thousands of years ago. Tea was first used as a medicine about 1000 B.C. and was later used as a beverage. During the period around A.D. 700, Lu Yu wrote his classic works on tea cultivation and preparation, which probably led to its acceptance as the national beverage. With the introduction of the stone roller between 1000 and 700 B.C., wheat became a popular crop in northern China. As a result, wheat flour replaced rice as the staple food and noodles, steamed buns, pastries, and dumplings became popular in the North.

The Chinese diet is based mainly on foods of plant origin. This is partially due to the large numbers of people being dependent on limited food resources—

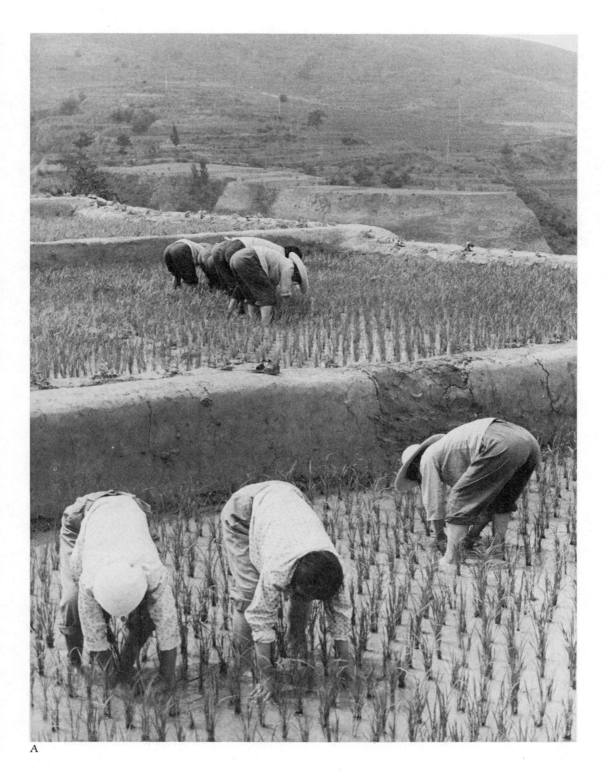

A

FIG. 30-2.
A. Hill rice paddies in the People's Republic of China. (FAO photo by H. Henle.)
B. In China, fishermen and their families are assured a balanced diet rich in protein thanks to their fishing activities and the traditional bowl of rice. (FAO photo by P. A. Pittet.)

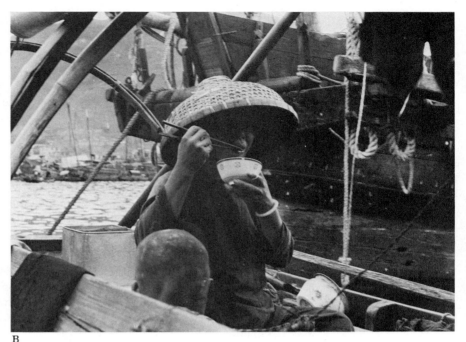

B

scarce amounts of workable land that can be used more effectively for crop cultivation than for raising livestock (Fig. 30-2A). In the South, rice is the staple food (Fig. 30-2B).

Milk and milk products have traditionally been absent from the Chinese diet, although recently ice cream has become a favorite treat in mainland China. Nondairy sources of calcium include fish and poultry bones that have become soft with slow cooking and vinegar marinade.

Fruits and vegetables are used extensively in the Chinese diet—fresh (when in season), preserved, or dried. The traditional methods of preservation are still the most popular and include pickling, salting, and drying. Unless preserved, vegetables used in menu preparation are usually very fresh. The stir-fry and steaming methods of cooking that are most frequently used not only retain color and texture, but most of the nutrients as well. The Chinese also make ingenious use of edible flower buds and petals, roots, bark, seeds, sprouts, and fungi in their cooking. Popular fruits include pears, plums, pineapples, loquats, and lichees, often as part of the main dish or used in desserts or snacks.

Meat and meat products are used sparingly due to cost and distribution limitations. Pork, beef, poultry, and fish are used, usually cut into thin strips or small cubes so they can be cooked quickly with fresh vegetables. Pork could probably be considered the staple meat of China due to its popularity. In the North, lamb and mutton are favored because sheepherding is common. Fish and poultry are often purchased live to ensure maximum freshness in preparation. Other fre-

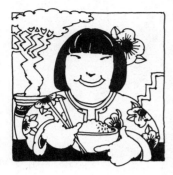

quently used protein foods include eggs (used in omelets, soups, as batters, and in custards) and soybeans. Soybeans are used in a wide variety of forms, including soy sauce, milk, spaghetti (bean thread or Chinese vermicelli), bean curd, and as a paste. Nuts and seeds, which contribute amino acids and other nutrients to dishes, are also used creatively by the Chinese.

Rice is the backbone of the Chinese diet. Steamed long-grain is used with the main meal; glutinous rice is used mostly with desserts; and rice flour is a favorite thickener for soups and sauces.

Although the amount and type may vary from region to region, the Chinese do season their dishes using a variety of condiments. Some of the more popular seasonings include fresh ginger root, sesame seeds and oil, garlic, black pepper, anise, cloves, red pepper, and combination spices such as five-spice powder (cinnamon, clove, anise, fennel, and Szechwan hot pepper).

Teas and wines are the most popular beverages.

MEAL PATTERNS

Chinese breakfast usually consists of a hot rice cereal served with side dishes and tea. Steamed noodles, steamed buns, or dumplings are more typical of a Northern breakfast. Lunch is usually a lighter version of dinner, and may range from a bowl of seasoned noodles to soup, rice, vegetables, and meat plus tea. Dinner is the main meal, often beginning with cold appetizers or soup. A variety of main dishes may be served, with each participant using chopsticks to eat directly off central platters or to place morsels on his or her own bowl of steamed rice. Preserved fruits may be served for dessert.

SPECIAL OCCASIONS

In China certain days are special occasions for specific family members only, or for an entire community. The New Year celebration is perhaps the most celebrated occasion, traditionally ushered in by family feasting, gifts of money, and visiting. The Moon Festival, centered around sacrifices to the moon for arranging marriages, is marked by giving mooncakes (round, filled pastries) and paper lanterns. Many other special occasions of the Chinese are also celebrated with foods.

England

As a general rule, Britons prefer simple foods that are well-cooked and sparsely seasoned. Meats (particularly beef and game), pork, and seafood, together with well-cooked vegetables, usually comprise the main dish. Breads, in the form of rolls, quickbreads, cakes, and pies, form a large part of the diet. Fruits are served as preserves, marmalades, and cooked desserts rather than fresh. Cheeses are favorites and are eaten before or after a meal, or as a snack.

Milk is usually served fresh with tea, creamed soups, or in puddings. Clotted cream is eaten with bread and jam at tea time. Several cheeses are produced locally, including Cheddar, Stilton, and Cheshire.

Many homes in the English countryside have small gardens which provide a variety of fruits and vegetables. Although some fruits are eaten fresh, most, such as quince, apricots, cherries, pears, and berries, are cooked and sweetened first and served as jams, preserves, marmalades, and chutneys. The most popular vegetables include potatoes, cabbage, turnips, and brussels sprouts; salads are not as well liked.

Beef (particularly steak) is used extensively in the British diet, in addition to chops, mutton, lamb, and seasonal game. Stews and sausages are also popular, as well as grilled or fried cuts. Seafood also constitutes a large portion of the typical diet, particularly batter-fried, smoked, pickled, or poached varieties. Herring, flounder, haddock, salmon, sole, oysters, crabs, and prawns are all readily available. Eggs are also used frequently, scrambled with bacon or sausage at breakfast, fried with meat for lunch, and as a component of puddings, custards, and batters.

White breads, rolls, and oatmeal are among the favorite breads and cereals of the Britons. Toast is eaten cold and spread with butter, preserves, or marmalade. Baked goods are very popular, as are sweets of all types, including pastries, hard candies, and very sweet tea.

The most frequently used spices in an English kitchen include salt and pepper, thyme, sage, rosemary, and onions. Tea is a very important beverage for the English, and it is served several times a day with milk and sugar. Draft beer is a popular beverage at local public houses, or pubs, where sandwiches and lunch platters are also served.

MEAL PATTERNS

Breakfast in England is usually tea with some type of bread or buns. A midmorning break for tea may also include bread of some sort. In the cities lunch may be taken at a local pub, and include a sandwich and draft beer or ale. Tea time usually occurs between 4 P.M. and 7 P.M., and is termed "high tea" if the accompanying food is substantial. A typical evening supper might include beef, vegetables, steamed or baked pudding, and tea.

SPECIAL OCCASIONS

Many special occasions in England are celebrated with foods and specific customs. The ancient Druid rite of bonfires and human sacrifices has been replaced by the consumption of gingerbread men while still watching roaring bonfires. In the autumn, All Soul's Eve is celebrated by households by setting out wine and buns to satisfy wandering souls. During the Lent and Easter season, simnel cakes and hot cross buns mark this occasion with special symbolism. Christmas in England is celebrated with many traditional foods, including roast goose and sausage stuffing, mince pie, flaming Christmas pudding, and rum-drenched fruit cake.

Finland

Only about 8 percent of the total land surface in Finland is fertile. This portion lies mostly along the coast, while the remainder of the country is composed of stony fields or forests. As a result, the production of crops is limited, and fish supply much of the food. Some of the principal crops include wheat, barley, oats, rye, and potatoes. The sauna, while enjoyed by the Finnish people for its pleasurable, relaxing qualities, is also used to smoke-cure ham, bacon, and lamb. Because of the short growing season, fresh produce is scarce, with the majority of the fruits and vegetables being pickled and preserved for use during the winter.

Dairy products are very popular in Finland. Milk is consumed fresh, clabbered, or as buttermilk. A wide variety of aged and unripened cheeses, cream, and sour cream are also used.

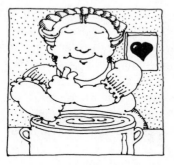

Fresh fruits and vegetables are enjoyed seasonally. Berries, such as strawberries, blueberries, raspberries, cranberries, and gooseberries, are frequently made into preserves and used with meats, as fillings in pastries, as part of puddings, tart fruit soups, or just eaten plain. The traditional vegetables, potatoes and cauliflower, are usually eaten in casseroles. Mushrooms are eaten fresh and preserved.

A wide variety of meats are included in the Finnish diet, such as beef, pork, veal, lamb, reindeer, bear, elk, and other game. Herring is the staple fish, although salmon, sardines, flounder, pike, and whitefish are also enjoyed.

Breads and whole grains are part of almost every meal in the form of porridges, baked goods, and often with berries.

Most Finns do not have a "sweet tooth," preferring the natural flavor of wholesome ingredients. A sour flavor is preferred over sweet, as evidenced by their preference for sour rye bread, soured (clabbered) milk, and tart fruits and desserts. Onion, garlic, dill, and smoked flavoring are typical seasonings. The most popular beverage is coffee, although a variety of alcoholic and nonalcoholic beverages are also enjoyed such as beer, vodka, cognac, tea, milk, and buttermilk.

MEAL PATTERNS

Breakfast in Finland may consist of coffee and a yeast bread, or meat and cheese sandwiches, or coffee alone. Lunch may be cooked cereal or a more substantial meal of meat or fish, potatoes, gravy, cheese, and bread and butter. An afternoon break provides coffee and cake or cookies, or open-faced sandwiches. Dinner may be a baked casserole of meat and potatoes served with fruit or vegetable preserves and bread and butter. An evening snack might consist of coffee and cake or cookies.

Smörgåsbord, which translates as "bread and butter table," is a buffet-type of dining, which may present as many as 60 selections at one time (such as that served at Stockholm's Operakällaren Restaurant) [1]. The first plate taken from the table is traditionally filled with herring selections. The second plate usually includes other fish dishes, such as smoked salmon and eel, and may be served with a cold cucumber and vinegar salad. Meats and salads follow on the third plate, and include such delicacies as calf's liver pâté, ham, roast beef, and assorted cold cuts with pickled onions and gherkins, and a cold salad, such as tomatoes vinaigrette. The hot dishes are served on the fourth plate, and include such selections as Swedish meatballs, hot vegetable dishes, and croquette of fowls. A dessert of cheese or fruit salad follows.

SPECIAL OCCASIONS

Most of the population of Finland are Lutheran; therefore, religious holidays are celebrated nationally. May Day marks the end of the long winter and is celebrated with special cookies and a fermented lemon drink. Easter has its own special food traditions in Finland—yeast breads, special cheeses, and puddings just for the occasion. Christmas also has its foods, including vegetable casseroles, baked hams with dried fruits, rice pudding, and special Christmas cookies.

Germany

The cuisine of Germany has been influenced by numerous other cultures in a history marked by wars and conflicts. Steak tartar and sauerkraut are just two examples of this influence, both coming from the Tartars' experiences in Mongolia and China. France and England also influenced Germany's history and culinary development. The staple foods of Germany today are pork, potatoes, black bread, beer, and sauerkraut. Germany is known for its fine beers, perhaps the best in the world.

Fresh whole milk as a beverage is used mostly by children and during pregnancy and lactation. Sour cream, milk, buttermilk, and unripened and aged cheeses are used in baking and in various recipes. Coffee is taken with canned milk. Imported cheeses are often enjoyed as a dessert, particularly after a cold meal.

Germany is known for its vineyards and fine grapes, but other fruits are also cultivated. Plums, pears, cherries, and apples are eaten fresh or made into cooked compotes or pastry fillings. Dried fruits are also widely used. The most popular vegetables include cabbage, potatoes, white asparagus, mushrooms, cauliflower, turnips, and carrots.

Pork is the favorite meat of Germany and is used as sausages, chops, or roasts. Beef, poultry, wild game, and fowl are also widely used. Sausages (würste), of all varieties, are popular. Herring, lobster, eel, flounder, and many other types of seafood are found in the German menu. Eggs are used plain or in baking and cooking. Legumes, such as peas and beans, are eaten in side dishes, soups, or one-meal dishes.

A wide variety of breads are served in Germany, ranging from the dark rye breads to white rolls and breads with salt, seeds, or wheat grains on the crusts. Hot cereals may be served for breakfast, particularly to children.

In addition to fine wines, succulent pork and potato dishes, and delectable beer, the Germans are also known for their sweets. Sugar is used liberally in coffee, fruit dishes, as a seasoning of meats, and in baked goods. Many other seasonings are also popular in Germany, including dill, caraway, sesame, poppy, onions, and garlic. As mentioned earlier, beer is the favorite beverage of Germany, although rich coffee also has an important place.

MEAL PATTERNS

Breakfast is usually a light meal of coffee with milk and sugar and bread or rolls with butter and preserves. A midmorning break might include meat or cheese sandwiches. Lunch may be the largest meal of the day, consisting of soup, a meat and vegetable dish, and dessert. A midafternoon snack of coffee and pastry is usual. Dinner may be served late and consists of soup, cold meats and cheeses, and dessert. Dining out is very popular in Germany; there are restaurants catering to various cuisines.

SPECIAL OCCASIONS

Germany contains about an equal number of Protestants and Catholics, each with their own set of special religious holidays. Other well-known national celebrations include Munich's Oktoberfest, a 16-day festival of beer, sausages, and roasted chickens, dancing, and singing. New Year's Eve is heralded in with the traditional dish of whole poached carp, with a sauce of beer, ginger, lemon, almonds, and raisins. Christmas in Germany has its own special food traditions, including rich cakes, cookies, and breads.

Greece

The birthplace of some of the world's greatest philosophy, drama, and literature, Greece today has a cultural heritage unlike that of any other country. The closeness of the Greek family and the strength of the Greek Orthodox Church are two factors behind the character of these people. From a history marked with domination and conflicts, the Greeks, and their cuisine, have managed to survive and flourish. The male and female roles are clearly defined for all but the upper classes of Greek society. Women are expected to run the household and not be concerned with outside matters, while the men have complete, unquestioned freedom. Because nearly everyone in Greece is a member of the Greek Orthodox Church, the feasts and fasts of daily life are usually religious in nature.

Yogurt and cheese are the preferred dairy foods in Greece; both are used in cooking and as snacks. Many cheeses are made fresh, ranging from unripened ones resembling cottage cheese to aged varieties that are grated. Some are used as pastry filling or in salads.

Fruits are abundant in Greece and are enjoyed fresh or preserved with thick, sweet syrup. Several unique types of melons are found in this Mediterranean country, as are grapes, figs, apricots, cherries, quinces, apples, plums, and peaches. Fresh or cooked vegetables are served with most meals; potatoes, carrots, zucchini, and eggplant are among the staples. Some vegetables are batter-dipped and deep-fried, while others, like olives, are enjoyed fresh in salads.

Lamb is the traditional meat of Greece. It is cooked with a variety of seasonings, including cinnamon, rosemary, oregano, yogurt, and lemon. Other meat sources include pork, chicken, and fish. A wide variety of nuts and seeds are used creatively in Greek cooking. Lentils and beans are also used, particularly on fast days when meats are forbidden.

White breads made from wheat flour and sprinkled with sesame seeds appear with all meals. Pasta and rice are also used, mostly in soups and casserole dishes. Phyllo dough is prepared commercially and is made into savory pastries and desserts.

Many of the traditional Greek pastries come drenched in a thick syrup, and always are served with water or coffee. Fresh or preserved fruits also may be served for dessert. Common seasonings in Greek dishes include cinnamon, yogurt, lemon, green dill, garlic, onions, mint, and oregano. Ouzo and retsina are two of the popular alcoholic beverages.

MEAL PATTERNS

Hospitality is a cornerstone of Greek tradition; men and women alike take pride and honor in receiving guests. Preserved fruits with water or ouzo and small pastries are usually served to guests between meals. Breakfast may be only coffee or juice. Lunch is a more substantial meal, perhaps of hot soup, bread and cheese, a salad of fresh produce, and fresh fruit or pastry. Dinner would be similar to lunch, only with a meat dish added on nonfasting days. Midmorning or afternoon snacks of coffee and pastry are common. Taverns abound, frequented mostly by men, offering anything from a single drink to a complete meal of bread, meat, vegetables, and wine.

SPECIAL OCCASIONS

Since nearly every Greek belongs to the Greek Orthodox Church, the special occasions and foods which help mark them are almost always religious. See the following section on Christianity for more details about the Greek Orthodox religion.

Italy

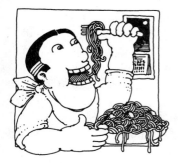

This ancient country also has felt the influences of many nations through its history, including Europe, the Middle East, the Spanish, Muslims, and Austrians. Even today, the influence of ancient Roman food customs can still be seen in many parts of Italy. Many of the poor in Italy still live in earthen huts with open fireplaces. This country has distinctive regional preferences in food customs and preparation. In the North, rice, butter, cornmeal, and milk predominate, while in the South, olive oil, wine, and pasta are more popular. Cheese, vegetables, and cereals are the staples of the Italian diet. Breads and pastas are made from rice, wheat, and corn. Fresh vegetables are plentiful; among the most popular are eggplant, zucchini, greens, squash, peas, and beans. Cheeses are produced locally and are used in salads, soups, with pasta, as fillings, and for snacks and appetizers. Meats and seafoods are used creatively, although in small amounts, because of their cost and limited availability. Fresh fruits and cheeses are typical desserts, although elaborate pastries are made for special occasions. Italy is also known for its wide variety of fine wines, which are part of daily meals.

MEAL PATTERNS

A typical urban breakfast might include tea, coffee, or hot chocolate with bread and jam. Lunch and dinner are similar, differing only in the number of courses. Appetizers and soup may precede a rice or pasta dish, a fish course followed by a meat course, then cheese, fruit, and dessert.

SPECIAL OCCASIONS

Italy is mostly Roman Catholic; the food traditions and customs are centered around religious days. Christmas is perhaps the most important holiday, celebrated with numerous special pastries, honey cakes, chocolate dishes, family specialties of pasta, fish and seafood, fowl, pork, and brandied fruits. Easter has its own food traditions, including lamb, yeast breads, and fruited buns.

Russia

This country encompasses more than 240 million inhabitants speaking more than 200 languages and spreading over two continents. No one cuisine can be truly called "Russian" since so many different ethnic groups make up this country. Foods have been adapted from the cuisine of neighboring countries, such as noodles and tea from China, sausages and pickled cabbage from Germany, wine from Greece, and pastas from Italy. The staple foods of Russia are breads and meats. Rye is the major grain of the North, wheat in the South, and corn in the Southwest. Since the majority of church-going Russians belong to the Russian Orthodox Church, with its rules against eating meats with blood and the meatless days, fish and dairy products are also popular.

Sour cream is used widely in Russian cooking, as are sour milk, pot cheese, cottage cheese, and local varieties. Whole, fresh milk and cream are also used in cooking and baking.

In season, fresh berries are particularly enjoyed. Due to the harsh and long winters, most fruits must be imported. Fruits are eaten fresh, preserved, or used as fillings or sweet desserts. The most popular vegetables include cabbage, onions, potatoes, turnips, squash, and beets. Sauerkraut and pickled cucumbers are also popular. Cold vegetable salads may be served with sour cream.

Pork, beef, poultry, veal, and game are all used, as are fish and seafood. Caviar is a special delicacy. Eggs are used in baking, in pastries, or as appetizers.

Most breads are from dark, coarse grains and are baked into a variety of shapes. Noodles and yeast dough are used to make dumplings, pastries, and rolls.

Sweets are common in Russia, such as sweet preserves with tea, candied fruits, or baked desserts. The most common seasonings include sweet and sour (such as dill, onion, vinegar). Butter is a favorite topping. Tea, brewed in the traditional samovar, and vodka are the most popular beverages of Russia.

MEAL PATTERNS

Breakfast and lunch are usually light meals. Breakfast consists of tea, breads, and perhaps an egg, while lunch may be a hot meat or fish dish with milk and stewed fruit. Dinner is the main meal, preceded by vodka and appetizers, followed by soup, meat and vegetables, and then dessert.

SPECIAL OCCASIONS

Although Russian Orthodox is the predominant religion, Soviet rule has altered church importance in daily life. Easter is one of the most celebrated holidays, perhaps because it follows the long winter. Dough-filled pastries, known as blintzes, are flavored with sour cream, fruit preserves, or herring. Traditional Easter foods include ham, herring, cream cheese with fruits and nuts, decorated eggs, and fruited breads. Christmas is another favorite holiday. A traditional dish of boiled grains, sugar, honey, nuts, and raisins is served by Orthodox Russians on Christmas Eve and to mourners at an Orthodox funeral. Wedding cakes are often topped with a container of salt to symbolize welcome.

Spain

Spain is another ancient country whose history has helped shape its present-day customs and traditions. Influenced by Arabs, Moors, Berbers, and the countries of Europe, Spain remains a unique combination of old and new, poverty and wealth. Spanish cooking is noted for its use of fresh ingredients and minimal amount of seasonings. Wine and olive oil are the backbones of Spanish cooking, along with the staples of onions, tomatoes, and garlic.

Dairy products in the form of cheeses are preferred in Spain. Another favorite is the pudding dessert, caramel flan. Canned and fresh milk are used in baking and cooking.

Many tropical fresh fruits are enjoyed daily, either alone as a snack or dessert or with meat or fish. Among the most popular are oranges, lemons, melons, grapes, apricots, peaches, and berries. Vegetables are mostly served cooked or pickled, with an oil and vinegar dressing. Most are available all year, including zucchini, eggplant, potatoes, peas, cauliflower, tomatoes, peppers, and onions.

Fish and seafood are very popular and are prepared in numerous ways. Pork, lamb, and many types of game are also widely used. A traditional Spanish dish, paella Valenciana, combines fish and seafood with tomatoes and other vegetables, and is served over rice.

Breads are used with all meals, and are usually the crusty wheat types. In some areas, corn or cornmeal is also used.

Sweets are common in the Spanish diet, perhaps reflecting the Muslim influence. Candied fruits, sweet pastries, and honey-drenched cakes are favorites. The most common seasonings include saffron (which colors rice a brilliant yellow), onions, and garlic. Coffee and hot chocolate are popular beverages. The red wines are sherries from Jerez and are world famous.

MEAL PATTERNS

Breakfast in Spain often begins with coffee or hot chocolate and bread or pastry. Lunch may be a meal of meat or fish and vegetables, crusty bread, and wine. Gazpacho, a cold soup made from tomatoes, garlic, cucumbers, and water-soaked bread might be a main course. Dinner may be eaten late, particularly in Madrid.

SPECIAL OCCASIONS

A country of predominantly Roman Catholics, Spain has almost daily festivals and celebrations to honor local and national saints and special rituals. Most of the major celebrations are religious ones, including Easter and Christmas.

The United States of America

Because the United States is a land of people from many different countries, no one dietary pattern is representative of the entire nation. This diversity is one of the most interesting things about America and makes the dining experience so unique in this country. When traveling throughout the United States, certain regional preferences do become apparent and they are discussed below. One of the best ways to explore the regional dishes of an area is to search out recipes and cookbooks from that particular city, town, or state. Often local groups, such as churches, 4-H clubs, or the Junior League, will produce collections of recipes, some of which may have been passed down from earlier generations and may reflect ethnic origins.

Despite the differences discussed below, all Americans share in the celebration of certain holidays, including New Year's Eve and Day, Saint Valentine's Day, Saint Patrick's Day, Mother's Day, Father's Day, Memorial Day, Independence Day (the Fourth of July), Labor Day, and Thanksgiving. Christian Americans also celebrate Easter and Christmas; Jewish Americans celebrate Yom Kippur, Rosh Hashanah, and Hannuka. Most of these holidays have their own special foods used in the festivities; in others, a certain color predominates. For example, champagne is the traditional beverage with which to greet the New Year; the color red and sweets are traditional for Valentine's Day; the color green for Saint Patrick's Day. Both Memorial Day and Independence Day are usually celebrated with outdoor picnics, since they both occur in the summertime; the latter is also celebrated with fireworks and sparklers. Thanksgiving is usually celebrated with feasting, as the Pilgrims did to mark their first harvest hundreds of years ago. Roasted turkey, cranberry sauce, apple, pumpkin, and mincemeat pies are all traditional foods for this holiday, although regional and ethnic foods are also common to mark present-day thanks for the bounty of America. Christmas is also celebrated throughout the country, with its common spirit of brotherhood crossing all religious boundaries. It is a season of giving and caring, and the food traditions reflect this. Candies (particularly candy canes) are traditional, as are gingerbread cookies and other sweets that uniquely express family origins. When describing the foods of America, one is really talking about how the food traditions of other countries have been blended and adapted to this land for which most of us are immigrants. The result is a unique and wonderful cuisine that is really thousands of cuisines, each offering its own interpretation of what is American.

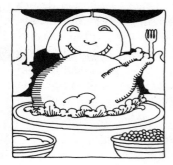

THE SOUTH

The dietary patterns of the South reflect the influence of its history, including the large Black slave population in the 1700s and 1800s, the French presence in Louisiana, and the Indian influence on the earliest American settlers in Virginia.

Among the dairy products preferred are buttermilk, dried milk, and canned evaporated milk, although fresh whole milk is also enjoyed.

Fresh fruits and vegetables are abundant, although the long cooking of the latter results in loss of some nutrients. The "pot liquor," or cooking liquid, saves some of these nutrients when it is used in making soups. Black-eyed peas and kidney beans are used frequently, as are all types of greens, which are usually cooked with salt pork.

Pork, chicken, local small game, and fish are used extensively. Many of the foods discarded by the Southern slave owners during the pre–Civil War period were creatively turned into savory dishes in slave kitchens. Some of these dishes are still favored today as "soul cooking"—chitlins, chicken wings, pork snout, and pig's feet.

Grits (a cereal made from corn), cornmeal, hominy, rice, and biscuits are preferred in the South.

THE NORTHEAST

History has left its mark on the food habits and traditions of the Americans of the Northeast. Some of the earliest settlers (the Pilgrims) came to this area, and many of their dishes are still served, particularly during Thanksgiving. Some of the customs of the New England region include clam chowder (made with milk), baked beans, fish cakes and lobster, and baked breads. Many of the large cities in this area of the country have restaurants and food shops that reflect the cultural presence of different groups.

THE MIDWEST

This area of the country is known for its fertile and bountiful land to which large numbers of Europeans immigrated in the 1800s, including the Germans, Scandinavians, Swiss, and English. These immigrants at first preserved their food traditions, but succeeding generations integrated them into local habits, preparing purely native dishes on traditional holidays. The Midwest, ranging from the Great Lakes to Ohio, produces much of the corn, wheat, and other agriculture for the nation. Known for state fairs where livestock, produce, and home cooking are displayed with pride, the Midwest is a blend of many cultures.

THE SOUTHWEST

The influence of several cultures is evident in this part of the country, including the Spanish, Mexicans, Chinese, Japanese, and the Native American Indians. Corn, in the form of tortillas or cornbread, is popular. Spicy foods, such as chili and tamales, include hot red peppers, onions, and garlic. Along the seacoast, shrimp, crab, and fish of all sorts are popular, as are avocados, olives, and citrus fruits.

Role of Religion in Dietary Practices

Religion plays an important role in the dietary practices of many people [1]. The regular participation of abstinence from a particular food item is a symbolic way of expressing devotion and faith. Five major religions encompass about 60 percent of the world's population. These include Christianity, Judaism, Islam, Hinduism, and Buddhism. The main dietary observances of each of these five religions are presented here.

CHRISTIANITY

Christianity is one of the most widespread religions. In 1975 it numbered about 954 million, or one out of every four people in the world. Of this figure, 57 percent were Roman Catholic, 34 percent were Protestant, and 9 percent were Eastern Orthodox. One of the most well-known practices of the Roman Catholic Church was the abstinence from eating meat on Fridays in remembrance of the sacrificial death of Christ. This church law was abolished by the United States Catholic Conference in 1966; now Catholics are required to abstain from eating meat only on Fridays during Lent. In addition, Catholics observe a number of fast days.

Followers of the Adventist movement have more dietary practices as part of their religious beliefs than any other group of Protestants. The Adventist movement, those who believe in the imminent second coming of Christ, includes the Seventh-Day Adventists. This group believes that diet, exercise, and rest are the way to maintain and preserve health and that one's life-style should be aimed at achieving these goals. Most Seventh-Day Adventists are lacto-ova vegetarians; some are strict vegetarians (no eggs, meat, or dairy), while others do eat meat. Coffee, tea, tobacco, and alcoholic beverages are all considered harmful to one's health because of their stimulating effects on the body. Water is the preferred beverage and is taken before or after meals. Most spices are avoided because they are thought to be harmful to the digestive tract. Breakfast is usually a substantial meal. Lunch is the largest meal of the day; dinner is light. To allow proper time for digestion and assimilation of foods, it is suggested that meals be eaten about 5 to 6 hours apart.

The Eastern Orthodox Church has its foundation in the Middle East, the Balkans, Russia, and the northeastern Mediterranean area. In 1975 the estimated world membership numbered about 87 million, with 4.1 million residing in the United States. In the Greek Orthodox religion, there are numerous fast days in which one can demonstrate devotion—every Wednesday and Friday to commemorate the betrayal of Christ and His death on the cross; the 40-day fast called the Great Lent, which precedes Easter; the 40-day fast called Advent, which begins in November; and two shorter fasts in June and August. During these fast periods no meat, fish (except shellfish), or animal products may be eaten; olive oil also is not used. A common meal in Greece during a fast day is dried bean and lentil soup.

Easter is the most important holiday in the Eastern Orthodox Church, occurring after the Jewish Passover. Several important periods precede Easter. The first is a 3-week pre-Lenten period of preparation and repentance. The third Sunday of this period is called the *Meat Fare Sunday* during which all meat in the house is consumed or disposed of on this day and during the following week. On the next Sunday, termed *Cheese Fare Sunday*, all cheese, eggs, and butter in the household is consumed. The next day, termed *Clean Monday*, marks the beginning of the Great Lent and the abstinence from all animal foods until Easter Sunday. On Palm Sunday and the Annunciation Day of the Virgin Mary, fish is allowed. To symbolize the tears of the Virgin Mary, lentil soup is always eaten on Good Friday. It is often served with vinegar to recall that when Christ was on the cross, he was given vinegar instead of the water he had requested. The Easter fast is traditionally broken on Easter Sunday with a soup made from the internal organs of the lamb. Round, leavened loaves of bread decorated with hard-boiled eggs dyed red are also traditional. The red color is symbolic of the blood of Christ, and the egg, a symbol of his tomb. The breaking open of the eggs on Easter morning symbolizes the opening of the tomb and the belief in the resurrection of Christ.

The laywomen of the Eastern Orthodox Church are actively involved in the preparation of the altar bread, which must be made from the purest ingredients, free from all shortening, milk, sugar, and eggs. Boiled whole-grain wheat serves a role in memorial services for the dead, being offered at the altar periodically after the death of a family member. It is considered to be a symbol of the resurrection of Christ and everlasting life. The wheat is mixed with raisins and pomegranate seeds (as symbols of sweetness and plenty), and other ingredients, then placed on a silver tray and sprinkled with powdered sugar (to wish the departed a sweet life in heaven). The mixture is blessed at the mourning services and later distributed to friends of the deceased.

JUDAISM

The origins of Judaism were set down in the five books of the Old Testament and began with God's covenant with Abraham and Moses. The most sacred writings are in the Torah, composed of the books of Genesis, Exodus, Leviticus, Numbers, and Deuteronomy. These writings contain the basic laws expressing the will of God to the Jews. The Talmud, another sacred book, was written later as rabbis tried to interpret the teachings of the Torah to make them more meaningful in daily life.

The Torah makes a distinction between "clean" and "unclean" animals; only the former are fit to eat. Animals that are considered clean are those that chew their cud and whose hooves are cloven (divided); to be acceptable, an animal must meet both of these criteria. Pigs, shellfish, eels, winged insects, reptiles, and birds of prey are forbidden in the diet of the Orthodox Jew. The blood and internal fat of an animal also are considered taboo.

Meat and dairy foods must not be eaten together, nor even be prepared or served on the same dishes. Two sets of dishes, silverware, and cooking utensils must be kept in an Orthodox Jewish home, one for meats and the other for dairy products. Six hours must lapse between eating meat and milk, but only 1 hour for eating meat after milk. *Kosher* refers to foods that are permitted by the Bible and processed and prepared in the prescribed manner. A rabbi must supervise the slaughtering of animals for them to be considered kosher. The animal's throat is slit, which humanely renders it unconscious while permitting as much blood to drain out as possible. The animal is then inspected carefully and stamped with the seal of the shocket (the actual butcher) to signify its ritual purity. The meat is further treated to completely remove all the blood. It is soaked in cold water for 30 minutes, drained, sprinkled with salt, and allowed to stand for 1 hour, then washed in cold water. The meat is now ready to be cooked. Many processed foods may be purchased with a "U" or "K", indicating that they have been prepared according to the Laws of Kashrut and are kosher.

Sabbath, which begins at sundown Friday and continues until sundown Saturday, is considered a day of rest and spiritual reunion. Friday is usually spent preparing for the Sabbath, including cooking all the food that will be eaten on that day. *Challah* is a traditional bread served on the Sabbath; usually two loaves are on the table. This is to signify the double portion of Manna given to the Israelites by God for the Sabbath during the 40 years they spent wandering in the wilderness.

Rosh Hashanah (the Day of Judgment) through Yom Kippur (the Day of Atonement) mark the 10 most solemn holy days of the Jewish year. On Rosh Hashanah, the challah is decorated with a ladder or birds to symbolize the prayers of the family to heaven. Slices of apples and bread dipped in honey are eaten as a symbolic wish for sweetness in the coming new year. Yom Kippur is a day of fasting for everyone except children.

During the 8-day Festival of Pesach (Passover), which commemorates the flight of the Israelites from Egypt, specially prepared foods must be used (Kasher L'Pesach, or Kosher for Passover). The unleavened bread used during this time is called *matzo*, and is prepared in sufficient quantities ahead of time to last the 8 days of the festival. Detailed instructions for its preparation are given in the Talmud.

The Orthodox Jews have retained all the rituals and customs of the Talmud and Laws of Kashrut. The Reform Jews consider the dietary laws outdated and do not practice any of the restrictions or obey the Laws of Kashrut. The Conservative Jews fall somewhere in the middle, obeying some of the laws, including eating only kosher foods, but not following many of the ancient practices and rituals.

ISLAM

Although Islam is the youngest major religion in the world, it is the second largest, with over 538 million followers. It is both a religion and a way of life. This religion was founded by Mohammed, who was born in Mecca, Saudi Arabia in A.D. 751. Through visions of the Archangel Gabriel, Mohammed became convinced that he was a prophet of Allah, the one true God. The most sacred Islam writing is the Koran, thought to be the words spoken to Mohammed by Allah. This book is composed of 14 chapters, or suras; the second sura contains, among other things, instructions on dietary practices and the need for fasting.

During the ninth month of the lunar Muslim year all faithful Muslims are expected to observe the fast of Ramadan, in which no food or water is taken from sunrise to sunset. This fast is considered to be a yearly reaffirmation of one's allegiance to Islam. Exempt from the fast are those traveling, and women who are pregnant or nursing, but these individuals must make up the missed days at a later time.

Many of the dietary practices of Islam are similar to those of the Jewish religion. For example, the consumption of both blood and pork is forbidden. Animal flesh is considered fit to eat only if it is slaughtered according to proper ritual, similar to that of the Jews.

HINDUISM

This is the oldest known religion in the world, thought to have originated in India about 4000 years ago and having about 524 million followers. The religion is centered around Brahman, the Universal Spirit. The caste system, an integral part of the Hindu way of life, has definite rules and regulations about how members of each caste should marry and socialize, as well as what foods they may eat. Originally there were four castes. The *Brahmans*, the highest caste, pursued study and religious teachings and were supported by the lower castes; the *Kshatriyas*, the warriors and rulers, protected the Brahmans and the most sacred animal to the Hindu, the cow; the *Vaisyas* were merchants, farmers, and traders whose duty included improving the economic situation of the country; and the *Sudras* were menial laborers whose moral duty was to serve the three higher classes. Individuals born outside these four castes were called outcastes or untouchables. This group used to be considered so lowly as to not even be allowed to enter a town or village. Outcastes were not allowed to own land or build houses. Through the efforts of Gandhi, the designation of untouchability was declared illegal in 1949. The Indian government also expressed opposition to the caste system at that time.

The most religious Hindus are strict vegetarians, although this practice is less enforced in the lower castes. All animals are considered to be part of Brahman, but the cow is particularly sacred. They wander at will through towns and countrysides, unharmed. Unfortunately, they often consume or destroy crops needed by the people.

Since both milk and clarified butter (ghee) come from cows, they are considered to be sacred foods. Unlike other foods, they cannot be contaminated by the touch of someone from a lower caste. Coconuts are also considered to be a sacred food. In addition to meat, other foods are also forbidden for the Hindu of the upper castes, including onions, garlic, mushrooms, and turnips.

BUDDHISM

This religion originated in India during the sixth century B.C. Siddhartha Gautama, who was later to become Buddha, The Enlightened One, had been raised a Hindu. Discontented with his luxurious life, he abandoned it at the age of 29 and wandered India in search of the cause of misery and its solution. One evening while meditating, legend has it that he passed into mystic rapture and was transformed into the Buddha.

In Buddhism it is believed that each individual comes into the world with a debt, or *karma*, which he tries to reduce during his lifetime. Each succeeding life can reduce this debt; wrong actions such as injury to others, lying, and stealing can add to it. By acquiring merit in this life, an individual can help himself progress toward a higher existence in the next life. Part of this life of merit includes the selfless giving of voluntary gifts, including food, to beggars and the Buddhist monks. These latter individuals are completely dependent on voluntary contributions for their support. The very best food of the household is given to the monks.

Application to the Health Professions

Individuals working in the health professions should have an intimate knowledge of people's beliefs, attitudes, knowledge, and behavior before attempting to introduce any change. This is particularly true of food customs and traditions, which may carry with them the sacred memories of childhood, home life, family, religion, and national pride. Anyone attempting to alter the diet of a group must take into consideration what the food and its preparation symbolize. Sensitivity, diplomacy, but above all respect for another's beliefs must prevail if transcultural nutrition education is to be effective and successful.

References

1. Lowenberg, M. E., et al.   Food, People, and Religion. In M. E. Lowenberg, et al. (eds.), *Food and People* (3rd ed.). New York: Wiley, 1979.

Suggested Readings
NUTRITION

Armstrong, B. K., et al.   Hematological, vitamin B_{12}, and folate studies on Seventh-Day Adventist vegetarians. *Am. J. Clin. Nutr.* 27:712, 1974.

Cavaiani, M., Urbashich, M., and Nielson, F.   *Simplified Quantity Ethnic Recipes.* Rochelle Park, N.J.: Hayden, 1980.

Chang, B.   Some dietary beliefs in Chinese folk culture. *J. Am. Diet. Assoc.* 65:436, 1974.

Crane, N. T., and Green, N. R.   Food habits and food preferences of Vietnamese refugees living in northern Florida. *J. Am. Diet. Assoc.* 76:591, 1980.

Gibson, L. D.   The psychology of food: Why we eat what we eat when we eat it. *Food Technol.* 35:54, 1981.

Gomes, J.   Bridging the gap: Southeast Asian children and school lunch. *School Food Serv. J.* 35:70, 1981.

Grivetti, L. E., and Pangborn, R. M.   Origin of selected Old Testament dietary prohibitions. *J. Am. Diet. Assoc.* 65:634, 1974.

Grivetti, L. E., and Paquette, M. B.   Nontraditional ethnic food choices among first generation Chinese in California. *J. Nutr. Educ.* 10:109, 1978.

Harris, R. S., et al.   The composition of Chinese foods. *J. Am. Diet. Assoc.* 25:28, 1949.

Harwood, A.   The hot-cold theory of disease. *J.A.M.A.* 216:1153, 1971.

Hertzler, A. A., Wenkam, N., and Standal, B.   Classifying cultural food habits and meanings. *J. Am. Diet. Assoc.* 80:421, 1982.

Hou, H. C.   Egg preservation in China. *Food Nutr. Bull.* 3:17, 1981.

Hubbard, D. W.   Immigrants' special: Our nutritional heritage. *School Food Serv. J.* October, 1976.

James, S. M.   When your patient is black West Indian. *Am. J. Nurs.* 78:1908, 1978.

Jerome, N. W.   The U.S. dietary pattern from an anthropological perspective. *Food Technol.* 35:37, 1981.

Jerome, N. W., Kandel, R. F., and Pelto, G. H. (eds.).   *Nutritional Anthropology: Contemporary Approaches to Diet and Culture.* Pleasantville, N.Y.: Redgrave, 1980.

Judd, J. E.   Century-old dietary taboos in 20th century Japan.   *J. Am. Diet. Assoc.* 33:489, 1957.

Kuhnlein, H. V., and Calloway, D. H.   Contemporary Hopi food intake patterns. *Ecology of Food and Nutr.* 6:159, 1977.

Lang, M. E.   Cultural super-foods. *Prof. Nutr.* 12:1, 1980.

Martin, M.   Native American medicine. *J.A.M.A.* 245:141, 1981.

Meleis, A. I.   The Arab American in the health care system. *Am. J. Nurs.* 81:1180, 1981.

Nalbandian, A., Bergan, J. G., and Brown, P. T.   Three generations of Armenians: Food habits and dietary status. *J. Am. Diet. Assoc.* 79:694, 1981.

Newman, J. M., Contento, I., and Kris, E.   Perspectives on food and nutrition in the People's Republic of China. *J. Nutr. Educ.* 13:43, 1981.

Olawacz, L., and El-Beheri, B.   Kreplach, kasha, and knishes. *Diabetes Forecast* 33:30, 1980.

Outpatient diets match cultural background. *Hospitals* 45:70, 1971.

Phillips, M. G., and Dunn, M. M.   Toward better understanding of other lands and other people: Their folkways and foods. *Nurs. Outlook* 9:498, 1961.

Root, W.   *Food: An Authoritative and Visual History and Directory of the Foods of the World.* New York: Simon & Schuster, 1980.

Rosanoff, A., and Calloway, D. H.   Calcium source in Indochinese immigrants. *N. Engl. J. Med.* 306:240, 1982.

Sakr, A. H.   Fasting in Islam. *J. Am. Diet. Assoc.* 67:17, 1975.

Sanjur, D.   *Social and Cultural Perspectives in Nutrition.* Englewood Cliffs, N.J.: Prentice-Hall, 1981.

Schaefer, A. E.   Immigrants: Diets and dietary problems. *School Food Serv. J.* October, 1976.

Selected references on the hot/cold theory of disease. *Med. Anthropol. Newsletter* 6:8, 1975.

Stephenson, S.   Treasures from China. *Food Manage.* 16:52, 1981.

Toma, R. B., and Curry, M. L.   North Dakota Indians' traditional foods. *J. Am. Diet. Assoc.* 76:589, 1970.

Wallace, J. Y. (ed.).   *The American Quantity Cookbook: Tracing Our Food Traditions.* Boston: Cahners, 1976.

Williams, C. D.   Cultural and other barriers in the implementation of health programs. *Am. J. Clin. Nutr.* 31:2037, 1978.

FOODS AND COOKING

Bancroft, A.   *Religions of the East.* New York: St. Martin's Press, 1974.

Bar-David, M. L.   *The Israeli Cookbook.* New York: Crown, 1973.

Candler, T. G.   *The Northern Italian Cookbook.* New York: McGraw-Hill, 1977.

Castle, C., et al.   *Peasant Cooking of Many Lands.* San Francisco: 101 Productions, 1972.

Clairborne, C., and Lee, V.   *The Chinese Cookbook.* Philadelphia: Lippincott, 1972.

DeLeon, J. V.   *Mexican Cookbook.* Mexico City: Culinary Arts Institute, 1971.

Fitzgibbon, T.   *A Taste of Rome: Traditional Food.* Boston: Houghton Mifflin, 1975.

Iny, D.   *The Best of Baghdad Cooking.* Toronto: Clark, Irwin, 1976.

Kahler, E.   *The Germans.* Princeton, N.J.: Princeton University Press, 1974.

Lang, G.   *The Cuisine of Hungary.* New York: Atheneum, 1971.

Langseth-Christensen, L.   The Cuisines of Germany. *Gourmet*, June, 1973.

Lianides, L.   Easter in Greece. *Gourmet*, April, 1974.

Mendes, H.   *The African Heritage Cookbook.* New York: Macmillan, 1971.

Nelson, K. S.   *The Eastern European Cookbook.* Chicago: Henry Regnery, 1973.

Ovstedal, B.   *Norway.* London: Batsford, 1974.

Paradissus, C. *The Best of Greek Cookery.* Athens: Estathiadis Bros., 1972.

Pike, M. *Food and Society.* London: John Murray, 1971.

Polvay, M. Cuisines of Russia. *Gourmet,* February, 1974.

Priestly, J. B. *The English.* New York: Viking Press, 1973.

Simoons, F. J. *Eat Not This Flesh.* Madison, Wisconsin: University of Wisconsin Press, 1961.

Tannahill, R. *Food in History.* New York: Stein & Day, 1974.

Zane, E. *Middle Eastern Cookery.* San Francisco: 101 Productions, 1974.

Chapter 31

NUTRITION EDUCATION AND THE ECONOMICS OF FOOD

Nutrition education and the economics of food are grouped together in this chapter for the simple reason that they are so closely associated in daily life. Walking down a supermarket aisle, the choices the consumer makes are influenced by economics (how much money is available to spend on food that day) and one's knowledge of nutrition. Both of these factors must be taken into consideration when purchasing foods, but many other variables influence the final decisions. Examples of some variables include *culture* (must the foods purchased be kosher?); *life-style* (is the consumer planning a dinner party for twenty or buying foods for brown-bag lunches for the week?); *medical conditions* (must the foods be low-sodium or low-fat?), to name a few. If today is payday, the food choices might be more extravagant than if the shopping were done on the last day before the check arrives. Food choices made on the way home from work, when the consumer may be very hungry, will probably be based more on taste than any other factors.

This chapter will explore nutrition education, how this education influences consumer behavior, and the role of economics.

Nutrition Education

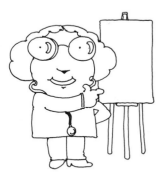

The purpose of nutrition education is to affect change in behavior that will result in nutritionally sound food practices. Permanent change is probably the most difficult to bring about in adults, whose food habits have become set with the passage of time. When a change in diet is part of a therapeutic regimen, the sick adult may be more receptive and motivated to alter his or her eating habits, although experience has shown that this change is often short-lived. Despite this, nutrition education continues to be stressed by physicians, nutritionists, public health workers, nurses, and industry in the hopes of beneficially changing nutrition behavior.

Children and younger adults have been found to be more receptive to nutrition education, perhaps because their food habits and life-styles have not yet become rigid. Federal programs, such as School Lunch and School Breakfast, include an education component, in addition to providing nutritious, well-balanced meals free or at greatly reduced costs to children from financially eligible families. The Special Supplemental Feeding Program for Women, Infants, and Children (WIC) provides foods for pregnant, lactating, and postpartum women and children from birth to age five. The program also provides nutrition education to women and their families.

The following sections present some of the strategies at the national and international level aimed at providing nutrition education.

NATIONAL PROGRAMS

In 1969 the White House Conference on Food, Nutrition, and Health was held. It recognized that malnutrition and hunger affected millions of Americans who,

TABLE 31-1. Growth of USDA's food assistance programs

Program	Budget and number of consumers (1968)	Budget and number of consumers (1979)
Food Stamp Program	$288 million; 2.8 million	$6 billion; 16 million
School Lunch Program (partial subsidy)	$42 million; 3 million	$1.2 billion; 12 million $600 million; 26 million
School Breakfast Program	$5.5 million; 300,000	$200 million; 3 million
Child Care and Summer Food Service for Children	$3.2 million; 140,000	$250 million; 3 million
Supplemental Feeding Program for Women, Infants and Children (WIC)	$14 million; 206,000 (1974)	$550 million; 1.5 million
Nutrition for the Elderly	?; $41,000 (1974)	$202 million; 2.3 million

Source: N. Katz, *Hunger in America: The Federal Response*, New York: Field Foundation, 1979.

because of poverty, could not afford an adequate diet. The Conference also acknowledged that sufficient income alone does not guarantee an adequate diet; nutrition education, choosing the proper foods, is also needed if malnutrition and hunger are to be eradicated [1].

In the 10 years following the Conference, the United States Department of Agriculture (USDA) expanded its food assistance programs to low-income groups to meet this challenge, as summarized in Table 31-1. Although some reductions or reallocations may have occurred since 1979, federal contributions are still substantial. In 1978, expenditures by the USDA for nutrition research exceeded $28.6 million, of which $10 million was spent on nutrition education [2]. The USDA provides a variety of nutrition information and educational materials for use by educators, researchers, and the general public; some of these are listed at the end of this chapter.

Nutrition education is a vital component of each program administrated by the USDA. The Cooperative Extension Service, the oldest government nutrition education program, has been in existence since 1914, providing families with education and information about food and nutrition (Fig. 31-1). Another part of the Cooperative Extension Service are the 4-H projects, which in 1978 included nearly 2 million youths in food and nutrition education projects. Nutrition education is also a component of the Food Stamp Program, aimed at providing recipients with a better understanding of good nutrition and how to apply this understanding. Nutrition education was legislated into the Special Supplemental Feeding Program for Women, Infants, and Children (WIC) in 1977 [3]. Individual and group counseling stresses the importance of good maternal nutrition for the development of the unborn child, adequate diet during breast-feeding, and proper infant nutrition. Children are a special target for the USDAs educational programs. In 1977 the Food and Agriculture Act appropriated $26 million to fund state education programs in nutrition, with a major emphasis on educating

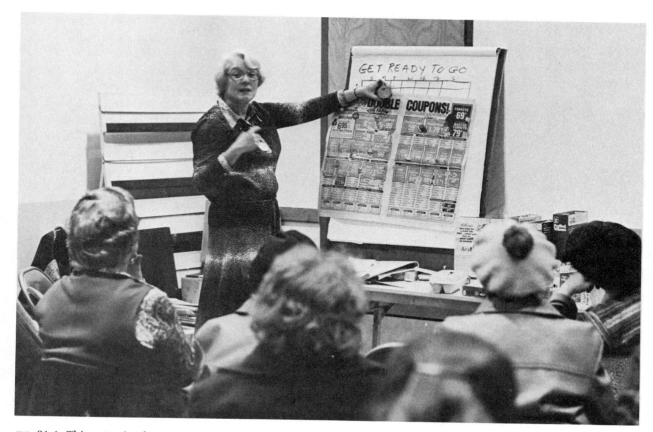

FIG. 31-1. This extension home economist is explaining how to take advantage of coupon offers to save on food expenses. She is one of 3000 such home economists extending information to families and groups across the country. (USDA photo by Fred Witte.)

children [4]. This act included education of foodservice personnel and educators. The USDA also has developed a nationwide nutrition education effort for children through the mass media.

In addition to the USDA, there are numerous other agencies, both public and private, that are concerned with nutrition education. State departments of health, welfare, and agriculture, state universities, boards of education, and educational, social, and civic groups all contribute directly or indirectly to nutrition education through services, programs, fund raising, or by campaigns to make the consumer more aware of the principles of good nutrition. Scores of government and voluntary agencies on the national level are also concerned with nutrition, ranging from the American Red Cross to the Bureau of Indian Affairs to the Nutrition Foundation.

Because family income often parallels the nutritional quality of the diet, much of the nutrition programming, including education, is aimed at the poor. In trying to achieve the goal of improved nutrition, most programs have made the twofold effort of improving the amount of food available (either through providing free or reduced-cost foods or by increasing the buying power of available food dollars) and providing nutrition education.

INTERNATIONAL
PROGRAMS

Several international agencies are directly concerned with nutrition, including the Food and Agriculture Organization (FAO), the World Health Organization (WHO), the United Nations Children's Fund (UNICEF), and the Food for Freedom Program. The FAO, founded in 1945, aims to improve the standard of living and the nutrition of people of all countries, and to increase the efficiency and productivity of fisheries, forestry, and farming. It provides technical assistance in nutrition, agriculture, economics, forestry, and fisheries to member nations in response to requests for assistance. Some of these services include developing better agricultural practices, improved strains of plants, and protein mixtures of high nutritional value. The WHO, formed in 1948, is the authority for international health work. The major goals of this agency are to eradicate disease and improve sanitary standards of food and water. Originally conceived in 1947 to continue emergency feeding in the European countries devastated by war, UNICEF has come to be known for its distribution of milk throughout the world in school feeding, emergency relief, and maternal and infant health centers. The Food for Freedom Program was enacted by Congress in 1954 as a means for channeling surplus agricultural products to the world's needy. It is administered through the Department of State and the Agency for International Development.

Economics of Food
AMERICA'S FOOD SHOPPING
HABITS

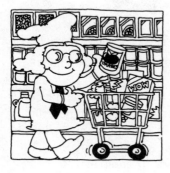

Since 1894, the U.S. Department of Agriculture has been monitoring food consumption patterns in the United States [5]. The first national survey was done in 1930; the most recent was in 1978 and included 15,000 households and 34,000 individuals. Information was obtained through interviews and covered a 7-day period. A number of factors make the food choices of Americans today vastly different from 10, 20, or 100 years ago. More women are presently employed outside the home; therefore, they spend less time preparing meals. There is a greater demand for fast, uniform foods, as evidenced by the growing fast-food chains (see Chap. 23 for more details). The average consumer is more aware of the relation of diet to weight control, disease, and general health. The Government has also contributed to changing food consumption patterns, through such programs as Food Stamps, School Lunch, and WIC for pregnant and nursing women.

The most recent survey showed that more of the household food dollar is being spent for meals and snacks outside the home, although this varied with family income. The consumption of meat, fish, and poultry was up; consumption of pork, luncheon meat, eggs, and dry beans was down. The average intake of citrus fruits and green, leafy vegetables was also increased.

FOOD BUDGETS

Food economists and nutritionists at the U.S. Department of Agriculture (USDA) have devised four different food plans to aid the consumer in planning and purchasing foods for a well-balanced diet within a budget [6]. The four food plans are thrifty, low-cost, moderate-cost, and liberal, and are based on the amount of money an individual or family has to spend on food. The thrifty plan is

TABLE 31-2. The food plan for the family

Income (before taxes)	1-person family	2-person family	3-person family	4-person family	5-person family	6-person family
$ 2500–5000	T* or LC	T* or LC	T*	T*	T*	T*
$ 5001–10,000	MC	LC	T* or LC	T*	T*	T*
$10,001–15,000	L	MC	LC or MC	LC	T or LC	T*
$15,001–20,000	L	L	MC	LC or MC	LC	T or LC
$20,001–30,000	L	L	MC or L	MC	LC or MC	LC
$30,001–40,000	L	L	L	MC or L	MC or L	MC
$40,001 or more	L	L	L	L	L	MC or L

T = thrifty; LC = low-cost; MC = moderate-cost; L = liberal.
*Many families of this size and income are eligible for assistance through the Food Stamp Program.
Source: USDA *Your Money's Worth in Foods*. Home and Garden Bulletin No. 183, Science and Education Administration (revised), 1979.

the guide for families with the smallest food budget, and is used as the basis for the coupon allotment in the Food Stamp Program.

The first step in planning a food budget is to determine which of the four plans best suits the individual's or family's situation. Factors to evaluate include income, family size, and the importance of food in relation to other family needs. In 1979, the estimated weekly food bills for a family of four with elementary school children was set by the USDA to be $46 for thrifty; $60 for low-cost; $75 for moderate-cost; and $90 for the liberal food plan. Suggested food plans by family size and income are given in Table 31-2.

MEAL PLANNING

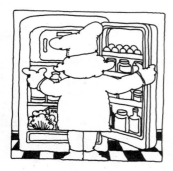

The purpose of meal planning is to serve food that the family will eat and enjoy; to provide a balanced diet; and to stay within the time/budget/energy limitations of the family. Once the amount of money for the food budget has been determined, it takes careful planning to provide nutritious, well-balanced meals within that monetary framework, particularly if the food plan is thrifty or low-cost. Only variety can provide all the essential nutrients needed for growth, repair, and maintenance. The daily meal plan should include the following, modified for different age groups (see Section VI, Nutritional Needs Through the Life Cycle, for specific meal plans): 2 or more *meat* servings (2 to 3 oz meat or 1 egg/serving); 2 to 4 *milk* servings (8 oz milk or 1 oz cheese or ½ cup yogurt/ serving); 4 or more *fruits and vegetables,* including at least one serving each of a good source of vitamin A and of vitamin C; 4 or more *bread* servings (1 slice bread or 1 oz cereal or ½ to ¾ cup rice or noodles/serving).

Life-style considerations are important in distributing these servings throughout the day. For example, college students may need late-night snacks to fit their study habits; young children need to eat smaller meals more frequently; a working parent may depend more on casseroles prepared ahead of time; a homemaker may prepare all the family's meals from scratch.

Each meal (and most snacks) should provide protein and carbohydrate, with fat as needed for taste and calories. The servings from each food group should be distributed throughout the day's meals, rather than all breads and cereals, for example, being served at dinner. Table 31-3 gives an example of a week's menus, showing how to distribute servings from each food group.

The next step in meal planning is to actually plan menus. This can be done for a few days or up to a week. When planning dishes to prepare, keep in mind the possibility of substituting a less expensive item for the one suggested in the recipe (see Tables 31-4, 31-5, and 31-6). Another way of maximizing savings is to plan the week's menus around advertised specials or using items previously purchased on sale. Watch newspaper ads; clip coupons; be flexible (Fig. 31-2). Make sure the other members of the household will eat what is planned—no food is a bargain if it is thrown away! Another factor to consider when choosing recipes is the skill of the person who will prepare them; time is important, as is the cost of extra servings that might be wasted.

The remaining step is to make up a shopping list. Impulse buying can upset the budget. Individual items should be purchased in the largest quantity that can be stored properly and will not result in waste. Compare cost per ounce and determine if the larger size is really a bargain.

FOOD SHOPPING

Check food prices at several stores, then decide which offers the most reasonable prices plus other features, such as parking, variety, and use of credit cards. Using several stores far apart from each other may result in wasting any savings on additional gasoline or bus fare.

The following sections present tips on the most economical ways to shop.

BREADS AND CEREALS

This food group provides essential vitamins, particularly thiamin and riboflavin, iron, calcium, and protein, while at the same time being versatile and very economical. Enriched and whole-grain breads and cereals provide three to four times the amounts of iron, thiamin, riboflavin, and niacin as unenriched products, usually at comparable prices. Always compare prices of *equal* weights of bread to find the best buy as larger loaves do not always weigh more. Cereals with fruit or sugar added are usually more expensive and provide less nutrients per ounce than whole-grain or less processed types. Ready-to-serve and hot cereals packaged in individual packages are much more expensive than the same cereal in large boxes. Parboiled, instant, or processed rice is more expensive than regular rice. Rice mixes are much more expensive than regular rice with seasonings added in the home. Ready-baked products may or may not be less expensive than baked goods made at home; by pricing the cost of the ingredients for home preparation, a better comparison can be made.

FRUITS AND VEGETABLES

These foods can be purchased fresh, canned, frozen, or dehydrated. The season and supply influence the price of fresh produce, whereas the cost of frozen,

TABLE 31-3. Sample menu planning

	Sunday	Monday	Tuesday	Wednesday	Thursday	Friday	Saturday
BREAKFAST	Fresh grapefruit Scrambled eggs Fresh milk English muffin	Orange juice Peanut butter Yogurt Toast	Tomato juice Cheese Yogurt Muffins	Orange slices Walnuts and raisins Cottage cheese Toast	Pineapple juice Hard-boiled eggs Cottage cheese Farina	Orange juice Sliced ham Grated cheese Farina	Tomato juice Omelet Fresh milk English muffin
LUNCH	Fresh orange Tunafish sandwich Cole slaw Ice cream	Apple Cheeseburger on a bun Lettuce and tomato	Apple Bologna sandwich Sliced tomato Milk shake	Pear Tunafish sandwich Lettuce Milk	Canned peaches Peanut butter sandwich Carrot sticks Milk	Pear Bologna sandwich Salad Yogurt	Canned pears Hamburger on bun Sliced tomato Yogurt
SNACK	Crackers Fresh milk	Oatmeal cookies Ice cream	Oatmeal cookies Yogurt	Graham crackers Milk	Date-nut bars Yogurt	Graham crackers Fresh milk	Date-nut bars Ice cream
DINNER	Beef stew on rice Garden salad Fresh milk	Broiled chicken Broccoli Baked potato Fresh milk	Broiled fish Macaroni Spinach Iced tea	Roast beef Baked squash Brussels sprouts Hot tea	Spaghetti with meat sauce Green beans Coffee	Tuna-noodle casserole Garden salad Iced tea	Grilled pork chops Applesauce Garden salad Lemonade

TABLE 31-4. Comparing costs of grains, fruits, and vegetables

	Special factors to consider when comparing cost	Relative cost	
		Usually more economical	Usually more expensive
Grains	Compare cost of bakery products and cereal by weight rather than by volume	Day-old bread	Fresh bread Rolls, buns
	Compare servings per pound when comparing cost of to-be-cooked and ready-to-eat cereals	White enriched bread products	Whole grain
	Whole grain and enriched products have more nutrients than unenriched products	To-be-cooked cereal	Ready-to-eat cereal
	Bran cereals provide extra fiber	Unsweetened cereal	Presweetened cereal
	Wheat germ adds extra nutrients to a grain dish	Plain rice and pasta	Seasoned rice and pasta
		Regular rice	Parboiled and instant rice
Fruits and vegetables (fresh)	Consider freshness and quality; it may affect nutritive value	Fresh produce in season and in abundant supply	Fresh produce out of season and in limited quantities
	Avoid produce with large bruises, cuts, or spots of decay		
	Buy only amount that can be used before spoiling	Locally grown produce	Produce transported a long distance
	Consider amount of waste (e.g., inedible peel, outer leaves, core, pit, tough stalks, green areas on potatoes)		
	Oversized vegetables may be tough		
Fruits and vegetables (canned and frozen)	Graded A, B, C; all grades approximately equal in wholesomeness and nutritive value	Cut up or sliced	Whole
		Diced or short cut	Fancy cut
		Mixed sizes	All same size
	Canned produce contains some cooking fluid, which accounts for a percent of weight	Fruits in light syrup	Fruits in heavy syrup
	Frozen produce has little or no waste	Frozen orange juice	Whole oranges
		Plain vegetables	Mixed vegetables or vegetables in sauces

Source: C. Suitor and M. Hunter, *Nutrition: Principles and Application in Health Promotion*. Philadelphia: Lippincott, 1980.

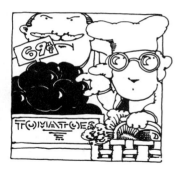

canned, or dehydrated fruits and vegetables varies by grade, brand, item, and type of processing.

To find the best buys, compare the costs for single servings. This can be done by dividing the price of a pound, a can, or package by the number of servings it provides. Buying fresh produce in season is usually the best buy, although certain items may still be too high for some food budgets. Compare different forms of the same food—fresh, frozen, canned, or dehydrated—to see which is priced lowest. Limit the purchase of fresh, perishable produce to the amount that can be used without waste. Stock up on canned or frozen produce when on sale, if space is available to store them properly. Lower-priced store brands may be of the same quality as better-known products; purchase by grade rather than brand (see Chap. 13 for more discussion on grade).

MILK AND DAIRY PRODUCTS

The form in which milk is purchased can result in a wide variance in price. Some of the factors that determine the selling price of milk include whether it is fresh, canned, cultured, or dried; whether part or all of the fat has been removed; and whether milk solids, vitamins, and minerals have been added. Where the milk is purchased, if it is home delivered, and the size of the container are also contributing factors.

To minimize costs, it is best to buy fresh fluid milk at a food or retail dairy store; home delivery or small special-service stores usually charge more. As a general rule, the larger the container, the lower the cost per serving, if buying the larger size does not result in increased waste. Nonfat dry milk is the least expensive form of milk and the easiest to transport since all the fluid has been removed. To add to the savings, nonfat dry milk should be purchased in as large a package as possible that can be stored and used without waste.

Other milk products can be used to replace part or all of the daily milk requirement, although at a greater cost. To replace ½ cup of fluid milk, ¾ cup ice cream or ½ cup plain yogurt would cost three times as much. Generally, the harder, aged cheeses are more expensive than the unripened cheeses. This is partially true because the latter contain more moisture and, therefore, less nutrients per ounce. Cheeses that are grated usually cost more than an equal amount purchased in bulk. Larger containers of dairy products usually cost less per pound than smaller containers. Cottage cheese with fruit and cheeses with nuts or wine cost more than plain versions.

MEAT

This food group takes the largest portion of the average food budget, about one-third as estimated by the USDA. Since the range of costs, quality of cuts, and varieties are great, considerable savings can be made with careful shopping.

The price per pound is not always the best indicator of the best buy or the number of servings a cut will provide. A high-priced cut with little fat, bone, or waste is actually a better value than a lower-priced cut with substantial amounts

TABLE 31-5. Comparing costs of protein foods and dairy products

Type of food	Relative cost	Nutrition information	Palatability
Meats (beef, veal, lamb, and pork)	Among the most expensive types of food Cost for edible portion (EP) rises if meat contains high percent of bone, fat, gristle Generally 450 gm (1 lb) uncooked meat yields 3–4 servings (3 oz each); if percent of inedible portion is high, yield is less; cooked meat with no waste may yield more Ground meat may be made from a variety of cuts Ground beef (hamburger) usually has most fat, costs less than ground beef with less fat	High grades—well marbled with fat Low grades—lower in fat Tough cuts equal in nutritive value to tender ones (EP) *Different* types of meats (e.g., veal, pork) are similar in nutritive value; pork is highest in thiamin Organ meats higher in vitamins and minerals; lower in fats but higher in cholesterol Some meat products (bologna, hot dogs) high in fat; low in protein and micronutrients	Graded—prime, choice, good, standard Cut affects tenderness more than grade does Meat usually most palatable when cooked in manner suggested for it Tough cuts can be more flavorful than tender cuts in dishes such as stew, pot roast Tough cuts can be cooked in several appetizing ways to make them tender
Poultry	Whole birds usually cost less than parts Well-fleshed large birds have larger EP than small birds	Less iron than meats but still a good source	May be graded (e.g., Grade A) Young poultry more tender than mature poultry (fowl, hen, stewing chicken) Mature poultry suitable for stewing, soups, salads, casseroles
Fish	Cost of fish varies with season and region Fresh fish usually more expensive than frozen Fillet and steaks yield greatest EP, dressed fish yields less EP, whole fish has lowest EP Some shellfish more expensive than other fish Canned fish has high EP Canned flaked or grated less expensive than solid or chunk	Most fish is low in fat Regular canned fish usually has much higher sodium content than fresh or frozen Federal inspection of fish and fishery products is voluntary Less iron than meats but still a good source	Fresh fish usually has more desirable flavor Frozen fish may have rancid taste, texture variable Some fish bony

Eggs	Inexpensive form of protein and minerals Sizes—peewee, small, medium, large, extra large, and jumbo Difference in sizes about 10% by weight. Buy larger-size eggs when their price is less than 10% higher than next smaller size (e.g., buy large eggs at 97¢ per dozen when medium eggs cost 89¢ per dozen—89¢ + 9¢ [10% of 89] = 98¢)	White and brown shelled eggs are equally nutritious Difference in color of yolk not significant in terms of nutritive value Size and grade have no relation to nutritive value An egg substitute is equivalent to an egg in some, but not all, nutrients	Graded AA, A, B Grade A eggs are firm, good for all uses, especially if appearance is important Grade B eggs have a thin white, which spreads; the flavor is not as delicate as grade A; they are satisfactory for general cooking
Dairy products	Nonfat dry milk least expensive, fortified skim milk next, whole milk most expensive Yogurt, cottage cheese, and ice cream or ice milk more expensive than milk Aged or sharp natural cheese more expensive than mild natural cheese Imported cheese more costly than domestic Pasteurized processed cheese usually costs less than natural cheese Individually wrapped sliced and grated more expensive than wedges Mild cheddar, swiss, and cottage cheese relatively inexpensive Compare cost of a pound of cheese to a pound of meat; it may serve as a meat substitute occasionally	Fortified nonfat dry milk has most of protein, vitamins, and minerals of whole milk, only water and fat have been removed Milk has approximately twice as much calcium as ice cream Imitation milk products are not comparable to milk in nutritive value Most processed cheeses have a higher sodium content than natural cheeses Cheese does not provide iron, which meat does	To make instant dry milk tastier: (1) mix a few hours before using, (2) serve ice cold, (3) mix equal parts of reconstituted dry milk with whole milk Canned and dry milk can be used satisfactorily in cooking and baking Cottage cheese spoils more quickly than other varieties of cheese

Source: C. Suitor and M. Hunter, Nutrition: Principles and Application in Health Promotion. Philadelphia: Lippincott, 1980.

TABLE 31-6. Menu planning within two budgets

Meal pattern	Lower cost (plan I)*	Higher cost (plan II)*
BREAKFAST		
Fruit or juice	Orange juice (frozen)	Melon (fresh)
Main dish or cereal with milk	Oatmeal with milk	Cheese and mushroom omelet
Bread	Toast with jelly	English muffin
Beverage	Milk (nonfat dry)	Milk (fresh)
LUNCH		
Main dish	Cheese sandwich	Boiled ham on roll
Vegetable or fruit	Celery sticks, banana	Lettuce and tomato
		Broccoli in butter sauce
Bread	Bread (in sandwich)	Bread (in sandwich)
Beverage	Milk (nonfat dry)	Milk (fresh)
SNACK		
Fruit or cookies	Cookies (homemade)	Pear (fresh)
Beverage	Apple juice (canned)	Chocolate milk (fresh)
DINNER		
Main dish	Baked chicken	Beef round roast
Vegetables	Carrots, mashed potatoes	Asparagus (frozen)
		Au gratin potatoes (frozen)
Bread	Bread	Dinner rolls (bakery)
Dessert	Apple pie (homemade)	Banana nut cake (frozen)
Beverage	Milk (nonfat dry)	Milk (fresh)

*Estimated cost for family of four with two schoolchildren (Washington, D.C., Fall, 1978) for Plan I, $7.50; for Plan II, $17.00.
Source: USDA Home and Garden Bulletin 183. *Your Money's Worth in Foods.* 1979. P. 8.

of bone, gristle, or fat. Equal portions of lean meats of different types or cuts generally provide similar food value.

To get the best buys, select the cuts and types of meat, poultry, and fish that provide the most lean for the money. Proper methods of preparation can make almost any cut appetizing and tender. Watch for special sales, particularly of more expensive cuts. When buying in larger quantities, always be sure the meat can be stored properly, or wastage will result. Use smaller servings of meat and rely on more economical foods to add protein, such as cottage cheese, eggs, beans, or legumes. Use all of the meat for the best buys—leftovers in casseroles; meat bones in soups; drippngs in gravies.

Conclusions

The attainment of adequate nutrition has many obstacles in its path—disease, poverty, inadequate technology, and ignorance, to name just a few. In the past 100 years, during which most of the nutrition discoveries have taken place, great progress has been made in overturning these obstacles. The focus of clinical nutrition was previously aimed at the deficiency diseases; it has now shifted to the role of diet in the causation of the chronic degenerative diseases. Years ago

FIG. 31-2. Clipping coupons and watching for advertised specials requires time and work but the results in savings can be substantial. Also, newspapers sometimes run monthly price surveys of selected foods to show what are the current bargains. (USDA photo by Murray M. Berman.)

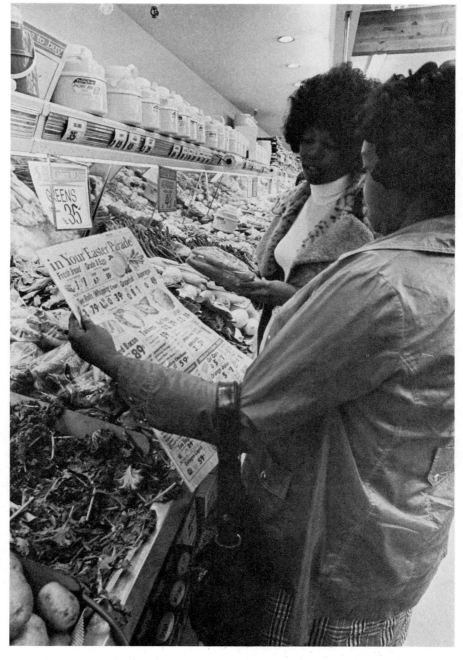

the major emphasis was on improving sanitary conditions and infection control. With technologic advantages, programs to combat poverty, and health and nutrition education programs at all levels both nationally and internationally, tomorrow's challenge will be the prevention of disease and the continued advancement of the health and welfare of the world's population.

References

1. White House Conference on Food, Nutrition and Health. *Final Report*. Washington, D.C.: U.S. Government Printing Office, 1970.
2. Cross, A. T. USDA's strategies for the 80's: Nutrition education. *J. Am. Diet. Assoc.* 76:333, 1980.
3. Child Nutrition Act of 1966, Section 17(d), as amended, 42, U.S.C. 1786(d).
4. National School Lunch Act, Section 15, Child Nutrition Amendments of 1977, 42, U.S.C. 1788.
5. A peek into America's shopping bag. *FDA Consumer* 14:4, 1980.
6. Science and Education Administration, USDA *Your Money's Worth in Foods.* Home and Garden Bulletin No. 183, revised, April 1979.

Suggested Readings

Bell, A. C., et al. A method for describing food beliefs which may predict personal food choice. *J. Nutr. Educ.* 13:22, 1981.

Block, J. R. Federal focus on nutrition and dietetics. *J. Am. Diet. Assoc.* 79:643, 1981.

Board of the National Nutrition Consortium. Statement of nutrition education policy. *J. Nutr. Educ.* 12:138, 1980.

Boren, A. R., Dixon, P. N., and Harden, M. L. Innovations in nutrition education. *J. Am. Diet. Assoc.* 80:148, 1982.

Chapman, N. Incorporating nutrition into family planning services. *J. Nutr. Educ.* 10:129, 1978.

Contento, I. Children's thinking about food and eating: A Piagetian-based study. *J. Nutr. Educ.* 13 [Suppl.]:86, 1981.

Cuffaro, C., and Shymko, D. L. Games and audiovisual aids in preadolescent nutrition education. *J. Nutr. Educ.* 12:162, 1980.

Dixon, G., and Pickard, K. Nutrition education for young patients. *Children Today* Jan./ Feb. 1975. Pp. 7–11.

Dombrow, C. A. Good beginnings: A nutrition education program for preschoolers. *J. Can. Diet. Assoc.* 42:32, 1981.

Duyff, R. L., et al. Soup-to-nuts: A television approach to nutrition education. *J. Am. Diet. Assoc.* 80:157, 1982.

Dwyer, J. National conference on nutrition education: Directions for the 1980s. *J. Nutr. Educ.* 12 [Suppl.]:1, 1980.

Fleming, P. L., and Brown, J. E. Using market research approaches in nutrition education. *J. Nutr. Educ.* 13:4, 1981.

Gussow, J. D. The science and politics of nutrition education. *J. Nutr. Educ.* 12:140, 1980.

Industrial food in the family economy. *Nutr. Rev.* 40 [Suppl.]:18, 1982.

Karvetti, R.-L. Effects of nutrition education. *J. Am. Diet. Assoc.* 79:660, 1981.

Keith, J. E. The economics of nutrition planning. *J. Am. Diet. Assoc.* 79:649, 1981.

Kirk, T. R. Appraisal of the effectiveness of nutrition education in the context of infant feeding. *J. Hum. Nutr.* 34:429, 1980.

Leveille, G. A.   A nutrition scientist's view of food and nutrition education needs. *Food Technol.* 34:56, 1980.

McLaren, D. S. (ed.).   *Nutrition in the Community.* New York: Wiley, 1976.

Nutrition education announcements spark interest. *School Food Serv. J.* 35:16, 1981.

O'Hayan, C., et al.   Computer games for teaching nutrition. *J. Nutr. Educ.* 12:190, 1980.

Pelto, G. H.   Anthropological contributions to nutrition education research. *J. Nutr. Educ.* 13 [Suppl.]:2, 1981.

Popkin, B. M., and Haines, P. S.   Factors affecting food selection: The role of economics. *J. Am. Diet. Assoc.* 79:419, 1981.

Ritenbaugh, C.   An anthropological perspective on nutrition. *J. Nutr. Educ.* 13 [Suppl.]:12, 1981.

Shannon, B., and Smiciklas-Wright, H.   Nutrition education in relation to the needs of the elderly. *J. Nutr. Educ.* 11:85, 1979.

Tonon, M.   Models for educational interventions in malnourished populations. *Am. J. Clin. Nutr.* 31:2279, 1978.

PUBLICATIONS BY THE
USDA

Nutrition: Food at Work for You
Nutritive Value of Foods (Agriculture Handbook #8)
Your Money's Worth in Foods
Facts About Nutrition
The Thing the Professor Forgot
Patient Education Materials for Ostomates
Public and Patient Cancer Education Materials in Spanish

Chapter 32

NUTRITION AND ATHLETICS

The influence of diet on athletic performance has been known since ancient times. Each society has held its own beliefs as to which foods confer added strength and endurance, and which weaken the body and spirit. To this day, many trainers and coaches insist on a pregame meal of red meat and honey in the belief that it will improve athletic performance during competition.

The following chapter outlines what is currently known about nutrition and athletics, including the physiology of exercise, factors in optimal performance, ideal body weight and diet, the preevent meal, and glycogen loading. Diet alone is not the key to athletic excellence—it must be combined with a regimen of training and psychological discipline, built on a framework of overall good health.

Physiology of Exercise
MUSCLE ACTION AND METABOLISM

Muscles are composed of filamentous cells or fibers. Within the individual muscle cells are parallel rows of contractile proteins, *actin* and *myosin*. Muscle works by the sliding, or shortening, of these two elements. Also within the cells are mitochondria, the chemical "powerhouses" of the body, which burn metabolic fuels (glucose and fatty acids); and cytoplasm, which contains glycogen (storage form of carbohydrate) and the enzymes needed for converting nutrients into fuel. Glucose and fatty acids are supplied to the muscle cells via the blood. Oxygen combines with these fuels in a series of steps regulated by enzymes to produce energy, *ATP* (adenosine triphosphate), and the waste products of carbon dioxide and water. A combination of oxygen, fatty acids, and glucose make ATP, the fuel needed for actin and myosin filaments to shorten (or for the muscle to contract) (Fig. 32-1). ATP is not stored in muscle and therefore must be constantly regenerated from foods. Fatty acids are stored in the body's fat cells; glucose is stored as glycogen (many glucose molecules linked together) within the muscle. Glycogen stores are depleted during exercise, especially during periods of intense or prolonged activity such as sprinting, running, swimming, or cross-country skiing. There is a direct relationship between glycogen stores and the duration of physical exercise.

The limits of human endurance have been associated with the ability to consume oxygen maximally (VO_2 *max*). Normal, active males have maximum O_2 uptakes (VO_2 *max*) of 35–50 ml/kg/min. Among those athletes with the highest VO_2 max values are distance runners and marathoners. These athletes have oxygen uptake capacities nearly 50 percent greater than normally active individuals [1], between 65 and 80 ml/kg/min. *Endurance training* is defined as repeated activity without becoming breathless, with an expenditure of 75 percent or less of maximum O_2 uptake. This type of training can increase the size of mitochondria; the number of capillaries bringing oxygen, glucose, and fatty acids to cells; the enzyme systems; and the amount of glycogen stored per unit of muscle weight. The muscle itself also becomes more efficient, and there is an

FIG. 32-1. Action of voluntary or skeletal muscles.

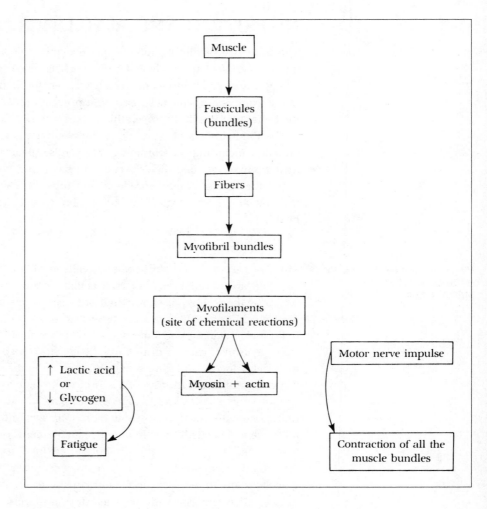

increase in the number of *slow-twitch fibers.* These fibers have a large number of mitochondria, prefer to use fatty acids (rather than glucose) as the energy source for ATP production, and are utilized when oxygen is available, as during endurance training. *Sprint training* is opposite to endurance training; it requires exerting maximum effort, with breathlessness following if carried on for more than a few seconds. It results in an increased number of *fast-twitch fibers*, those muscle cells with fewer mitochondria, increased contractile fibers, and increased enzymes to utilize glycogen. These fibers are utilized when there is little oxygen, as with short bursts of energy.

FACTORS IN OPTIMAL PERFORMANCE

The ability to utilize a large fraction of the *aerobic capacity* (%VO_2 max) during competition is an important factor in optimal performance. The availability and utilization of *energy resources* also influence athletic performance. Early in an endurance competition, about 90 percent of energy is supplied by carbohydrate

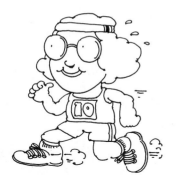

and about 10 percent by fat; by the end, 95 to 98 percent is derived from fat (free fatty acids). The *thermoregulatory response* also affects the efficiency of muscle metabolism; the circulatory system must transfer metabolically produced heat from the active muscle to the body surface, where it is dissipated by evaporation of sweat to the environment. Body temperature during a marathon race is directly dependent on metabolic rate or body weight or both (lower temperature with lighter weight); the average body temperature is between 104 and 105°F. *Body fluid loss* is the final factor directly affecting athletic performance. The dissipation of body heat by sweat evaporation results in large body water losses. During marathons as much as 4 to 6 kg (8.8 to 13.2 lb) of weight loss from fluids are usual. Most of this fluid loss is drawn from the intracellular spaces, not plasma volume (see Chap. 8 for details). This explains why marathon runners can tolerate such large losses without circulatory problems. When the fluid loss is greater than 3 percent, however, the body temperature begins to rise. Runners are usually unable to ingest enough fluids during competition to offset the large losses and some may become dehydrated.

DEHYDRATION SYNDROME AND HEAT STROKE

Dehydration syndrome can occur when there is as little as 3 percent loss of total body water. Appetite and capacity for work decrease, and both heart rate and body temperature increase with even slight activity. With a 5 percent loss, there is evidence of heat exhaustion and the capacity for hard, muscular work decreases by 20 to 30 percent [1]. A 7 percent loss results in hallucinations, and 10 percent can lead to heat stroke, circulatory collapse, and eventually death.

It is not possible to replace more than 800 ml per hour by drinking fluids; this is insufficient to meet needs during hard, long-term competition since losses average more than 2000 ml per hour. To avoid dehydration syndrome and heat stroke, it is advised that the athlete be well hydrated before competition. Small portions of chilled, dilute glucose with 20 to 30 mEq/liter of sodium should be taken at frequent intervals (not to exceed 1 liter per hour, to avoid risk of gastric overfilling) [1].

Heat stroke is caused by physical exertion and inadequate fluid intake. The major predisposing factors include high temperature, high humidity, poor body ventilation, and several hours of water deprivation preceding intense physical activity [2]. Without food, humans can survive about 30 days, but only 5 or 6 without water. About 3 pints of water per day are lost in the expired air, urine, sweat, and stools from a 70-kg male (154 lb) in a temperate climate. In a warm environment, this loss, accomplished by the evaporation of sweat, is the only means for lowering body heat. During physical exercise, body heat production is greatly increased. Without water available for perspiration, the body temperature increases above normal, resulting in overheating. Heat stroke is characterized by a high body temperature (106 to 110°F), deep coma, convulsions, absence of sweating, and failure to form urine. To avoid the symptoms of heat stroke, fluid intake must be adjusted as activity level and environmental temperature increase.

Ideal Body Weight
TYPE OF SPORT

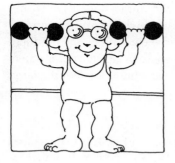

The ideal body weight for an athlete varies with the physical demands of the individual sport. In events such as weight lifting and shot put, additional weight may actually improve balance and stability. For swimmers, extra weight, particularly fat, aids in buoyance and insulation. Runners, especially marathoners, tend to be short and very lean. Marathon runners tend to have 5 to 7 percent body fat, or 9 to 12 percent less than normally active men. The average height of all the Boston Marathon Champions from 1897 to 1965 was only 67.1″, and average weight was 135.4 pounds [3]. Since skeletal structures and fat are dead weight in running, it is easy to see why the most successful runners are so built (Fig. 32-2).

The ideal body weight for an athlete provides maximum strength and endurance per pound, with body fat reduced to a minimal level compatible with health and optimal energy. With less body fat there is increased efficiency, although a minimal amount is vital for normal body functioning. In weight-matched events, such as lightweight rowing or wrestling, the athlete with the greatest muscle mass and least fat content has a competitive advantage. In events requiring almost continuous body movement, any additional body fat can limit both speed and endurance. The amount of body weight present as fat can be easily assessed by skinfold calipers, as described in Chapters 22 and 29. A triceps skinfold measurement less than 8 mm is considered to be lean for an athlete; 8 to 15 mm, acceptable; and greater than 15 mm, overweight [4].

WEIGHT REDUCTION

Weight loss in the athlete should be accomplished through a modest reduction in diet and a moderate increase in exercise; the rate of loss should not exceed 2 to 3 pounds per week. More rapid loss by starvation or dehydration compromises health and athletic performance. A weight-reduction diet during athletic training should provide no less than 1800 to 2200 calories per day for men, and 1600 to 2000 calories per day for women [5]. Since each pound of body weight represents 3500 calories, a daily caloric deficit of 1000 calories will result in a loss of 2 pounds per week.

SPECIAL PROBLEMS OF
FEMALE ATHLETES

It has been found that a minimal level of stored energy is necessary for ovulation and menstrual cycles in the female; this has been termed the *critical lean/fat ratio* [6]. When the total body fat content drops below 9 to 10 percent (normal is 20 to 22 percent), female athletes experience *secondary amenorrhea* (three or less menstrual cycles in 1 year), or if prepubescent, have *delayed menarche* [7, 8]. For runners, the frequency of amenorrhea is positively correlated with the number of miles run per week. An alternate explanation for the cessation of regular cycles in highly trained female athletes is the metabolic and hormonal effects of stress resulting from arduous training and competition. One of the side effects of amenorrhea is a higher hematocrit (volume percentage of red blood cells in the blood), which may explain the better endurance performance in these female athletes [8].

FIG. 32-2. This runner's training program probably includes
a nutritious and well-planned
diet in addition to daily 5- to
10-mile jaunts. (Photo by Jeffrey
Grosscup)

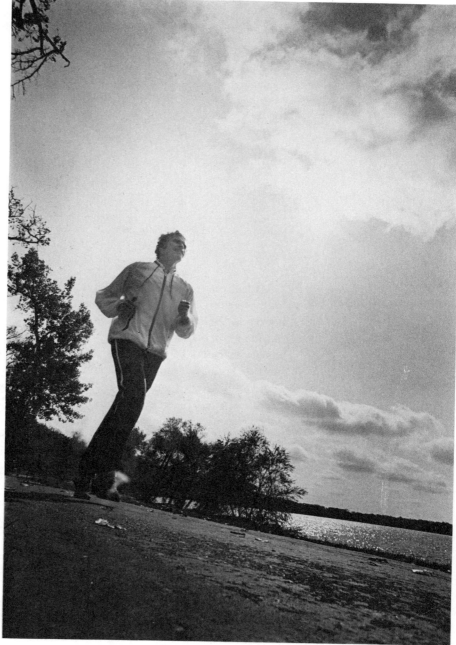

TABLE 32-1. Caloric cost of exercise per minute

Sport	Kcal/min
Long distance running	19.4
Wrestling	14.2
Swimming	11.2
Basketball	8.6
Bicycling	8.2
Tennis	7.1
Gymnastics	6.5
Walking at 3.5 mph	5.2
Baseball	4.7
Volleyball	3.5
Reclining	1.3

Source: S. H. Vitovsek, Is more better? (Nutrition aspects of athletic performance II.) *Nutrition Today*, Nov/Dec 1979. Pp. 10–17.

Ideal Diet
PROPORTION OF CALORIES AND NUTRIENTS

The ideal diet for training and competition is one that maintains an efficient body weight while meeting the increased energy requirements. The caloric cost of exercise depends on the athlete's size and metabolic rate, and the intensity and duration of the sport. The energy expended can be measured by the amount of oxygen consumed; both increase with increases in body weight, speed, and number of muscle contractions, and decrease with improved skill. The position and ease of lung expansion also affects energy expenditure. Table 32-1 outlines the caloric cost of exercise per minute; Table 32-2 shows caloric requirements for participation in athletic events.

The proper proportion of nutrients in an athlete's diet should be divided as 15 percent of calories from protein, 30 to 35 percent from fat, and 50 to 55 percent from carbohydrate. These proportions differ from the average American diet by being lower in protein and fat (20 percent and 40 percent, respectively), and higher in carbohydrate (40 percent). The lower proportion of protein is contrary to the misconception that athletes need more protein to build muscles; the size of the muscle depends on the physical demands placed on it. Carbohydrate is the most efficiently utilized fuel, and is more readily available when needs are increased during training and competition. These guidelines have been translated into servings per day in Table 32-3.

The protein foods in an athlete's diet should be of high biologic value, containing all eight of the essential amino acids needed to build and repair tissues. Such proteins are also vital for the production of hormones, antibodies, and enzymes—all essential for optimal performance. Excessive amounts of dietary protein, however, increase the work of the liver and kidney, for its metabolism and elimination of its by-products. Also, by increasing the amount of protein in the diet, consumption of carbohydrate, a more valuable and efficient fuel, will be reduced.

TABLE 32-2. Determining caloric requirements for participation in athletic events

Sport	Reference athlete		Daily caloric requirement for maintenance + light work (kcal)	Calories expended per minute of activity	Minutes of activity per event	Calories expended per event	Approximate daily caloric requirement for maintenance + light work + event participation (kcal)
	Height	Weight (lb)					
MEN							
Football	6'2"	195	2700	10.2	10	102	2800
Wrestling	6'3"	218	3000	14.2	8	114	3100
Gymnastics (apparatus)	5'10"	153	2100	6.5	6	39	2100
Hockey	6'3"	195	2700	11.5	15	173	2900
Long-distance running (5 miles)	5'9"	155	2100	14.4	25	360	2600
Swimming	6'1"	174	2400	11.0	20	220	2600
Tennis	5'10"	160	2200	7.1	45	320	2500
Baseball	6'1"	200	2700	4.7	60	282	3000
Basketball	6'3"	175	2400	8.6	40	344	2800
WOMEN							
Swimming	5'4"	137	1800	11.0	25	275	2100
Tennis	5'5"	115	1600	7.1	60	420	2000
Gymnastics (apparatus)	5'7"	120	1600	5.0	4.5	23	1625
Basketball	5'10"	160	2200	8.6	32	275	2500
Running (1 mile)	5'7"	120	1600	10.6	5.5	58	1700

Source: D. M. Huse and R. A. Nelson, Basic balanced diet meets requirements of athletes. *Physician and Sports Medicine* 5:52, 1977.

TABLE 32-3. Daily food plan (3000 kcal) for athletic training

MEAT OR SUBSTITUTE (10 oz daily)
1 oz of meat or its equivalent contains 7 gm protein, 5 gm fat, and 73 calories. Meat or substitutes include beef, veal, lamb, pork, fish, fowl, cold cuts,* cheese,* cottage cheese, egg,* shellfish,* and peanut butter.*

MILK (3 cups daily)
One cup of skim milk contains 8 gm protein, 12 gm carbohydrate, and 80 calories. Milk substitutes include whole,* 2%,* skim, evaporated milk,* or ice cream.*

BREAD OR SUBSTITUTE (12 servings daily)
One serving of bread or its equivalent contains 2 gm protein, 15 gm carbohydrate, and 68 calories. Bread or substitutes include bread, dinner rolls, biscuits, cereal, pancake,* waffle,* crackers, potato, rice, macaroni, noodles, popcorn, or pretzels.

FAT (12 servings daily)
One serving of fat contains 5 gm fat and 45 calories. Fats or oils include butter,* margarine, oils, salad dressing, gravy,* bacon,* and cream.*

VEGETABLES (3–4 servings daily)
One serving of vegetable contains 2 gm protein, 7 gm carbohydrate, and 36 calories. Vegetables may be fresh, frozen, cooked, or canned.

FRUIT OR FRUIT JUICE (6 servings daily)
One serving of fruit contains 10 gm carbohydrate and 40 calories. Fruits may be fresh, frozen, cooked, or canned.

DESSERT (1 serving daily)
One serving contains 3 gm protein, 5 gm fat, 30 gm carbohydrate, and 200 calories. Desserts include pie, sweet roll, cookies, cake, or chocolate.

SUGARS AND SWEETS (4 servings daily)
One serving contains 15 gm carbohydrate and 60 calories. Sugars and sweets include sugar, jelly, honey, syrup, hard candy, and carbonated beverage.

*Omit from diet to reduce cholesterol and/or saturated fat.
Source: D. M. Huse and R. A. Nelson, Basic balanced diet meets requirements of athletes. *Physician and Sports Medicine* 5:52, 1977.

Fat is the most frequently used fuel to power muscles. With moderate energy expenditure (60 to 70 percent of maximum), about half the energy is supplied by carbohydrate and half by fat. The body requires more oxygen to burn fat as a fuel than to burn carbohydrate; therefore, fat is preferentially used when oxygen supplies are ample. With exercise or workloads greater than 90 percent of maximum effort (or O_2 consumption), almost all of the energy is derived from carbohydrate, since oxygen supplies are reduced.

Metabolism appears to be disturbed when carbohydrate levels are low or nonexistent. Production of ketone bodies (end product of fat breakdown) increases, along with the development of fatigue, negative water and electrolyte negative balances, and an increased excretion of nitrogen. About 100 to 150 gm of carbohydrates per day is necessary to avoid ketosis and amino acid use. Both fats and carbohydrates serve as energy fuels, the proportion depends on the level of work and dietary intake, as discussed above. During prolonged exercise of 40 to 60 percent VO_2 max uptakes, one of the main determinants for work capacity is the concentration of muscle glycogen. It is not known if it is due to the maintenance of a higher blood glucose level or increased efficiency in muscular work. Up to 70 percent VO_2 max, the blood supplies sufficient carbohydrate; above this level, the muscle glycogen stores affect endurance [9].

FLUIDS, ELECTROLYTES, AND VITAMINS

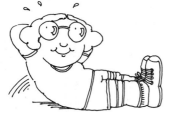

Fluids are needed to regulate body temperature and prevent dehydration, which could lead to *hyperthermia* and heat stroke. If fluids are taken during exercise, they should be dilute enough to be emptied rapidly from the stomach; concentrated fluids cause cramping by drawing the body's fluids into the gastrointestinal tract. If the athlete is healthy, electrolyte supplements should not be necessary since the kidneys will naturally compensate by conserving sodium and potassium. Sodium supplements are necessary only when perspiration losses are heavy during hot weather and when exercise is done over a long period of time. Sodium supplements can actually be potentially dangerous because, if not taken with sufficient fluids, they can lead to dehydration (by requiring extra fluids for their dilution and excretion). Potassium levels may be low in some athletes after exercise, due to hemodilution rather than depletion. Potassium is actually liberated into the bloodstream from cells as glycogen is broken down.

During exercise, there is no additional vitamin requirement other than the levels found in a balanced diet of adequate calories. Excessive amounts of vitamins do not improve performance, although deficiencies may decrease it. High intakes of vitamin C, thought to enhance collagen synthesis and repair, have been associated with the development of kidney stones and vitamin B_{12} deficiency (see Chap. 33, Self-Prescribed Regimens). Other side effects of high doses of vitamin C include a rebound deficiency, diarrhea, and a tendency to develop scurvy when the high dosages are discontinued [10].

Athlete's anemia is the term for borderline low level of hemoglobin found among many endurance athletes. Because it is resistant to iron supplements, athlete's anemia is probably not of nutritional origin. Some iron is lost in perspiration, but not enough to cause iron deficiency. Athletes should be aware that large doses of iron may cause nausea, constipation, gastrointestinal upset, and deposition in tissues in genetically predisposed individuals.

PREEVENT MEAL

Timing of the preevent meal is of increased importance in middle-duration and long-duration events because its content is a source of energy. Timing is also important in contact sports where there is an increased risk of trauma; surgery and anesthesia are less dangerous for an individual with an empty stomach. It is recommended that the meal be eaten at least 3 hours before most events, to allow time for gastric emptying. Gastric emptying is slowed by fear, worry, anger, excitement, or any strong emotion. Normal emptying of the stomach averages 3 to 4 hours; with pregame tension it may be delayed up to as much as 6 hours. Fatty foods also delay gastric emptying and digestion. When food is present in the stomach or intestines, both digestion and muscular activity are compromised since the blood supply must be divided between the two functions. Liquids and semisolid foods require little gastric digestion and are absorbed quickly; blood glucose values at 1, 2, and 3 hours are increased [11].

The meal prior to a short-duration event has much less effect on performance since the energy to be used during the event comes from food metabolized long before the competition. For long-duration or average-duration events (which require an aerobic or steady-state type of metabolism), the preevent meal should be relatively high in carbohydrates for the following reasons [4]:

1. There is increased utilization of carbohydrates as a fuel because it is the most efficient source of energy.
2. By increasing the amount of carbohydrate in the preevent meal, the proportions of fat and protein are decreased. Fat takes longer to digest and protein may place a strain on the kidneys, especially since blood flow to the kidneys is decreased during exercise.
3. More glycogen is stored in muscles by high carbohydrate diets.

Foods to avoid include coffee and tea, due to their diuretic effect, and alcohol, because it impairs fine motor coordination.

Glycogen Loading

The amount of stored glycogen affects the intensity and duration of physical exercise and is the limiting factor in endurance exercise. The purpose of glycogen loading is to supersaturate muscles with glycogen for optimal competitive performance. When fed a high-carbohydrate diet for 3 days before competition, runners had twice the glycogen stores and faster running times than controls [12]. Such activities as crew, ice hockey, tournament tennis, cross-country skiing, long-distance swimming and cycling, and distance running may be enhanced by glycogen loading.

During heavy exercise, glycogen (storage form of carbohydrate) is utilized as the main energy source, at the rate of 2 to 3 gm per minute [13]. Normally about 300 to 400 gm of glycogen are stored in the liver and muscle, but a glycogen-loading regimen can double this amount. There is a correlation between increasing glycogen levels and prolonging endurance, but this does not necessarily increase speed of competitive performance. As glycogen stores approach zero, speed and endurance also decline. Therefore, endurance is ultimately affected by the minimal level of glycogen present and the rate of glycogen utilization. The ingestion of small amounts of carbohydrate during exercise may decrease the rate of glycogen utilization and increase endurance. With training, there is more efficient metabolism of free fatty acids and therefore less depletion of glycogen stores.

The method of glycogen loading involves three phases. *Phase I*, the depletion phase, occurs on days 7 to 4 before the athletic event. The muscles are depleted of glycogen by exercising to exhaustion by the same activity as performed during the event. After depleting the muscles of glycogen, a high-fat, high-protein, low-carbohydrate diet is given for 3 days. The carbohydrate intake during this phase should be about 100 gm per day to prevent muscle proteins from being broken down to meet energy needs and to avoid ketosis. Because of the low carbohydrate intake, the individual may feel tired, irritable, nervous, or nauseated. *Phase II,* the supersaturation phase, occurs on days 3 to 1 before the event. The caloric intake is the same as in Phase I, but 250 to 525 gm of carbohydrate are taken (1000 to 2100 calories from carbohydrate), supersaturating the muscles with glycogen [14]. It is recommended that little or no exercise be done during this phase because it will diminish the glycogen stores. *Phase III* is the day of the event. Any diet may be taken that is tolerated, but the preevent meal should be eaten 4 to 6 hours prior so that the stomach and intestines are empty during competition. A shorter method, using only Phase II and III can be used for shorter events to fill, not supersaturate, glycogen stores. The individual should exercise to exhaustion 4 days before, then have 3 days on a high-carbohydrate diet. On a regular, mixed diet, the level of muscle glycogen is about 1.5 gm per 100 gm of muscle; with 3 days on a high-carbohydrate diet it is about 2.5 gm; on the short method it is about 4.0 gm; and with the full regimen it is 5.0 gm [4].

The effects of overloading muscle with glycogen may not be completely beneficial; it is not known what effect it has on the heart. Also, for every gram of glycogen stored in muscle or liver, 2.7 gm of water are also bound. This may result in an additional 2.5 to 3.5 kg of body weight as bound water when glycogen stores are supersaturated, contributing to a feeling of stiffness and heaviness in the muscles [13]. This additional fluid may be viewed as an impediment to optimal performance, or as a water reserve readily utilized during physical exercise. A summary of recommendations for athletes involved in training or competition is given in Table 32-4.

TABLE 32-4. Recommendations for athletes involved in training or competition

1. Meet increased caloric and nutrient needs by increasing the number of selections from the "calories-plus-nutrients" foods.
2. Maintain a hydrated state by consuming fluid before, during, and after exercise.
3. Meet needs for additional electrolytes from foods ordinarily consumed.
4. Electrolyte supplements should be used only on the advice of the team physician.
5. A high-carbohydrate intake prior to competition can be beneficial to some athletes engaging in endurance events.
6. The use of beer, wine, or distilled alcoholic beverages as a source of calories, as a muscle relaxant, or as an ergogenic aid is not advocated.
7. Recommendation that a light pregame meal be eaten 3 to 4 hours prior to the competition.

8. Athletes not currently involved in training or competition should reduce their caloric intake to balance their energy expenditure.

Source: Nutrition and physical fitness: A statement by the American Dietetic Association. *Journal of the American Dietetic Association* 76:437, 1980.

Conclusions

Optimal athletic performance results from a combination of several factors, one of the most important being proper diet. As with other states of health, variety and balance is the key, with modifications at special times during training and competition. No single food or food group holds the secret to outstanding performance; this results only from hard training, proper diet, psychological discipline, and good health.

References

1. Bergstrom, J., and Hultman, E. Nutrition for maximal sports performance. *J.A.M.A.* 221:999, 1972.
2. National Academy of Science–National Research Council. Water deprivation and performance of athletes. *Nutr. Rev.* 32:314, 1974.
3. Costill, D. L. Physiology of marathon running. *J.A.M.A.* 221:1024, 1972.
4. Vitovsek, S. H. Is more better? (Nutrition aspects of athletic performance II.) *Nutr. Today* Nov./Dec. 1979. Pp. 10–17.
5. Smith, N. J. Excessive weight loss and food aversion in athletes simulating anorexia nervosa. *Pediatrics* 66:139, 1980.
6. Frisch, R. E., and McArthur, J. W. Menstrual cycles: Fatness as a determinant of minimum weight for height necessary for their maintenance or onset. *Science* 185:949, 1974.
7. Frisch, R. E., Wyshak, G., and Vincent, L. Delayed menarche and amenorrhea in ballet dancers. *N. Engl. J. Med.* 303:17, 1980.
8. Feicht, C. B., et al. Secondary amenorrhea in athletes. *Lancet* 2:1145, 1978.
9. Consolazio, F., and Johnson, H. L. Dietary carbohydrate and work capacity. *Am. J. Clin. Nutr.* 25:85, 1972.
10. Hoyt, C. J. Diarrhea from vitamin C (letters to the editor). *J.A.M.A.* 244:1674, 1980.
11. Macaraeg, P. V. J. High carbohydrate, low fat liquid meal for athletes. *J. Sports Med.* 14:259, 1974.
12. Karlsson, J., and Saltin, B. Diet, muscle glycogen and endurance performance. *J. Appl. Physiol.* 31:203, 1971.
13. Olson, K.-E., and Saltin, B. Diet and fluids in training and competition. *Scand. J. Rehab. Med.* 3:31, 1971.
14. Forgac, M. T. Carbohydrate loading: A review. *J. Am. Diet. Assoc.* 75:42, 1979.

Suggested Readings

Bailey, R. R., et al. What the urine contains following athletic competition. *N.Z. Med. J.* 83:309, 1976.

Buxbaum, R., and Michelli, L. J. *Sports for Life: Fitness Training, Injury Prevention, and Nutrition.* Boston: Beacon Press, 1979. P. 204.

Chapman, C. B., and Mitchell, J. H. The physiology of exercise. *Sci. Am.* 212:88, 1965.

Clark, N. *The Athlete's Kitchen: A Nutrition Guide and Cookbook.* Boston: CBI Publishing, 1981.

Darden, E. *Nutrition and Athletic Performance.* Pasadena, Calif.: Athletic Press, 1976. P. 208.

Fluid replacement in the athlete; the pregame meal; nutritional faddism and athletics. *Nutr. & M.D.* December 1977.

Fogoros, R. N. "Runner's trots": Gastrointestinal disturbances in runners. *J.A.M.A.* 243:1743, 1980.

Frisch, R. E., et al. Delayed menarche and amenorrhea of college athletes in relation to age of onset of training. *J.A.M.A.* 246:1559, 1981.

Hanley, D. F.   Athletic training: And how diet affects it. *Nutr. Today* Nov./Dec. 1979. Pp. 5–9.

Hanley, D. F.   Basic diet guidance for athletes. *Nutr. Today* Nov./Dec. 1979. Pp. 22–23.

Hartung, G. H., et al.   Relation of diet to high-density lipoprotein cholesterol in middle-aged marathon runners, joggers, and inactive men. *N. Engl. J. Med.* 302:357, 1980.

Hursh, L. M.   Practical hints about feeding athletes. *Nutr. Today* Nov./Dec. 1979. Pp. 18–20.

Jetté, M., et al.   The nutritional and metabolic effects of a carbohydrate-rich diet in a glycogen super-compensation training regime. *Am. J. Clin. Nutr.* 31:2140, 1978.

Martin, B., Robinson, S., and Robertshaw, D.   Influence of diet on leg uptake during heavy exercise. *Am. J. Clin. Nutr.* 31:62, 1978.

Milkereit, J., and Higdon, H.   *Runner's Cookbook*. Mountain View, Calif.: World Publications, 1979. P. 331.

Nutrition and athletic performance. *Dairy Counc. Dig.* vol. 46, 1975.

Rebar, R. W., and Cumming, D. C.   Reproductive function in women athletes. *J.A.M.A.* 246:1590, 1981.

Serfass, R. C.   Nutrition for the athlete, update, 1982. *Contemp. Nutr.* vol. 7, 1982.

Smith, N. J.   *Food for Sport*. Palo Alto, Calif.: Bull Publishing, 1976. P. 188.

Smith, N. J.   Gaining and losing weight in athletics. *J.A.M.A.* 236:149, 1976.

Spence, H. A.   Dietary requirements of ultra-long distance runners. *Food Nutr. Notes Rev.* 34:172, 1977.

Sullivan, S. N.   The gastrointestinal symptoms of running. *N. Engl. J. Med.* 304:915, 1981.

Travis, S. P. L., and Templer, M. J.   "Carboloading" and dehydration. *Lancet* 1:1370, 1981.

Williams, M. H.   *Nutritional Aspects of Human Physical and Athletic Performance*. Springfield, Ill.: Thomas, 1976.

Chapter 33

SELF-PRESCRIBED REGIMENS

This chapter presents some of the more common "self-prescribed regimens," ranging from megavitamin therapy to the use of laetrile to treat cancer. The topics presented represent only the tip of the iceberg, only a fraction of the unproven, unscientific, unsafe, and even lethal therapies in current use by many Americans.

The reasons for the popularity of some of these regimens may stem from misinformation or misinterpretation of inadequate information. Food fads and medical quackery become dangerous when they prevent the consumer from seeking proper medical or nutritional treatment that might have spared them unnecessary suffering or even saved their lives. Some of the regimens, such as high doses of certain vitamins advocated by so-called experts, have resulted in permanent birth defects.

Freedom of choice in the United States can be a dual-edged sword. Americans have the choice to follow the advice of anyone they choose, including medical and nutrition quacks and charlatans, many of whom make great profits off the gullability of the consumer. The ready access of high doses of vitamins and minerals over the counter make implementing many of the food fads very easy. Although the only true cure for health quackery is consumer education, perhaps there is something deep inside everyone that believes in miracles, and perhaps that one of the current fads may finally be just that [1].

Megavitamins
GENERAL CONSIDERATIONS

Many Americans feel that if a little is good, a lot must be better. In today's health-and-nutrition-conscious society, thousands apply this myth to the use of vitamins, in the hope of warding off colds, clearing up acne, improving their sex lives, or just for coping with that "rundown feeling." Many of these unsubstantiated claims are based on extrapolations from animal studies, human studies consisting of extremely small groups, or poorly designed and controlled experiments. Many supposed nutrition "experts" advocate the use of large doses of various vitamins; the results are dangerous or even catastrophic [2]. The Food and Drug Administration's National Clearinghouse for Poison Control Centers have over 4000 cases of vitamin poisoning reported to them each year, 3200 involving children [3].

Some of the myths about vitamins have been around for so long that it is difficult to distinguish them from fact. For example, many people believe that additional vitamins provide extra energy. Vitamins do aid in the conversion of food to energy (usually as cofactors), but amounts in excess of the recommended daily allowances (RDA) are merely wasted. Certain rare medical conditions may require specific vitamins in additional amounts, but the diagnosis and treatment of these disorders should always be done by a medical doctor.

The daily use of a multivitamin supplement as an insurance for good health is another commonly accepted (and widely advertised) myth. A balanced diet from

FIG. 33-1. Vitamin "therapy" has become a multimillion dollar business. This drug store window, like many around the country, advertises a large and varied inventory of vitamin and mineral supplements. (Photo by Paul Wissel.)

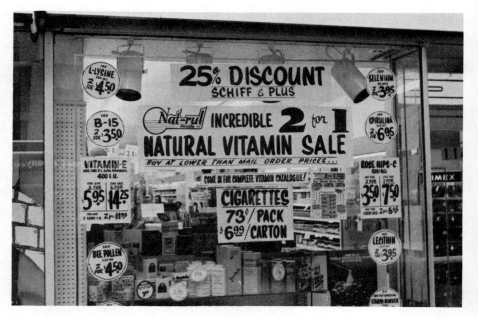

a variety of foods will usually meet the RDA for all nutrients without the need for vitamin or mineral supplements. In addition, food tastes better than pills (Fig. 33-1).

Large doses of individual vitamins, in amounts far greater than physiologic requirements, have been advocated for a variety of conditions. The use of vitamins in amounts 10 times the RDA is called *megavitamin therapy*. Of particular danger are the fat-soluble vitamins that are stored in the body, usually the liver. The following discussion presents some of the more popular regimens and their possible side effects. See Tables 33-1 and 33-2 for the toxic effects of vitamins and minerals.

VITAMIN E

This vitamin has been one of the most intensely studied over the past few years. At present, vitamin E supplementation is indicated in only two conditions—for premature infants who may not have received adequate amounts before birth and to prevent eye damage to this same group of infants when they are given oxygen therapy; and for individuals with intestinal disorders in which fats are poorly absorbed. Some of the interest in this vitamin has been based on misinterpretations of animal research; male rats placed on a vitamin E–deficient diet became sterile. Large doses of vitamin E have not been proven to be effective in humans, however, in treating sterility or infertility.

Vitamin E acts as an antioxidant, but its precise role in metabolism is still unclear. Toxic effects have been demonstrated in animals, including decreased growth rate, hematocrit, thyroid function, and bone calcification, but skin rash to vitamin E aerosol deodorant has been the only toxic effect reported in humans

TABLE 33-1. Toxic effects of dietary and supplemental excesses of vitamins

Vitamin	Toxic range	Symptoms
Vitamin A	>50,000 IU/day	Irritability; nerve lesions; headaches; insomnia; painful bones and joints; hepatosplenomegaly; abnormal bone growth; jaundice; anorexia; decreased clotting time
Vitamin D	>4000 IU/day	*This is the most toxic of all vitamins when used in excess.* Symptoms include anorexia, nausea, thirst, diarrhea, renal failure, polyuria, muscular weakness, joint pains, resorption of bones, and calcification of soft tissues.
Vitamin E	Unknown	High blood pressure; allergies; GI distress; nausea; derangements of iron metabolism
Vitamin K	Unknown	Possible thrombosis; vomiting; porphyrinuria; and kernicterus
Vitamin B_1 (thiamin)	>6000 mg/day	Edema; nervousness; sweating; tachycardia; tremors; allergies; fatty liver; vascular hypotension
Vitamin B_2 (riboflavin)	Unknown	Paresthesia; itching
Vitamin B_6	>1000 mg/day	Limited toxicity
Vitamin B_{12} (cyanocobalamin)	Unknown	Polycythemia (increased number of red blood cells)
Vitamin C (ascorbic acid)	Unknown	Possible kidney stones in gouty individuals; possible damage to beta cells in the pancreas; decreased insulin production; possible diarrhea; allergies; reproductive failure; thrombosis; aciduria (oxalic, folic, or uric); B_{12} inactivation
Biotin	Unknown	Essentially nontoxic
Folic acid	Unknown	No toxicity reported
Niacin	>50 gm/day	Burning; itching; peripheral vasodilation; decreased serum cholesterol; fatty liver; stimulated central nervous system; increased pulse rate, respiratory rate, and cerebral blood flow; decreased blood pressure
Pantothenic acid	Unknown	Increased blood histamine; increased sensitivity of skeletal joints

Source: Adapted from R. J. Kutsky, *Handbook of Vitamins, Minerals and Hormones* (2nd ed.). New York: Van Nostrand Reinhold, 1981.

[4]. Other drug interactions include increased requirements of this vitamin with oral contraceptive use, and the need to reduce digitalis with high vitamin E usage [5, 6].

VITAMIN A

Vitamin A, as discussed in Chap. 7, is an essential nutrient necessary for the maintenance of tissue, optimal growth, and normal visual function. A deficiency of this vitamin causes impaired dark adaptation and night blindness. Recent nutrition surveys in the United States indicate that a significant proportion of the population has a low intake of vitamin A and low plasma vitamin A levels.

Dietary sources of vitamin A include carotenoids, which are converted to vitamin A in the intestines, or preformed sources, as in foods from animal sources. There is no danger of excessive intake when the vitamin A is in the form of carotenoids. The recommended dietary allowances for vitamin A are 2000 IU (400 retinol equivalents) for infants and children; 5000 IU (1000 retinol equivalents) for adult males; and 4000 IU (800 retinol equivalents) for adult females.

Excessive intakes of preformed vitamin A may result in potentially toxic side

TABLE 33-2. Toxic effects of dietary and supplemental excesses of minerals and trace elements

Substance	Toxic range	Effects	
		Acute	Chronic
Phosphorus	Unknown	Hyperphosphatemia, hypocalcemia, hypomagnesemia, tetany, laxative effects	Secondary hyperparathyroidism, bone resorption, calcification of heart and kidney, hypocalcemia
Calcium	Unknown	Calcium salts are practically nontoxic except for calcium arsenate (arsenic toxicity), calcium molybdate (molybdenum toxicity), calcium chloride (gastric irritant), hypercalcemia (hyperthyroid individuals), vitamin D overdosage	Practically nontoxic except for the three acute effects
Magnesium	>15 gm/day	Purgative, nausea, malaise, muscular weakness and paralysis, paralysis of respiratory cardiovascular, and CNS	Muscle weakness, hypotension, ECG changes, sedation, confusion
Sodium	>18 gm/day, or 30 gm/day as NaCl	Animals: excessive water intake, diarrhea, stiff gait, salivation, muscular fibrillation, exhaustion, respiratory failure, encephalopathy, congestion of organs, death (terminally)	Animals: inhibition of growth, increased water intake, increased urinary volume, massive edema, hypertension, anemia, lipemia, hypoproteinemia, azotemia, death (terminally)
Potassium	>12 gm/day, or 25 gm/day as KCl	Animals: convulsions, CNS paralysis, diarrhea, diuresis, dehydration, fever, congestive heart failure, cardiac arrhythmias, respiratory failure	Cardiac and CNS depression, mental confusion, weakness, vomiting, numbness, tingling
Zinc	>1 gm/day	Diarrhea, CNS depression, tremors, paralysis of the extremities	Poor growth, anemia, anorexia, symptoms of calcium and iron deficiencies
Iron	>100 mg/day	Shock, rapid increase in pulse and respiration, hypotension, pallor, drowsiness in 6–8 hours, prostration, coma and death from cardiac failure in 36 hours	Prolonged clotting time, metabolic acidosis, hemorrhaging

Mineral	Dose		
Cobalt	>490 mcg/day	Nausea, vomiting, diarrhea, paralysis, hypotension, hypothermia, death	Thyroid dysfunction, goiter, congestive heart failure, damage to alpha cells of the pancreas, cancer
Copper	>250 mg/day	Fever, tachycardia, hypotension, anemia, oliguria, uremia, coma, cardiovascular collapse, death	Nausea, vomiting, diarrhea, dizziness, general debility, jaundice
Chromium	>500 mg/day	Cr^{6+}: GI ulceration, CNS symptoms; Cr^{3+}: little or no effect	Animals: Cr^{6+}: depressed growth, damaged liver and kidney; Cr^{3+}: vomiting and diarrhea; humans: no reports of toxicity
Manganese	>1 gm/day	Animals: retarded growth; humans: calcium loss in feces, severe rickets, anorexia, impotency, muscle fatigue	Manganism (similar to Parkinson's disease), nephritis, cirrhosis, anorexia, muscle fatigue, anemia, tremors, hallucinations, insomnia, slurred speech, mental confusion
Iodine	>1000 mcg/day	GI irritation, hemorrhage	Iodism: brassy taste, burning sensation, of mouth and throat, head cold symptoms, pulmonary edema, skin lesions, gastric irritation, diarrhea
Fluoride	>80 mg/day; lethal dose: 2 gm/day	Weakness, GI symptoms, salivation, nausea, abdominal pain, diarrhea, hypocalcemia, irritability, convulsions, death from paralysis or cardiac failure	Mottled teeth, calcification of ligaments
Selenium	>0.4 mcg/day	Animals: blindness, abdominal pain, salivation, anorexia, weakness	Dental caries, loss of weight and hair, anemia, birth defects
Molybdenum	>1000 mcg/day	Severe diarrhea	Gout

Source: Adapted from R. J. Kutsky, *Handbook of Vitamins, Minerals and Hormones* (2nd ed.). New York: Van Nostrand Reinhold, 1981.

effects. Because of the easy availability of large doses of vitamin A without a prescription and the accumulation of this drug by the body, toxic levels can be reached within short periods. Teratogenic effects of vitamin A have been demonstrated in animals, including cleft-palate, central nervous system malformations, and heart and kidney defects. Renal malformations have been reported in humans [7]. High doses of vitamin A given to children have resulted in edema of the extremities and face, rash, bone pain, hypercalcemia, and signs of increased intracranial pressure [8].

VITAMIN D

This vitamin is involved in the regulation of calcium and phosphate metabolism, and is essential for the prevention of rickets in children and osteomalacia in adults. The two sources of inactivated vitamin D include the intestinal absorption from the diet or food supplements with dietary fats, and from the conversion of 7-dehydrocholesterol in the skin by ultraviolet light. Four hundred IUs of vitamin D per day is the recommended daily allowance for infants and children; this amount can usually be met by the consumption of 1 quart of fortified formula or milk per day. This requirement decreases to 300 IU during adolescence and to 200 IU during adulthood.

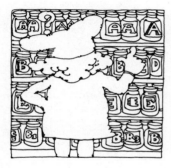

Toxic effects of this vitamin are manifest by alterations in calcium metabolism. In the past, large and prolonged doses of vitamin D were used to treat arthritis. More recently, large doses have been inappropriately used during infancy, pregnancy, and in renal disease. In England during World War II, when diets of infants were oversupplemented with vitamin D, the incidence of infantile hypercalcemia rose [9]. This syndrome includes renal, cardiovascular, and cerebral damage.

Some of the few diseases that do require increased dosages of vitamin D include hypoparathyroidism and epilepsy treated with long-term phenytoin therapy [10, 11].

VITAMIN C

This vitamin has received much interest recently concerning its use as a prophylactic measure against the common cold [12]. The effectiveness of large doses of this vitamin are still being disputed.

Vitamin C is essential for wound healing and the integrity of capillary structure, among other functions. The RDAs for adults, set at 60 mg per day in 1980, have been challenged as being too low, adequate only to prevent scurvy, the deficiency disease caused by lack of this vitamin.

Large doses of vitamin C may cause diarrhea and acidification of the urine. This latter effect may lead to the precipitation of cystine or oxalate stones in the urinary tract. When healthy adults become conditioned to high doses of this vitamin, they develop scurvylike symptoms when returning to a normal intake. Infants born to women who took high doses of vitamin C during pregnancy have been shown to develop scurvy when removed from this high vitamin level at birth [13]. High levels of vitamin C have also been shown to destroy substantial amounts of vitamin B_{12}, which could eventually lead to the development of megaloblastic anemia; high doses may cause the precipitation of gouty arthritis or renal calculi in susceptible individuals [14, 15].

Organic Foods

Many consumers hold beliefs about nutrition that are based more on custom, fashion, and fantasy than on fact. There is a growing interest on the part of consumers in the safety and nutritional quality of the American diet. Much of this interest, however, is influenced by misleading information that the American food supply is unsafe, tainted, or in some way nutritionally inadequate.

Products that are labeled "natural" or "organic" are usually promoted as being purer and nutritionally superior to those products that are conventionally grown and marketed. The majority of these claims are not supported by scientific evidence, but it is often difficult for the public to separate fact from fantasy, particularly when the term "natural" is used. If a false or misleading claim is made on the label of a food product, the Food and Drug Administration (FDA) can take legal steps against the company on the grounds that the product is misbranded or mislabeled. The Federal Trade Commission can take legal action if false claims are made in promotional materials or advertisements for the product. However, indirect promotion of a product, such as false claims made in a speech, magazine article, or book are protected by the First Amendment of the United States Constitution—free speech and a free press.

One of the basic alleged differences between organically and conventionally grown food is that organic food has more nutrients and is grown without the use of "harmful" pesticides. Plants take what they need from the soil for their own metabolism; if the nutrients are not present in the soil, the plant will not grow. The amount of nutrients in any given plant is genetically determined. Various plants can be bred to have more of a given nutrient, but this cannot be achieved by simply changing the type of fertilizer used. Actually, organically grown foods are more likely to be contaminated with *Salmonella*, an organism that causes a common form of food poisoning. The FDA monitors the level of residual pesticide present in foods, using extremely conservative international standards. (See Chap. 20 for a more detailed discussion of how the FDA monitors pesticide residues in foods.) These levels have always been much lower than what is considered unsafe. Small amounts of pesticides may be stored in the body, where they are harmless, but the majority are metabolized by the liver and excreted.

The decision to use pesticides is made by balancing known or suspected risks against benefits. Without pesticides, the USDA estimates that every second or third crop of potatoes or tomatoes would be wiped out, and commercial production of apples, oranges, and grapefruit would be impossible [16]. Actually, the traces of pesticides that appear in both organic and nonorganic food may come from drifting sprays used for roadside weeds or forest protection, or from rainfall runoff from nearby farms.

Despite the futility of trying to keep organically grown foods free from pesticide residue and richer in various nutrients, perhaps the only true difference between organic and conventional foods is their cost. The USDA estimates that organic foods can cost twice as much at the supermarket as regular foods. In 1972, organic food retail sales totaled $500 million; by 1980, this figure had reached $3 billion [17].

The consumer would profit more by using the additional money it costs to buy organic foods to purchase a wider variety of conventionally grown foods, or more fresh produce. Variety is the key to good nutrition, ensuring an adequate intake of all nutrients.

Vegetarian Diets

In recent years there has been a trend toward vegetarian diets by individuals and groups. Some types of vegetarian diets are based on religious, life-style, or ecologic concerns, such as the Zen macrobiotics. Basically, there are three types of vegetarian diets—pure or strict vegetarian; lacto-ovo vegetarian; and lacto-vegetarian. The first type excludes all foods of animal origin, including fish, meat, poultry, eggs, and all dairy products. The second type excludes meat, fish, and poultry but includes eggs and all dairy products. The third type is the same as the second, except that it also excludes eggs.

A vegetarian diet can be nutritionally sound and well-balanced, if planned properly. The more liberal the diet, the better the chances are for nutritional adequacy. Nuts, seeds, legumes, and grains supply essential and nonessential amino acids, iron, and B-complex vitamins. By combining them within a meal, an adequate intake of the essential amino acids is ensured. Fruits and vegetables supply vitamins A and C, needed minerals, and fiber. Milk and milk products provide complete protein (all the essential amino acids), vitamins A, D, and B_{12}. Eggs also contribute complete protein and iron (Fig. 33-2).

The vegetarian diet, particularly if it is of the pure or strict type, is apt to be lacking in several nutrients, particularly calcium, iodine, and vitamins D, B_{12}, and riboflavin. The best and most concentrated dietary sources of calcium are milk and milk products. When these sources are excluded from the diet, it is more difficult to obtain an adequate intake of this essential nutrient. Some dark green leafy vegetables do contribute substantial amounts of calcium, such as collards, dandelion greens, mustard greens, kale, and turnip greens, but they may also contain oxalic acid, which binds calcium in an insoluble form. Calcium is also present in some legumes, dried fruits, nuts, broccoli, cabbage, okra, and rutabaga. Children and pregnant and lactating women should include milk or milk products in their diets because of their greater needs and the difficulty of meeting those needs with alternative sources of calcium. This essential nutrient is required for the clotting of blood, normal muscle and nerve function, and the formation of healthy bones and teeth.

Iodine is another essential nutrient required for normal metabolism. It is needed for the production of thyroxine by the thyroid gland; its absence from the diet results in hypertrophy of that gland, a condition known as goiter. The soil

FIG. 33-2. Vegetarian diets can be well-balanced and nutritious. By combining foods that contain different amino acids (to make complete protein) and a variety of vitamins, all the necessary elements for a healthy meal are provided. (Courtesy of the National Dairy Council.)

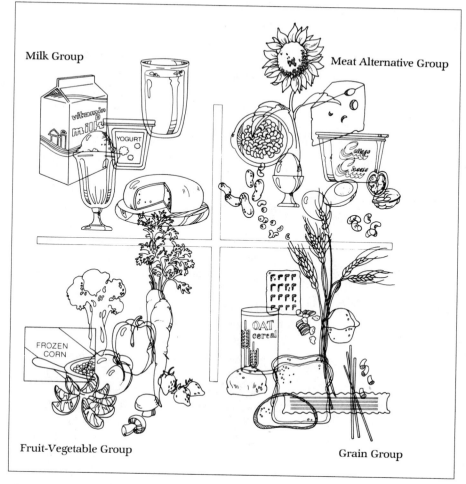

along seacoast areas is usually rich in this nutrient, which is picked up by foods grown there. Foods grown in soil away from the seacoast may be deficient in iodine. The use of iodized table salt ensures an adequate intake of this nutrient.

Vitamin D occurs naturally, although only in limited amounts in several foods of animal origin (fish, egg yolk, butter, and liver). Fortified foods contribute a substantial amount of this essential nutrient, and may include breakfast cereals, margarine, and milk. With adequate exposure to sunlight, vitamin D is formed within the skin. When all dietary sources of vitamin D are removed from the diet, fish liver oils or a vitamin D supplement should be used. This is particularly true for infants, children, and pregnant and lactating women, and during the winter months when exposure to sunlight is minimal. Caution must be used with these preparations because excessive amounts of vitamin D can be toxic. This vitamin is essential in calcium and phosphorus metabolism, including the normal development of bones and teeth.

Vitamin B_{12} is found only in foods of animal origin; a pure vegetarian diet lacks this nutrient. Some foods may be fortified with vitamin B_{12} such as some breakfast cereals; if these foods are not included in the diet, this vitamin should be taken as a supplement. Since vitamin B_{12} is essential for normal blood cell formation and nerve function, a deficiency of this vitamin may cause nerve damage and, eventually, anemia.

The richest dietary sources of riboflavin are milk and meat. When these two food groups are removed from the diet, it becomes more difficult to obtain an adequate intake of this vitamin. Dried yeast, eggs, green leafy vegetables, broccoli, winter squash, legumes, nuts, seeds, whole grains, and enriched breads contribute fair amounts. If needs cannot be met through dietary sources, supplementation is necessary.

Another common problem with most vegetarian diets is that they may be so high in bulk that they do not meet caloric requirements [18]. As a result, protein is utilized for energy instead of being used for tissue growth and repair. An adequate intake of complete protein and sufficient calories is essential for good nutrition.

As with any other type of diet, variety helps ensure an adequate intake of most, if not all, essential nutrients. The more restrictive the diet, the greater the likelihood of nutrient deficiencies. Legumes provide amino acids, B-complex vitamins, and iron. Nuts and seeds also contain amino acids, fat, an important source of concentrated calories, iron, and B vitamins. Whole grains and cereals contribute trace minerals, B vitamins, iron, carbohydrates, and amino acids. Dark green leafy vegetables add vitamins and calcium.

The Zen macrobiotic diet is an extreme form of vegetarianism, created by the Japanese Georges Ohsawa. The philosophy behind this diet and the attendant life-style is outlined in his two books—*Zen Macrobiotics* and *Philosophy of Oriental Medicine*. The main goals of this rigid nutritional system are mostly spiritual. There are 10 stages of dietary restrictions, from -3 to $+7$, gradually eliminating animal products, fruits, vegetables, and fluids. The lower-level diets can meet nutritional needs, but since the higher-level diets consist solely of cereals, they are nutritionally imbalanced. In addition, the caloric intake is usually low. Strict adherence to the higher-level diets can cause scurvy, anemia, severe tissue wasting, and even death. Poor growth has been reported in children and infants placed on the Zen macrobiotic regimen of Kokoh, a food mixture for infant feeding. Parents may be more accepting of nutritional advice for their children than for themselves, and if informed of the infant's poor growth and detrimental long-term consequences, they may adopt a lower, more nutritionally adequate step of the diet.

Weight-Reduction Diets   The majority of the popular weight-reducing diets utilize a low carbohydrate intake to cause rapid weight loss [19]. Although this may seem effective on a short-term basis, it does not really represent a true loss of weight. The body's reserves of carbohydrate, found mostly in muscle and the liver, are stored with water—2.7 gm for every gram of glycogen (stored carbohydrate). When carbohydrate reserves are depleted by a low- or no-carbohydrate intake, almost 3 gm of water is lost for every gram of glycogen mobilized, resulting in diuresis (water loss) and an apparent rapid weight loss.

After the carbohydrate reserves become depleted (about 12 hours in most individuals), the body is forced to use fat stores for energy. The fat stores are metabolized to yield two carbon units, which are then either used for energy production, or if present in excess quantities, condensed into carbon fragments termed *ketone bodies* and excreted in the urine. Ketosis, when these ketone bodies are present in the blood and urine, can produce a number of undesirable side effects, including calcium depletion, dehydration, muscle weakness, nausea, gout or gouty arthritis, kidney failure or stones, and possibly the development of atherosclerosis in susceptible individuals.

Low-carbohydrate, ketogenic diets such as those currently popularized by Dr. Stillman and Dr. Atkins are neither new nor innovative. Over 100 years ago an English surgeon, William Harvey, designed a diet for obesity that excluded sweet and starchy foods while permitting meat ad libitum [20]. Variations of this diet have appeared periodically, particularly during the past 30 years, all with the same major features in common—low to absent carbohydrate content; unrestricted protein and fat; and unrestricted calories. Among the versions that have been published since 1950 include Pennington [21], Air Force Diet [22], Taller [23], the Drinking Man's Diet [24], Stillman [25], and Atkins [26].

This type of dietary regimen is without any scientific merit and is actually contrary to the laws of thermodynamics; that is, energy intake always equals energy output. The main philosophy of the diet is that when a sufficiently low carbohydrate level is reached, enough ketone bodies will be generated to cause large and rapid weight loss despite a high caloric intake (unrestricted protein and fat intake). Dietary carbohydrates are viewed as "poisons" that lead to diabetes, cardiovascular disease, hypoglycemia, and obesity.

Contrary to the above theory, any weight-reducing regimen can be effective only if the number of calories (from any dietary source) is decreased to a level less than that required by the individual. Weight loss on the low-carbohydrate regimen may actually be due to a reduction of total intake, since most individuals are not accustomed to eating a diet limited to proteins and fats.

Perhaps the safest and most nutritionally sound reducing diet publicized today is that designed by Weight Watcher's International. The program provides reducing, leveling, and maintenance diets for teenagers and adults based on a food-exchange system of a variety and balance of foods. Deficient only in calories, their dietary plans provide all other nutrients in sufficient amounts. In addition, the social and educational stimuli provided aid in weight loss and maintenance.

Diet and Hyperactivity

The role of diet in maintaining physical health is fairly well understood, but its influence on psychological states is not as clear. Recently, claims have been made suggesting that certain chemicals found in foods (some present naturally and others added during processing) may be responsible for hyperactivity seen in some children [27, 28]. There is much debate over the term *hyperactivity*, a diagnosis that may also include minimal brain dysfunction or hyperkinetic syndrome. Hyperactivity is basically a symptom, which may be caused by any one of a variety of factors including subclinical seizure disorders, a child's basic personality, or it may reflect a true hyperkinetic state. One of the most ardent proponents of the theory that diet can cause hyperactivity is Dr. Benjamin Feingold, emeritus director of the Laboratory of Medical Entomology of the Kaiser Foundation Research Institute. His theory is that behavioral disturbances and learning disabilities are caused by "salicylatelike" natural compounds in foods, "low-molecular-weight food additives," and artificial food flavors and colors in particular [29, 30]. His therapy for hyperactivity, a diet in which a wide variety of natural and processed foods have been eliminated, has supposedly produced dramatic improvements in many patients. His treatment involves the exclusion of 21 fruits and vegetables, which, according to Feingold, contain "natural salicylates," all foods that contain artificial flavors, and a wide variety of nonfood items that contain the compounds he lists (some prescription drugs, over the counter medications, toothpastes, mouthwashes, cough drops, and perfumes, to mention a few).

To evaluate Dr. Feingold's theory, an expert panel of scientists was assembled by the Nutrition Foundation. They evaluated the evidence; their conclusions, based on the most current knowledge about hyperactivity and food additives in children, were presented in 1975 [31]. At that time the experts in food, medicine, and behavior found that no controlled studies had demonstrated that hyperkinesis was related to the intake of food additives; the claims that hyperactive children improve on this diet had not been confirmed; and the nutritional qualities of the diet may not meet the long-term nutrient needs of children. Subsequent research has not supported Dr. Feingold's theories.

One reason why Dr. Feingold's regimen may work with some children is that it involves the entire family. For example, parents are instructed to spend a weekend morning making additive-free cake and candy with their children. Hyperactive behavior is often associated with family problems, and the changes in family dynamics may produce more benefits than any supposed inclusion or exclusion from the diet.

Laetrile

Because of the emotional and psychological impact of the diagnosis of cancer, and the perceived and real side effects of therapy, many individuals with this diagnosis have sought out alternative, unconventional therapies. One of the most lethal of these is laetrile, a cyanide poison naturally present in the kernels of apricot pits and a number of other stone fruits and nuts.

Laetrile was first conceived by Ernst T. Krebs, Sr., a California physician who tried apricot pits as a cancer remedy while searching for an enzyme that would hasten the aging of bootleg whiskey [32]. His son developed an injectable form of the substance. According to their theory, which is not supported by any scientific evidence, laetrile works by releasing cyanide and poisoning the cancer cells; normal cells are protected by an enzyme not found in the cancer cells. When taken in tablet form, it is broken down in the gastrointestinal tract, where the cyanide is released and can cause poisoning. The cyanide in laetrile can also be released by the presence of the enzyme beta-glucosidase, heat, mineral acids, or by megadoses of vitamin C, especially in the presence of blood [33].

Laetrile's advocates have failed to obtain FDA approval for its sale in interstate commerce, since the Federal Food, Drug, and Cosmetic Act requires that any drug must be proven effective and safe before it can be marketed, and laetrile has not. In studies by the National Cancer Institute and numerous independent cancer research centers, all evidence indicates that laetrile does not prevent, cure, or even slow down cancer. In an attempt to circumvent the need for drug approval, laetrile promoters have tried marketing their product as a vitamin (vitamin B_{17}), suggesting that cancer is really caused by a deficiency of this vitamin. Laetrile is not a vitamin, and there is no such thing as vitamin B_{17}. Actually, the most effective anticancer drugs work by depriving tumors from getting the vitamins that they need!

The tragedy of laetrile is twofold; first, the promoters of this often fatal "cure" are reaping great wealth at the expense of cancer victims and their families; second, the lure of a miracle cure raises false hopes and induces potentially curable cancer patients to delay or forsake all conventional treatment. This is one of the saddest and most tragic areas of medical and nutritional quackery.

References

1. Bruch, H.   The allure of food cults and nutrition quackery. *Nutr. Rev.* 32 [Suppl.]:62, 1974.
2. DiPalma, J. R., and Ritchie, D. M.   Vitamin toxicity. *Ann. Rev. Pharmacol. Toxicol.* 17:133, 1977.
3. Heenan, J.   Myths of vitamins. *FDA Consumer*, March, 1974.
4. Aeling, J. L., Panagotacos, P. J., and Andreozzi, R. J.   Allergic contact dermatitis to vitamin E aerosol deodorant. *Arch. Dermatol.* 108:579, 1973.
5. Vogelsang, A.   Twenty-four years using alpha tocopherol in degenerative cardiovascular disease. *Angiology* 21:275, 1970.
6. Aftergood, L., and Alfin-Slater, R. B.   Oral contraceptive–alpha tocopherol interrelationships. *Lipids* 9:91, 1974.
7. Bernhardt, I. B., and Dorsey, D. J.   Hypervitaminosis A and congenital renal anomalies in human infant. *Obstet. Gynecol.* 43:750, 1974.
8. Lippe, B., et al.   Chronic vitamin A intoxication. *Am. J. Dis. Child.* 135:634, 1981.
9. Seelig, M. S.   Vitamin D and cardiovascular, renal and brain damage in infancy and childhood. *Ann. N.Y. Acad. Sci.* 147:537, 1969.
10. Pak, C. Y. C., et al.   Treatment of vitamin D–resistant hypoparathyroidism with 25–hydroxycholecalciferol. *Arch. Intern. Med.* 126:239, 1970.
11. Rowe, D. J. F., and Stamp, T. C. B.   Anticonvulsant osteomalacia and vitamin D. *Br. Med. J.* 1:392, 1974.
12. Pauling, L. C.   *Vitamin C and the Common Cold.* San Francisco: Freeman, 1970.

13. Cochrane, W. A.   Overnutrition in prenatal and neonatal life: A problem? *Can. Med. Assoc. J.* 93:893, 1965.

14. Hines, J. D.   Ascorbic acid and vitamin B_{12} deficiency. *J.A.M.A.* 234:24, 1975.

15. Stein, H. B., Hasan, A., and Fox, I. R.   Ascorbic acid–induced uricosuria. *Ann. Intern. Med.* 84:385, 1976.

16. Deutsch, R.   Where you should be shopping for your family. *Nutr. Rev.* 32 [Suppl.]:48, 1974.

17. Stephenson, M.   The confusing world of health foods. *FDA Consumer* 12:18, 1978.

18. Barness, L. A.   Nutritional aspects of vegetarianism, health foods, and fad diets. *Nutr. Rev.* 35:153, 1977.

19. American Medical Association Council on Foods and Nutrition: A critique of low-carbohydrate ketogenic weight reduction regimes. *Nutr. Rev.* 32 [Suppl.]:15, 1974.

20. Harvey, W.   *On Corpulence in Relation to Disease.* London: Henry Renshaw, 1872. Pp. 109, 122.

21. Pennington, A. W.   Treatment of obesity with calorically unrestricted diets. *J. Clin. Nutr.* 1:343, 1953.

22. *Air Force Diet.* Toronto: Air Force Diet Publishers, 1960.

23. Taller, H.   *Calories Don't Count.* New York: Simon & Schuster, 1961.

24. Jameson, G., and Williams, E.   *The Drinking Man's Diet.* San Francisco: Cameron, 1964.

25. Stillman, I. M., and Baker, S. S.   *The Doctor's Quick Weight Loss Diet.* Englewood Cliffs, N.J.: Prentice-Hall, 1967.

26. Atkins, R. C.   *Dr. Atkin's Diet Revolution: The High Calorie Way to Stay Thin Forever.* New York: David McKay, 1972.

27. Diet and hyperactivity: any connection? A scientific status summary by the Institute of Food Technologists' Expert Panel of Food Safety and Nutrition and the Committee on Public Information. April, 1976.

28. Feingold, B. F.   *Why Your Child Is Hyperactive.* New York: Random House, 1975.

29. Feingold, B. F., et al.   Adverse reaction to food additives. Paper presented at Annual Convention, American Medical Association, 1973.

30. Feingold, B. F.   Food additives and child development (editorial). *Hosp. Prac.* October, 1973. P. 11.

31. National Advisory Committee on Hyperkinesis and Food Additives.   Report to the Nutrition Foundation. New York: Nutrition Foundation, 1975.

32. Lehmann, P.   Laetrile: the fatal "cure." *FDA Consumer* 11:10, 1977.

33. Herbert, V.   Laetrile: The cult of cyanide, promoting poison for profit. *Am. J. Clin. Nutr.* 32:1121, 1979.

Suggested Readings

Abdulla, M., et al.   Nutrient intake and health status of vegans. *Am. J. Clin. Nutr.* 34:2464, 1981.

American Academy of Pediatrics, Committee on Nutrition.   Nutritional aspects of vegetarianism, health foods, and fad diets. *Pediatrics* 59:460, 1977.

American Dietetic Association.   *Vitamin-Mineral Safety, Toxicity, and Misuse.* Chicago: ADA, 1978.

Arnrich, L.   Toxic Effects of Megadoses of Fat-soluble Vitamins. In J. N. Hathcock and J. Coon (eds.), *Nutrition and Drug Interrelations.* New York: Academic Press, 1978.

Bean, W. B.   Some Aspects of Pharmacologic Use and Abuse of Water-soluble Vitamins. In J. N. Hathcock and J. Coon (eds.), *Nutrition and Drug Interrelations.* New York: Academic Press, 1978.

Dickerson, J. W. T., and Pepler, F.   Diet and hyperactivity. *J. Hum. Nutr.* 34:167, 1980.

Dwyer, J. T., et al.   Size, obesity, and leanness in vegetarian preschool children. *J. Am. Diet. Assoc.* 77:434, 1980.

Dykes, M. H. M., and Meier, P.   Ascorbic acid and the common cold: evaluation of its efficacy and toxicity. *J.A.M.A.* 231:1073, 1975.

Ferguson, H. B., Rapoport, J. L., and Weingarten, H.   Food dyes and impairment of performance in hyperactive children. *Science* 211:410, 1981.

Food additives and hyperactivity. *Lancet* 1:662, 1982.

Forbes, G. B.   Food fads: Safe feeding of children. *Pediatr. Rev.* 1:207, 1980.

Fulton, J. R., Hutton, C. W., and Stitt, K. R.   Preschool vegetarian children. *J. Am. Diet. Assoc.* 76:360, 1980.

Growth of vegetarian children. *Nutr. Rev.* 37:108, 1979.

Harmer, I. C., and Foiles, R. A. L.   Effect of Feingold's K–P diet on a residential, mentally handicapped population. *J. Am. Diet. Assoc.* 76:575, 1980.

Heenan, J.   Myths of vitamins. *FDA Consumer* March, 1974.

Herbert, V.   Megavitamin therapy. *Contemp. Nutr.* October, 1977.

Herbert, V.   *Nutrition Cultism: Facts and Fictions.* Philadelphia: Stickley, 1980.

Herbert, V.   The nutritionally and metabolically destructive "nutritional and metabolic antineoplastic diet" of laetrile proponents. *Am. J. Clin. Nutr.* 32:96, 1979.

Herbert, V.   Pangamic acid ("vitamin B_{15}"). *Am. J. Clin. Nutr.* 32:1534, 1979.

Hopkins, H.   Regulating vitamins and minerals. *FDA Consumer* July/August 1976. Pp. 10–11.

How vitamin C really works . . . or does it? *Nutr. Today* Sept./Oct. 1979. Pp. 6–19.

Infant cult diet. *Nutr. & M.D.* Feb., 1982.

Jukes, T. H.   Megavitamins and food fads. In R. E. Hodges (ed.), *Nutrition: Metabolic and Clinical Applications.* New York: Plenum, 1979.

Nutrition Misinformation. *Dairy Counc. Dig.* July/August 1981.

Oski, F. A.   Vitamin E: A radical defense. *N. Engl. J. Med.* 303:454, 1980.

Pearce, J. R.   Nutrition beliefs: More fashion than fact. *FDA Consumer* June 1976. Pp. 25–27.

Peto, R., et al.   Can dietary beta carotene materially reduce human cancer rates? *Nature* 290:201, 1981.

Position paper on the vegetarian approach to eating. *J. Am. Dietet. Assoc.* 77:61, 1980.

Robb, P.   Cooking for Hyperactive and Allergic Children. Fort Wayne, Ind.: Cedar Creek Publishers, 1980.

Roberts, H. J.   Perspective on vitamin E as therapy. *J.A.M.A.* 246:129, 1981.

Siegel, R. K.   Ginseng abuse syndrome: Problems with the panacea. *J.A.M.A.* 241:1614, 1979.

Spannhake, E. B.   *Eye It Before You Diet: A Nutritional Analysis of Nine Popular Diets.* Washington, D.C.: The Sugar Association, 1977.

Stare, F. J., Whelan, E. M., and Sheridan, M. J.   Diet and hyperkinesis: Is there a relationship? *Nutr. & M.D.* January, 1980.

The Scarsdale Diet. *Nutr. & M.D.* October, 1980.

Tsai, A. C., et al.   Study on the effect of megavitamin E supplementation in man. *Am. J. Clin. Nutr.* 31:831, 1978.

Young, J. H.   *The Medical Messiahs: A Social History of Health Quackery in Twentieth-Century America.* Princeton, N.J.: Princeton University Press, 1967.

Young, J. H.   *The Toadstool Millionaires: A Social History of Patent Medicines in America Before Federal Regulation.* Princeton, N.J.: Princeton University Press, 1961.

Part 4

THERAPEUTIC APPLICATION OF NUTRITION

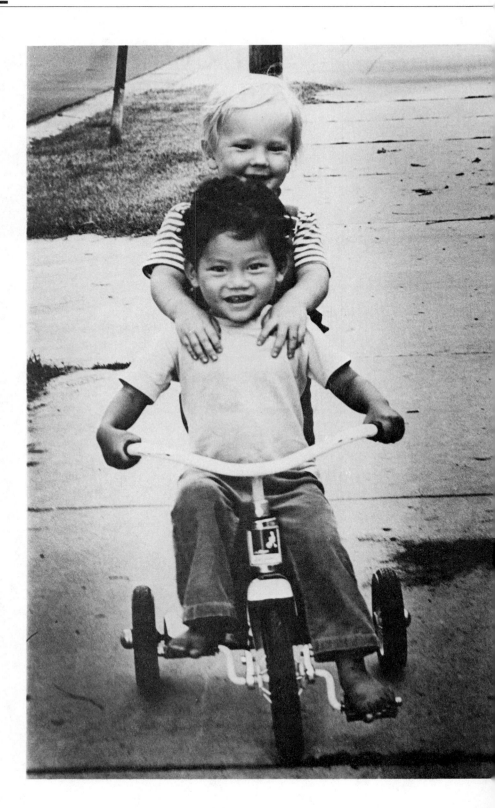

PRINCIPLES OF DIET THERAPY

Since most of the discoveries in biochemistry and nutrition have taken place during this century, diet therapy might be considered a relatively new science. However, people have been practicing diet therapy in one form or another for centuries, although prior to World War I it was based more on empirical knowledge and experience than on sound scientific facts. As discussed in Chapter 37, many foods have been used as drugs for hundreds, even thousands, of years. Only recently have the active ingredients in many of these traditional, ancient therapies been refined and utilized by modern medicine.

The four chapters in this section provide the background principles for diet therapy. Chapter 34, Malnutrition, discusses the effects of primary malnutrition, due to a deficiency of calories or protein and calories. The prevalence and treatment of these deficiency diseases (starvation, marasmus, and kwashiorkor) and their short-term and long-term consequences are discussed. Chapter 35, Principles of Parenteral Nutrition, presents one of the newest and most valuable tools available in dietetics today. From its development in the late 1960s, parenteral nutrition has become a valuable adjunct in the acute and chronic treatment of patients whose complications, disease conditions, or metabolic needs preclude adequate oral nutrient intake. The composition of parenteral fluids, indications, complications, and hazards are presented. In Chapter 36, Physiologic Stress, the hormonal and metabolic responses to serious trauma, infection, sepsis, and burn injuries are discussed. Special emphasis is on the evaluation and nutritional management of the burn patient. Chapter 37, Drugs, Nutrients, and Nutritional Status, presents the interrelationships between food and the ever-expanding therapeutic use of pharmacologic agents. The effect of drugs on nutrient absorption and metabolism, taste and appetite, and resultant nutrient imbalances is discussed, as is the effect of food on drug metabolism.

Since one or more of the principles presented in these chapters will be utilized in Section IX, Nutritional Therapy in Disease, it is important that the student have a thorough understanding of Section VIII.

Chapter 34

MALNUTRITION AND PRIMARY NUTRITIONAL DISEASES

Malnutrition actually means "defective" nutrition. The term can be interpreted to mean overnutrition, as seen in obesity, or undernutrition, such as starvation. An individual who is obese may still be malnourished by having low stores of iron, deficiencies of various vitamins, and a reduced immune response. Malnutrition in this chapter, however, is limited to the conditions of fasting, starvation, and protein-calorie deficiency. These are conditions of *primary* malnutrition, caused solely by an inadequate dietary intake such as during famine, drought, or when a child is weaned too early. Malnutrition may also be caused by any number of other factors, including malabsorption from the gastrointestinal tract or interference with nutrient utilization by drugs, alcohol, or metabolic disease; this is termed *secondary* malnutrition. There can be psychological factors behind a special type of starvation that can occur even when adequate food is readily available. This type of malnutrition is termed anorexia nervosa and is also discussed in this chapter.

Starvation, marasmus, and kwashiorkor (forms of primary malnutrition) and their effects on behavior, intelligence, and the immune system will be covered in this chapter. A comparison of various forms of malnutrition is given in Table 34-1.

Fasting and Starvation
METABOLIC ALTERATIONS

BRIEF FASTING

The human brain requires a constant supply of glucose as fuel. About two-thirds of the total circulating glucose is used by the brain; the remaining one-third goes to the red blood cells and skeletal muscles. A sudden drop in the blood glucose level causes confusion, behavioral changes, coma, and if prolonged, death.

The brain requires between 100 and 150 gm of glucose per day. Less than 100 gm is derived from the stored carbohydrate, glycogen, in the liver. Between meals and during fasting for short periods, some tissue proteins (the glucogenic amino acids) are broken down and converted into glucose by the liver (gluconeogenesis). The kidney also synthesizes a small amount of glucose during this time.

During brief periods of fasting, the red blood cells, white blood cells, bone marrow, renal medulla, and peripheral nerves all metabolize glucose for energy. The glucose is converted primarily to lactate and pyruvate, which are then transported back to the liver and kidney where they are reconverted to glucose (this process is termed the *Cori cycle*). The energy needed for the conversion of two molecules of lactate to glucose is supplied by the oxidation of fat. The remaining tissues (heart, renal cortex, and skeletal muscle) utilize either fatty acids released directly into the circulation or the products of partially oxidized fatty acids (acetoacetate or betahydroxybutyrate). In the liver, glycerol (derived

TABLE 34-1. A comparison of some forms of malnutrition

Characteristics	Starvation	Anorexia nervosa	Kwashiorkor	Marasmus
Primary deficiency	Calories	Calories	Protein	Calories
Age	Any age	10–30	At weaning	Children
Sex	Both	90% female	Both	Both
Growth retardation			Slight	Significant
Body water	Decreased	Decreased	Increased	Decreased
Subcutaneous fat	Decreased	Decreased	May be normal	Decreased
Skin and hair lesions			Increased	Absent
Edema	Late	Late	Present	None
Diarrhea	Late	None	Present	Marked
Weight loss	Marked	Marked	Mild or absent	Marked
Serum albumin	Normal	Normal	Decreased	Normal
Hemoglobin	Normal	Normal	Decreased	Normal
Magnesium	Decreased	Decreased		Decreased
Liver	Normal	Normal	Enlarged and fatty	Normal
Pancreatic enzymes			Decreased	Normal

Source: J. A. Bray, Nutritional Factors in Disease. In W. A. Sodeman and T. M. Sodeman (eds.), *Pathologic Physiology* (6th ed.). Philadelphia: Saunders, 1979. P. 981.

from adipose tissue), lactate, pyruvate, and the glucogenic amino acids are all converted to glucose. The energy for these processes is derived from fatty acid oxidation.

To summarize, in the fasting individual there are two sources of energy—muscle protein and adipose tissue; and three sites of fuel utilization—terminal glucose combustion mainly in the brain, the breakdown and recycling of glucose primarily in the red blood cells, and fatty acid and ketone utilization by the remainder of the body [1]. The liver is the main control point, synthesizing glucose from a variety of precursors and utilizing fatty acid oxidation as its energy source. A summary of the metabolic substrate cycles and fuel metabolism during fasting is presented in Figs. 34-1A and B.

Alanine is the principal amino acid substrate for the hepatic synthesis of glucose. Because alanine makes up only about 6 to 8 percent of the total cell content of amino acids, most of it must first be synthesized from its precursor, pyruvic acid, by the addition of an amino group from the breakdown of other amino acids. During brief periods of fasting, about 66 gm of protein are catabolized daily to provide energy for metabolism.

PROLONGED FASTING OR STARVATION

During prolonged fasting or starvation, adaptive mechanisms help reduce the breakdown of tissue protein to about 20 gm per day after 5 or 6 weeks [1]. These metabolic adaptations are aimed at deriving energy from adipose tissue and conserving protein reserves as efficiently as possible. In addition, several mea-

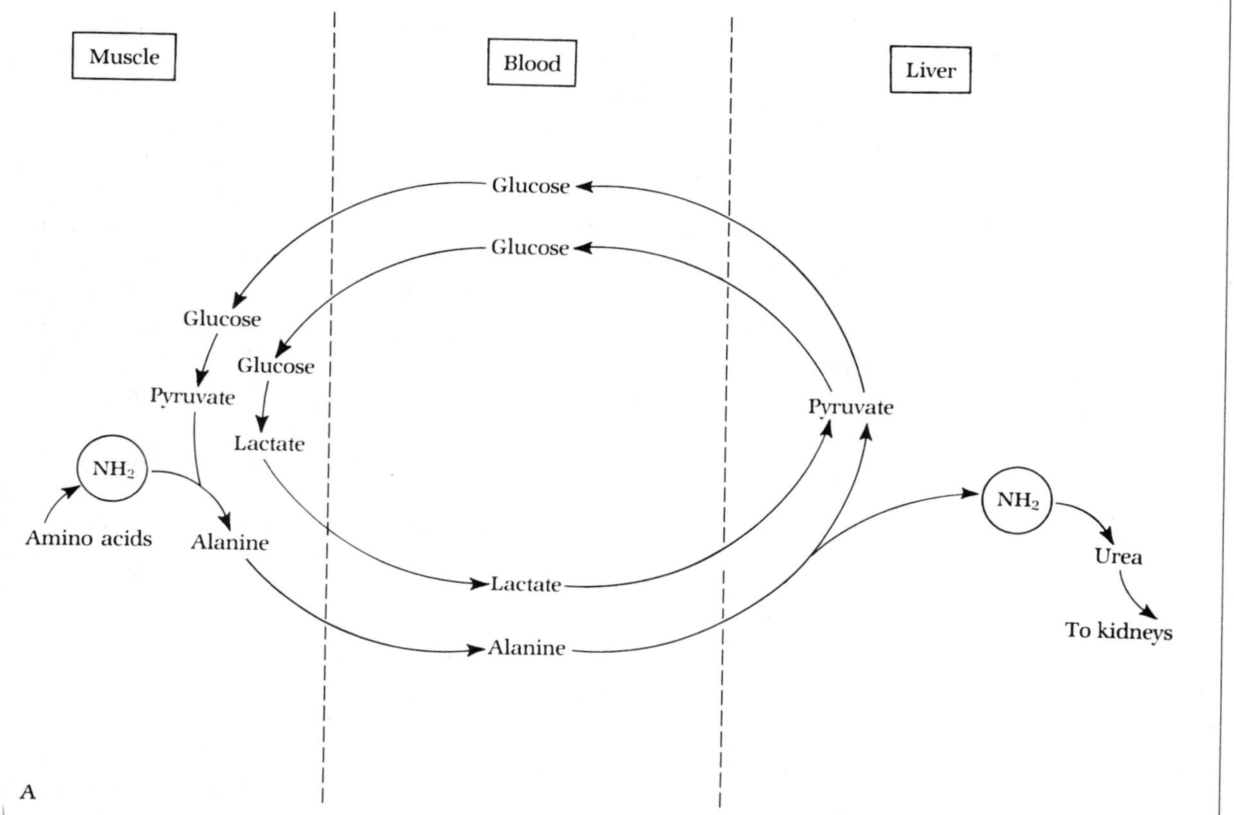

PURPOSES To derive energy from adipose tissue
To conserve protein reserves as efficiently as possible

MECHANISMS
1. The utilization of free fatty acids instead of glucose as fuel for the majority of the body's tissues
2. The Cori cycle—the shuttling of lipid-derived calories as glucose to the glycolytic tissues, where it is broken down to lactate and sent back to the liver to be resynthesized to glucose
3. Adaptation of the brain to using fatty acids and the products of their partial oxidation for energy

B

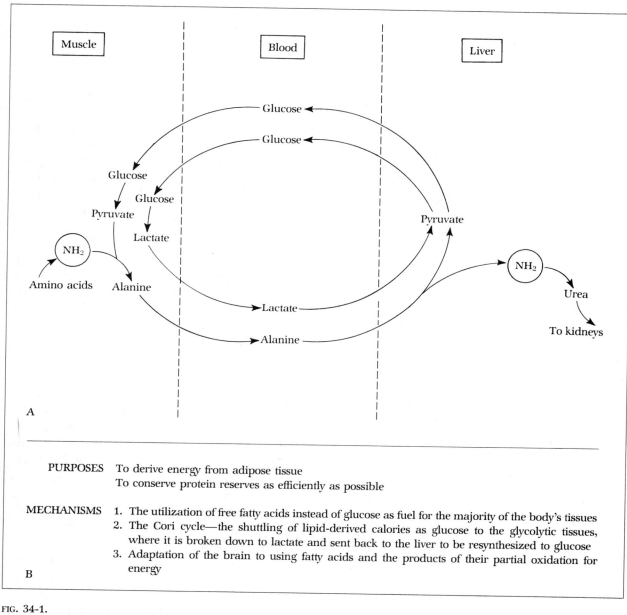

FIG. 34-1.
A. Metabolic substrate cycles. (From V. R. Young and N. S. Scrimshaw, The physiology of starvation. *Scientific American* 225:14, 1971.)
B. Metabolic adaptations to prolonged fasting or starvation.

sures tend to conserve available energy, including a reduction in the basal metabolic rate, a loss of metabolically active tissue, and a reduction in energy expenditure. The release of alanine from skeletal muscle decreases, causing a slowdown in gluconeogenesis by the liver. The brain adapts to an alternate source of energy (the ketone bodies) derived from the fatty tissues. The ketone bodies are acetoacetic acid and its two derivatives, acetone and betahydroxybutyrate.

During starvation fatty acids are released from adipose tissue and oxidized in the liver to acetoacetic acid, which is then transported to the tissues as an energy source. When the level of acetoacetic acid, acetone, and betahydroxybutyrate reach high enough blood levels, enzymes in the brain capable of utilizing them for energy are activated. As a consequence, less glucose is needed.

Protein continues to be lost from the body along with urea and ammonia, which are excreted in the urine. Less fluid is needed since the amount of nitrogen excreted in the urine is reduced. The ammonia is formed from amino acids to maintain acid-base balance; in the process glucose is produced. The change in the acid-base balance of the blood, caused by the body's increased production of ketone bodies during prolonged starvation, causes the kidney to synthesize more glucose than the liver. Therefore, after prolonged fasting, the majority of the reduced gluconeogenesis occurs in the kidney.

The initial loss of weight is due to the utilization of carbohydrate stores (glycogen) and the fluid stored with them. Each gram of glycogen is stored with 2.7 gm of water (see Chap. 32). When glycogen is broken down and utilized for energy, the water is freed and excreted in the urine, causing a rapid weight loss. With depletion of glycogen stores and a conversion to fat catabolism, the rate of weight loss is slowed. With continued fasting or starvation, a greater proportion of weight loss is derived from the body's fat stores. Because fat contributes more calories (energy) per gram than does carbohydrate or protein, and is stored in a nearly anhydrous (water-free) state, the rate of loss is slowed. Except with particularly large losses of body fat, only the size of the individual fat cells decreases while the total number remains unchanged.

The loss of fluid is greatest during the first week, is small during the second, and by the end of the third week it is nonexistent. As the tissues begin to waste, intracellular fluid is lost, causing the size of the extracellular fluid compartment to be greater in proportion. This, in turn, results in edema (*famine edema*). The causes of famine edema include loss of elasticity of the skin, causing seepage of fluid from the blood to the interstitial spaces; reduction in the glomerular filtration rate, resulting in delayed fluid excretion; and a fall in the concentration of plasma albumin, altering the osmotic pressure of the blood and causing a shift of fluid from the blood to the tissues (see Chap. 10 for more detail).

With tissue catabolism and the loss of intracellular fluid, there is also a profound loss of potassium. This element is stored with glycogen and with nitrogen (in muscle protein). With the breakdown of glycogen and muscle protein, the intracellular potassium is transferred to the extracellular fluid, where it is quickly removed by the kidneys. As much as one-third of the potassium may be lost, contributing to the deficiency symptoms of weakness, irritability, paralysis, and tachycardia (rapid heart rate).

HORMONAL CHANGES

The level of insulin falls during starvation since amino acids and glucose, which stimulate its secretion, are not being absorbed. The plasma levels of both pituitary growth hormone and glucagon are increased, favoring fat mobilization. Thyroid hormone is decreased, causing an adaptive lowering of the basal metabolic rate. Amenorrhea (cessation of menstruation), delayed puberty, loss of libido (sexual drive), and impotence seen during periods of starvation are all symptoms of reduced levels of testosterone, estrogen, and progesterone.

ANATOMIC CHANGES

Wasting of the tissue is the most characteristic feature of prolonged starvation. All tissues of the body, except the brain, have been shown to atrophy during starvation. All or nearly all of the adipose tissue has been mobilized, leaving the skin loose and flabby. The skeletal muscles also atrophy as a result of tissue catabolism. As starvation continues and more muscle mass is utilized for gluconeogenesis, the intercostal and upper abdominal muscles may become so compromised that they can no longer perform the task of breathing. Respiratory failure due to loss of muscle mass may result. In addition to muscle proteins being utilized, rapidly turning over, newly synthesized proteins (including the enzymatic proteins of the liver and kidney) are also diverted for energy needs. This may explain why kidney failure is often the final cause of death in starvation.

The heart atrophies in proportion to or slightly less than the body weight [2, 3]. There is actual shrinkage of the muscle fibers by as much as 50 percent. Atrophy this severe is often irreversible and subsequent heart failure is frequently the cause of death, even during the period of nutritional rehabilitation. If there is concurrent anemia, hypertension, or hypermetabolic condition (fever or sepsis), there is less cardiac atrophy [3].

With starvation there is also wasting of the muscular walls and mucous membrane lining the small intestine. As a consequence, the ability to absorb nutrients is greatly impaired. The type of foods given during the early rehabilitation period are very important. If foods are too high in bulk or fiber or too difficult to digest, the individual may die from diarrhea or malabsorption.

Other effects of starvation include wound disruption, poor healing, and an increased tendency to phlebitis and skin breakdown. Nonspecific effects on the central nervous system include personality changes, decreased awareness, and irritability. It is not known whether these effects are caused by a lack of nutrients to the brain or by the toxic accumulation of the products of muscle breakdown.

TREATMENT

Intravenous feedings are the preferred initial therapy, but may not be available. Only bland, diluted foods can be tolerated by the thin-walled, atrophied small intestine. Frequent small feedings of skim milk, diluted to 10 to 15 percent strength, are recommended [4]. Fats may also be used, being valuable for their high caloric content. Semisolid foods may be introduced as the individual begins to recover.

Intractable diarrhea is commonly the precipitating cause of death in starvation. It may be caused by improper foods, such as the desperate eating of roots and leaves whose roughage is too difficult for the atrophied intestine to absorb. It may also be caused by an intestinal infection or a combination of factors. Once it has begun, the loss of fluids and the resultant electrolyte imbalance quickly result in death.

Anorexia Nervosa

Anorexia nervosa is a self-induced aversion to food, causing a unique type of malnutrition. It is seen most often in young, single women, between puberty through the thirties, and is often viewed by the patient as a solution of psychic conflicts.

The symptoms, in addition to severe weight loss, include a low basal metabolic rate. Many of these patients weigh as little as 70 lb, having maintained themselves on 1000 calories per day or less for many months. Vomiting is usual if food is forced, or may even be self-induced. Constipation and other vague gastrointestinal complaints are common. Blood pressure, pulse, and temperature are all lower than normal. Skin and hair are dry and edema of the ankles may be present; amenorrhea is also common. Ironically, despite the severe and prolonged dietary restrictions, these patients usually do not exhibit any gross nutritional imbalances. Lowered zinc and copper levels have been reported [5].

Patients with anorexia nervosa often go to extreme lengths to preserve their emaciation, including constant exercise. They consider their weight appropriate and have a real fear of gaining weight. They will resort to any number of devious methods to dispose of food when under supervision. These patients may perceive that some other family member is not eating enough and that they certainly are.

An estimated 5 to 20 percent of all patients with anorexia nervosa die, either from infections, cardiac failure, or other related causes [6]. Many of those who survive later develop chronic mental illness. Prognosis is better when the patient can be hospitalized during the early phases of therapy. Family visits must be limited and a disciplined, but sympathetic, regimen established for the patient. Both the family and the patient should be made to understand that this disease can be fatal if allowed to continue. Psychiatric consultation is imperative. The diet should be augmented by approximately 300 to 400 calories per day, each day, until an intake of 3400 to 3600 calories is attained. By discharge, the weight gain should be slow but steady. Continued psychiatric support, if possible, may help prevent recurrences.

Protein-Calorie Malnutrition
BACKGROUND

Protein-calorie malnutrition among children is the most important and widespread nutritional problem in the world today. Protein and calorie deficiency occurs in children as two distinct clinical diseases—*marasmus* and *kwashior-*

kor. Although each may be found as a separate syndrome, it is common to see a gradation from one type to the other. The term *marasmus* comes from the Greek *marasmos*, meaning wasting or withering. It is a type of malnutrition caused primarily by a deficiency of protein and calories. Marasmus in children is equivalent to starvation in adults. *Kwashiorkor*, a disease caused by protein deficiency when the weaned child is given starchy, low-protein foods, is a term first used by the Ga tribe in Ghana describing the illness the older child gets when the next baby is born. The term was first introduced into medicine by the pediatrician Cicely Williams in 1933. Both types of malnutrition usually occur in children under 5 years of age, since the requirement for protein and calories are greatest for this age group. Marasmus occurs more frequently in infants under 1 year of age and in urban settings; kwashiorkor is seen mostly in the second year of life and in more rural areas.

Most of the changes discussed under the heading of starvation also occur to some degree with marasmus, kwashiorkor, and the syndrome between the two, marasmic kwashiorkor. Marked wasting of the skeletal muscles and atrophy of the heart and intestinal mucosa are common findings. Death may be due to organ failure, infection, or dehydration and electrolyte imbalance caused by diarrhea.

The length of hospitalization and degree of nutritional rehabilitation are currently areas of debate among clinicians [7]. Some argue that the child should achieve 85 to 90 percent of his or her expected weight for height before discharge, while others suggest an attainment of only 75 percent [8, 9]. In either case, the risk of death is highest for infants below 80 percent of their weight-for-age and for children 12 to 36 months, below 70 percent [10].

MARASMUS

ETIOLOGY

The causes of marasmus most often stem from poverty in the urban setting and lack of adequate nutritional knowledge. It may also occur in grossly neglected children; secondary to prematurity or such diseases as cystic fibrosis and celiac disease; or from overwhelming infections, diarrhea, or malabsorption.

Early cessation of breast-feeding in developing countries has been cited as the single most common precipitating factor leading to the development of marasmus. The early cessation of breast-feeding may be due to failure of lactation, death of the mother, separation of the mother from the infant, or, more commonly, a desire of the mother to feed her infant formula from a bottle rather than breast-feeding. She may be influenced by advertising and pressures from outside cultures. She may stop breast-feeding because she has become pregnant again, and it is the belief among many of the poor and uneducated that the milk of a pregnant woman is bad for her child.

Formula feeding does not automatically lead to marasmus, but among the poor, especially in developing countries, it does pose an added risk. Many mothers do not have sufficient income to purchase enough formula; as a result, they tend to overdilute it with water, decreasing the formula's nutritional density.

Often, too, the water supply used is unsafe and facilities are inadequate for refrigeration and bottle sterilization, compounding the problem with gastrointestinal infections. A common treatment for such sick infants is the withholding of food, or a diet of rice water or plain water for long periods. Thus, the vicious cycle of marasmus begins.

CLINICAL FINDINGS

In all cases of marasmus growth failure is clearly evident. Advanced cases present an unforgettable picture. There is extreme wasting of the muscles; the limbs are very thin, while the belly may be protuberant. Weight is far below standard for the child's age, and if the disease is of long duration, his length is also below normal. He may be dehydrated, with little or no subcutaneous fat. The skin is dry, atrophic, and loose, hanging in wrinkles, especially around the thighs and buttocks. Anemia, diarrhea, hair changes, and signs of vitamin deficiencies may be present. The serum protein concentration is reduced, but not as severely as in kwashiorkor. The liver is not infiltrated with fat. In contrast to children with kwashiorkor who tend to be irritable or disinterested, the mental state of the marasmic child appears to be unaffected.

TREATMENT

The response to severe marasmus is slow, and prolonged hospitalization may be necessary. Treatment may have to be approached gradually, initiated with intravenous feedings, followed by the gradual introduction of protein-containing foods, and then a high-protein diet. Figures 34-2A and B show a child with severe marasmus and the same child after 10 months of nutritional rehabilitation. An adequate intake of both protein and calories is mandatory to allow for weight gain and growth. Dried skim milk is frequently used, with vegetable oil added to provide additional calories. The complications and concurrent illnesses, such as anemia, diarrhea, infections, dehydration, and vitamin deficiencies, should also be treated.

It is important that the child not be discharged from the hospital only to return to the same environment and circumstances that led to the development of the disease initially. An adequate diet is essential for recovery and continued growth.

KWASHIORKOR

ETIOLOGY

Kwashiorkor mostly affects children, between 1 and 3 years of age, whose diets are grossly deficient in protein. This type of malnutrition is common in many of the developing countries, but it is also seen in association with poverty in the United States and Europe. It is most frequently seen during the weaning period, when the child's diet is changed from breast milk to a diet high in starch and low in protein (see Fig. 34-3).

Many factors contribute to the rapid development of kwashiorkor among young children—their rapid growth and relatively high protein requirements;

FIG. 34-2.
A. Child with severe maras-
   mus. (FAO photo.)
B. Same child after 10 months
   of nutritional rehabilitation.
   (Photo courtesy of Public
   Health Department, Iran;
   issued by FAO.)

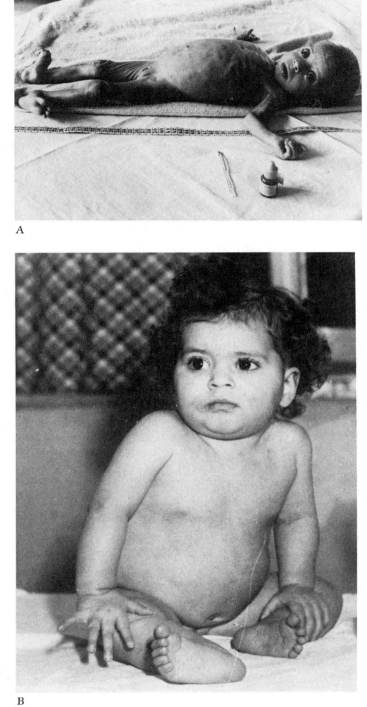

A

B

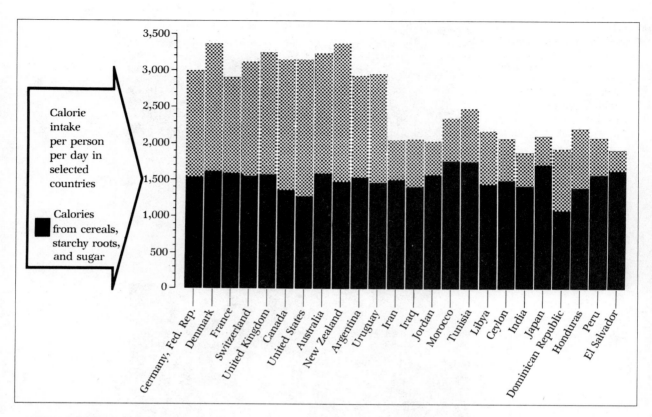

FIG. 34-3. Calorie intake per person per day in selected countries. (FAO photo.)

the lack of high-protein foods in their daily diets; the cultural distribution of foods that are available (that is, adults and older children usually receive most of the protein-rich foods); seasonal food shortages; concurrent poverty; ignorance to dietary needs by the parents; infections; and illnesses.

CLINICAL FINDINGS

As with marasmus, growth failure is always evident; both height and weight are affected. There is wasting of the muscles, but it may be masked by edema. The edema may be slight or severe, depending on the degree of protein deficiency, but it always occurs and is an important feature of the disease (Fig. 34-4). It may be present all over the body, including the face, but is usually more marked in the lower limbs. Characteristic changes in the skin may occur. The dermatosis of kwashiorkor consists of areas of depigmentation and other areas of deeper pigmentation. These latter patches may desquamate like blistered paint ("flaky-paint dermatosis"). Ulcers and deep cracks in the skin may also be seen, compounded by lesions caused by vitamin deficiencies. Hair changes also characteristic of this disease are common. The hair loses its curl and becomes sparse, thin, and soft. Black hair loses its pigmentation and may become streaked with gray, red, or blond color. Hair can be an indicator of earlier nutritional

FIG. 34-4. Child with kwashiorkor. (FAO photo.)

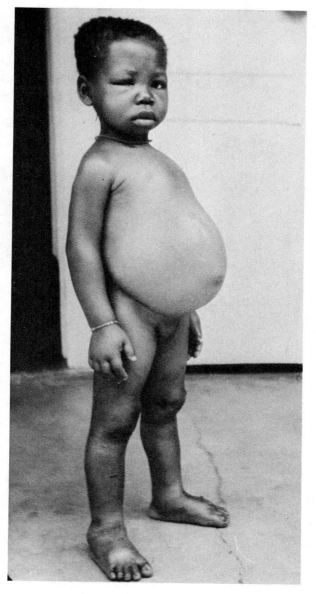

experiences; parallel strips of discolored hair are known as the "flag sign" (Fig.
34-5). Anemia is common, caused by a deficiency of protein, and compounded
by a lack of iron, vitamin C, B_{12}, and folic acid. There are reductions in the serum
albumin and globulin content of the blood due to failure of synthesis in the liver.
Diarrhea, occasionally bloody, is also a common finding. The liver is always
enlarged (hepatomegaly) and infiltrated with fat in this disease. Symptoms of
vitamin deficiencies may also be found, such as lesions of the mouth and tongue

FIG. 34-5. "Flag sign" in a malnourished child. (FAO photo by Marcel Ganzin.)

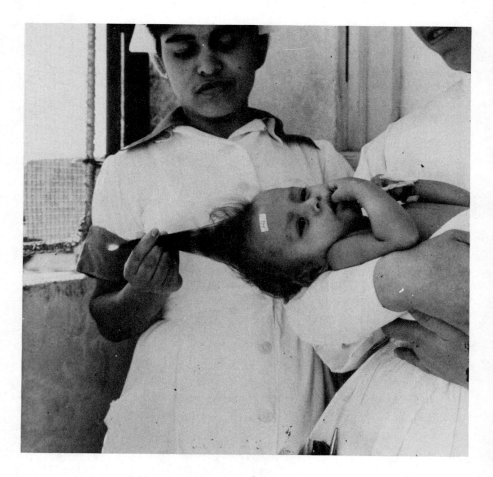

(lack of B vitamins) and eye changes (lack of vitamin A) (Fig. 34-6). Apathy is typical in kwashiorkor; the child is uninterested in his surroundings and irritable when being moved or bathed.

TREATMENT

As with marasmus, dried skim milk with vegetable oil is recommended. Potassium and additional fluids may be necessary if the diarrhea is severe. Infections, anemia, and vitamin deficiencies should all be treated with the appropriate measures. As the child recovers, the diet can be advanced to include more varied protein-rich foods. The cooperation of the mother is important if relapses and repeated admissions are to be avoided.

Neurologic Development

Severe malnutrition in children under 5 years of age can have profound, permanent adverse effects on brain development and subsequent learning and behavior. As shown in Table 34-2, by the end of the first postnatal year the human

FIG. 34-6. Skin changes and mouth lesions of malnutrition. (Photograph of the Kenya Information Services; issued by FAO.)

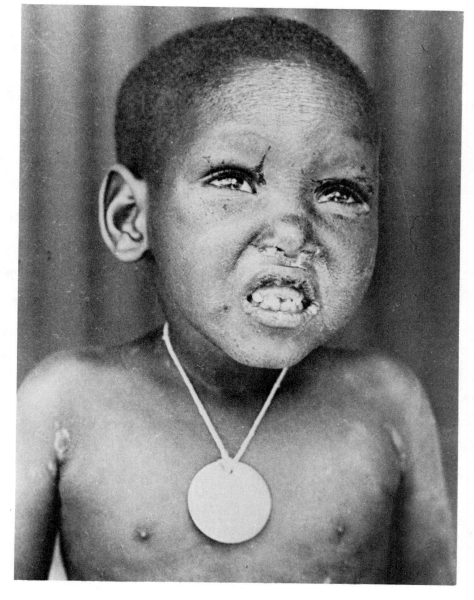

brain has grown to about 70 percent of its adult size, as compared to the total body weight, which has reached only about 15 percent of its final adult total. Because brain growth is accomplished largely through protein synthesis, a deficiency of this essential nutrient will adversely affect this process.

NORMAL BRAIN DEVELOPMENT

Brain development begins early in fetal life, with spurts of growth during which it is most vulnerable to nutritional insults. The major portion of brain growth

TABLE 34-2. Chronologic order of brain development

Time period	Physiologic event (brain growth spurt)
In utero	
Conception	
10–18 weeks	Multiplication of neuroblasts
	Oligodendroglial population established
	Myelination begins
	Brain growth spurt begins
26 weeks	First peak of DNA synthesis
	Peak rate of neuronal division
Birth	Second peak of DNA synthesis
	Peak rate of glial division
	Total neuronal number attained
	25% of adult brain weight achieved
3 months	Total lipid deposition in gray matter completed
6 months	DNA content stops increasing
	Head circumference stops increasing
12 months	DNA synthesis stops in brainstem
	Total oligodendroglial cells attained 70% of adult brain weight achieved
24 months	90% of total lipid deposited in white matter
3–4 years	Myelination completed
10 years	Total lipid deposition in white matter completed

Source: B. Luke, Nutritional Influence on Brain Development and Behavior. In B. Luke, *Maternal Nutrition.* Boston: Little, Brown, 1979. P. 125.

begins at midgestation (10 to 18 weeks after conception) and ends by the third or fourth postnatal year, making at least five-sixths of the human brain growth spurt postnatal [11]. Normal cellular growth in the brain is composed of two phases—the early *proliferative phase* when cell division is dominant and the quantity of protein and lipid remain constant; and the later *hypertrophic phase* when cell division slows and finally stops, and there is an increased rate of myelin synthesis. The DNA content of the brain reflects the total cell number. The head circumference and DNA content of the brain parallel each other, both increasing until about 6 months of age. Both brain weight and protein content increase linearly through the first year.

The brain is composed of a variety of cells, many of which contain large amounts of lipid. Since most of the lipid is within cell membranes (e.g., myelin sheaths), changes in this component constitute a change in myelination. The total lipid content of the brain changes little during the first months of gestation; thereafter, lipid deposition proceeds rapidly. By 2 years of age, 90 percent of the total lipid is deposited, and by 10 years, adult values are attained. Lipids represent about 75 percent of the dry weight of human myelin. After myelination, synaptic connections and dendritic branching are established, which extend well into the third postnatal year and beyond.

Structural Effects of Malnutrition

The major effect of malnutrition is interference with cellular growth. The results of nutritional deprivation depend on the duration, severity, and stage of brain development. Malnutrition imposed on the human infant during the first 8 months of life causes a reduction in the number of glia (the fibrous, nonnervous supporting elements of the nervous system) and in myelination. If continued, cell size is reduced, including a decrease in the number of neurons, the length of processes, or both, plus curtailed myelination [12]. During the proliferative phase of brain growth, cell division is retarded; during the hypertrophic phase, the enlargement of cells is affected. The magnitude of the effect produced by the nutritional insult on cell division is related to the rate of division and the timing of the restriction. Data indicate that marasmic infants, who died of malnutrition during the first year of life, had reduced brain weight, nucleic acid, and protein content [13, 14]. This indicates a decreased rate of DNA synthesis and cell division, resulting in a reduction in the total number of brain cells. The brains of older children, who were presumably well-nourished during the first year of life and died of kwashiorkor, did not show a reduction in cell number, but rather in cell size (protein/DNA ratio). A decrease in cell number is reflected by both reduced brain weight and by smaller head circumference.

Intellectual Effects of Malnutrition

Chronic subnutrition and severe malnutrition in children demonstrate the relationship of growth achievement to intellectual performance. Studies done in Guatemala, Mexico, and India have shown that taller children (height being used as an indicator of long-term nutrition) had higher levels of neurointegrative competence in processing information [15–17]. This is important because of the demonstrated association between such competence and the ability to acquire primary reading skills [18–20]. An association has also been established between children suffering from severe nutritional illnesses and delayed language acquisition [21]. Severely malnourished children begin to lag behind in language at about 6 months of age. Children who had been undernourished during infancy remained stunted in both language development and concept formation even after age 3 [22]. Other researchers have observed a decreased IQ in children who were hospitalized for malnutrition before 12 months of age [23]. These researchers have found a correlation between the severity of the child's illness on admission (as estimated by his deficit of expected weight-for-age on admission) and decreased IQ in the school years.

Malnutrition directly affects the developing central nervous system. It may also cause intellectual deficits as a result of the child's loss of learning time while hospitalized. Only with adequate diet, teaching, love, and stimulation can this intelligence gap caused by malnutrition even begin to be overcome.

Immune Status

One hundred million children are affected by malnutrition, mostly in Asia, Africa, and South America where it is responsible for half of the deaths that occur before 5 years of age [24]. Many of these deaths are precipitated by an overwhelming infection, such as intractable diarrhea, measles, whooping cough, or pneumonia. Malnutrition, particularly in children, increases susceptibility to disease, lowers resistance to infection, and increases severity of the infection.

NORMAL IMMUNITY

EXTERNAL DEFENSES

The skin, the epithelial linings of the gastrointestinal, respiratory, and genitourinary tracts, and the cornea of the eye are all natural barriers restricting the entrance of microorganisms into the body. In addition, the secretions in which many of the epithelial tissues are bathed have bactericidal properties. The acid secretions of the stomach, the lysozymes present in tears, and the sebum of the skin all give added defense against microbial invasion. Any dietary deficiency that results in altered integrity of epithelial surfaces or production of the protective secretions increases the body's susceptibility to infection. Once an organism has gained entrance to the body, it encounters the internal defenses.

INTERNAL DEFENSES

The human body has two main defense systems—*humoral* and *cellular*. Both react to foreign proteins (antigens). Humoral immunity is due to circulating antibodies in the gamma globulin fraction of plasma proteins. Cellular immunity is responsible for delayed allergic reactions, the rejection of tissue transplants, and the rejection of tumor cells. Cellular immunity is also the major defense against infections due to viruses, fungi, and certain bacteria. The body may react to a microorganism by developing a fever. This indicates an increase in metabolic activity and may create an environment unfavorable for the survival of the invading organism.

Humoral Response

The protein of the invading microorganism is foreign to the body and acts as an *antigen*, stimulating antibody production by plasma cells. *Antibodies* are immunoglobulins that react with specific antigens, destroying them. A bacterial toxin (a substance released from the bacteria) may also stimulate antibody production. Antibodies may persist in the blood for many years, preventing a second infection with the same organism or causing a repeat infection to be less severe.

Cellular Response

The body may also respond to a foreign microorganism by the production of specialized cells in the bone marrow that migrate to the sites of infection to ingest and destroy the invading microorganism (phagocytosis). Different microorganisms evoke the production of different cell types.

GRANULOCYTES. The bone marrow is stimulated to produce and release large numbers of white blood cells, which include granulocytes, monocytes, and lymphocytes. The granulocytes (also termed *polymorphonuclear leukocytes*) are the most numerous. Granulocytes mature into three types of cells—neutrophils, basophils, and eosinophils. All granulocytes contain the enzyme myeloperoxidase, which aids in the destruction of ingested bacteria. Neutrophils are the body's first line of defense; they seek out, ingest, and destroy bacteria. The monocytes constitute the second line of defense, following the neutrophils into the area of infection to phagocytose bacteria, other foreign matter, and dead cells. The eosinophils phagocytose antigen–antibody complexes. The basophils contain histamine and heparin; they are the least prevalent of the granulocytes.

MONOCYTES. Monocytes enter the circulation from the bone marrow; after 24 hours they enter the tissues to become *macrophages* (also termed the *reticuloendothelial system*). Like the granulocytes, they contain peroxidase and lysosomal enzymes and are actively phagocytic. Bacterial products interact with factors in the plasma to produce agents that attract phagocytic cells to the area. Monocytes migrate to these areas in response to this chemical stimuli, engulfing and destroying bacteria in a manner similar to that of the granulocytes. Under nonpathologic conditions, macrophages normally remove worn-out red blood cells from the circulation (mainly in the liver and spleen), and store iron.

LYMPHOCYTES. Lymphocytes are formed in the lymph glands, thymus, spleen, and bone marrow, and enter the bloodstream from the lymphatics. Lymphocytes have special receptors on their surfaces for particular antigens. After the antigen binds to the lymphocyte, the latter divides. Its daughter cells are transformed into plasma cells, which then secrete large amounts of antibodies into the circulation. These antibodies are termed *immunoglobulins*. There are five general types of immunoglobulin antibodies produced by the lymphocyte-plasma cell system— IgG, IgA, IgM, IgD, and IgE. They are capable of great variation in structure, which explains how there can be a unique antibody for each antigen. The level of antibodies may be acquired directly from the mother through the placenta, or in the colostrum of breast milk. They also can be acquired through repeated exposure to small doses of the infecting organism or from protective inoculations.

Effects of Malnutrition

Malnutrition may increase the body's susceptibility and decrease its resistance to infection. Once an infection is established, the individual's previous state of nutrition is of great importance in determining the eventual outcome. Malnourished individuals are less able to withstand the toxic effects of infection, particularly on the heart, liver, and kidneys. The increased metabolism and breakdown of tissues caused by infectious diseases can have a more devastating effect in the malnourished individual. If the diet during convalescence is inadequate in protein and calories, it makes the individual, especially a child, more prone to repeated infections. This cycle is seen in the development of kwashiorkor.

In animals, diets deficient in various nutrients have been shown to cause a reduction in the cellular immune response to infection and a decrease in the production of antibodies [25]. This has also been demonstrated, to a lesser degree, in humans [26]. Pyridoxine deficiency leads to impaired protein and DNA synthesis. In humans, this has resulted in reduced antibody responses to vaccines. A deficiency of pantothenic acid also reduces antibody response to immunization, but through inhibiting plasma cells from producing new immunoglobulins [25]. Vitamin B_{12} deficiency and pernicious anemia result in impaired lymphocyte response and a decrease in the bactericidal and phagocytic capacity of neutrophils [27]. Folic acid deficiency also depresses immune function. Iron-deficient individuals show defective macrophage and neutrophil functioning. Zinc deficiency causes abnormalities in cellular and humoral immunity as well as atrophy of lymphoid tissue. Adequate plasma and tissue levels of the fat-soluble vitamins, particularly A and E, help resist infection by maintaining the integrity and composition of external cell membranes. Large doses of vitamin E have actually been shown to suppress immune function [28].

An interesting phenomena of uncomplicated famine is often *anorexia*, loss of the desire to eat. Animal experiments have shown that virus infections appear to be mitigated by starvation. In humans this paradox has been summarized by Murray and Murray [29]

". . . increased resistance to viral infection and at least some bacterial infections exist in the face of an apparent decrease in immune function with the important corollary that increased susceptibility to infection occurs with refeeding when immune function might be expected to be on the mend."

Anorexia, and the resultant nutrient deficiencies, may be nature's method of creating an unfavorable environment for the invading microorganism.

Conclusion

The high incidence of infectious diseases among the poorer populations throughout the world may be due more to overcrowding, poor sanitary conditions, and increased risks of cross-infection (the passage of microorganisms from person to person) than to any nutritional effect on the functioning of the immune system. Health programs in these areas should recognize these factors and approach the problem of infectious diseases and malnutrition through the improvement of nutrition, housing, sanitation, and health education. The cycle of malnutrition and its devastating effects can be overcome.

References

1. Cahill, J. F. Starvation in man. *N. Engl. J. Med.* 282:668, 1970.
2. Nutter, D. O., et al. Cardiac dynamics and myocardial contractility in chronic protein-calorie undernutrition. *Clin. Res.* 26:256A, 1978.
3. Heymsfield, S. B., et al. Cardiac abnormalities in cachectic patients before and during nutritional rehabilitation. *Am. Heart J.* 95:584, 1978.

4. Davidson, S., et al. *Human Nutrition and Dietetics* (6th ed.). London: Churchill Livingstone, 1975. P. 287.
5. Casper, R. C., et al. An evaluation of trace metals, vitamins, and taste function in anorexia nervosa. *Am. J. Clin. Nutr.* 33:1801, 1980.
6. Schleimer, K. Anorexia nervosa. *Nutr. Rev.* 39:99, 1981.
7. Rehabilitation of malnourished children. *Lancet* 1:1350, 1981.
8. Landman, J., et al. A catch-up growth chart. *J. Trop. Pediatr.* 27:47, 1981.
9. Cooper, E., Headden, G., and Lawrence, C. Caribbean children, thriving and failing in and out of hospital. *J. Trop. Pediatr.* 26:232, 1980.
10. Kielmann, A. A., and McCord, C. Weight-for-age as an index of risk of death in children. *Lancet* 1:1247, 1978.
11. Stoch, M. B., and Smythe, P. M. Does undernutrition during infancy inhibit brain growth and subsequent intellectual development? *Arch. Dis. Child.* 38:546, 1968.
12. Winick, M., Brasel, J. A., and Rosso, P. Nutrition and Cell Growth. In M. Winick (ed.), *Nutrition and Development.* New York: Wiley, 1972. Pp. 49–97.
13. Davison, A. N., and Dobbing, J. Myelination as a vulnerable period in brain development. *Br. Med. Bull.* 22:40, 1966.
14. Winick, M., and Rosso, P. The effect of severe early malnutrition on cellular growth of human brain. *Pediatr. Res.* 3:181, 1969.
15. Birch, H. G. Malnutrition, learning and intelligence. *Am. J. Public Health* 62:773, 1972.
16. Cravioto, J., and DeLicardie, E. R. Intersensory Development in School Age Children. In N. S. Scrimshaw and J. E. Gordon (eds.), *Malnutrition, Learning, and Behavior.* Boston: M.I.T. Press, 1968. Pp. 252–269.
17. Champakam, S., Srikantia, S. G., and Gopalan, C. Kwashiorkor and mental development. *Am. J. Clin. Nutr.* 21:844, 1968.
18. Birch, H. G., and Belmont, L. Auditory-visual integration in normal and retarded readers. *Am. J. Orthopsychiatry* 44:852, 1964.
19. Birch, H. G., and Belmont, L. Auditory-visual integration, intelligence and reading ability in school children. *Percept. Mot. Skills* 20:295, 1965.
20. Kahn, D., and Birch, H. G. Development of auditory-visual integration and reading achievement. *Percept. Mot. Skills* 27:459, 1968.
21. Waterlow, J. C., Cravioto, J., and Stephen, J. K. L. Protein Malnutrition in Man. In M. L. Anson, et al. (eds.), *Advances in Protein Chemistry.* New York: Academic, 1960.
22. Energy-protein malnutrition and behavior. *Nutr. Rev.* 38:164, 1980.
23. Cabak, V., and Najdanvic, R. Effect of undernutrition in early life on physical and mental development. *Arch. Dis. Child.* 40:532, 1965.
24. Suskind, R. M., et al. The Malnourished Child: Clinical, Biochemical and Hematologic Changes. In R. M. Suskind (ed.), *Malnutrition and the Immune Response.* New York: Raven Press, 1977. Pp. 1–8.
25. Axelrod, A. E. Immune processes in vitamin deficiency states. *Am. J. Clin. Nutr.* 24:265, 1971.
26. Smythe, P. M., et al. Thymolymphatic deficiency and depression of cell-mediated immunity in protein-calorie malnutrition. *Lancet* 2:931, 1971.
27. Beisel, W. R., et al. Single-nutrient effects on immunologic functions. *J.A.M.A.* 245:53, 1981.
28. Prasad, J. S. Effect of vitamin E supplementation on leukocyte function. *Am. J. Clin. Nutr.* 33:606, 1980.
29. Murray, J., and Murray, A. Suppression of infection by famine and its activation by refeeding: A paradox? *Persp. Biol. Med.* 20:471, 1977.

Suggested Readings

Ashworth, A.   Practical aspects of dietary management during rehabilitation from severe protein-energy malnutrition. *J. Hum. Nutr.* 34:360, 1980.

Barac-Nieto, M., et al.   Body composition in chronic undernutrition. *Am. J. Clin. Nutr.* 31:23, 1978.

Barnet, A. B., et al.   Abnormal auditory evoked potentials in early infancy malnutrition. *Science* 201:450, 1978.

Bartel, P. R., et al.   Long-term effects of kwashiorkor on the electroencephalogram. *Am. J. Clin. Nutr.* 32:753, 1979.

Beisel, W. R.   Effects of infection on nutritional status and immunity. *Fed. Proc.* 39:3105, 1980.

Beumont, P. J. V., et al.   The diet composition and nutritional knowledge of patients with anorexia nervosa. *J. Hum. Nutr.* 35:265, 1981.

Brain growth in kwashiorkor. *Nutr. Rev.* 33:107, 1975.

Bruch, H.   *The Golden Cage: The Enigma of Anorexia Nervosa.* Cambridge, Mass.: Harvard University Press, 1978. Pp. 150.

Butterworth, C. E.   The skeleton in the hospital closet. *Nutr. Today* March/April 1974. Pp. 4–8.

Chandra, R. K.   Cell-mediated immunity in nutritional imbalance. *Fed. Proc.* 39:3088, 1980.

Chandra, R. K.   Trace elements and immunity: A synopsis of current knowledge. *Food Nutr. Bull.* 3:39, 1981.

Chandra, R. K., and Newberne, P. M.   *Nutrition, Immunity and Infection.* New York: Plenum, 1977.

Chen, L. C., Chowdbury, A. K. M., and Huffman, S. L.   Anthropometric assessment of energy-protein malnutrition and subsequent risk of mortality among preschool aged children. *Am. J. Clin. Nutr.* 33:1836, 1980.

Ciseaux, A.   Anorexia nervosa: A view from the mirror. *Am. J. Nurs.* 80:1468, 1980.

Cravioto, J.   Nutrition, stimulation, mental development, and learning. *Nutr. Today* 16:4, 1981.

Devadas, R. P., et al.   A study on the incidence, infestation, and its interrelationship with malnutrition among children. *Indian J. Nutr. Diet.* 17:1, 1980.

Faulk, W. P., and Edsall, G.   Vaccines and vaccination programs: Special emphasis in malnutrition. *Am. J. Clin. Nutr.* 31:2237, 1978.

Garrow, J. S.   Dietary management of obesity and anorexia nervosa. *J. Hum. Nutr.* 34:131, 1980.

Good, R. A., West, A., and Fernandes, G.   Nutritional modulation of immune responses. *Fed. Proc.* 39:3098, 1980.

Hansen, L. P., et al.   The development of high-protein rice flour for early childhood feeding. *Food Technol.* 35:38, 1981.

Heymsfield, S. B., and Nutter, D. O.   The Heart in Protein-calorie Undernutrition. In J. W. Hurst (ed.), *Update I: The Heart.* New York: McGraw-Hill, 1979.

Iatrogenic kwashiorkor in California. *Nutr. Rev.* 39:397, 1981.

Infections and undernutrition. *Nutr. Rev.* 40:119, 1982.

Interaction of infection and nutrition in children: Two studies from Bangladesh. *Nutr. Rev.* 39:394, 1981.

Jackson, A.   Hospital management of malnutrition. *Cajanus* 13:146, 1980.

Koster, F., Gaffar, A., and Jackson, T. M.   Recovery of cellular immune competence during treatment of protein-calorie malnutrition. *Am. J. Clin. Nutr.* 34:887, 1981.

Latham, M. C.   Protein-calorie malnutrition in children and its relation to psychological development and behavior. *Physiol. Rev.* 54:541, 1974.

Marshall, M. H.   Anorexia nervosa: Dietary treatment and re-establishment of body weight in 20 cases studied on a metabolic unit. *J. Hum. Nutr.* 32:349, 1978.

Medical news: Closing in on the nutrition-immunity link. *J.A.M.A.* 244:2715, 1980.

Minuchin, S., Rosman, B. L., and Baker, L. *Psychosomatic Families: Anorexia Nervosa in Context.* Cambridge, Mass.: Harvard University Press, 1978. P. 351.

Prohaska, J. R., and Lukasewycz, O. A. Copper deficiency suppresses the immune response in mice. *Science* 213:559, 1981.

Single nutrients and immunity. *Am. J. Clin. Nutr.* 35 [Suppl.]:417, 1982.

Slater, L. E. Food shortage by the year 2000? *Food Eng.* 53:55, 1981.

Steffee, W. P. Malnutrition in hospitalized patients. *J.A.M.A.* 244:2630, 1980.

Stiehm, E. R. Humoral immunity in malnutrition. *Fed. Proc.* 39:3093, 1980.

Waterlow, J. C. Classification and definition of protein-calorie malnutrition. *Br. Med. J.* 3:366, 1972.

Whitehead, R. J. Infection and the development of kwashiorkor and marasmus in Africa. *Am. J. Clin. Nutr.* 30:1281, 1977.

Chapter 35

PRINCIPLES OF PARENTERAL NUTRITION

Since 1616, when William Harvey first discovered that blood circulates, numerous attempts have been made to use the vascular system for intravenous therapy. Forty years after Harvey's discovery, Sir Christopher Wren, the famous English architect and astronomer, first introduced such substances as wine, ale, and opium into the veins of dogs, using a goose quill and pig's bladder [1]. In the 1660s, experiments continued with intravenous injections and blood transfusions, including the first documented blood transfusion from a lamb to a human in Paris in 1667 [1]. Legal and religious constraints were soon placed on attempts at blood transfusions as the number of deaths and complications increased, resulting from ignorance of microorganisms, sterilization, blood-typing, and cross-matching.

In the mid 1800s, sugar solutions were first infused into animals and, before the turn of the century, into humans. In the late 1800s, an intravenously administered saline solution was first used in the treatment of surgical shock in a man. With the discovery of microbiology by Pasteur and the application of the principles of asepsis by Lister, the intravenous administration of solutions became safer and more practical.

Several problems limited the administration of nutrients by vein [2]. First, the amount of fluid a sick adult can safely handle is only about 35 to 50 ml/kg body weight, or about 3 to 3½ liters per day. Next is the limitation set by the caloric density of the nutrients themselves—4 calories per gram of carbohydrate or protein, and 9 calories per gram of fat. The third problem is the concentration of the solution that can be safely administered into a peripheral vein; the highest concentration tolerated without causing irritation to the vessel is a 5 to 10% dextrose solution, or about twice the isotonicity of blood. Three liters of a 5% dextrose solution would provide only about 600 calories in a day, hardly enough to meet energy requirements even during health, and void of protein, vitamins, minerals, and essential fatty acids needed for metabolism, wound healing, and repair.

Intravenous hyperalimentation, or *total parenteral nutrition (TPN)*, is the intravenous administration of nutrients in sufficient quantity and concentration to maintain metabolism and tissue synthesis when oral feedings are either inadequate or not possible. In 1944, the first documented report of success of total parenteral nutrition was published by Helfrick and Abelson [3]. An infant was fed for 5 days via an ankle vein. Their success was not duplicated for over 2 decades because of the need for frequent changing of intravenous sites, or because the calories provided were insufficient to spare the amino acid mixtures for anabolism.

In the late 1960s, Stanley Dudrick and his coworkers devised a technique that was to make parenteral nutrition a practical reality. They suggested that a catheter be implanted and maintained in the superior vena cava for long periods at a time (Fig. 35-1). Because of the high blood flow in this central vein, a hyperos-

FIG. 35-1. Placement of catheter in superior vena cava. Concentrated nutrient solution is infused through a catheter directly into the superior vena cava, the 1-in. vein that returns blood to the heart from the upper part of the body. The high volume of blood flow in this large vein quickly dilutes the solution to a safe level. The catheter is inserted into the right subclavian vein and pushed along until the tip of the catheter is in the superior vena cava. The catheter can also be inserted through the left subclavian vein or one of the jugular veins. If the nutrient solution is continuously infused for 24 hours a day, the patient will receive enough nourishment for him to be able to gain weight. (From S. J. Dudrick and J. E. Rhoads, Total intravenous feeding. *Scientific American* 226:73, 1972.)

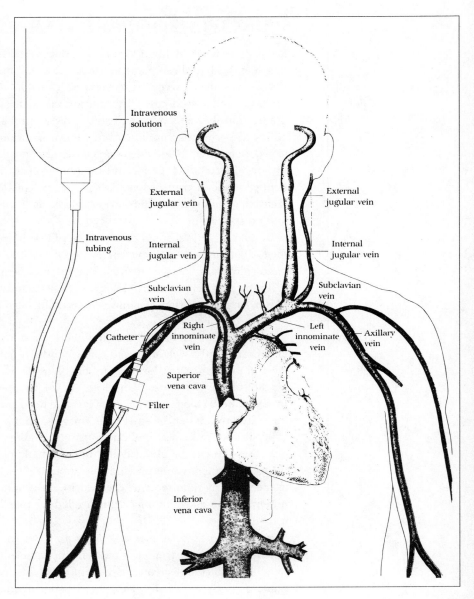

molar nutritive fluid would be quickly diluted, avoiding damage to the vein. By using a hypertonic glucose-protein hydrolysate fluid with electrolytes, vitamins, and minerals, Dudrick and his coworkers were able to demonstrate good growth and development, first in beagle puppies, and later in a human infant [4, 5]. Over the past 15 years, this procedure has been perfected through their efforts and those of many others, and has proved to be a valuable diet therapy tool. It has reduced morbidity and mortality in patients whose complications, disease conditions, or metabolic needs preclude adequate oral nutrient intake, and can actually promote wound healing, growth, and weight gain. As a result of its widespread use and acceptance, the American Society of Parenteral and Enteral Nutrition (ASPEN) was organized to educate the health care team to provide adequate support to the patient on parenteral nutrition.

Indications and Patient Selection

Any patient whose disease condition, complications, or metabolic demands hinder adequate oral nutrient intake may profit from parenteral nutrition. Some specific examples include [6]

1. *Preoperative preparation of malnourished patients* (e.g., patients with stricture or carcinoma of the esophagus, carcinoma of the stomach, or severe peptic ulcer with gastric outlet obstruction)
2. *Postoperative surgical complications* (e.g., prolonged ileus, enterocutaneous fistulae, peritoneal sepsis, and biliary or pancreatic fistulae)
3. *Inflammatory bowel disease* (e.g., regional enteritis, transmural and mucosal colitis, diverticulitis, and intractable gastroenteritis)
4. *Inadequate oral intake or absorption* (hypermetabolic states, e.g., following major trauma or burns; malignant neoplasms being treated with chemotherapy or radiation; pancreatitis; short bowel syndrome; coma; and anorexia nervosa)

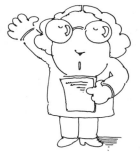

Parenteral nutrition should be initiated in any patient with protein-calorie malnutrition or with signs of its development. Two rough indicators would be patients who have had poor oral intake for 7 or more days or those who have lost 7 to 10 percent or more of their body weight. An assessment of nutritional status is important in potential candidates of parenteral nutrition, both to establish the degree of malnutrition and to provide baseline information used to judge the progress of nutritional therapy.

Nutritional Assessment

A thorough nutritional assessment done before initiating therapy and repeated at set intervals will provide useful parameters on which to base initial and subsequent diet therapies. Listed below are several indicators of nutritional status; these have all been discussed in detail in Chap. 22.

1. Evaluation of skeletal muscle: Measure the midarm muscle circumference.
2. Evaluation of lean body mass: Measure the creatinine/height index.
3. Evaluation of degree of depletion of visceral protein, during stress: Measure the degree of depression of the secretory proteins—serum albumin, transferrin, and total iron-binding capacity (TIBC).
4. Evaluation of the cellular immune system: Estimated by total lymphocyte count and delayed cutaneous hypersensitivity to common recall antigens. The skin tests are read at 24 and 48 hours; wheals greater than 5 mm are considered positive. One positive test indicates intact immunity.

FIG. 35-2. Harris-Benedict equations for calculation of basal energy expenditure (BEE). (From J. A. Harris and F. G. Benedict, *A Biometric Study of Basal Metabolism in Man.* Washington, D.C.: Carnegie Institution, 1919. [Carnegie Institution of Washington, Publ. No. 279].)

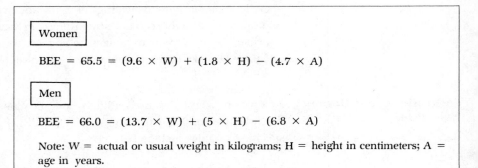

Women

$$BEE = 65.5 = (9.6 \times W) + (1.8 \times H) - (4.7 \times A)$$

Men

$$BEE = 66.0 = (13.7 \times W) + (5 \times H) - (6.8 \times A)$$

Note: W = actual or usual weight in kilograms; H = height in centimeters; A = age in years.

5. Evaluation of fat reserves: Measure triceps skinfold.
6. Rate of metabolism: Estimate the basal caloric requirement or basal energy expenditure (BEE). This can be calculated from the Harris-Benedict equation derived from the results of indirect calorimetry (see Fig. 35-2). During stress, between 12 and 16 percent of the total caloric expenditure is from the oxidation of amino acids; this is reflected in the urine as urinary urea nitrogen (gm/day). There is a direct relationship between urinary urea nitrogen excretion (as estimated from a 24-hour urine collection) and oxygen consumption (energy expenditure) (see Fig. 35-3).
7. Nitrogen balance: Nitrogen balance can also be determined from the same 24-hour urine collection used to estimate urinary urea nitrogen excretion and rate of metabolism [6].

Nitrogen balance = (nitrogen intake in grams) − (urinary urea nitrogen + 4*)

Example

Nitrogen intake: 2 liters of solution with 5 gm of nitrogen per liter

                                       = 10 gm nitrogen intake

Nitrogen out: 2400 ml urine output in 24 hours,

                              containing 6 gm of nitrogen per liter.

$$\frac{6 \text{ gm nitrogen}}{\text{liter}} \times 2.4 \text{ liters} = 14.4 \text{ gm urinary urea nitrogen}$$

14.4 gm + 4 gm constant = 18.4 gm nitrogen out

Nitrogen balance = (10 gm nitrogen intake) − (18.4 gm nitrogen out)

                         = −8.4 gm nitrogen (negative nitrogen balance)

*4 = constant for skin + fecal + urinary nonurea nitrogen

FIG. 35-3. Rates of hypermetabolism estimated from urinary urea nitrogen excretion. (From J. Duke et al., *Surgery* 68:168–174, 1970; P. Rutten et al., *Journal of Surgical Research* 18:477–483, 1975.)

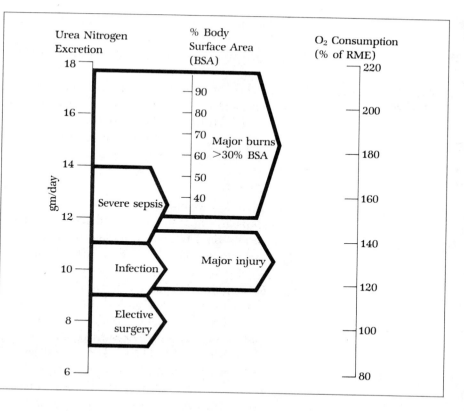

Other baseline measurements that need to be monitored periodically are given in Table 35-1.

Composition of Parenteral Nutrition Fluids

PERIPHERAL PARENTERAL NUTRITION

When oral intake is slightly insufficient (up to 1500 calories/day) or when intake is compromised for no more than 2 weeks, parenteral nutrition may be delivered via a peripheral vein. It has been suggested that a solution containing 3 to 4% amino acids mixed with 5 to 10% dextrose be given simultaneously with a fat emulsion to deliver between 1100 to 1800 calories and 0.8 to 1.0 gm of amino

TABLE 35-1. Baseline laboratory measurements

CBC	Phosphorus	Cholesterol
Glucose	Magnesium	Total protein
BUN	SGOT	Albumin
Creatinine	SGPT	Transferrin or TIBC
Electrolytes (Na, K, Cl)	Alkaline phosphatase	Triglycerides
Calcium	Bilirubin	

Source: M. V. Kaminski, W. A. Burke, and G. L. Blackburn, *Intravenous Hyperalimentation in Modern Hospital Practice.* Tuckahoe, N.Y.: USV Laboratories, 1977.

acids per kilogram body weight daily [7]. When nutrients can only be taken by the intravenous route, and if more than 2000 calories/day are required for longer than 2 weeks, parenteral nutrition via a central vein is necessary.

TOTAL PARENTERAL
NUTRITION

The primary purpose of total parenteral nutrition is to maintain an adequate nutritional state or to improve the nutritional state in a previously malnourished individual [8]. It is indicated only when oral or tube feeding is contraindicated or is inadequate, and when peripheral parenteral nutrition no longer meets the nutritional needs of the patient.

PROTEIN

With a massive injury, there is a shift in the source of energy from carbohydrates to protein, with a larger proportion of needs being derived from the latter. This is due to several factors, including the inability of the tissues to take up glucose from the plasma. The protein of lean muscle then becomes the most readily available source of calories for survival. Proteins are broken down to ketone bodies in the liver and utilized as energy by the brain and muscle. With simple fasting, about 75 gm of protein per day is broken down (6.25 gm of protein = 1 gm of nitrogen). This catabolic process is accelerated in patients stressed by trauma, surgery, sepsis, or other conditions.

Positive nitrogen balance requires sufficient essential and nonessential amino acids together with adequate calories to avoid utilization of amino acids to meet caloric needs. The two types of nitrogen sources available include hydrolysates of fibrin, or casein, or a mixture of pure crystalline amino acids. Only about half of the amino acids in the hydrolysates are in the free form, while the other half are present as short peptides. The metabolic fate of this second group (peptides) is unknown. The recommended amino acid intakes for various groups are as follows:

INFANTS [9]	2.5–4.0 gm/kg/day
ADULTS [7]	
Nondepleted postoperative	0.8–1.0 gm/kg/day
Nutritionally depleted	1.5–1.8 gm/kg/day
Hypermetabolic	2 gm/kg/day

The amount of amino acids given should be high enough to promote positive nitrogen balance, yet low enough to avoid azotemia (the presence of excessive amounts of nitrogen in the blood). The amino acid requirements reflect metabolic and physiologic conditions, increasing with the degree of protein catabolism. Two guidelines to be followed in the composition of the amino acid mixture include [10]—in children, the essential amino acids should be patterned after the needs of the growing child; and the essential to nonessential amino acid ratio should be about 1:1.5.

CALORIES

The direct effects of injury or major surgery, including fever, blood, plasma and protein loss, tissue damage, and the metabolic requirements for clearance of damaged tissues, also increase caloric needs. Fever causes the most profound effect on caloric requirements, with each degree (°F) of fever causing a 7 to 8 percent increase in caloric needs.

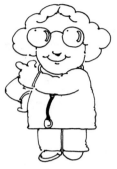

The energy (in calories) supplied must meet requirements including resting metabolism, physical activity, the patient's condition and disease state. To ensure that infused amino acids are utilized for tissue synthesis and not for caloric requirements, an optimal nitrogen/calorie ratio must be maintained—1 gm of nitrogen: 150 to 250 calories. The minimum daily energy expenditure required to maintain a healthy adult in a basal metabolic state is about 600 calories/day. An average healthy adult who is ambulatory has a basal requirement of about 1500 to 1800 calories/day (see Fig. 35-2). For the nondepleted, postoperative patient, the basal energy expenditure (BEE) is increased about 20 percent; for a major skeletal injury, 10 to 30 percent; for the nutritionally depleted patient, about 50 percent; and for the hypermetabolic patient, it is increased about 100 percent [7]. The BEE of hypermetabolic patients is increased by stress, sepsis, trauma, or severe burns; additionally, they are hypercatabolic because of increased loss of lean tissue, resulting in increased nitrogen excretion (1 gm of nitrogen corresponds to 32 gm of lean tissue) [11].

CARBOHYDRATES AND FATS

Glucose is the carbohydrate of choice for parenteral feedings, although substitutes such as fructose, maltose, sorbitol, and ethanol have been tried. A minimum of 100 gm of carbohydrate per day is needed to prevent ketosis and utilization of protein for energy needs. It is difficult to obtain sufficient calories in the form of carbohydrates. Recently, fat emulsions in combination with at least 20 percent of the calories from carbohydrates have been used to help meet the demand for energy. The fat emulsions contain either soybean or cottonseed oil with egg yolk or soybean phospholipids as emulsifiers. Glycerol, sorbitol, or xylitol is also added to make the emulsion isotonic with the blood. Fat emulsions provide essential fatty acids and a concentrated source of energy (1.1 cal/ml or 9 cal/gm). Because their osmolarity is so similar to that of blood (280 mOsm/liter for fat emulsion, 300 mOsm/liter for blood), they can be administered via a peripheral vein. Intravenous fat has been shown to be as effective as glucose in sparing protein and promoting positive nitrogen balance [12]. The administration of 500 ml of fat emulsion every other day will both prevent and correct essential fatty acid deficiency. The nonprotein calories should be provided as 50 percent fat and 50 percent carbohydrate, which prevents problems related to infusing large amounts of glucose while avoiding hyperlipidemia and fatty acid deficiency. Contraindications to the use of fat emulsions include hyperlipidemia,

TABLE 35-2. Amino acid and dextrose concentrations of various parenteral formulations

Parenteral formulation	Amino acids (%)	Dextrose (%)
Peripheral formulation	3–4	5–10
Central formulation	4–5	25
Renal formulation	1.7 (essential amino acids only)	45
Cardiac formulation	3.5	40

Source: L. Michel, A. Serrano, and R. A. Malt. Nutritional support of hospitalized patients. *New England Journal of Medicine* 304:1147, 1981.

liver injury, allergies, and coagulation disturbances. The amino acid and dextrose concentrations of various parenteral formulations are given in Table 35-2.

VITAMINS, MINERALS, AND FLUIDS

Vitamin requirements are elevated due to the increased metabolic demands associated with fever, infection, and injury. Vitamins are also needed in higher amounts to reverse prior depletion and to compensate for excessive urinary losses. To prevent vitamin deficiencies, it is recommended that B-complex vitamins, 0.5 mg folic acid, and 550 mg ascorbic acid be added to each liter of parenteral solution. It is also recommended that 3.5 ml of a multivitamin preparation (B vitamins plus vitamins A, D, and E) be added weekly to the solution, and that 10 mg of vitamin K and 150 μg of vitamin B_{12} be given intramuscularly [7].

It is difficult to estimate mineral needs when there are abnormal mineral losses due to loss of body fluids or breakdown of body tissues. Trace elements must be included in any mineral supplementation to avoid the development of deficiencies. Plasma electrolyte levels must be monitored to provide a basis for adjusting dosages (see Table 35-2).

FLUID LOSSES

Many factors influence fluid losses in any individual patient. Careful monitoring of intake and output and clinical evaluation should provide reasonable estimates. For a normal, healthy adult, the amount of water needed daily for excretion, insensible water loss, and proper tissue hydration is about 100 ml per 100 calories [13], or about 35 ml/kg for adults and 100 ml/kg for infants [14]. Such factors as high fever, renal failure, cardiac decompensation, and excessive water loss from the gastrointestinal tract modify fluid requirements.

Complications and Hazards

A typical fat-free parenteral nutrition fluid has a total osmolarity nearly six times the isotonic value of blood; therefore, a slow infusion in a central vein is necessary to avoid damage to the vein and to maintain constant glucose and electrolyte levels. The composition of the parenteral nutrition fluid is an excellent culture media for microorganisms, making meticulous aseptic techniques mandatory to avoid contamination and the risk of sepsis. Also, because the parenteral nutrition fluid is a chemically complex mixture, interactions among its constituents may occur.

METABOLIC COMPLICATIONS

The high osmolarity of nutritive fluid can cause complications such as coma, due to hyperosmolar nonketotic *hyperglycemia;* convulsions, secondary to acute osmotic changes; and osmotic diuresis with sodium loss and dehydration. *Hypoglycemia* may also occur as a result of the sudden cessation of the glucose load, as when the catheter becomes dislodged or the total parenteral nutrition is abruptly stopped. *Hypophosphatemia* (low blood phosphate) can also result because of the low content of phosphate in the fluid, although the nitrogen source may contribute some phosphate (i.e., casein is a phosphoprotein). This disorder may affect circulating erythrocytes, platelets, and leukocytes, causing them to have a decreased lifespan and diminished function. *Hyperammonemia* may also result, especially when the nitrogen sources used are protein hydrolysates, since they contain some preformed ammonia. This complication can be prevented by the administration of the amino acids arginine and/or ornithine, since there may be low levels of these in the protein hydrolysate. *Hypovitaminosis* and *hypervitaminosis* may result from the administration of inadequate or excess amounts of vitamins. Present knowledge is imprecise regarding parenteral requirements, especially the potentially toxic vitamins such as A and D. The minimum daily requirement for many trace elements, such as cesium, cadmium, molybdenum, rubidium, and arsenic, are not yet known, and deficiencies of these elements may soon be recognized.

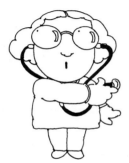

Essential fatty acid deficiency usually occurs after 2 or more weeks of fat-free parenteral nutrition in adults [15]. This deficiency may produce lesions in the skin and hair, growth failure, and an increase in the metabolic rate. Essential fatty acids are important components of cell membranes; their deficiency may cause irreversible damage to the brain and other nervous tissue. Studies in animals have shown that prenatal and postnatal essential fatty acid deficiency results in retardation of brain development and a reduction in some of the myelin (nerve sheath) components [16].

Many of these metabolic complications may be corrected early by changes in the parenteral nutrition fluid, although this requires that the patient be continuously monitored (see Table 35-3).

SURGICAL COMPLICATIONS

Surgical complications are due to the presence of the central venous catheter, and most often include *sepsis, thrombosis,* and *dislodgment* of the catheter. Strict aseptic technique in the insertion and care of the catheter, in frequent dressing changes, and in the mixing of the parenteral nutrition fluids is mandatory. *Infection* is the greatest hazard associated with indwelling catheters. With aseptic technique and proper insertion, an indwelling catheter may remain safely in place for weeks or months.

TABLE 35-3. Metabolic problems associated with total parenteral nutrition

	Problem	Diagnosis	Possible causes	Treatment
Glucose metabolism	Hyperglycemia	Increased blood sugar Glycosuria	Excessive rate of infusion Inadequate insulin	Adjust rate of infusion Administer regular insulin
	Hyperosmolar nonketotic coma	Increased blood sugar Increased serum and urine osmolality Glycosuria Coma	Excessive total glucose load or rate of infusion: inadequate insulin, glucocorticoids, latent diabetes, sepsis, pancreatic disease, acute or chronic renal failure	Appropriate fluids and insulin therapy
	Ketoacidosis in the diabetic	Increased blood sugar Acidosis Ketones	Inadequate endogenous insulin response: inadequate exogenous insulin therapy	Appropriate fluids and insulin
	Postinfusion hypoglycemia	Confusion Coma Decreased blood sugar	Unusual in nondiabetic patient; seen in patients with liver depleted of glycogen who have been in severe negative nitrogen balance	Gradually taper glucose infusion prior to termination
			Persistence of endogenous insulin production by stimulated islet cells	
Amino acid metabolism	Hyperchloremic metabolic acidosis	Increased serum chloride Acidosis	Excessive chloride and monohydrochloride content of certain crystalline amino acid solutions	Provide a portion of sodium and potassium as lactate salts rather than chlorides

	Hyperammonemia	Increased blood ammonia Lethargy	Pediatric age group and patients with cirrhosis are at high risk. May be due to relative arginine deficiency which decreases effectiveness of urea cycle: ornithine, aspartic, and/or glutamic acid deficiencies have been implicated	Add 2 mM/kg/day of arginine glutamate or 3 mM/kg/day of arginine hydrochloride
	Prerenal azotemia	Increased BUN	Excessive protein hydrolysate or amino acid infusion	Adjust rate of administration
Essential fatty acid deficiency		Dermatitis, hair loss, thrombocytopenia, poor wound healing	Abnormal plasma lipid patterns, serum deficiency of phospholipid linoleic and/or arachidonic acids	Infusion of intralipid Vitamin E administration
Calcium phosphorus metabolism		Hypophosphatemia 1. decreased erythrocyte 2,3-DPG 2. increased affinity of hemoglobin for oxygen 3. aberrations of erythrocyte metabolism	Inadequate phosphorus administration, redistribution of serum phosphorus into cells and bone	Add phosphorus to TPN regimen
	Hypocalcemia	Decreased serum calcium Tetany, muscle spasm	Inadequate calcium administration Profound in patients who have phosphorus replacement without calcium replacement Hypoalbuminemia	Add adequate calcium to TPN regimen

Source: S. Papper and G. R. Williams, *Manual of Medical Care of the Surgical Patient.* Boston: Little, Brown, 1981.

Summary

Total parenteral nutrition has opened the doors to a new and dramatic form of diet therapy as a useful adjunct to medicine. With more research, total parenteral nutrition will also help better define nutritional needs of various metabolic and disease states, as well as requirements for some of the lesser-known trace elements.

Case Studies

1. Mrs. Johnson is being admitted for elective surgery. She weighs 50 kg (110 lb), is 157.5 cm in height (62 in.), and is 24 years old. Calculate her basal energy expenditure (BEE) before and after surgery.

2. Eloise, a 3-month-old girl, has been on fat-free, total parenteral nutrition for 6 weeks. She has stopped gaining weight and has developed lesions on her skin and hair. These are signs of what type of deficiency? Why does it appear so much quicker in children than in adults?

3. Mr. Allen, a 30-year-old male, was involved in an automobile accident. He suffered multiple broken bones, and underwent emergency surgery for a ruptured spleen and a collapsed lung. Because of his extensive injuries and surgery, he is considered a hypermetabolic patient and is to be placed on total parenteral nutrition. Assuming he is 6 feet in height (183 cm), and weighs 200 lb (90.9 kg), calculate his BEE both before and after the accident, how much protein he now requires, and assuming a 50 to 50 percent division of nonprotein calories between carbohydrate and fat, calculate the amount of grams of each he should receive daily.

4. Mrs. Haviland, a 90-year-old woman, is recovering from hip surgery after having sustained a fracture while ice skating. Her BEE before the injury and surgery was 900 cal/day, increased now 30 percent by the major skeletal injury. The surgical site has become infected and she has a fever of 104.6°F (40°C). Calculate her BEE after the injury and surgery and during her febrile period.

References

1. Annan, G. L. An exhibition of books on the growth of our knowledge of blood transfusions. *Bull. N.Y. Acad. Med.* 15:622, 1939.
2. Dudrick, S. J., and Rhoads, J. E. New horizons for intravenous feeding. *J.A.M.A.* 215:939, 1971.
3. Helfrick, F. W., and Abelson, N. M. Intravenous feeding of a complete diet in a child: Report of a case. *J. Pediatr.* 25:400, 1944.
4. Dudrick, S. J., et al. Long-term total parenteral nutrition with growth, development, and positive nitrogen balance. *Surgery* 64:134, 1968.
5. Wilmore, D. W., and Dudrick, S. J. Growth and development of an infant receiving all nutrients by vein. *J.A.M.A.* 203:860, 1968.
6. Kaminski, M. V., Burke, W. A., and Blackburn, G. L. *Intravenous Hyperalimentation in Modern Hospital Practice.* Tuckahoe, N.Y.: USV Laboratories, 1977.
7. Michel, L., Serrano, A., and Malt, R. A. Nutritional support of hospitalized patients. *N. Engl. J. Med.* 304:1147, 1981.
8. Shils, M. E. Guidelines for parenteral nutrition. *J.A.M.A.* 220:1721, 1972.

9. Heird, W. C., and Winters, R. W.   Total parenteral nutrition: The state of the art. *J. Pediatr.* 86:2, 1975.

10. Parenteral nutrition. *Dairy Counc. Dig.* March/April 1979.

11. Elwyn, D. H.   Nutritional requirements of adult surgical patients. *Crit. Care Med.* 8:9, 1980.

12. Jeejeebhoy, K. N., et al.   Metabolic studies in total parenteral nutrition with lipid in man: Comparison with glucose. *J. Clin. Invest.* 57:125, 1976.

13. Meng, H. C.   Parenteral nutrition: Principles, nutrient requirements, and techniques. *Geriatrics* 30:97, 1975.

14. Dudrick, S. J., and Ruberg, R. L.   Principles and practice of parenteral nutrition. *Gastroenterology* 61:901, 1971.

15. Goodgame, J. T., Lowry, S. F., and Brennan, M. F.   Essential fatty acid deficiency in total parenteral nutrition: Time course of development and suggestions for therapy. *Surgery* 84:271, 1978.

16. McKenna, M. C., and Campagnoni, A. T.   Effect of pre- and postnatal essential fatty acid deficiency on brain development and myelination. *J. Nutr.* 109:1195, 1979.

Suggested Readings

Ausman, R. K.   A standardized approach to parenteral nutrition for the geriatric patient. *J. Am. Geriatr. Soc.* 29:172, 1981.

Blackburn, G. L., et al.   Protein sparing therapy during periods of starvation with sepsis or trauma. *Ann. Surg.* 177:588, 1973.

Borgen, L.   Total parenteral nutrition in adults. *Am. J. Nurs.* 78:224, 1978.

Candy, D. C. A.   Parenteral nutrition in paediatric practice: A review. *J. Hum. Nutr.* 34:287, 1980.

Chernoff, R.   Nutritional support: Formulas and delivery of enteral feeding. I. Enteral formulas. *J. Am. Diet. Assoc.* 79:426, 1981.

Dudrick, S. J., and Rhoads, J. E.   Total intravenous feeding. *Sci. Am.* 226:73, 1972.

Duke, J. H., et al.   Contribution of protein to caloric expenditure following injury. *Surgery* 68:168, 1970.

Fischer, J.   *Total Parenteral Nutrition.* Boston: Little, Brown, 1976.

Grant, J. P.   *Handbook of Total Parenteral Nutrition.* Philadelphia: Saunders, 1980. P. 197.

Grundfest, S., and Steiger, E.   Home parenteral nutrition. *J.A.M.A.* 244:1701, 1980.

Heird, W. C., and Winters, R. W.   Total intravenous alimentation. *Am. J. Dis. Child.* 126:287, 1973.

Johnston, I. D. A.   Parenteral nutrition in the cancer patient. *J. Hum. Nutr.* 33:189, 1979.

Kaminski, M. V.   Humanism in hyperalimentation. *J. Parent. Ent. Nutr.* 5:1, 1981.

Matol, J. R., and Jeffrey, L. P.   Formulation of a trace element solution for long-term parenteral nutrition. *Am. J. Hosp. Pharm.* 35:165, 1978.

McCamman, S., Beyer, P. L., and Rhoads, J. E.   A comparison of three defined formula diets in normal volunteers. *Am. J. Clin. Nutr.* 30:1655, 1977.

Phillips, G. D., and Garnys, V. P.   Trace element balance in adults receiving parenteral nutrition: Preliminary data. *J. Parent. Ent. Nutr.* 5:11, 1981.

Plumer, A.   *Principles and Practice of Intravenous Therapy* (3rd ed.). Boston: Little, Brown, 1982.

Rutten, P., et al.   Determination of optimal hyperalimentation infusion rate. *J. Surg. Res.* 18:477, 1975.

Sailer, D., and Muller, M.   Medium chain triglycerides in parenteral nutrition. *J. Parent. Ent. Nutr.* 5:115, 1981.

Weinsier, R. L., and Krumdieck, C. L.   Death resulting from overzealous total parenteral nutrition: The refeeding syndrome revisited. *Am. J. Clin. Nutr.* 34:393, 1981.

Chapter 36

PHYSIOLOGIC STRESS

Physiologic stress represents an abnormal state of hypermetabolism and negative nitrogen balance. It may be caused by infection, trauma, burn injury, or overwhelming illness. The metabolic adjustments that result from serious stress are hormonally mediated and are essential for survival.

This chapter will present the physiologic and metabolic adjustments to periods of acute stress, with special emphasis on burn injuries. Nutrition is discussed comparing prestress and poststress states.

General Considerations

HORMONAL ADJUSTMENTS

The hormonally mediated adjustments made by the body in response to severe physical stress are essential for survival. The major mediator of the metabolic response following injury or infection is the increase in adrenal gland activity, producing catecholamines (adrenalin, epinephrine, and norepinephrine) and glucocorticoids. This latter group affects the metabolism of protein and carbohydrate and augments the action of the catecholamines during stress.

Catecholamines are essential for maintaining body homeostasis. The release of catecholamines has also been termed the *fight or flight* response, since the metabolic changes it causes allow maximum physiologic response. This response is characterized by an increase in heart rate (tachycardia), alterations in skin and muscle blood flow, increased respiratory rate, sodium and water retention, and an outpouring of glucose and free fatty acids into the bloodstream. Catecholamines facilitate neuromuscular transmission due to their ability to increase the release of acetylcholine from nerve endings. At the time of an injury, there may be a delayed physiologic response to the hormonal discharge termed the *ebb phase*. If the individual survives the initial injury, there is an increase in metabolic reactions to provide for the inflammatory response and tissue repair (the *flow phase*).

The catecholamines affect cardiac function, circulation, and respiration. These hormones have a direct effect on the liver, increasing the conversion of glycogen to glucose and the conversion of the deaminated carbon skeletons of amino acids to glucose. They also cause the mobilization of muscle glycogen, converting it to lactic acid, which is then transported to the liver to be synthesized into glucose (the Cori cycle). The catecholamines suppress the release of insulin, which in turn favors the mobilization of free fatty acids. In addition, the release of glucagon is stimulated, further augmenting hepatic gluconeogenesis (see Chap. 35, for more detail).

METABOLIC RESPONSES

The metabolic responses to severe physical stress include hypermetabolism, negative nitrogen balance, and altered sources of energy. During the hypermetabolic phase of severe stress, an elevation in temperature and oxygen consumption occurs, which is related to the extent and severity of the insult. For each degree Celsius elevation, there is a 10 to 13 percent increase in metabolic demands [1]. Patients with mild infections may only have a 10 to 15 percent increase in metabolism; those with long-bone fractures, a 15 to 30 percent increase. Those with multiple injuries or more extensive infections may have metabolic rates 25 to 50 percent above normal. Patients with extensive trauma who require respirators have increased metabolic activity from 50 to 75 percent [2]. Severe burns produce the greatest elevation, accounting for as much as a twofold increase as a consequence of hypermetabolism. With resolution of the infection or when wound healing is achieved, the metabolic rate returns to normal.

PROTEIN LOSS

The most characteristic metabolic response after severe physical stress is negative nitrogen balance. An acceleration in protein catabolism is a metabolic consequence of injury. The amount of nitrogen lost is related to the previous nutritional state of the patient and the severity of the stress. There are also increased losses of sulfur, phosphorus, potassium, magnesium, zinc, and creatinine. The nitrogen lost does not arise from the site of the trauma or infection, but rather represents the proteolytic (protein breakdown) response of tissue proteins [3, 4]. Amino acids are broken down from the muscles and transferred to the liver where the deaminated carbon skeleton is converted to glucose. The nitrogen (the deaminated component of the amino acids) is utilized for nonessential amino acid synthesis or converted to urea and excreted in the urine. The rate of ureagenesis parallels that of gluconeogenesis.

The loss of nitrogen is related to the size of the injury or extent of the infection. It decreases with time and becomes positive with resolution of the stress. Nitrogen contributes 15 to 20 percent of the metabolic fuel oxidized during stress; fat makes up the remaining 80 to 85 percent [5]. This figure is increased by bed rest; it is decreased with muscular exercise, a decreased temperature, anesthesia, and poor nutritional intake.

A summary of the effects of stress on metabolism are given in Fig. 36-1.

ALTERATIONS IN BODY WEIGHT/MASS

After severe physical stress, such as serious trauma, infection, sepsis, or a burn injury, the body undergoes a series of metabolic changes. One of the most obvious and dramatic is the loss of body mass resulting from anorexia (loss of appetite), gastrointestinal dysfunction, hypermetabolism, and an increased loss of nitrogen. The loss of weight is directly related to the extent and severity of the stress, and may reach 30 percent or more. A loss of 10 percent of the normal body mass causes a rapid deterioration in maximal work performance. It is believed that the rate of loss affects performance more than the absolute amount lost. Weight losses of 40 to 50 percent of body mass are almost always fatal, representing a concurrent loss of between one-fourth to one-third of the body's protein mass.

Patients who experience extensive loss of weight often have low serum protein levels, resulting in poor wound healing, increased skin breakdown, diminished homeostatic responses to hemorrhage, decreased resistance to infection, and

FIG. 36-1. Effects of stress on metabolism.

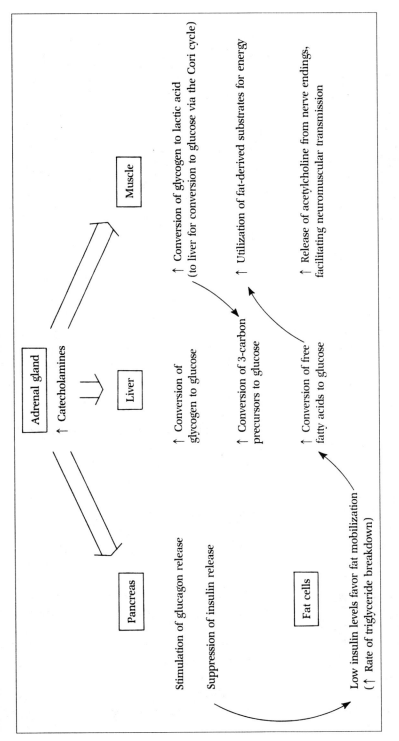

FIG. 36-2. Survival rates in burn injuries by age and area burned. Sigmoid curves showing survival of humans as function of total percent of body surface burned and age. Survival curves estimated by probit analysis for five different age categories. (From I. Flora, J. D. Feller, and R. Bawol, Baseline results of therapy for burned patients. *J.A.M.A.* 236:1943, 1976.)

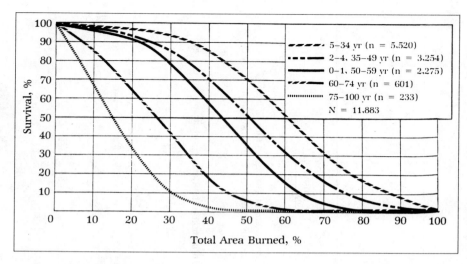

increased morbidity and mortality. There is a reversal of these pathologic states with improved nutritional status and positive nitrogen balance.

A loss of no more than 10 percent in body weight is usually tolerated in patients with severe physical stress who had previously normal body composition. In those with previously depleted body mass, nutritional therapy is more vigorous and initiated earlier.

Burns

A major burn injury presents the greatest known state of accelerated tissue breakdown, loss of body mass, and depletion of protein and energy reserves. The hypermetabolism, acute weight loss, and severe protein wasting that characterize the metabolic response all dramatically increase nutritional needs. Anorexia, loss of appetite, is a common consequence of a burn injury, compounding the problem of nutritional imbalance.

This section will present the major metabolic derangements that occur following a burn injury and the diet therapy utilized during treatment.

PHYSICAL ASSESSMENT

Before therapy is initiated, the burn injury should be evaluated for depth of the burn wound and percent of total body surface (TBS) involved. These two factors have the greatest influence on survival. Other factors that also affect survival include age, sex, complicating injuries, and past medical history (Fig. 36-2). Males generally have a higher survival rate than females.

The depth of the burn wound is classified as *partial-thickness* or *full-thickness*. Partial-thickness burn injuries include *first-degree*, involving only the epidermis; and *second-degree*, extending through the epidermis into the corium (Fig. 36-3). Full-thickness burns, also known as *third-degree*, are those in which all the dermal elements are destroyed and skin grafting is required.

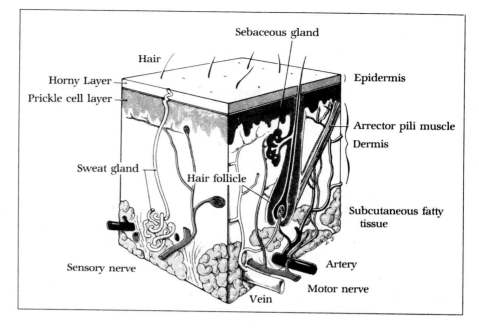

For second-degree and third-degree burns the area involved is estimated as the percentage of the TBS (total body surface) area. This can be roughly determined by using the "rule of nines" (Fig. 36-4 and Table 36-1).

PHYSIOLOGIC RESPONSE

In a burn injury, the increase in metabolic rate is directly related to the depth and severity of the insult, although it may be altered by the patient's age, sex, preburn nutritional status, medical history, and physical condition.

Weight loss and wasting of tissues are natural sequelae of moderate and severe burns due to the complications of the injury and the additional caloric demands imposed by the wound-healing process. Patients with greater than 40 percent TBS burn can lose more than 20 percent of their initial body weight if vigorous nutritional support is not instituted early enough [6].

The loss of the protective epithelium is one of the main causes for the increased caloric requirement with burns. With the destruction of epithelium, there is a resultant increase in water loss from the tissues through evaporation (hypo-osmolar fluid loss) [7]. The increased caloric requirement parallels the fluid loss; for every liter of fluid lost, 576 additional calories are utilized by the evaporation process [7]. A burn wound 1 square meter in size could result in the loss of 4 to 5 liters of fluid in 24 hours, and the utilization of 2300 to 2900 additional calories. The increased fluid loss from the wound site causes surface cooling, which may stimulate metabolic heat production to maintain body temperature. It is also thought that patients with severe burns have a higher internal temperature and that the increased evaporative water loss is a route for the release of heat produced by increased hormonal activity.

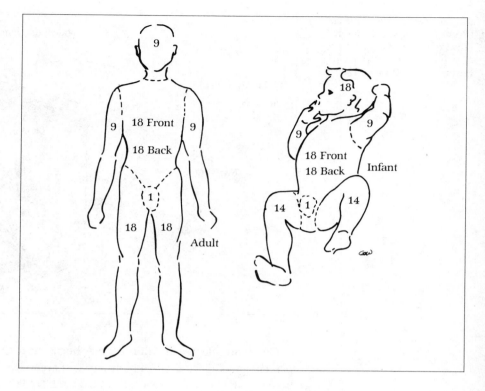

The wound healing process and epithelization and vascularization of an autograft also utilize additional calories. If complications develop, such as fever or infections, they add further to the caloric cost. Anorexia, the loss of appetite, is a common consequence following a burn injury, compounding the problem of increased caloric need. It has been postulated that the anorexia that accompanies infection, fever, burns, or other severe stress may actually be an adaptive mechanism for survival and, in a sense, may be starving out invading organisms [8, 9].

During the early postburn period, the loss of protein from the open wound accounts for as much as 20 to 25 percent of the total nitrogen lost from the body. These losses decrease with time and return to normal with closure of the burn wound.

TABLE 36-1. Rule of nines

Head and neck = 9%	9%
Each arm = 9% (× 2)	18%
Anterior trunk = 18%	18%
Posterior trunk = 18%	18%
Each leg = 18% (× 2)	36%
Perineum = 1%	1%
Total Body Surface (TBS)	100%

The body's requirement for albumin may become excessive if the burn injury is large and/or severe. It is lost through exudation at the wound and is also utilized in increased amounts for the healing process. Because of this, the liver's capacity to form albumin may not be able to keep pace with the body's demand for it. Low serum levels of albumin (hypoalbuminemia) cause a loss of the intravascular oncotic pressure and lead to sequestration of fluids and edema formation (seepage of fluid from the blood into the tissues). Fluid may seep into the lungs, causing a diminished diffusion of oxygen. Hypoalbuminemia may also cause sodium retention and potassium loss.

The serum albumin level should be maintained at greater than 2 gm%. If it drops below this level intravenous replacement therapy is indicated. It should be administered at a slow, steady rate of 1 to 2 gm/kg body weight/24 hours [7].

NUTRITIONAL MANAGEMENT

ENERGY

The following formula for determining the ideal caloric intake for adult burn patients takes into account both body size and the magnitude of the injury (percent of body surface burn) [10]:

$$\text{Ideal caloric intake} = [25 \times \text{weight (kg)}] + [40 \times \% \text{ TBS burn}]$$

This figure may need to be adjusted according to other variables influencing caloric requirements, including level of physical activity, preburn nutritional status, and the environment (i.e., temperature and humidity).

PROTEIN

The protein requirement is increased two- to fourfold over preburn levels. Adequate fat and carbohydrates must also be supplied so the protein can be used for tissue repair and not as an energy source. Under normal conditions, the average adult requires about 0.8 mg protein per kilogram body weight per day. With a major burn, that amount is increased to 1.6 to 3.2 gm/kg body weight/day [11]. This amount of protein represents between 12.2 and 24.5 percent of the total caloric intake.

VITAMINS AND MINERALS

The exact levels of vitamins needed for burn injuries have not yet been established but are assumed to be in proportion to the caloric intake. During the early postburn period, sodium restriction may be necessary since the total body sodium content increases greatly. The opposite is true of potassium, which is lost with the breakdown of tissue proteins and glycogen. Supplementation may be necessary.

FEEDING METHODS

During the initial postburn period, parenteral feeding may be necessary due to nausea and vomiting and/or a nonfunctioning gastrointestinal tract. The solution

TABLE 36-2. The effects of nutritional support on the metabolic responses to injury and infection

Metabolic response	Effects of nutrition
Hypermetabolism	Minimal effects with usual caloric loads
Negative nitrogen balance	Reduced, abolished, or reversed*
Hepatic gluconeogenesis	Reduced
Skeletal muscle proteolysis	Reduced
Weight loss	Reduced, abolished, or reversed*
Diminished membrane transport	Improved

*The effect is related to the quantity of the calories and nitrogen provided.
Source: Panel report on nutritional support of patients with trauma or infection. *American Journal of Clinical Nutrition* 34:1213, 1981.

should contain glucose and nitrogen and should be given via a central vein (see Chap. 35). Care should be taken to avoid infection and the other metabolic complications that can occur with this feeding technique. As the gastrointestinal tract begins to function, the diet can be advanced to clear fluids, then full fluids, and finally, a full diet. Intravenous feeding may be continued since it is difficult to meet the increased nutritional demands through oral feedings alone.

With adequate nutritional support, there is a reversal of the pathologic changes associated with stress. Table 36-2 summarizes those effects.

Case Studies

1. Karen is a 24-year-old, 130-lb (59.0-kg) female who has been hospitalized with third-degree burns over both arms. Use the rule of nines and calculate her ideal caloric intake. If her diet provided the maximum amount of protein, how many grams should she get per day?

2. Mrs. O'Sullivan is a 96-year-old grandmother who experienced second-degree burns over her legs when her great-granddaughter accidently spilled a pot of hot tea on her. Her diet has been advanced to full fluids. Utilizing your knowledge of geriatrics (see Chap. 27), what foods would you suggest to her when she is filling out her menu?

3. Based on your knowledge of fluids and electrolytes (see Chap. 10), what symptoms would you be watching for in the severely-burned patient (third-degree burns over more than 40 percent of the total body surface area)?

References

1. Dubois, E. T. *Fever and the Regulation of Body Temperature.* Springfield, Ill.: Thomas, 1948.
2. Panel report on nutritional support of patients with trauma or infection. *Am. J. Clin. Nutr.* 34:1213, 1981.
3. Aulick, L. H., and Wilmore, D. W. Increased peripheral amino acids release following burn injury. *Surgery* 85:560, 1979.

4. Long, C. L., et al.   Contribution of skeletal muscle protein in elevated rates of whole body protein catabolism in trauma patients. *Am. J. Clin. Nutr.* 34:1087, 1981.

5. Duke, J. H., Jr., et al.   Contribution of protein to caloric expenditure following injury. *Surgery* 68:168, 1970.

6. Artz, C. P., Moncrief, J. A., and Pruitt, B. A. (eds.).   *Burns: A Team Approach.* Philadelphia: Saunders, 1979. P. 453.

7. Abston, S.   Burns in children. *Clin. Symp.* 28:14, 1976.

8. Murray, M. J., and Murray, A. B.   Anorexia of infection as a mechanism of host defense. *Am. J. Clin. Nutr.* 32:593, 1979.

9. Murray, M. J., and Murray, A. B.   Starvation suppression and refeeding activation of infection: An ecological necessity? *Lancet* 1:123, 1977.

10. Curreri, P. W., et al.   Dietary requirements of patients with major burns. *J. Am. Diet. Assoc.* 65:415, 1974.

11. *Major Body Burns: Dietary Modifications in Disease.* Columbus, OH: Ross Labs, 1978. P. 9.

Suggested Readings

Atkins, E., and Bodel, P.   Fever. *N. Engl. J. Med.* 286:27, 1972.

Brodribb, A. J. M., and Ricketts, C. R.   The effect of zinc in the healing of burns. *Injury* 3:25, 1971.

Christopher, K. L.   The use of a model for hemodynamic balance to describe burn shock. *Nurs. Clin. North Am.* 15:617, 1980.

Curreri, P. W., and Luterman, A.   Nutritional support of the burned patient. *Surg. Clin. North Am.* 58:1151, 1978.

Holli, B. B., and Oakes, J. B.   Feeding the burned child. *J. Am. Diet. Assoc.* 67:240, 1975.

King, S. L., and Parham, E. S.   The diet-stress connection. *J. Home Econ.* 73:25, 1981.

Larkin, J. M., and Moylan, J. A.   Complete enteral support of terminally injured patients. *Am. J. Surg.* 131:722, 1976.

Liljedahl, S. O., and Birke, G.   The nutrition of patients with extensive burns. *Nutr. Metab.* 14 [Suppl.]:110, 1972.

Long, C. L.   Energy balance and carbohydrate metabolism in infection and sepsis. *Am. J. Clin. Nutr.* 30:1301, 1977.

Long, C. L., et al.   Whole body protein synthesis and catabolism in septic man. *Am. J. Clin. Nutr.* 30:1340, 1977.

Long, C. L., Kinney, J. M., and Geiger, J. W.   Nonsuppressibility of gluconeogenesis by glucose in septic man. *Metabolism* 25:193, 1976.

Pennisi, V. M.   Monitoring the nutritional care of burned patients. *J. Am. Diet. Assoc.* 69:531, 1976.

Pruitt, B. A., Jr.   Fluid and electrolyte replacement in the burned patient. *Surg. Clin. North Am.* 58:1291, 1978.

Shangraw, R. E., and Turnisky, J.   Local response of muscle to burns: Relationship of glycolysis and amino acid release. *J. Parent. Ent. Nutr.* 5:193, 1981.

Wilmore, D. W.   Carbohydrate metabolism in trauma. *Clin. Endocrin. Metab.* 5:731, 1976.

Wilmore, D. W.   Nutrition and metabolism following thermal injury. *Clin. Plast. Surg.* 1:603, 1974.

Wilmore, D. W., and Aulick, L. H.   Metabolic changes in burned patients. *Surg. Clin. North Am.* 58:1173, 1978.

Chapter 37

DRUGS, NUTRIENTS, AND NUTRITIONAL STATUS

During the past 20 years the therapeutic use of drugs has increased greatly, causing some nutritional side effects not previously encountered. As the type and variety of drugs prescribed continue to expand, it will become increasingly more important to anticipate and correct nutritional imbalances caused by their use.

The degree of interaction between food and drugs is dependent on the individual's state of health, nutritional status, age, sex, concomitant use of other medications, and drug dosage. Drugs may affect nutritional status by altering appetite, nutrient absorption, or nutrient metabolism. (See chapter appendix.) The converse is also true; nutritional status, specific nutrients, and other compounds present in foods can alter drug metabolism. In addition, certain foods, when used in sufficient quantity, may act as drugs.

This chapter will discuss the interaction between drugs and diet and the mechanisms behind the clinical manifestations. When specific drugs are discussed, both their generic (or chemical) name and trade names will be given (the latter in parentheses). When a drug is usually known by only one name, such as digitalis or phenobarbital, only that name will be used.

Absorption

The oral route is the most common mode of administration for most drugs; therefore, factors influencing absorption are most likely to occur within the gastrointestinal tract. The presence or absence of food in the gastrointestinal tract can cause changes in pH (acidity or alkalinity), gastric motility, and secretions. These effects can influence the degree of ionization, solubility, stability, gastric and intestinal transit time, and therefore the amount of drug absorbed.

DECREASED ABSORPTION

A drug may interfere with nutrient absorption by acting as a solution in which nutrients become dissolved. This is the case with mineral oil, which is used as a laxative. By creating a physical barrier at the mucosal surface, it impairs micelle formation and because the fat-soluble vitamins are soluble in mineral oil, it hampers their absorption. As a consequence, rickets and osteomalacia have been documented as the result of excessive intake of this drug.

The absorption of most drugs is diminished by the presence of food in the gastrointestinal tract. Of special note are the antibiotics, tetracycline (Achromycin or Sumyoin) and demeclocycline (Declomycin), whose absorption is particularly impaired when the individual drinks milk or eats dairy products. The calcium present in these foods combines with the antibiotics to form insoluble compounds (calcium chelates), which are not absorbed from the gastrointestinal tract. The simultaneous ingestion of high doses of iron salts, such as ferrous sulfate, has a similar effect in reducing absorption of these antibiotics. This is a two-way mechanism, resulting in malabsorption of calcium or iron and the antibiotic.

Certain drugs can interfere with the absorption of nutrients. Cholestyramine (Questran), a drug used to lower the plasma level of cholesterol, is a good example. As a nonabsorbable resin, cholestyramine indirectly lowers plasma cholesterol by binding bile acids and preventing their reabsorption and recycling in the enterohepatic circulation (see Chap. 11). With a decrease in the enterohepatic cycling of bile acids, there is an increased hepatic conversion of cholesterol to bile acids and a fall in the plasma level of cholesterol. While cholestyramine's binding action is desirable in hypercholesterolemia, the resin also interferes with the absorption of a variety of other drugs, including chlorothiazide (Diuril), phenobarbital, levothyroxine (Synthroid), anticoagulants, and digitalis, by the same mechanisms [1]. Cholestyramine also interferes with the absorption of fat, fat-soluble vitamins, and folic acid [2].

INCREASED ABSORPTION

The absorption of a few drugs is actually enhanced by the presence of food in the gastrointestinal tract. This may be due to the increased degree of dissolution of drug tablets by prolonged contact with the gastric contents and improved drug absorption brought about by the delay in gastric emptying [3]. The absorption of quinine is actually enhanced by antacids and calcium-rich foods, since these factors increase the percentage of the drug present in the nonionized and more absorbable form.

Changes in the pH of the gastrointestinal tract affect the rate of absorption of ionizable drugs. The absorption of medicinal iron can be enhanced by taking it with fruit or fruit juices that contain ascorbic acid. Vitamin C aids in the conversion of ferric iron (Fe^{3+}) to ferrous iron (Fe^{2+}). Both fructose (fruit sugar) and ascorbic acid form soluble complexes with iron, enhancing its absorption (see Chap. 7). The altered pH may adversely affect the metabolism of other drugs. Carbonated beverages and many fruit or vegetable juices can result in excessive acidity. As a result, certain drugs dissolve in the stomach (instead of the intestines) where they are more readily absorbed into the bloodstream.

Drugs whose side effects include slowing the rate of gastric emptying, such as codeine, morphine, atropine, and chloroquine, also decrease the rate of absorption of other drugs and nutrients.

Structural changes in the gastric mucosa and binding of bile acids required for fat absorption are side effects of the gut-sterilizing antibiotic, neomycin. The drug colchicine, used for the treatment of gout (painful deposits of uric acid in the joints), alters the mucosal transport system and, therefore, impairs nutrient absorption. Such drugs as colchicine, neomycin, and the oral antidiabetic agents can impair the absorption of vitamin B_{12}. Table 37-1 summarizes the primary intestinal absorption defects induced by drugs.

Taste and Appetite

Appetite is a vital function for the survival of a species and is controlled by a variety of oral, gastric, intestinal, and hormonal processes (see Chaps. 11 and 29). The influence of a drug on taste or appetite can be its primary (desirable) action

TABLE 37-1. Primary intestinal absorption defects induced by drugs

Drug	Usage	Malabsorption or fecal nutrient loss	Mechanism
Mineral oil	Laxative	Carotene, vitamins A, D, and K	Physical barrier Nutrients dissolve in mineral oil and are lost Decreased micelle formation
Phenolphthalein	Laxative	Vitamin D, calcium	Potassium depletion Loss of structural integrity
Neomycin	Antibiotic to "sterilize" gut	Fat, nitrogen, sodium, potassium, calcium, iron, lactose, sucrose, vitamin B_{12}	Structural defect Decreased pancreatic lipase Binding of bile acids
Cholestyramine	Hypocholesterolemic agent Bile acid sequestrant	Fat, iron, vitamins A, K, B_{12}, and D	Binding of bile acids and nutrients
Potassium chloride	Potassium repletion	Vitamin B_{12}	Decreased ileal pH
Colchicine	Anti-inflammatory agent in gout	Fat, carotene, sodium, potassium, lactose, vitamin B_{12}	Mitotic arrest Structural defect Enzyme damage
Biguanides Metformin Phenformin	Hypoglycemic agents	Vitamin B_{12}	Competitive inhibition of vitamin B_{12} absorption
Para-amino salicylic acid	Antituberculosis agent	Fat, folate, vitamin B_{12}	Mucosal block in folate uptake
Sulfasalazine (Azulfidine)	Anti-inflammatory agent in ulcerative colitis and regional enteritis	Folate	Mucosal block in folate uptake

Source: D. A. Roe, *Drug-Induced Nutritional Deficiencies.* Westport, Conn.: AVI Publications, 1976. P. 130.

or its secondary (undesirable) action or side effect. Drugs whose primary action is to suppress appetite are termed *anorectics;* those which stimulate it are *orectics.* The anorectic and orectic groups of drugs exert their respective actions by influencing the neural regulation of food intake. The anorectic drugs act on the ventromedial hypothalamus (the "satiety center" of the brain) whereas the orectic drugs exert their action on the lateral hypothalamus (the "feeding center" of the brain). These drugs stimulate or suppress the appetite by altering the chemical environment of the hypothalamus.

The secondary action of tranquilizers, antidepressants, steroids, and oral contraceptives has been reported to be an increase in appetite.

Drugs whose side effects include nausea and vomiting often cause a decrease in appetite and food intake. Drugs in this category include cancer chemotherapeutic agents, digitalis, anticonvulsants, and an excess of alcohol, sedatives, and tranquilizers.

Cancer chemotherapeutic agents cause a loss of appetite and resultant decrease in food intake due to systemic effects of the drug. These effects include alterations in sense of taste, soreness of the mouth and throat, abdominal pain or diarrhea after eating, and general malaise. An aversion to food is common, particularly to meat (see Chap. 44, Neoplastic Diseases).

Digitalis, the heart medication used to increase the force of contraction, can also cause a loss of appetite when high dosages are taken over long periods of time.

Tranquilizers, such as diazepam (Valium), chlordiazepoxide HCl (Librium), and chlorpromazine (Thorazine), can have a variable effect on appetite, depending on the circumstances under which they are taken. When given to agitated, psychotic patients, the effect is an increase in food intake due to the decreased level of agitation. These drugs can have the opposite effect when given to the elderly patient, causing a decreased level of consciousness and a reduction in food intake.

When amphetamines are used in the management of hyperactive children, growth retardation may occur due to decreased appetite, resulting in diminished food intake.

Some drugs, such as griseofulvin (Grifulvin), penicillamine, thiamazole, and lincomycin (Lincocin), have been reported to decrease taste acuity (as a side effect) by complexing with zinc or copper [4].

Drugs and drug groups that affect food intake are summarized in Table 37-2.

Drug-Induced Nutrient Imbalances
ORAL DIURETICS

Diuretics are a group of drugs that increase the production of urine by enhancing the urinary excretion of sodium and water. This is accomplished by decreasing sodium reabsorption in the renal tubules. There are basically three groups of diuretics—thiazides or benzothiadiazides, potassium-sparing diuretics, and loop diuretics. The thiazides are the most frequently prescribed and act by decreasing the reabsorption of sodium in the loop of Henle and parts of the distal tubule, as well as increasing the urinary excretion of chloride, potassium, and bicarbonate ions. Some of the potential side effects and toxic manifestations of these drugs, which include chlorothiazide (Diuril), hydrochlorothiazide (Esidrix), chlorthalidone (Hygroton), and methyclothiazide (Enduron), are nausea, vomiting, and diarrhea; hypokalemia due to excessive potassium loss; metabolic alkalosis due to excessive chloride loss; hyponatremia; hyperuricemia; and hyperglycemia.

The potassium-sparing diuretics, which include spironolactone (Aldactone) and triamterene (Dyrenium), act on the distal portions of the nephron by blocking the sodium-retaining properties of aldosterone. These diuretics remove sodium and water without causing an excessive loss of potassium. Potential side effects of this group of diuretics include hyperkalemia, hyponatremia, megaloblastic anemia, hyperglycemia, and gastrointestinal irritation.

The loop diuretics include furosemide (Lasix) and ethacrynic acid (Edecrin).

TABLE 37-2. Drugs and drug groups that affect food intake

DRUGS THAT REDUCE FOOD INTAKE
    Intentional appetite-reducing drugs
        Amphetamines
        Methylphenidate
        Mazindol
        Bulk agents
    Drugs that produce adverse responses to food
        Digitalis and related alkaloids
        Cancer chemotherapeutic agents
        Anticonvulsants
        Alcohol (excess)
        Sedatives and tranquilizers (excess)

DRUGS THAT INCREASE FOOD INTAKE
    Intentional appetite-stimulating drugs
        Cyproheptadine
        Alcohol (small amount)
    Drugs with side effects of increasing appetite
        Corticosteroids
        Oral hypoglycemic agents
        Insulin
        Psychotropic agents
          Phenothiazines
          Benzodiazepines

Source: D. A. Roe, *Clinical Nutrition for the Health Scientist*. Boca Raton, Fla.: CRC Press, 1979. P. 91.

They block the active transport of chloride in Henle's loop and therefore interfere with the passive reabsorption of sodium. The possible side effects from this group of diuretics include hypokalemia, hyperglycemia, metabolic alkalosis, hyponatremia, hyperuricemia, blood abnormalities, and gastrointestinal irritation. The frequent side effects of diuretic therapy are given in Table 37-3.

ANTICONVULSANTS

The long-term use of anticonvulsants, including phenobarbital, diphenylhydantoin (Dilantin), and primidone (Mysoline), can cause deficiencies of folic acid and vitamins D and K. The precise mechanism involved is not clear, but it is thought that these drugs cause an increased rate of metabolism of these vitamins,

TABLE 37-3. Frequent side effects of diuretic therapy

Side effect	Thiazides	Loop	Potassium-sparing
Hypokalemia	Yes	Yes	No
Hyperkalemia	No	No	Yes
Hyponatremia	Yes	Yes	No
Hyperuricemia	Yes	Yes	No
Hyperglycemia	Yes	Yes	Yes
Low blood pressure	Yes	Yes	Yes

Source: G. Kemp and D. Kemp, Diuretics, *American Journal of Nursing* 78:1006, 1978.

as well as decreased absorption. Malformations in the infants of women who received Dilantin during pregnancy may be caused by drug-induced fetal malnutrition or vitamin deficiencies, or by direct toxic effects of the drug on the fetus.

ORAL CONTRACEPTIVES

The use of oral contraceptives alters certain aspects of metabolism, which in turn affects requirements and blood levels of several nutrients. The vitamins most commonly depleted include riboflavin, folic acid, B_6, and C. Clinical evidence of deficiency is rare. However, blood levels of other nutrients such as vitamin A, iron, and copper are actually increased by the use of contraceptive steroids [5]. The niacin requirement may be reduced in oral contraceptive users since this drug enhances the metabolic pathway by which tryptophan forms niacin.

Due to a decrease in menstrual blood flow, women on oral contraceptives are less likely to develop iron-deficiency anemia.

ALCOHOL

Alcohol not only causes a variety of interactions with drugs but also a unique form of malnutrition. In combination with antidepressants, tranquilizers, and antihistamines, alcohol causes excessive drowsiness, which can be particularly hazardous when operating machinery or driving a car. Alcohol also interacts with anticoagulants; antidiabetic agents, including insulin; sedatives; MAO inhibitors; and high blood pressure medications. Severe alcohol liver dysfunction can alter all hepatically metabolic drugs. Low *zinc* and *magnesium* levels are present in alcoholics, secondary to enhanced urinary losses and poor dietary intake.

Mineral Imbalances

The use of oral diuretics, alone or in combination with digitalis glycosides, can lead to increased urinary losses of magnesium and zinc, resulting in a deficiency of these elements if the losses are prolonged or severe. Oral diuretics also increase the urinary losses of *calcium*. Drug-induced *vitamin D* deficiency may be caused by anticonvulsants (diphenylhydantoin [Dilantin] and phenobarbital) and the sedative glutethimide (Doriden), resulting in *calcium* malabsorption.

Phosphate malabsorption and resultant depletion may be caused by antacids containing magnesium and aluminum hydroxides. The antacids bind phosphates in the gut; they are later excreted in the feces as magnesium and aluminum salts. With severe depletion, osteomalacia may result. In patients with renal disease, the phosphate-binding properties of certain antacids are actually beneficial, since excess phosphates cannot be eliminated by the diseased kidneys [6].

Hypokalemia (low serum potassium) may result from the excessive intake of *glycyrrhizic acid*, a substance found in some brands of licorice and certain types of chewing tobacco. Various other drugs that potentiate the potassium-depleting effects of licorice include para-aminosalicylic acid (PAS), used in the treatment of tuberculosis; oral diuretics, particularly thiazide diuretics; and alcohol. Glycyrrhizic acid may also cause an elevation in blood pressure. The excessive use of laxatives or cathartics may also cause potassium deficiency by excessive loss via the intestine.

Oral diuretics, particularly of the thiazide group, can also lead to potassium depletion. This risk is greatest in patients with a poor intake of potassium-rich foods or in those with an increased potassium excretion due to alcohol abuse or alcoholic cirrhosis [7]. Corticosteroids are another group of drugs that may also produce potassium depletion as well as increased urinary excretion of calcium.

Vitamin Imbalances

Folic acid is an essential vitamin needed for normal cell division and protein synthesis. Methotrexate (Amethopterin), a cancer chemotherapeutic agent, is a *folic acid antagonist*, which acts by inhibiting cell division in rapidly dividing normal tissue and in malignant cells. The tissues most affected include the gastrointestinal mucosa and the bone marrow. Methotrexate binds to the dihydrofolate reductase enzyme, which is required for the conversion of folate to its active enzyme form.

The *fluorinated pyrimidines*, such as fluorouracil (5-fluorouracil) and dactinomycin (Actinomycin-D), also produce changes in the bone marrow and gastrointestinal tract. Megaloblastic anemia is a common consequence of treatment with these agents.

Other drugs that exert an antifolate effect include the diuretics triamterene (Dyrenium), and pyrimethamine (Daraprim) used in treating malaria. Isoniazid (INH), used to treat tuberculosis, causes a deficiency of vitamin B_6.

Vitamin B_{12} absorption and metabolism may also be affected by a variety of drugs. Methotrexate (Amethopterin) can cause mucosal atrophy and impaired vitamin B_{12} absorption secondary to folate deficiency. Cholestyramine (Questran), used to bind bile acids, may also bind intrinsic factor and cause vitamin B_{12} deficiency. Several drugs cause an alteration in the gastrointestinal mucosa including colchicine, para-aminosalicylic acid (Para-aminosalicylic acid), and high intakes of alcohol. Treatment with slow-release potassium chloride may also cause vitamin B_{12} deficiency and megaloblastic anemia due to excessive acidification of the ileum.

Table 37-4 summarizes drug-induced vitamin imbalances.

Food-Related Drug Reactions

Specific chemical compounds present in or added to certain foods can react with different drugs to alter their efficacy. These reactions may range from mild to serious; they may also be fatal at times.

FOOD ADDITIVES

EDTA, the commonly used abbreviation for *ethylenediamine tetraacetic acid*, is an efficient food additive. The structure of this molecule is such that it traps positively charged metal ions, such as aluminum, nickel, zinc, copper, iron, and manganese, within its negatively charged interior. This is useful since foods become contaminated with trace amounts of these metals during processing,

TABLE 37-4. Drug-vitamin interactions

Drugs	Vitamins	Possible mechanisms	Possible manifestation
Anticonvulsants	Folacin	Decreased absorption Competitive inhibition of vitamin coenzymes Enzyme induction	Megaloblastic anemia
	Vitamin D	Enzyme induction	Rickets, osteomalacia
	Vitamin K	Enzyme induction	Neonatal hemorrhage
Cholestyramine	Folacin	Complexation of the vitamin	
	Vitamin B_{12}	Inhibition of intrinsic factor function	
	Vitamin A		
	Vitamin D	Binding of bile salts	
	Vitamin K		
Colchicine	Vitamin B_{12}	Absorptive enzyme damage Damage to the intestinal wall	
Coumarin anti-coagulants	Vitamin K	Unknown	Hemorrhage
Estrogen containing oral contraceptives	Folacin	Inhibition of absorptive enzymes Increased synthesis of folate-binding macroglobulin Enzyme induction	Megaloblastic anemia
	Vitamin B_{12}	Changes in tissue oxygenase distribution	
	Vitamin B_6	Induction of tryptophan enzyme Competition for vitamin-binding sites on apoenzyme	Depression
	Riboflavin	Unknown	
	Thiamin	Unknown	
	Vitamin C	Decreased absorption Increased ceruloplasmin concentration Increased concentration of reducing compounds Changes in tissue distribution	
Glutethimide	Vitamin D	Enzyme induction	Osteomalacia
Hydralazine	Vitamin B_6	Increased excretion of vitamin-drug complex	Peripheral neuropathy
Irritant cathartics	Vitamin D	Increased peristalsis Damage to the intestinal wall	Osteomalacia
Isoniazid	Vitamin B_6	Increased excretion of vitamin-drug complex	Peripheral neuropathy Generalized convulsion (infants) Anemia
	Niacin	Competitive inhibition of vitamin coenzymes Secondary to vitamin B_6 deficiency	Pellagra
Methotrexate	Folate	Inhibition of dihydrofolate reductase enzyme	Megaloblastic anemia
Mineral oil	Vitamin A		
	Vitamin D	Lipid solvent	Rickets
	Vitamin K		
Neomycin	Vitamin B_{12}	Damage to the intestinal wall Inhibition of intrinsic factor function	
	Vitamin A	Damage to the intestinal wall Inhibition of pancreatic lipase Binding of bile salts	
Para-aminosalicylic acid	Vitamin B_{12}	Decreased absorption	Megaloblastic anemia

TABLE 37-4 (CONTINUED)

Drugs	Vitamins	Possible mechanisms	Possible manifestation
Penicillamine	Vitamin B_6	Increased excretion of vitamin-drug complex	Peripheral neuropathy
Potassium chloride	Vitamin B_{12}	Decreased ileal pH	
Pyrimethamine	Folacin	Inhibition of dihydrofolate reductase enzyme	Megaloblastic anemia
Salicylates	Folacin	Decreased protein binding	
	Vitamin C	Decreased uptake in thrombocytes and leukocytes	
	Vitamin K	Unknown	
Sulfasalazine	Folacin	Decreased absorption	
Tetracycline	Vitamin C	Increased excretion	
Triamterene	Folacin	Inhibition of dihydrofolate reductase enzyme	Megaloblastic anemia
Trimethoprim	Folacin	Inhibition of dihydrofolate reductase enzyme	Megaloblastic anemia

Source: L. Ovesen, Drugs and vitamin deficiency. *Drugs* 18:278, 1979.

impairing the taste, odor, and appearance of food, as well as causing a health hazard. EDTA is used in mayonnaise and salad dressings to prevent oxidation of the oil component and resultant rancidity. It prevents the metal-catalyzed browning of processed fruits and vegetables and the oxidation of vitamin C in fruit juices. In beer, EDTA is used to trap trace amounts of iron and copper. It is also used to trap trace metals present in canned shellfish and in soft drinks to prevent artificial colors from fading.

In some individuals who have developed a sensitivity to this compound by previous exposure to cosmetics, deodorizers, detergents, liquid soaps, and industrial chemicals, the ingestion of foods containing EDTA can cause dermatitis (inflammation of the skin), usually of the face [8].

Salicylate is a naturally occurring substance in some fruits, such as plums. Also used as a flavoring, methyl salicylate is marketed under the name oil of wintergreen or teaberry. Salicylate is used in a wide variety of foods, such as gums; mints; jelly beans; root beer; apple, blueberry, and cherry turnovers; breakfast squares; and refrigerated cinnamon-sugar cookies [8]. In individuals who are allergic to aspirin (acetylsalicylic acid), the consumption of foods containing salicylates may cause the same reaction, usually urticaria (hives).

Tartrazine is another substance found in a variety of foods, including many breakfast cereals, various yellow and green candies, Coca-Cola, and other beverages. It is still used as a dye in many antibiotic and vitamin preparations. Like salicylates, tartrazine can lead to the development of urticaria in sensitized individuals, with the severity of the reaction being dependent on the degree of hypersensitivity and the amount ingested.

Other small-molecular-weight allergens occurring in foods include quinine, penicillin, and oleo resin. *Quinine*, in the form of quinine sulfate (the drug), in tonic water, Campari, quinine water, bitter lemon, and as a flavoring agent

TABLE 37-5. Food sources of tyramine and dopamine

DAIRY PRODUCTS	VEGETABLES
Sharp or aged cheeses	Avocado
Yogurt	Broad beans
Sour cream	Soy sauce
FISH	**FRUIT**
Salted, dried fish	Bananas
Pickled herring	Figs
	Raisins
MEAT	**BEVERAGES**
Meat extracts	Ale and beer
Beef liver	Chianti and sherry wines
Chicken liver	Cola beverages
Salami	Coffee
Pepperoni	Chocolate
Yeast	

in various gums and candies can cause purpura (hemorrhages in the skin) in susceptible individuals. Although current laws forbid the sale of milk from cows being treated for mastitis with penicillin, it would still be possible for an individual with a penicillin allergy to obtain milk from a farmer using this drug on his cattle. *Oleo resin* may be found on raw cashew nuts sold in health food stores or used in vegetarian restaurants. This substance causes a reaction similar to that of poison ivy in individuals sensitive to it.

Monamine Oxidase Inhibitors

One of the most serious and potentially lethal drug-nutrient interactions known is between the monamine oxidase inhibitor drugs and foods containing tyramine and dopamine. Monamine oxidase inhibitor (MAO) drugs include procarbazine (Matulane), used in the treatment of Hodgkin's disease (a type of cancer), and the antidepressants iproniazid, isocarboxazid (Marplan), nialamide, phenelzine (Nardil), and tranylcypromine (Parnate). These drugs block the oxidative deamination of endogenous and exogenous amines, including tyramine and dopamine, causing nausea, vomiting, headaches, and palpitations. Severe hypertensive attacks have also been known to occur, resulting in death from cerebral hemorrhage. The buildup of nonmetabolized tyramine or dopamine causes the release of the catecholamine norepinephrine from nerve endings and the resultant side effects. The degree of hypertension and the severity of the attack varies with the drug dosage and the amount of tyramine- or dopamine-containing food consumed. Common food sources of these amines include Chianti wine, aged cheese, chicken livers, pickled herring, broad beans, beer, and yeast or yeast extract. A complete list is given in Table 37-5.

Acetaldehyde Reactions

Tetraethylthiuram disulfide, also known as Antabuse or Disulfiram, is used to treat alcoholism. If alcohol is consumed while an individual is taking this drug, nausea and vomiting, a fall in blood pressure, chest pain, and a throbbing headache will occur within 5 to 15 minutes. Various other symptoms are also known to develop, all of which are related to the amount of alcohol consumed and the dosage of the drug.

These symptoms are due to the inhibition of the enzyme, aldehyde dehydrogenase, and the resultant increase in blood levels of acetaldehyde. Individuals taking tetraethylthiuram disulfide will experience this acetaldehyde reaction not only when they consume even small quantities of alcohol, but also when food containing liquor, beer, or wine is eaten, or when medications containing alcohol, such as Geritol or Nyquil, are used.

Other drugs that may produce acetaldehyde-type reactions when alcohol is taken include metronidazole (Flagyl) (used for the treatment of vaginal *Trichomonas* infections), oral antidiabetic agents of the sulfonylurea group, chloramphenicol (Chloromycetin) (an antibiotic), and tetrachloroethylene (used for the treatment of hookworm).

The intake of alcohol may have an adverse effect on diabetics taking oral antidiabetic drugs such as tolbutamide and other sulfonylurea agents. The drug-nutrient reaction in these individuals produces hypoglycemia (low blood sugar), characterized by faintness, depression, irrational behavior, and even coma.

Drug Metabolism and Nutritional Status

It has been demonstrated that changes in diet and nutritional status can alter drug metabolism. For example, individuals consuming a high-protein–low-carbohydrate diet metabolize the drugs antipyrine and theophylline (Aminophylline) faster than those on a low-protein–high-carbohydrate diet [9]. Compounds present in certain foods, such as indolic compounds present in cabbage and brussels sprouts, can also speed up drug metabolism [10]. Soybeans, rutabagas, turnips, kale, cabbage, and brussels sprouts contain substances known as goitrogens, which inhibit the production of thyroid hormone and therefore can produce goiter. Individuals taking thyroid medication should limit their intake of these foods. Changes in the microflora of the gastrointestinal tract, caused by alterations in the dietary content of fiber or animal protein, for example, can also influence the rate of drug metabolism. In individuals suffering from protein-calorie malnutrition, toxic levels of many drugs are reached sooner.

Smoking has recently been implicated as causing adverse interactions with many drugs. The 1979 Surgeon General's Smoking and Health Report states that smoking may result in increased risks with drug use, affect an individual's response to certain diagnostic tests, and interact with certain food constituents [11]. Because of this, smokers may have to take larger dosages of some drugs than nonsmokers. Among the drugs affected are theophylline (Aminophylline) (used for asthma), propoxyphene HCl (Darvon), and pentazocine HCl (Talwin) (analgesics), imipramine (Tofranil, Antipress) (an antidepressant), glutethimide (Doriden) (a sedative), furosemide (Lasix) (a diuretic), and propranolol (Inderal) (a heart medication).

FIG. 37-1. Herbal medicine garden in rural China. (FAO photo by F. Botts.)

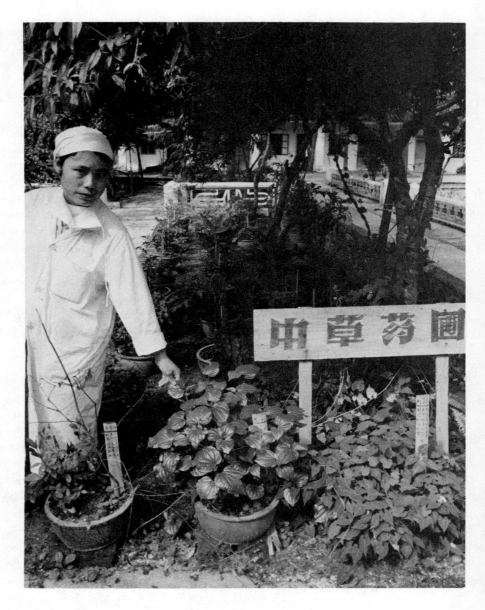

The Use of Foods as Drugs

Many foods of plant or animal origin have been used as drugs to treat a variety of illnesses for thousands of years [19]. For example, the Chinese have used rhubarb as a cathartic for over 5000 years; it is an ingredient found in many laxatives today. Ephedrine, obtained from a species of Ephedra, has been used to relieve asthma and hay fever for nearly 2700 years. The juice of the aloe plant has been used to treat burns for at least 2300 years; it is used today as an ingredient in ointments for the same purpose. The Rauwolfia root was used in India over

2000 years ago to treat such diseases as cholera, epilepsy, and insanity. From the active ingredients in this plant, the first modern tranquilizer and antihypertensive, reserpine, was produced. The foxglove plant has been used as a heart stimulant for about 1000 years; today its active ingredient, digitalis, is one of the most commonly prescribed heart medications. The bitter juice of the white willow tree has been used to relieve pain since the first century A.D.; its active ingredient, salicylic acid, or aspirin, is the most widely prescribed analgesic today. Quinine, still used today to treat malaria, was originally made from the bark of *Cinchona*, a flowering evergreen found on the slopes of the Andes (Fig. 37-1).

Poisons used by ancient civilizations in Africa and South America have also been put to therapeutic use by modern medicine. Strophanthin, used as an arrow poison by the natives of southeast Africa, has been found to be an effective, fast-acting heart remedy when used in very small doses. Curare, an arrow poison used by the South American Indians, causes muscle paralysis and death by asphyxiation. As a modern drug, curare is used as a muscle relaxant for patients undergoing surgery and those put on respirators.

Ergot, a fungus that infests rye and other grains, constricts the blood vessels and causes gangrene of the extremities. For centuries, midwives have used ergot preparations to control bleeding during childbirth. A derivative, ergotrate, is still used today to prevent and control postpartum hemorrhage. Several foods, when eaten in sufficient quantity, have been shown to inhibit platelet aggregation, or blood clots. Among them are onions, garlic, ginger, mackerel, salmon, and Black tree fungus [12–18]. This last food has long been used as a folk medicine to prevent postpartum thrombophlebitis and to promote longevity.

Conclusions

Interactions between foods and drugs can range from mild to severe to fatal. The cause-and-effect relationship is not always evident and may be masked by the use of several drugs or compounding factors. As the use of drugs expands, the possibilities of diet-drug interactions increase. Foods may exert pharmacologic actions when used in the correct amounts and should be considered when evaluating an unexpected side effect.

References

1. Levine, R. R. *Pharmacology: Drug Actions and Reactions* (3rd ed.). Boston: Little, Brown, 1983. P. 298.
2. Roe, D. A. Effects of drugs on nutrition. *Life Sci.* 15:1219, 1974.
3. Roe, D. A. *Clinical Nutrition for the Health Scientist.* Boca Raton, Fla.: CRC Press, 1979. P. 89.
4. Hanlon, D. P. Interaction of thiamazole with zinc and copper. *Lancet* 1:929, 1975.
5. Crews, M. G., Taper, L. J., and Ritchey, S. J. Effects of oral contraceptive agents on copper and zinc balance in young women. *Am. J. Clin. Nutr.* 33:1940, 1980.
6. Luke, B. Renal Disease. In B. Luke, *Case Studies in Therapeutic Nutrition*, Boston: Little, Brown, 1977. Pp. 3–22.

7. Hansten, P. D. *Drug Interactions* (2nd ed.). Philadelphia: Lea & Febiger, 1973. P. 357.

8. Roe, D. A. *Clinical Nutrition for the Health Scientist.* Boca Raton, Fla.: CRC Press, 1979. P. 85.

9. Kappas, A., et al. Influence of dietary protein and carbohydrate on antipyrine and theophylline metabolism in man. *Clin. Pharm. Ther.* 20:643, 1976.

10. Roe, D. A. *Clinical Nutrition for the Health Scientist.* Boca Raton, Fla.: CRC Press, 1979. P. 97.

11. Drug effects can go up in smoke. *FDA Consumer* March, 1979.

12. Baghurst, K. I., Raj, M. J., and Truswell, A. S. Onions and platelet aggregation. *Lancet* 1:101, 1977.

13. Phillips, C., and Poyser, N. L. Inhibition of platelet aggregation by onion extracts. *Lancet* 1:1051, 1978.

14. Makheja, A. N., Vanderhoek, J. Y., and Bailey, J. M. Inhibition of platelet aggregation and thromboxane synthesis by onion and garlic. *Lancet* 1:781, 1979.

15. Hammerschmidt, D. E. Szechwan purpura. *N. Engl. J. Med.* 302:1191, 1980.

16. Dorso, C. R., et al. Chinese food and platelets. (Letters to the editor.) *N. Engl. J. Med.* 303:756, 1980.

17. Siess, W., et al. Platelet-membrane fatty acids, platelet aggregation, and thromboxane formation during a mackerel diet. *Lancet* 1:441, 1980.

18. Goodnight, S. H., Harris, W. S., and Connor, W. E. The effect of W-3 fatty acids on platelet composition and function in man. *Clin. Res.* 23:312A, 1980.

19. DeVore, R. T. Our medical debt to the distant past. *FDA Consumer* 11:12, 1978.

Suggested Readings

Aftergood, L., and Alfin-Slater, R. B. Oral Contraceptives and Nutrient Requirements. In R. B. Alfin-Slater and D. Kritchevsky (eds.), *Nutrition and the Adult.* New York: Plenum Press, 1980. Pp. 367–395.

Barn, T. K. Interaction of drugs and nutrition. *J. Hum. Nutr.* 31:449, 1977.

Becking, G. C. Trace elements and drug metabolism. *Med. Clin. North Am.* 60:813, 1976.

Borgstedt, A. D., et al. Long-term administration of anti-epileptic drugs and the development of rickets. *J. Pediatr.* 81:9, 1972.

Campbell, T. C., and Hayes, J. R. Role of nutrition in drug-metabolizing enzyme system. *Pharmacol. Rev.* 26:171, 1974.

Clark, F. Drugs and vitamin deficiency. *J. Hum. Nutr.* 30:333, 1976.

Effect of drugs on food intake and nutrient absorption. *Nutr. M.D.* June 1981.

Faloon, W. W. (ed.). Symposium: Drug-nutrient relationships. *Am. J. Clin. Nutr.* 26:103, 1973.

Govoni, L. E., and Hayes, J. E. *Drugs and Nursing Implications* (4th ed.). New York: Appleton-Century-Crofts, 1982.

Halsted, C. H. Alcoholism and malnutrition. *Am. J. Clin. Nutr.* 33:2705, 1980.

Halsted, C. H. Folate deficiency in alcoholism. *Am. J. Clin. Nutr.* 33:2736, 1980.

Hartshorn, E. A. Food and drug interactions. *J. Am. Diet. Assoc.* 70:15, 1977.

Hathcock, J. N., and Coon, J. (eds.). *Nutrition and Drug Interrelations.* New York: Academic, 1978.

Hethcox, J. M., and Stanaszek, W. F. Interactions of drugs and diet. *Hosp. Pharm.* 9:373, 1974.

Kark, R. M. Medicinal Uses of Foods. In J. N. Hathcock and J. Coon (eds.), *Nutrition and Drug Interrelations.* New York: Academic Press, 1978. Pp. 821–835.

Lambert, M. L., Jr. Drug and diet interactions. *Am. J. Nurs.* 75:402, 1975.

Lehmann, P. Food and drug interactions. *FDA Consumer* March, 1978.

Lindenbaum, J., and Roman, M. J. Nutritional anemia in alcoholism. *Am. J. Clin. Nutr.* 33:2727, 1980.

Luke, B. Think "nutrition" if she's on the Pill. *RN* March, 1976. Pp. 33–37.

March, D. C. *Handbook: Interactions of Selected Drugs with Nutritional Status in Man.* Chicago: The American Dietetic Association, 1976.

Mezey, E. Alcoholic liver disease: Roles of alcohol and malnutrition. *Am. J. Clin. Nutr.* 33:2709, 1980.

Miller, O. N. (Chairman). Symposium on Nutrition and Drug Metabolism. *Fed. Proc. Fed. Am. Soc. Exp. Biol.* 35:2459, 1976.

Mueller, J. F. Drug-induced Interrelationships. In R. B. Alfin-Slater and D. Kritchevsky (eds.), *Nutrition and the Adult.* New York: Plenum Press, 1980. Pp. 351–365.

Ovesen, L. Drugs and vitamin deficiency. *Drugs* 18:278, 1979.

Revolutionary Health Committee of Hunan Province. *A Barefoot Doctor's Manual.* Seattle: Cloudburst Press, 1977.

Roe, D. A. *Drug-induced Nutritional Deficiencies.* Westport, Conn.: AVI Publications, 1976.

Spiller, G. A. (ed.). *Nutritional Pharmacology* (vol. 4). *Current Topics in Nutrition and Disease.* New York: Alan R. Liss, 1981.

Appendix

DRUGS MENTIONED IN CHAPTER 37

Chloramphenicol (Chloromycetin) This broad-spectrum antibiotic acts on a variety of gram-negative and gram-positive bacteria by interfering with protein synthesis within the bacteria. It also interferes with red blood cell maturation and may therefore cause a decreased response to folic acid, iron, and vitamin B_{12}.

Chlordiazepoxide hydrochloride (Librium) A minor tranquilizer, this drug also acts as a sedative, anticonvulsant, and muscle relaxant, and it exerts some appetite-stimulating and analgesic effects. Its use with alcohol potentiates its central nervous system depressant effects.

Chlorothiazide (Diuril) This drug acts as both a diuretic and antihypertensive agent, increasing the excretion of sodium, chloride, water, uric acid, potassium, and bicarbonate.

Chlorpromazine (Thorazine) Used in the management of acute and chronic psychoses (major tranquilizer) and as an antiemetic. Its absorption is decreased by antacids, while its effect may be potentiated by MAO inhibitors.

Chlorthalidone (Hygroton) A diuretic and antihypertensive agent that is structurally similar to Chlorothiazide, but is absorbed more slowly and has a longer duration of action.

Cholestyramine (Questran) This ion-exchange resin combines with intestinal bile salts to form an insoluble, nonabsorbable complex that is excreted in the feces. The increased fecal loss of bile salts results in an increased oxidation of serum cholesterol to bile acids, causing a drop in the blood levels of cholesterol and low-density lipoproteins. Because it binds bile acids in the gastrointestinal tract, this drug may interfere with calcium absorption and the normal absorption of fat and fat-soluble vitamins. It is used for the relief of pruritus associated with biliary stasis and as an adjunct to the diet therapy of type II hyperlipoproteinemia. It interferes with the absorption of iron and many other drugs.

Dactinomycin (Actinomycin D) This antineoplastic agent acts by interfering with protein synthesis and mitosis in rapidly dividing cancerous and normal cells.

Demeclocycline (Declomycin)   A tetracycline antibiotic, but excreted more slowly than other tetracyclines.

Dextrothyroxine sodium (D-Thyroxine)   This anticholesteremic agent acts by stimulating the liver to excrete cholesterol. It is used to treat hypothyroidism in patients with cardiac disease and as an adjunct to diet therapy in patients with type II hyperlipoproteinemia.

Diazepam (Valium)   This drug acts as a minor tranquilizer, anticonvulsant, and skeletal muscle relaxant, and produces retrograde amnesia when administered intravenously. Its actions are potentiated by alcohol, antihistamines, narcotics, and MAO inhibitors.

Digitalis   This cardiotonic agent is thought to act by promoting the passage of calcium, sodium, and potassium ions in the heart muscle. It is used for a variety of heart conditions, including congestive heart failure.

Ethacrynic acid (Edecrin)   A rapid-acting diuretic used with congestive heart failure, cirrhosis, and renal disease. It may potentiate the actions of alcohol.

Fluorouracil (5-Fluorouracil)   An antineoplastic agent that acts by blocking the enzymes essential to normal DNA and RNA synthesis. It is used in the treatment of inoperable cancers.

Furosemide (Lasix)   A rapidly-acting diuretic that enhances the excretion of potassium, sodium, chloride, phosphate, hydrogen, magnesium, calcium, ammonium, and bicarbonate.

Glutethimide (Doriden)   A sedative and hypnotic with pharmacologic actions similar to barbiturates. Alcohol enhances absorption and potentiates central nervous system depression when taken with this drug.

Griseofulvin (Grifulvin)   An antifungal agent that deposits in keratin precursor cells and diseased tissue. This drug potentiates the effects of alcohol.

Hydrochlorothiazide (Esidrix)   A diuretic and antihypertensive agent of similar action to Chlorothiazide, but produces more naturesis.

Imipramine (Antipress)   A tricyclic antidepressant whose exact action is unknown. Used in endogenous depression and occasionally with electroconvulsive therapy. Increased sedation and psychomotor impairment is seen when this drug is taken with alcohol.

Isocarboxazid (Marplan)   An antidepressant that is usually used only when tricyclic antidepressants or electroconvulsive therapy is ineffective.

Isoniazid (INH)   An antibacterial, tuberculostatic agent that acts against actively growing tubercle bacilli by interfering with the metabolism of bacterial proteins, nucleic acids, carbohydrates, and lipids. This drug also acts as a competitive antagonist of pyridoxine (vitamin B_6). The use of alcohol while taking this drug may increase the risk of hepatotoxicity. Absorption is delayed or decreased by the concurrent use of aluminum-containing antacids.

Lincomycin hydrochloride (Lincocin)   An antibacterial agent that acts primarily against gram-positive organisms by inhibiting protein synthesis. Used for serious infections caused by susceptible bacteria in penicillin-allergic individuals.

Methotrexate (Amethopterin)   This antineoplastic agent acts by blocking the participation of the active form of folic acid in nucleic acid synthesis, thereby interfering with the mitotic process. Used primarily in combination with other antineoplastic agents, it is also used as an immunosuppressant in kidney transplantation. Increased risk of hepatotoxicity when taken concurrently with alcohol.

Methyclothiazide (Enduron)   A diuretic and antihypertensive agent similar to Chlorothiazide but exerting much greater natriuretic activity.

Metronidazole (Flagyl)   This antiprotozoal agent is used in the treatment of trichomoniasis, intestinal amebiasis, and amebic liver abscess.

Neomycin sulfate (Mycifradin Sulfate)   A broad-spectrum antibiotic used to treat the severe diarrhea caused by *E. coli* and to inhibit nitrogen-forming bacteria in the gastrointestinal tract and in urinary tract infections. This drug may reduce the absorption of vitamin B_{12}.

Pentazocine hydrochloride (Talwin Hydrochloride)   This narcotic analgesic is used for the relief of moderate to severe pain, mainly for preoperative analgesia or sedation and in obstetrics.

Phenelzine sulfate (Nardil)   This antidepressant and MAO inhibitor is used in the management of depression. Its effects are due to irreversible inhibition of mitochondrial enzymes involved in the breakdown of sympathomimetic amines, resulting in increased concentrations of epinephrine, norepinephrine, dopamine, and serotonin within the nervous system.

Phenobarbital   This long-acting barbiturate is used as an anticonvulsant, sedative, and hypnotic. This drug also lowers the bilirubin level in the blood by increasing the flow and excretion of bile salts. Central nervous system depression is potentiated by the concurrent use of alcohol.

Phenytoin (Dilantin)   This anticonvulsant is chemically related to phenobarbital. It stimulates hepatic enzymes, which may affect the metabolism of other drugs. The drug also increases metabolic inactivation of vitamin D.

Primidone (Mysoline)   This anticonvulsant is structurally similar to the barbiturates and is used to control seizures.

Procarbazine hydrochloride (Matulane)   An antineoplastic agent that acts by suppressing mitosis and causing chromatin damage to rapidly proliferating cells. Used in the treatment of Hodgkin's disease and in cancers unresponsive to other forms of treatment. Central nervous system depression is potentiated when this drug is used with alcohol.

Propoxyphene hydrochloride (Darvon)   This analgesic is similar to methadone and codeine and is used for the relief of mild to moderate pain. Additive central nervous system depression may occur with the concurrent use of alcohol.

Propranolol (Inderal)   This cardiac depressant drug acts by competing with epinephrine and norepinephrine for available beta-receptor sites. As a result, it selectively blocks the cardiac effects of beta-adrenergic stimulation and causes a reduction in heart rate, myocardial irritability, and force of contraction.

Pyrimethamine (Daraprim)   An antimalarial agent that acts by selectively inhibiting dehydrofolic reductase in the parasite, thereby destroying its ability to metabolize folic acid. Used in the treatment of malaria due to susceptible strains of plasmodia and in conjunction with a sulfonamide in the treatment of toxoplasmosis. Its effects may be decreased by the concurrent use of folic acid.

Spironolactone (Aldactone)   This diuretic and aldosterone antagonist acts by competing with aldosterone for receptor sites in the kidney. It promotes the excretion of sodium and water without the concomitant loss of potassium. It is used in cirrhosis, edema, essential hypertension, nephrotic syndrome, and to potentiate other diuretics or antihypertensive agents.

Tetracycline (Achromycin)   This broad-spectrum antimicrobial agent is effective against a wide variety of gram-positive and gram-negative bacteria, as well as many mycoplasma, rickettsiae, and protozoa. It acts by inhibiting protein synthesis in susceptible microorganisms. When administered with iron preparations or antacids containing aluminum, calcium, or magnesium, insoluble chelates are formed, resulting in malabsorption. Gastrointestinal absorption is also inhibited by sodium bicarbonate and other alkalis.

Theophylline (Aminophylline)   This xanthine-derivative is a smooth muscle relaxant, exerting its action primarily on the vessels of the bronchi and pulmonary tract, resulting in increased vital capacity. It is used for the relief of bronchial asthma, bronchitis, and emphysema.

Tranylcypromine sulfate (Parnate)   This antidepressant and MAO inhibitor is structurally similar to amphetamine. Because of its potential toxic effects, its use is reserved for patients with severe mental depression who have not responded to other therapies.

Triamterene (Dyrenium)   A potassium-sparing diuretic that is structurally related to folic acid. It promotes the excretion of sodium, chloride, and carbonate, while preserving potassium. It is used in the treatment of the edema of cirrhosis, congestive heart failure, and the nephrotic syndrome.

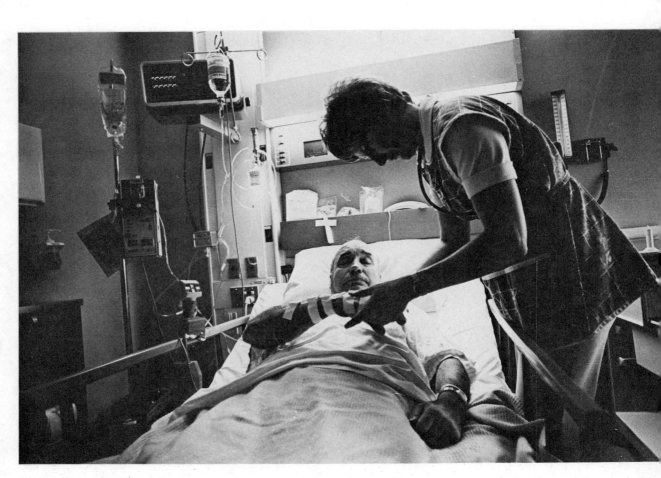

(Photo credit: Jeffrey Grosscup.)

NUTRITIONAL THERAPY IN DISEASE

In the following eight chapters nutrition will be presented in perhaps its most important role: in the treatment of disease states. The use of specific diet therapy ranges from controversial, as in Chapter 40, Cardiovascular Diseases, where there is still much debate over the relative importance of cholesterol intake, to a matter of life and death. This latter situation is discussed in Chapter 45, Congenital Metabolic Disorders, where, in certain diseases, a delay in initiating the appropriate diet therapy during the newborn period can result in death.

Problems of utilization of nutrients, such as altered absorption and its effect on nutritional status, are presented in Chapter 38, Diseases of the Gastrointestinal Tract. The short-term and long-term effects of insulin deficiency are discussed in detail in Chapter 39, Diabetes Mellitus. Another chapter devoted to the effects of one or more nutrient deficiencies is Chapter 41, The Anemias. Impairment of the normal renal excretory, regulatory, and endocrine abilities can have a profound effect on nutritional status and life, as discussed in Chapter 42, Renal Disease. Feeding difficulties, as the sequelae of other diseases or birth trauma, can present frustrations and challenges to the family and the health care team; these are presented in Chapter 43, Mental and Physical Handicaps.

Perhaps one of the most emotionally charged and potentially devastating diagnoses is that of cancer. Much has been learned about its treatment and the importance of nutrition as an adjunct to all forms of therapy. Chapter 44, Neoplastic Disease, discusses the nutritional effects of cancer, its treatments, methods of diet therapy, and possible theoretical dietary causes of this disease.

Before studying any of these chapters, a thorough understanding of the basics, Chapters 1 to 9, is essential. A knowledge of foods, Chapters 12 to 20, and nutrition during health, Chapters 23 to 29, is also helpful. The tools of diet therapy, Chapters 35 to 37, form the alphabet from which the language of dietetics is written. For all these reasons, this section was intentionally placed at the end of the book. For students who have not had the time or opportunity to read all sections before Section IX, suggested "chapters-to-review" are given before each of the chapters that follow. By reviewing at least the suggested chapters, the concepts presented will be more easily understood.

Chapter 38

DISEASES OF THE GASTROINTESTINAL TRACT

The gastrointestinal tract and its associated glands serve to obtain nutrients from ingested food for growth and maintenance of the body. This is accomplished by both mechanical and chemical means through the physical breakdown of food-stuffs by the action of the teeth and the churning of peristalsis, and the chemical breakdown by the various enzymes secreted into the lumen of the gastrointestinal tract. For a detailed presentation of normal physiology of the gastrointestinal tract and digestion, see Chap. 9.

Since the body is dependent on the gastrointestinal tract for all its nutrients, any abnormal functioning would cause systemic effects. Defects in absorption could be caused by tissue injury, drug effects, or inadequate secretion of digestive enzymes. This last cause may be due to mechanical blockage or vitamin deficiencies.

This chapter will present the most common diseases of the gastrointestinal tract, their causes, the clinical symptoms, and the recommended diet therapy. Case studies are given at the end of the chapter to illustrate the principles discussed.

Chapters to review: Section II, Chapters 11, 28, 34, 44.

Oral Cavity

Lesions in the mouth may be due to local irritation, medications, systemic disease, or nutritional deficiencies. This last group has been discussed in Chaps. 8, 9, 22, and 34. Any severe disease in the oral cavity can lead to serious dehydration and malnutrition.

TONGUE

Local irritation of the tongue may be caused by poorly fitting dentures, carious teeth, malignant disease, syphilis, or tuberculosis. An inflamed, painful tongue is most often due to an acute primary deficiency of one or more of the B-complex vitamins (acute glossitis). Iron-deficiency anemia of long duration or pernicious anemia in remission is reflected by a pale, smooth tongue (chronic atrophic glossitis). The treatment for each of these symptoms is correction of the underlying disorder.

TEETH AND GUMS

The etiology, signs, and symptoms of dental disease have already been presented in Chap. 28. Inflammation of the gums may be caused by a number of factors, including vitamin C deficiency (scurvy); infections with *Candida albicans* (thrush); various drugs, including iodides, salicylates, phenytoin; and several blood diseases (i.e., acute leukemia, aplastic anemia, and agranulocytosis). When the cause is nutritional, diet therapy will improve the lesions. If not, as with various drugs and in blood diseases, alternative supportive measures must be used.

Esophagus

Although less common than diseases of the stomach and colon, diseases of the esophagus can cause nutritional problems. The esophagus is susceptible to inflammation, trauma, or malignant disease, all three of which may result in stricture (a narrowing of the lumen opening). The primary clinical symptom is dysphagia, difficulty in swallowing. The patient first experiences difficulty in swallowing solid foods, then semisolids and, eventually, even fluids. Surgery, radiation, or the passage of a flexible tube are common treatments for esophageal stricture, depending on the etiology. Because malnutrition may have been progressive before medical attention was sought, it is advisable to build up nutritional stores before surgical therapy is initiated.

Plummer-Vinson syndrome is a disease of the esophagus with a nutritional etiology. It is most frequent among middle-aged women and is thought to be due to a deficiency of iron and the B-complex vitamins. The clinical symptoms include dysphagia, iron-deficiency anemia, glossitis, and achlorhydria (absence of hydrochloric acid). This disease may progress to carcinoma of the esophagus. Treatment includes correction of any nutritional deficiencies.

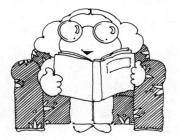

Herniation, the abnormal protrusion of an organ or a part through the containing wall of its cavity, can occur with the esophagus. Hiatus hernia and reflux esophagitis are often caused by obesity, chronic cough, and even by pregnancy, due to the increased bulk of the abdominal contents exerting more pressure on the hiatus (the opening in the diaphragm through which the esophagus passes). The action of the cardiac sphincter, the circular ring of muscle at the junction between the esophagus and the stomach, is lost, resulting in a reflux or regurgitation of gastric acid into the esophagus. The main symptom is heartburn, usually after meals and frequently with a change in posture (e.g., lifting and straining or bending over). Treatment is aimed at alleviating the primary cause, such as weight reduction in the obese individual, cure of the chronic cough, or delivery of the baby in the pregnant patient. The dietary treatment includes a bland diet with no solid foods taken within three hours before bedtime. If pain persists despite medical and dietary treatment, there may be some degree of ulceration or stricture that must be treated surgically.

Stomach

The main purpose of the stomach is to add fluid to the ingested food and initiate chemical digestion. The body and fundus of the stomach contain gastric glands that secrete mucus, digestive enzymes, and hydrochloric acid. The parietal cells of the stomach are the sole source of hydrochloric acid. These cells are also the site of production of intrinsic factor, the glycoprotein that binds to vitamin B_{12} and is required for its absorption by the ileum. The principal digestive action that occurs in the stomach is the hydrolysis of proteins, which can only take place in an acid environment.

Inflammation, irritation, ulceration, or surgery on the stomach results in a decrease in the quantity of digestive enzymes, incomplete hydrolysis of proteins, and the rapid movement of foodstuffs from the stomach to the intestines. The following section presents various common diseases of the stomach and the diet therapy.

PEPTIC ULCER

Peptic ulcer, an erosion in the mucosa of the stomach, duodenum, or lower end of the esophagus, is caused by an excessive secretion of acidic gastric juices. It develops due to the loss of the ability of the mucosa to withstand the digestive action of hydrochloric acid and pepsin. Ulceration may occur along any surface of the gastrointestinal tract that is exposed to acidic gastric juices. It most commonly occurs in the stomach or duodenum, but may also occur in the lower end of the esophagus or as Meckel's diverticulum, ectopic gastric mucosa. The cause of the ulceration is most likely due to the presence of an increased number of acid-secreting parietal cells in the gastric mucosa. In Zollinger-Ellison syndrome, a condition in which excessive amounts of gastrin are produced, the gastric hypersecretion results in intractable peptic ulceration.

In the past, patients with peptic ulcer disease were placed on a strict dietary regimen designed to decrease the secretion of gastric juice, neutralize gastric acidity, and decrease gastric motility. The most extreme of these regimens was the Sippy diet, which consisted of 3 oz of milk and cream every hour with neutralizing alkaline powders given in between. As the patient's condition improved, soft-boiled eggs, cooked cereals, creamed soups, and pureed vegetables were introduced. With continued relief from pain, the patient was maintained indefinitely on a bland diet, that is, one which is mechanically, thermally, and chemically nonirritating.

In recent years the value of this type of diet therapy has been challenged. In addition to the possible long-term harmful effects of a milk-rich or egg-rich diet, it has been observed that such factors as anxiety, emotional upsets, infections, fatigue, and alcohol contribute more to the development of a peptic ulcer than any dietary indiscretion [3]. Today, the long-term medical treatment of the peptic ulcer patient includes a diet selectively restrictive of the specific foods of which the patient is intolerant. In addition, such factors as smoking, alcohol, and caffeine-containing beverages, which stimulate gastric acid secretion, and the ulcerogenic drugs (i.e., aspirin, salicylates, reserpine, corticosteroids) are also avoided.

If the medical/dietary treatment of the peptic ulcer does not produce signs of healing, surgical treatment may be necessary. The surgical removal of all or part of the stomach (total or partial gastrectomy) is a common treatment for severe peptic ulcer, gastric cancer, or hemorrhage from peptic ulcer (Fig. 38-1). Depending on the type and extent of surgery, some degree of *maldigestion* (defective intraluminal hydrolysis of protein, fat, or carbohydrate) results. After this type of surgery, gastric digestion is never complete; the majority of digestion must then occur in the small intestine.

In surgery where the pylorus is removed, the duodenum is bypassed, and the stomach contents have direct access to the jejunum, several factors contribute to the problems that develop. The gastric phase of digestion is decreased, with a

FIG. 38-1. Gastric resection and reconstruction.
A. Partial gastrectomy.
B. Billroth I procedure (gastroduodenostomy).
C. Billroth II procedure (gastrojejunostomy). (From G. Nardi and G. Zuidema, *Surgery* [4th ed.]. Boston: Little, Brown, 1982.)

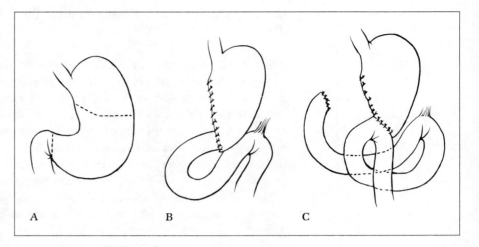

A   B   C

reduction in the volume of gastric acids, pepsin, and lipase. In addition, the stomach contents are inadequately mixed before entering the jejunum, causing decreased absorption. The normal hormonal factors that control gastric emptying no longer function since the pylorus has been removed. Normal release of bile and pancreatic secretions is disrupted by the rapid transit of food from the stomach to the jejunum. As a result, the presence of undigested food in the jejunum and lower small intestine permits bacterial decomposition causing diarrhea, loss of nutrients, and abdominal pain.

Depending on the type and extent of surgery, the patient may experience one or more of the following complications during the postsurgical period—hypoglycemia, weight loss, food intolerances, small-stomach syndrome, dumping syndrome, or jejunal ulceration. A feeling of distention and discomfort after a meal is experienced by about half of all patients having undergone gastric surgery (small-stomach syndrome). The treatment consists of smaller, more frequent meals. During the early postsurgical period most gastrectomy patients experience dumping syndrome within a short period after eating. This syndrome includes abdominal cramping, nausea, vomiting, diarrhea, and even hypotension and tachycardia within a few minutes after eating. These symptoms are caused by the rapid movement of the hyperosmolar gastric contents into the upper jejunum. The severity of the dumping syndrome usually decreases within 2 to 3 months after surgery. The dietary management during this period of adjustment includes small, frequent meals; liquids between meals only; and the use of complex carbohydrates and starches rather than simple sugars to decrease osmolarity.

GASTRITIS

Irritation of the gastric mucosa, gastritis, may be acute or chronic and is thought to be caused by alcohol, drugs, or other chemical irritants. It may also be a side effect of another disease, such as an immunologic or metabolic disorder. Gastric changes are seen in patients with iron-deficiency anemia and pernicious anemia.

The clinical symptoms range from mild anorexia and discomfort to nausea, vomiting, and heartburn. With acute gastritis, the treatment includes the appropriate use of antibiotics, gastric lavage, the withholding of all solid foods for 24 to 48 hours, and the replacement of fluid and electrolyte losses. With improvement, the diet is advanced to small feedings of milk and then a bland diet. In chronic atrophic gastritis, treatment is aimed at the underlying cause; the diet therapy is geared to individual intolerances.

CANCER OF THE STOMACH

This type of cancer is difficult to detect and may be diagnosed too late for surgery to be successful. The presenting symptoms include anorexia, weakness, abdominal pain, and iron-deficiency anemia. The goal of diet therapy is to maintain the patient in an optimal nutritional state while permitting the individual to choose foods he or she enjoys. Correction of the anemia and control of fluid and electrolyte imbalances, if present, are also important.

Small Intestines and Associated Organs

The small intestine is divided into three parts—the duodenum, the jejunum, and the ileum. After the chyme (the liquefied acid food mass) has passed from the pylorus of the stomach into the duodenum, the pancreatic and biliary secretions change the pH of the food mass to alkaline. This change in pH is necessary for the action of the enzymes contained within the intestinal and pancreatic juices. Because its long length (about 6 m) permits prolonged contact between digestive enzymes and the food mass, the majority of digestion and absorption occurs in this part of the gastrointestinal tract. Disease, inflammation, or surgery of the small intestine or its associated organs (liver, pancreas, gallbladder) can therefore have a profound effect on absorption and metabolism. The pancreas secretes six different proteolytic (protein-splitting) enzymes, three lipolytic (fat-splitting) enzymes, and pancreatic amylase, which hydrolyzes carbohydrates. Within the intestinal juices there are peptidases and carbohydrases, which hydrolyze proteins and carbohydrates, respectively. The liver produces bile, which is stored in the gallbladder and is necessary for the emulsification of fats and their subsequent absorption.

Malabsorption results when one or more of the processes of absorption or enzymatic digestion is impaired. This can result from pancreatic insufficiency, liver or gallbladder disease, disaccharidase deficiencies, drug or radiation therapy, or surgery.

MALABSORPTION SYNDROMES

Tropical sprue is a malabsorptive syndrome of the small intestine. It is the name given by the Dutch in Java to a tropical disease characterized by impaired absorption of carbohydrates, fats, fat-soluble nutrients, steatorrhea, weight loss, weakness, glossitis, and macrocytic anemia. These symptoms are associated with atrophy of the jejunal villi, which is similar to the changes seen in gluten enteropathy (celiac disease). The secretion of pancreatic enzymes and the absorption of dietary protein are normal. The primary cause of sprue is unknown. The treatment of sprue includes the use of broad-spectrum antibiotics; the administration of the appropriate vitamins to correct deficiencies (folic acid and vitamin B_{12}); and a low-fat, high-protein, high-carbohydrate, and high-calorie diet. During the acute stage, the diet should be bland and low in residue; most of the carbohydrate should be in the form of monosaccharides. Fat absorption may be enhanced by substituting medium-chain triglycerides. Calcium lactate for the low-serum calcium and tetany should be given; administration of vitamin K will help prevent bleeding.

In adults who develop sprue in nontropical environments, adult celiac disease should be suspected and the patient placed on a gluten-gliadin–restricted diet. The diet may be advanced as the patient recovers, although some degree of fat malabsorption may be permanent.

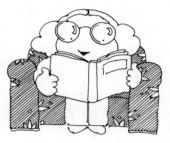

Celiac disease, also known as gluten-induced enteropathy, is an intestinal disorder found in children between the ages of 6 months and 6 years. The characteristic symptoms include loss of appetite, failure to thrive, steatorrhea, protuberant abdomen, and multiple nutritional deficiencies. The stools are characteristically large in volume, pale, and offensive due to free fatty acids; they are frothy because of the fermentation of unabsorbed carbohydrates. The pathology underlying this disorder is atrophy of the jejunal villi, resulting in malabsorption of fats and carbohydrates. Celiac disease usually runs in cycles of remissions and exacerbations; the disease improves gradually by age 6 or soon thereafter.

The causative factor in childhood celiac disease has been thought to be the hypersensitivity to two protein fractions, gluten and gliadin, found in wheat, rye, barley, and oats. More recently it has been demonstrated that it is the quantity of protein-bound glutamine in any given protein that is the offending agent. Wheat, rye, barley, and oats contain large amounts of protein-bound glutamine and, therefore, cause reactions in the hypersensitive child. Such foods as rice, corn, beef, fish, milk, eggs, and potatoes contain a smaller proportion of protein-bound glutamine and do not cause problems.

In adults, a syndrome previously known as *idiopathic steatorrhea* is now recognized to actually be a mild form of celiac disease first identified in adulthood. The clinical features of adult celiac disease are identical to those of sprue, except that the former responds to a gluten-gliadin–free diet.

The diet therapy for both childhood and adult celiac disease is the complete exclusion of all gluten and gliadin from the diet. This may be difficult since oats, barley, rye, and, particularly, wheat are present in such a wide variety of foods, such as breads, cakes, biscuits, pastries, macaroni, and spaghetti. They may also be used as a thickener or filler in many other foods. Figure 38-2 gives a list of foods to be omitted or included in the celiac disease diet. Within 1 month of starting on the diet, the stools often become normal and the clinical symptoms subside. In children, this intolerance usually disappears by age 6. In adults, complete recovery is not as frequent.

Iron-deficiency anemia and megaloblastic anemia may also be present with celiac disease or nontropical sprue and should be treated with iron and folic

FIG. 38-2. Gluten-gliadin–restricted diet for celiac disease. (From B. T. Burton, *Human Nutrition* [3rd ed.]. New York: McGraw-Hill, 1976.)

PERMISSIBLE FOODS	EXCLUDED FOODS
Skim milk, whole milk (as tolerated), soft drinks, cocoa and chocolate drinks that do not contain cereal thickeners, coffee made from ground coffee beans, tea	Cereal beverages (Postum, Ovaltine, malted milk), drinks containing cereal fillers or thickeners, beer and ale
Precooked infant cereal made from rice; refined cereals and cereal products made solely from rice or corn, if tolerated	All other cereal products
Bread or rolls made from potato flour, rice, corn, or soy, if tolerated	All other breads, rolls, biscuits, or cereal products
Meat, fish, fowl prepared as desired, but no gravies thickened with flour; no stuffing; no "breaded" cuts; no batter on the fowl; eggs; cheese	All other meats, meat loaf, luncheon meats, sausages, or any meat product or dish which contains cereal or flour
Potatoes, rice	Noodles, spaghetti, macaroni, or other flour-derived dishes
Butter, margarine, oils, and other fats, as tolerated	Salad dressings or mayonnaise made with flour thickeners
All pure vegetables (not creamed)	Creamed or breaded vegetables
All fruits and fruit juices	
Clear broths and vegetable soups; cream soups if thickened with corn-starch, cream, or potato flour	All soups containing flour, noodles, or other cereal derivatives
Jello, sherbet, homemade ice cream; rice or cornstarch puddings	Pastry, cakes, cookies, prepared mixes; most commercial puddings and ice cream; ice cream cones
Honey, jelly, jam, sugar, chocolate, homemade candy prepared without cereal derivatives	All candy containing cereal derivatives

acid. This will cure not only the anemia but the glossitis and stomatitis, if present.

INFLAMMATORY SYNDROMES

The term *enteritis* is from the Greek "enteron," meaning intestine, and "itis," denoting inflammation. There are a number of inflammatory small intestine disorders, including regional, tuberculous, or radiation enteritis; chronic ulcerative colitis; diverticulosis and diverticulitis; amyloidosis; scleroderma; lymphoma; tropical and nontropical sprue; and parasitic infections. The usual diet therapy includes a low-fiber diet, as given in Fig. 38-3. This philosophy has been changing over the past decade, however; a diet with moderate or even high fiber (residue) has recently been shown to be more effective.

Regional enteritis, also known as Crohn's disease, is an inflammatory process that may be confined to the lower ileum or may involve the colon, ileum, je-

FIG. 38-3. Bland low-fiber diet. (Adapted from Massachusetts General Hospital Dietary Department, *Diet Manual.* Boston: Little, Brown, 1976.)

	PERMISSIBLE FOODS	EXCLUDED FOODS
Milk	Whole, skim, buttermilk; yogurt; milk drinks flavored with moderate amounts of syrup, malt, or weak cocoa	Yogurt containing fruit or vegetable seeds and skins; beverages other than milk drinks
Eggs	Hard-cooked, pasteurized, and other *Salmonella*-free preparations	
Meats	Broiled, baked, boiled, roasted beef, lamb, veal, poultry, fresh pork, ham, bacon, fish, shellfish, liver, and other organ meats	Fried, highly seasoned, and pickled meats; frankfurters, sausages, cold cuts, sardines
Cheese	Mild cheese such as cottage, cream, American, Cheddar, Swiss	Strongly flavored, pungent cheese
Breads	Any plain bread, crackers, muffins, rolls	Those that contain whole grains, nuts, seeds; fried breads such as doughnuts
Cereals	Refined (ready-to-eat or cooked) cereals, such as farina, rice, cornmeal, cornflakes, oatmeal, noodles, macaroni, spaghetti	Coarse whole grains, bran, ready-to-eat cereals with raisins or berries
Vegetables	All tender-cooked or canned vegetables	Raw vegetables; highly seasoned or strongly flavored vegetables such as corn, dried beans, onions
Fruits	All tender-cooked or canned fruits, as tolerated; ripe bananas and fresh citrus fruit sections	Other raw fruits, dried fruits
Juices	Fresh, frozen, or canned juices, as tolerated	
Desserts	Simple puddings without nuts or fruits, such as custards, tapioca, gelatin; plain ice cream, sherbet, water ice, plain cake, cookies	Pastries, cakes, cookies, and puddings made with nuts or fruits containing seeds and skins
Soups	Lightly seasoned cream soups, chowders, bisques	Meat stock soups; highly seasoned or strongly flavored soups, such as bean soup
Fats	Butter, cream, cream cheese, bacon, mayonnaise, mayonnaise-type salad dressing	Olives, fried foods
Seasonings	Salt, sugar, clear jellies or fruit butters, honey, allspice, cinnamon, caraway seeds, mace, paprika, sage, thyme	Preserves containing seeds and skins, highly seasoned foods, other spices

junum, and even the duodenum and stomach. The cause of the inflammation is not known. Clinical symptoms include pain and cramping in the lower right quadrant, diarrhea, and a low-grade fever. Weight loss, anorexia, and malabsorption lead to the development of nutritional deficiencies. In addition, there may be a loss of blood, fluid, protein, and electrolytes from the inflamed mucosa.

The treatment of regional enteritis depends on the severity of the condition. With severe symptoms, the patient is hospitalized, given anti-inflammatory and antibiotic drug therapy, and the bowel permitted to rest by giving parenteral nutritional support. The diet is advanced to a low-residue, and, eventually, to a full, normal diet. The diet should also be geared to correcting any malnutrition or imbalances that may have developed during an exacerbation. The use of medium-chain triglycerides to aid fat absorption and the periodic administration of malabsorbed nutrients, such as iron, vitamin K, and vitamin B_{12}, may be useful.

Radiation enteritis is a side effect of the radiotherapy treatments used for cancer. Radiation affects the rapid renewal of mucosal cells lining the small intestine by impairing the synthesis of DNA. During therapy and 1 or 2 weeks immediately following, the mucosal cells begin to recover from the radiation therapy. During this time, the patient may experience nausea, vomiting, abdominal pain, diarrhea, and/or constipation. Radiation also affects the blood vessels supplying the mucosal cells by causing them to degenerate, which results in mucosal ulceration and necrosis. Weight loss and malabsorption of fat and bile acids may result and persist from 6 months to several years after the completion of therapy. The treatment depends on the severity of the damage. Low-residue oral feedings are frequently used, as are diets geared to individual tolerances. See Chap. 44, Neoplastic Diseases, for more detail.

A common complication of pulmonary tuberculosis is *tuberculous enteritis.* The causative agents are tubercle bacilli swallowed with sputum from the tuberculous lungs. The symptoms are similar to regional enteritis or ulcerative colitis. The diet therapy includes a bland diet, which is low in residue and high in protein.

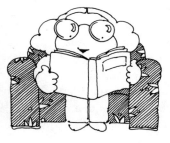

SHORT BOWEL SYNDROMES

Extensive resections of the small intestine may be necessary in some cases of acute regional enteritis, ulcerative colitis, or other irreversible pathologic disorders, sometimes leaving only inches of healthy small intestine intact. Intestinal bypass surgery has also been used to intentionally cause malabsorption and resultant weight loss in massive obesity. The complication rate and mortality are high for this type of elective surgery, as discussed in Chap. 29.

For whatever reason the surgery was performed, the postsurgical symptoms are similar [4]. Because the absorptive surface has been shortened, food passes through the small intestine more rapidly, causing malabsorption, diarrhea or steatorrhea, and fluid and electrolyte imbalances. With time, the remaining portion of the small intestine will hypertrophy to accommodate the additional work but in the interim, diet therapy may be useful in improving nutritional status and decreasing the severity of the complications. Protein in the form of casein hydrolysate, carbohydrate as sucrose or fructose, and fats in the form of MCT oil are more easily assimilated.

Hepatic Diseases

The liver has correctly been described as the chemist of the body. Its many and diverse metabolic processes affect every organ of the body. It accounts for 25 percent of the basal metabolism. This remarkable organ has enormous functional reserve and regenerative powers; if an adequate diet is maintained, normal hepatic functional efficiency can continue with as little as 15 percent of remaining hepatic tissue.

Because of the unique structure and internal architecture of the liver, its function can be affected by disturbances within the hepatocytes and by alterations in the biliary and circulatory systems. The causes of hepatic injury range from nutritional and metabolic to infectious, parasitic, toxic, obstructive, or malignant. Regardless of the cause, the degenerative changes that occur are similar, including fatty infiltration, fibrosis, necrosis, and cirrhosis. The liver may be damaged by malnutrition, such as poor protein intake, or by toxic substances such as alcohol, chemicals, or viruses. Once the liver is severely damaged, the nutritional status of the individual suffers. The nutritional disturbances may be due to a combination of factors including anorexia, malnutrition, impaired digestion and absorption of nutrients, or altered intermediary metabolism.

Infectious hepatitis (hepatitis A) is an acute viral infection of the liver spread by the oral-intestinal route. *Serum hepatitis* (hepatitis B) is caused by a similar virus, but is transmitted primarily via improperly sterilized needles or by blood transfusions from a donor who carries the virus. The treatment for both of these diseases includes bed rest; a diet high in protein, carbohydrate, and calories, and moderately low in fats; and prevention of further injury to the liver. Because of the disturbed liver function, plasma prothrombin levels may be low and may require supplemental vitamin K. A sample diet for hepatitis is given in Fig. 38-4.

With severely impaired liver function, as in advanced cirrhosis, *hepatic coma* may occur. This syndrome is characterized by progressive confusion, apathy, personality changes, coma, and, eventually, death. One of the major functions of the liver is the removal of ammonia from the blood by converting it to urea, which is then excreted by the kidneys. With severe hepatic damage, portal blood circulation decreases and collateral circulation develops, bypassing the liver. This means that ammonia-laden blood approaches the liver but is detoured through the collateral circulation. It reenters the systemic blood flow and produces ammonia intoxication of the central nervous system and coma. The ammonia is produced mainly as a result of digestion of dietary protein in the gastrointestinal tract. Other causes of toxic ammonia accumulation include production by intestinal bacteria and the action of bacteria on blood proteins from gastrointestinal bleeding. The treatment of hepatic coma includes sterilization of

FIG. 38-4. Sample diet for hepatitis. This diet contains approximately 105 gm protein, 40 gm fat, 600 gm carbohydrate, and 3180 kcal. (From B. Luke, Hepatic Disease. In *Case Studies in Therapeutic Nutrition.* Boston: Little, Brown, 1977.)

BREAKFAST
  2 soft-boiled eggs
  2 slices toast with 2 tbsp honey
  ½ fresh grapefruit
  8 oz skim milk

MIDMORNING
  8 oz orange juice with 3 tbsp honey

LUNCH
  Sandwich made with
    2 oz cheese
    2 slices whole-wheat bread
    Lettuce and tomato
  8 oz skim milk with 2 tbsp honey

MIDAFTERNOON
  8 oz orange juice with 3 tbsp honey

DINNER
  4 oz broiled chicken with 2 tbsp honey
  1 small baked potato
  ½ cup green peas
  2 slices whole-wheat bread
  8 oz skim milk

BEDTIME
  Milkshake made with
    8 oz orange juice
    8 oz skim milk
    3 tbsp honey
    Ice

the bowel with colonic lavage of antibiotics and a diet high in carbohydrates (to prevent protein catabolism), moderate in fat, and from low to no protein, depending on the patient's ammonia levels and mental status. Initial treatment may be directed at reducing the intestinal production of ammonia by bacteria. When antibiotic therapy is not sufficient or effective, protein restriction is warranted. A sample diet for hepatic coma is given in Fig. 38-5.

Biliary Diseases

The presence of sufficient quantities of bile in the intestine is necessary for the normal digestion and absorption of fats and fat-soluble nutrients. Bile is formed in the liver and stored and concentrated in the gallbladder. Between meals the gallbladder acts as an inactive reservoir for the bile. The presence of fats or fatty acids in the duodenum stimulates the sphincter of the common bile duct (the sphincter of Oddi) to relax and open and bile to flow into the duodenum. Pancreatic juices also mix with the bile, since they both enter into the duodenum via the common bile duct.

FIG. 38-5. Sample diet for hepatic coma. This diet contains approximately 15 gm protein, 25 gm fat, 320 gm carbohydrate, and 1580 kcal. (From B. Luke, Hepatic Disease. In *Case Studies in Therapeutic Nutrition*. Boston: Little, Brown, 1977.)

BREAKFAST
2 corn muffins with 2 tbsp jelly
½ fresh grapefruit
Coffee with 1 tbsp sugar

MIDMORNING
8 oz orange juice

LUNCH
Fruit salad with honey
Crackers
Frosted sponge cake
8 oz orange juice

DINNER
Buttered noodles
½ fresh cantaloupe
Steamed broccoli
Broiled tomatoes
Add protein by including 8 oz of milk (about 8 gm protein), or 1 oz of meat, fish, or poultry (about 7 gm protein).

The biliary tract is vulnerable to several disorders which may be viewed as different stages of the same pathologic progression. The simultaneous contraction of the gallbladder and relaxation of the sphincter is due to vagal stimulation; the opposite occurs with sympathetic stimulation. A disturbance in these reciprocal effects leads to functional disorders of the biliary tract, including *biliary dyskinesia* (spasm of the sphincter of Oddi) and *biliary achalasia* (failure of the sphincter to relax).

The most common biliary disorders include *gallstones* (cholelithiasis), *biliary calculi* (choledocholithiasis), and *acute* and *chronic cholecystitis*. Gallstones are the result of many factors, including altered cholesterol metabolism, biliary stasis, and a genetic predisposition. They are more common in women than men and more frequent in fair, obese, parous women above age 40. The presence of stones in the gallbladder is usually only discovered when they temporarily block a duct and produce a painful, colicky episode. The pain subsides when the stone drops back into the gallbladder. If the stone blocks the common bile duct, the obstruction may have to be corrected by surgery. With biliary calculi there may be transient jaundice, malabsorption of fats and fat-soluble vitamins, and the stools become clay-colored due to the absence of bile pigments. With the blockage of biliary flow into the duodenum, the resulting pressure and stasis may damage the liver parenchyma if the condition continues for long periods. Repeated attacks lead to acute and chronic cholecystitis.

Between attacks and before surgery, the diet therapy for each of these biliary disorders is a low-fat, low-calorie (if weight reduction is needed), high-protein, high-carbohydrate diet. Since fat is poorly digested due to the lack of bile, it is restricted in the diet. Supplemental fat-soluble vitamins, particularly vitamin K, may be necessary.

Pancreatic Insufficiency

Several diseases can result in pancreatic insufficiency, or the absence of all enzymes secreted by the pancreas. Among the most common are cancer of the pancreas with duct obstruction; pancreatic resection; cystic fibrosis; and chronic pancreatitis due to alcoholism, trauma, or gallbladder disease. With cancer of the pancreas, the maldigestion may be due to obstruction of the flow by the tumor or the cancer may cause local areas of inflammation. Although there is a large pancreatic reserve, as much as 80 percent of the pancreas may be surgically removed without impairing fat digestion [5]. With cystic fibrosis the pancreatic ducts, bile ducts, and the gallbladder become blocked with a thick, viscous material, which impedes the flow. The enzyme-secreting glands also become fibrous and nonfunctional in this hereditary disease. In chronic pancreatitis, there is a gradual fibrosis of the enzyme-secreting glands of the pancreas due to inflammation. This results in the passage of unhydrolyzed fat and protein into the colon where it is excreted, undigested, in the stool. The decreased insulin secretion by the pancreas causes glucose intolerance and, eventually, diabetes mellitus.

Regardless of the cause, the primary treatment for pancreatic insufficiency is replacement of pancreatic enzymes, which are usually taken with meals. To prevent their inactivation in the acid environment of the stomach, these enzymes are enhanced by the concomitant administration of sodium bicarbonate. Medications to decrease gastric acid output may also be helpful. Supplemental water-soluble preparations of vitamins A, D, K, and E, as well as restricting fat intake or using medium-chain triglycerides to improve fat digestion, may also be useful.

Disaccharidase Deficiencies

Unlike the pancreatic enzymes that are secreted, the disaccharidases exert their actions within the mucosal cells of the small intestine rather than in the intestinal lumen. Six disaccharidases have been isolated—two maltase enzymes, isomaltase, lactase, invertase, and trehalase. The disaccharides are hydrolyzed into monosaccharides, which are then transported across the intestinal mucosal cells into capillaries of the portal circulation to the liver. Glucose and galactose are absorbed by an active transport mechanism, that is, against a concentration gradient. This mechanism involves a sodium pump and a mobile carrier system, but the details are not fully understood.

A deficiency of disaccharidases may be *primary* (hereditary) or *secondary* (acquired). The two main types of primary disaccharidase deficiency include lactase deficiency and a combined invertase-isomaltase deficiency. Both of these diseases are very rare, but when present can cause severe symptoms. The lactose malabsorption may be secondary, due to malnutrition, mucosal injury (see Chap. 34), or just the normal decline in lactase activity known to occur in most adults. With glucose-galactose malabsorption, the mechanism for the active transport of glucose and galactose across the intestinal mucosa is not functioning.

The main symptom in all cases of sugar malabsorption is diarrhea. The unhydrolyzed sugar passes deep into the colon where it draws in water from the surrounding tissues. Bacteria normally present in the colon ferment the sugar and produce organic acids (lactic, pyruvic, and acetic), carbon dioxide, and hydrogen. The resulting clinical symptoms include abdominal cramps, bloating, diarrhea, and flatulence. With congenital lactose deficiency and congenital glucose-galactose malabsorption, the diarrhea starts soon after birth. With invertase-isomaltase deficiency, diarrhea begins when sucrose and starch are given as components of formula or supplementary food.

The main methods of treating sugar malabsorption include replacing the malabsorbed sugar with other carbohydrates and supplementation with the deficient enzymes. When lactase deficiency is present from birth, the newborn must be given formula containing sugars other than lactose (human milk contains about 7% lactose). Such formulas include Soybee, Mullsoy, and Nutromigen. With all types of lactose malabsorption, fermented dairy products are substituted for fresh ones, such as hard cheese for milk (see Table 38-1). In invertase-isomaltase deficiency, sucrose should be replaced by glucose. Food sources of sucrose are given in Table 38-2. Those that should be avoided include dates, bananas, apricots, oranges, melons, pineapples, and green peas. Because the enzyme amylase partially converts starch to isomaltose, patients with invertase-isomaltase deficiency should also limit their intake of starch, particularly potato and wheat products. Exogenous lactase is available, as are maltase and isomaltase.

Large Intestine

The main functions of the large intestine include water absorption and the production of mucus for lubrication. In addition, the large intestine absorbs the remaining digested food and its bacteria degrade some materials resistant to previous digestion [3]. These bacteria present in the colon also synthesize vitamin K (essential for the normal blood-clotting process) and, possibly, some B vitamins.

Inflammation, ulceration, obstruction, trauma, or surgery on this part of the lower gastrointestinal tract can influence fluid and electrolyte balance, protein metabolism, and the elimination of toxic waste products. As with inflammation and ulceration in any portion of the gastric lumen, fluids, proteins, blood, and electrolytes are lost as exudate and the mucosa's functional absorptive capacity is impaired. With surgery, the remaining portions of the intestines must hypertrophy to accommodate the increased workload. Until this is accomplished, malabsorption results.

Ulcerative colitis, the most common cause of chronic diarrhea in temperate climates, is characterized by inflammation and ulceration of the mucosa of the

TABLE 38-1. Composition and comparison of dairy products

Product and amount	Calories	Protein (gm)	Lactose (gm)	Lactose ratio to milk	Calcium (mg)	Calcium ratio to milk
Sandwich cheese (2 oz)						
American	210	12.6	0.96	0.09:1	364	1.4:1
Cheddar	230	14.2	1.18	0.11:1	386	1.5:1
Cream cheese	196	4.8	1.14	0.11:1	40	0.15:1
Swiss	210	15.6	0.96	0.09:1	522	2.0:1
Cottage cheese (4 oz)						
Plain, creamed	108	14.0	2.4	0.23:1	68	0.3:1
Lowfat (2%)	96	15.6	3.7	0.36:1	100	0.4:1
Uncreamed	92	21.2	0.8	0.08:1	28	0.1:1
Ice cream (4 oz)						
Vanilla (12%)	254	4.4	8.0	0.77:1	164	0.6:1
Ice milk (4 oz)						
Vanilla	166	4.4	8.4	0.8:1	156	0.6:1
Milk (8 oz)						
Whole milk (3.5% fat)	141	7.3	10.4	1:1	260	1:1
Chocolate drink	136	7.3	9.6	0.9:1	247	0.95:1
Eggnog (6% fat)	304	10.4	12.8	1.2:1	343	1.3:1
Skimmed	73	7.3	10.4	1:1	266	1:1
Yogurt (8 oz)						
Blueberry	257	9.6	10.4	1:1	282	1:1
Plain	134	12.0	13.6	1.3:1	362	1.4:1
Strawberry	232	10.4	12.0	1.2:1	314	1.2:1
Vanilla	195	11.2	12.8	1.2:1	336	1.3:1
Milk (reconstituted) (8 oz)						
Nonfat dry	80	8.0	12.4	1.2:1	300	1.2:1
Evaporated whole	174	8.8	12.5	1.2:1	325	1.3:1
Evaporated skim	96	9.6	13.9	1.3:1	350	1.4:1
Liquid breakfast mix (1-serving envelope)						
Vanilla	130	7.0	12.2	1.2:1	50	2:1

Source: B. Luke, *Maternal Nutrition*. Boston: Little, Brown, 1979. Pp. 94–95.

TABLE 38-2. Sugars in selected foods (grams/100 gm edible portion)

Food	Fructose	Glucose	Reducing sugar*	Sucrose
Apple	5.0	1.7	8.3	3.1
Apricot	0.4	1.9		5.5
Banana				
Yellow green			5.0	5.1
Yellow			8.4	8.9
Dates				
Deglet Noor			16.2	45.4
Egyptian			35.8	48.5
Mango			3.4	11.6
Melon				
Cantaloupe	0.9	1.2	2.3	4.4
Honeydew				
Vine ripened			3.3	7.4
Picked green			3.6	3.3
Yellow	1.5	2.1		1.4
Orange	1.8	2.5	5.0	4.6
Pineapple				
Ripened on plant	1.4	2.3	4.2	7.9
Picked green			1.3	2.4
Plums				
Italian prune			4.6	5.4
Sweet	2.9	4.5	7.4	4.4
Watermelon			3.8	4.0
Parsnips, fresh				3.5
Peas, green				5.5
Potatoes, white	0.1	0.1	0.8	0.1
Sweet potato				
Raw	0.3	0.4	0.8	4.1
Baked			14.5	7.2
Soybeans			1.6	7.2
Garden pea				6.7

*Mainly monosaccharides plus maltose and lactose.
Source: M. G. Hardinge, J. B. Swarner, and H. Crooks, Carbohydrates in foods. *Journal of the American Dietetic Association* 46:197, 1965.

large intestine. Clinical symptoms include the presence of blood and mucus in the stool, marked weight loss, anemia, weakness, and nutritional deficiencies. The specific etiology is unknown but allergic, psychogenic, immune, and microbial factors have been implicated. The main objectives of the diet therapy include bowel rest and correction of nutritional deficiencies. The medical treatment includes psychotherapy and steroid therapy. Surgery is indicated for those individuals who do not respond to medical treatment or who relapse frequently. The two most common procedures include *ileostomy* (the surgical formation of an opening through the abdominal wall into the ileum) or *colectomy* (excision of all or part of the colon). Besides the need for additional diet therapy after such surgery, due to the loss of the fluid-absorbing function of the large intestine, these patients should also receive special support for their change in bowel function and altered body image.

The diet for chronic ulcerative colitis should be high in protein, calories, vitamins, and minerals while still being bland and low in residue. The high-protein allowance is needed to replace blood losses and the protein lost as exudate from the open ulcerous areas of the colon, and because of the increase in protein catabolism that accompanies fever, if present. Milk should not be used to fulfill this protein requirement for several reasons—it is not a low-residue food; the individual may have primary or secondary lactose intolerance; and the high-fat content may aggravate the diarrhea. Other sources of protein, such as meat, fish, and poultry, should be emphasized.

Diverticulosis and Diverticulitis

Diverticula (from the Latin *devertere*, to turn aside) are herniations or blind pouches of the mucous membrane through weak areas or gaps in the circular muscle of the gut. They may be found in the esophagus, stomach, or large or small intestine and may be congenital or acquired. The presence of diverticula is known as *diverticulosis;* when inflamed, the condition is termed *diverticulitis.* They most commonly appear in the distal portions of the colon and are more prevalent among the elderly. It has been suggested that the irritable bowel syndrome is a forerunner of diverticulosis. When the intestinal herniations become infected and inflamed, ulceration and perforation may result. When perforation has occurred, surgery is indicated. Repeated attacks of diverticulitis result in adhesions (abnormal fibrous areas) and eventual narrowing of the lumen.

The traditional diet for diverticulosis has been low-residue, but this philosophy has been challenged in recent years. The use of fiber in the diet therapy of these patients has been shown to decrease symptoms and the frequency of relapses [2]. In areas of the world where individuals consume diets high in fiber, the incidence of this disease is low, suggesting a causal relationship [1]. For a more detailed discussion of fiber and its effect on health, see Chap. 25.

Case Studies

1. Mrs. Jones is a 43-year-old mother of three. She is overweight and has been told that her serum cholesterol is elevated. After a Sunday meal of deep-fried chicken, potato salad, and ice cream, she experienced an episode of sharp, colicky pain. Her physician told her she has gallstones. What foods could have precipitated the attack? What type of diet should she follow? Why do you think she has been bruising so easily; does it have any relationship to her condition?

2. Two years after a total gastrectomy, Mr. Smith's physician discovered that his patient had developed megaloblastic anemia. Mr. Smith had complained of a sore tongue (glossitis), loss of appetite, and recent weight loss. What is the relationship between the surgery and the development of the anemia?

3. Two-month-old Jimmy has just been diagnosed as having celiac disease. What would be a good choice for his first cereal at age 6 months? What would be appropriate desserts for him from ages 2 to 6? What foods would cause problems?

References

1. Brodribb, A. J. M.   Dietary fiber in diverticular disease of the colon. In G. A. Spiller and R. M. Kay (eds.), *Medical Aspects of Dietary Fiber.* New York: Plenum Press, 1980. Pp. 43–66.
2. Brodribb, A. J. M.   The treatment of diverticular disease with dietary fiber. *Lancet* 1:664, 1977.
3. Burton, B. T.   *Human Nutrition* (3rd ed.). New York: McGraw-Hill, 1976. P. 9.
4. Luke, B.   *Case Studies in Therapeutic Nutrition.* Boston: Little, Brown, 1977. Pp. 97–110.
5. Gastrointestinal diseases.   *Dietary Modifications in Disease.* Columbus, Ohio: Ross Labs, 1978. P. 9.

Suggested Readings

Allen, R., et al.   Crohn's disease involving the colon. *Gastroenterology* 73:723, 1977.
Almy, T. P.   The dietary fiber hypothesis. *Am. J. Clin. Nutr.* 34:432, 1981.
Ashkenazi, A., Levin, S., and Mishkin, A.   Immunoglobulin levels in children with celiac disease: Variations with age and diet. *Isr. J. Med. Sci.* 16:843, 1980.
Bliss, C. M.   Fat absorption and malabsorption. *Arch. Intern. Med.* 141:1213, 1981.
Burkitt, D. B.   Hiatus hernia: Is it preventable? *Am. J. Clin. Nutr.* 34:428, 1981.
Burkitt, D. B.   The role of dietary fiber. *Nutr. Today* 11:6, 1976.
Chandra, R. K., and Sahni, S.   Immunological aspects of gluten intolerance. *Nutr. Rev.* 39:117, 1981.
Chernoff, R., and Dean, J. A.   Medical and nutritional aspects of intractable diarrhea. *J. Am. Diet. Assoc.* 76:161, 1980.
Connell, A.   Dietary fiber and diverticular disease. *Hosp. Pract.* 11:119, 1976.
Graham, S., and Mettlin, C.   Diet and colon cancer. *Am. J. Epidemiol.* 109:1, 1979.
Gryboski, J.   False security of a gluten-free diet. *Am. J. Clin. Nutr.* 135:110, 1981.
Kirsner, J. B.   The irritable bowel syndrome. *Arch. Intern. Med.* 141:635, 1981.
Newmark, S. R.   The role of nutritional support in the treatment of gastrointestinal disease. *Surg. Clin. North Am.* 59:761, 1979.
Panel report on nutritional support of patients with gastrointestinal diseases.   *Am. J. Clin. Nutr.* 34:1206, 1981.
Rosenberg, I. H., Solomons, N. W., and Schneider, R. E.   Malabsorption associated with diarrhea and intestinal infections. *Am. J. Clin. Nutr.* 30:1248, 1977.
Samborsky, V.   Drug therapy for peptic ulcer. *Am. J. Nurs.* 78:2064, 1978.
Spiller, G. A., and Freeman, H. J.   Recent advances in dietary fiber and colorectal diseases. *Am. J. Clin. Nutr.* 34:1145, 1981.
Sturniolo, G. C., et al.   Zinc absorption in Crohn's disease. *Gut.* 21:387, 1980.

Thornton, J. R., Emmett, P. M., and Heaton, K. W.   Diet and Crohn's disease: Characteristics of the pre-illness diet. *Br. Med. J.* 2:762, 1979.

Thornton, J. R., Emmett, P. M., and Heaton, K. W.   Diet and ulcerative colitis. *Br. Med. J.* 1:293, 1980.

Thorpe, C. J., and Caprini, J. A.   Gallbladder disease: Current trends and treatments. *Am. J. Nurs.* 80:2181, 1980.

Werlin, S. L.   Growth failure in Crohn's disease: An approach to treatment. *J. Parent. and Ent. Nutr.* 5:250, 1981.

Zinc deficiency in Crohn's disease. *Nutr. Rev.* 40:109, 1982.

Chapter 39

DIABETES MELLITUS

Diabetes mellitus is a universal health problem affecting at least 30 million individuals throughout the world [1]. It is characterized by disorders in the metabolism of insulin, carbohydrate, fat, and protein, and by alterations in the structure and function of blood vessels and nerve tissue. The early symptoms of the disease are related to the metabolic effects; later, the findings are linked with complications from vascular changes.

Diabetes may be of two types. Type I, also known as *juvenile*, growth-onset, or ketosis-prone diabetes, accounts for about 5 percent of all cases; and type II, or *adult-onset* diabetes, accounts for approximately 95 percent of all cases. In juvenile diabetes, the primary abnormality is an absolute deficiency of insulin; in adult-onset, it is related more to a delayed release of endogenous insulin. The characteristics of these two types are compared in Table 39-1.

In this chapter, the normal function of insulin and the results when there are alterations in the production or utilization of this hormone will be presented. The drug and dietary treatment of diabetes will be discussed as well as the acute and chronic complications.

Chapters to review: Section II, Chapters 4, 36.

Insulin

The pancreas is composed of two different types of tissue—the *acinar cells*, which produce digestive enzymes, and the *islet cells* (also termed the *islets of Langerhans*). This second group of cells is present as several types—*alpha* cells, which produce glucagon; *C* cells and *delta* cells, of unknown function; and the *beta* cells, which constitute 60 to 80 percent of the cells of each islet and produce, store, and secrete insulin. The islet cells are surrounded by capillaries, which provide the insulin with a direct route into the bloodstream.

Special staining techniques make the alpha cells appear pink or red when viewed under the microscope; the insulin-containing granules of the beta cells appear deep bluish-purple. An injection of glucose into the bloodstream causes a depletion of the insulin granules of the beta cells within one-half hour. The abundance of the insulin granules is the result of demand and production. Glucagon, the hormone produced by the alpha cells, causes a rise in blood glucose, an action opposite to that of insulin (see Chap. 3, for more detail).

STRUCTURE

The hormone, insulin, is composed of two polypeptide chains (A and B) and has a molecular weight of about 6000. The A chain is composed of 21 amino acids and contains an internal disulfide bridge between two cystine molecules. The B chain contains 30 amino acids and is linked to the A chain by two disulfide bridges between molecules of cystine (see Fig. 39-1). The sequence of amino acids in each chain is unique to each species; differences occur primarily at positions 8, 9, and 10 on the A chain and at position 30 on the B chain. Pork, dog, and human insulin have the same amino acid sequence in the A chain, including identical amino acids at positions 8, 9, and 10. In the B chain, pork

TABLE 39-1. A comparison of essential features of type I and II diabetes

Features	Type I	Type II
Other names	Juvenile, growth-onset, ketosis-prone	Adult-onset, maturity-onset, ketosis-resistant
Age of onset	Usually under 35	Usually over 35
Type of onset	Abrupt (days to weeks)	Usually gradual (weeks to months)
Nutritional status at onset	Usually undernourished	Usually obese
Symptoms	Polydipsia, polyphagia, and polyuria	Frequently none
Ketosis	Frequent, unless diet, insulin, and exercise are properly coordinated	Infrequent, except in the presence of infection or stress
Endogenous insulin	Negligible to absent	Present; may be in excess but relatively ineffective because of obesity
Associated lipid abnormalities	Hypercholesterolemia frequent, particularly when control is suboptimal; all lipid fractions elevated in ketoacidosis	Cholesterol and triglycerides frequently elevated and related to obesity
Insulin	Needed for all patients	Necessary in only 20–30% of patients
Oral agents	Rarely efficacious, should not be used	Efficacious
Diet	Mandatory along with insulin for blood glucose control	Diet alone frequently sufficient to control blood glucose

Source: *Diabetes Mellitus.* Indianapolis: Eli Lilly, 1980. P. 2.

and dog insulin contain a different amino acid at position 30. Commercial preparations of insulin are frequently made from a combination of beef and pork zinc-insulin crystals. The differences in the amino acid sequences of insulin from different species do not affect its physiologic action in humans. To avoid the action of digestive enzymes, insulin must be injected subcutaneously.

FUNCTION

The main function of insulin is to promote the transfer of glucose across certain cell membranes. Many tissues, including skeletal and cardiac muscle, fibroblasts, and the cells of adipose tissue, do not permit the free entry of glucose into the cells. For these tissues (and others, as listed in Table 39-2), insulin reacts with key molecules of unknown identity on the surface and allows the entry of glucose into the cell. Other cells, such as red blood cells, brain cells, kidney, liver, and the cells of the intestinal mucosa, do not require insulin for the passage of glucose.

HISTORY AND TYPES

Drs. Charles H. Best and Frederick G. Banting discovered insulin in 1921 while working in a laboratory in Toronto. Within 2 years, commercially prepared insulin became available for individual use. The first insulin made available was amorphous insulin, followed by regular insulin. This latter type is made from zinc-insulin crystals. Regular insulin has its peak action from one-half to two hours after its administration.

Protamine zinc insulin was the result of research to prolong the glucose-lowering effect of regular insulin. In contrast to regular insulin, which is completely soluble at the pH of the body fluids, protamine zinc insulin has a very low solubility at that pH and is, therefore, absorbed much more slowly. The addition of protamine aids in the slow absorption. Protamine zinc insulin has a duration of action of about 14 to 24 hours or longer.

NPH insulin (also known as *Isophane*) is a combination of regular and protamine zinc insulin in a ratio of 2:1. This type of insulin incorporates some of the advantages of regular insulin and eliminates some of the disadvantages of protamine zinc insulin. The term *NPH* was derived from *N* for neutral; *P* for protamine; and *H* for Hagedorn, its discoverer.

It has been known for some time that zinc exerted a delaying action on the

FIG. 39-1. Primary structure of bovine insulin. (From I. Danishefsky, *Biochemistry for Medical Sciences.* Boston: Little, Brown, 1980.)

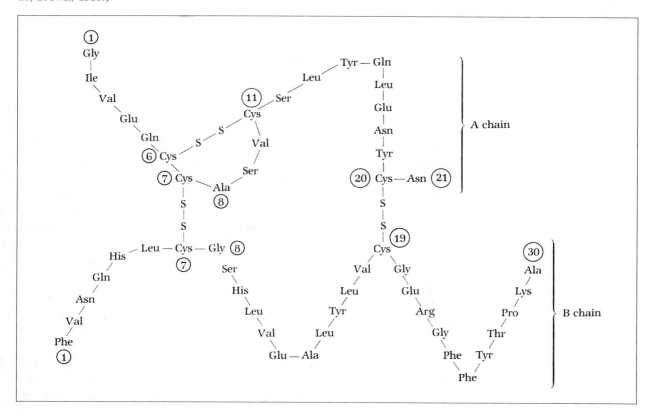

TABLE 39-2. Sensitivity of different tissues to insulin

INSULIN-SENSITIVE[a]	NOT INSULIN-SENSITIVE[b]
Muscle	Nerve tissues
Skeletal	Erythrocytes
Cardiac	Intestinal mucosa cells
Fibroblast	Kidney tubules
Mammary gland	Liver
Anterior pituitary	
Lens of the eye	
Aorta	

[a] Requires insulin for transfer of glucose.
[b] Does not require insulin for transfer of glucose.
Source: *Diabetes Mellitus*. Indianapolis: Eli Lilly, 1980. P. 23.

TABLE 39-3. Summary of available insulins

Type	Action	Peak activity (hours)	Duration (hours)
Regular	Rapid	2–4	5–7
NPH	Intermediate	6–12	24–28
Protamine zinc	Prolonged	14–24	36+
Semilente	Rapid	2–4	12–16
Lente	Intermediate	6–12	24–28
Ultralente	Prolonged	18–24	36+

Source: Lilly Preparations Used in the United States. In *Diabetes Mellitus*. Indianapolis: Eli Lilly, 1980. P. 42.

absorption of insulin, but it was not until 1951 that the exact mechanism was clarified. By increasing the amount of zinc in the insulin preparation, it was made even more insoluble at the pH of the body fluids. Three new types of insulin were created by varying the amount of added zinc. These include *ultralente*, the very long-acting crystalline form; *semilente*, the shorter-acting amorphous form; and *lente*, made of 70% ultralente and 30% semilente. This last type of insulin has almost identical characteristics to NPH insulin, but is free of the foreign modifying protein, protamine. The peak activity and duration of the lente insulins and others is given in Table 39-3. Recently, scientists have successfully produced biologic carbon copies of human insulin from bacteria. *Humulin* is a biosynthetic product manufactured using *E. coli* produced by recombinant DNA technology [2]. One bacterial form synthesizes the A chain, the other the B chain. Disulfide bridges are then formed chemically. This new type of insulin is available as regular, NPH, Humulin R (duration of 6–8 hours), and Humulin N (duration about 24 hours). Biosynthetic human insulin may be useful in those individuals who might develop allergies to animal insulin. The future implications of this exciting breakthrough have yet to be fully appreciated [3].

Classifications

Prediabetes is a period before overt clinical signs of diabetes, such as hyperglycemia, can be detected, but during which time subtle changes are taking place that eventually progress to the full disease. Individuals in whom these changes occur are usually members of the families of known diabetics, indicating that diabetes is most likely a hereditary disease.

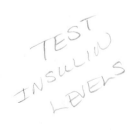

Insulin levels tend to be higher and blood glucose levels lower in prediabetics. Also, substances that inhibit the action of insulin have been found in the plasma of both prediabetics and diabetics. Insulin circulates in at least two forms, free and bound, or typical and atypical. The diabetic and prediabetic have more of the bound or atypical form than the nondiabetic individual. Long before any functional abnormality is present, the basement membrane in the glomerular capillaries of the kidneys shows a thickening in prediabetics. The pattern and size of the conjunctival blood vessels (the mucous membrane covering the anterior portion of the eyeball) is different in diabetics and prediabetics.

It is now evident that the prediabetic is actually a diabetic before the metabolic abnormalities become apparent. With time, the secretion of insulin by the beta cells of the pancreas becomes inadequate, resulting in metabolic diabetes.

Juvenile diabetes (type I or insulin-dependent) is the term used to describe the appearance of metabolic diabetes that first occurs any time from birth to age 20. During the early stages, there may be hypertrophy of the beta cells, which causes hypernormal insulinlike activity in the plasma. The first symptom may be an acute crisis, such as coma. During this time, the insulin requirement will usually be very high. Remission may take place after several months of treatment, during which time the insulin requirement may be drastically reduced or even eliminated for many months. With time, however, the beta cells eventually atrophy, resulting in a lifelong need for exogenous insulin.

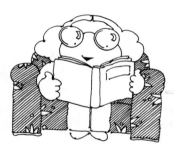

Juvenile diabetes is characterized by being "brittle," or unstable. Small changes in insulin dosages can cause ketosis with coma or hypoglycemia and the danger of brain damage. In addition, the daily routine of a child tends to fluctuate between sedentary schoolwork and rigorous exercise, causing wide fluctuations in insulin requirements. Because a child is still growing, the diet for the juvenile diabetic must be changed frequently to provide for normal growth.

Maturity-onset (type II or non-insulin-dependent) diabetes is usually much milder than the juvenile form. It is frequently due to the delayed release of endogenous insulin, as compared to the absolute insulin deficiency seen in growth-onset diabetes. This type of diabetes may often be controlled by oral antidiabetic agents, such as acetohexamide (Dymelor), chlorpropamide (Diabinese), tolbutamide (Orinase), or tolazamide (Tolinase), which stimulate the pancreas to release insulin and a regulated diabetic diet. See the appendix at the end of this chapter for more information on those drugs.

Metabolic Alterations

The term *diabetes mellitus* comes from the Greek, *diabetes*, meaning siphon, and from the Latin, *mel*, meaning honey. This disease is a hereditary metabolic disorder characterized by a decrease in or absence of endogenous insulin pro-

TABLE 39-4. Symptoms of diabetes mellitus

Clinical symptoms	Pathophysiology
Polydipsia (excessive thirst)	Renal threshold for sugar exceeded, secondary to increased osmolarity of the urine (glycosuria)
Polyphagia (excessive eating)	Metabolic attempt to compensate for nutrients lost in the urine
Polyuria (excessive urination)	Water passively excreted, secondary to increased osmolarity of the urine
Weight loss	Poor utilization of ingested nutrients, secondary to insulin deficiency
Weakness	Loss of nutrients in the urine (glycosuria)
Urinary infections	Secondary to the glycosuria, providing a medium for bacterial growth
Pruritus (itching)	Secondary to glycosuria, irritating the skin

duction and/or utilization. Insulin deficiency results in altered carbohydrate metabolism, including impaired intracellular glucose breakdown, decreased conversion to fat, and defective glycogen formation. The clinical manifestations of this alteration in carbohydrate metabolism include the accumulation of glucose in the blood (hyperglycemia) and the spillage of glucose in the urine (glycosuria) (see Table 39-4 for a summary of the symptoms of diabetes mellitus). Since glucose cannot be used effectively without adequate insulin, the body breaks down fat to supply metabolic fuel. This results in an abnormal accumulation of the end products of incomplete fat metabolism. These end products are acetoacetic acid, hydroxybutyric acid, and acetone, known collectively as ketones. The accumulation of ketones in the blood leads to ketosis and acidosis, and, eventually, acidotic coma. The metabolic alterations secondary to diabetes mellitus are related to changes in capillaries and small blood vessels, accelerated changes in larger blood vessels, and damage to nervous tissue. Manifestations of these changes are seen in the form of renal and neurologic complications, obstruction of the circulation in the extremities, and progressive blood vessel damage in the retina of the eye (see Table 39-5).

Complications
INSULIN SHOCK

The two most serious acute complications of diabetes mellitus include *hypoglycemic reactions* and *diabetic coma*. Hypoglycemic reactions, also known as *insulin shock*, are caused by an overdose of insulin; a delay in eating; vomiting or diarrhea; or an increase in exercise without a decrease in insulin dosage or increase in food intake. The progression to insulin shock can be rapid, within minutes for the diabetic on regular insulin or within hours for those using modified insulin or oral agents. The individual may feel weak, nervous, hungry, dizzy, or faint. Nausea and vomiting may follow and, if not treated, insulin shock may progress to coma and, eventually, death. The urine is usually negative for glucose or acetone; the blood glucose level may be 60 mg per 100 ml or less. The immediate treatment for insulin shock is any readily available carbohydrate. If

TABLE 39-5. Manifestations of the complications of diabetes

Eyes	Retinopathy, cataract formation, glaucoma, and extraocular muscle palsies
Mouth	Gingivitis, increased incidence of dental caries, periodontal disease, and greater resorption of alveolar bone
Pregnancy	Increased incidence of large babies, stillbirths, miscarriages, neonatal deaths, and congenital defects
Nervous system	Motor, sensory, and autonomic neuropathy
Vascular system	Large-vessel disease and microangiopathy
Skin	Xanthoma diabeticorum, necrobiosis lipoidica diabeticorum, furunculosis, mycosis, and pruritus
Kidneys	Diabetic glomerulosclerosis, arteriolar nephrosclerosis, and pyelonephritis

Source: *Diabetes Mellitus.* Indianapolis: Eli Lilly, 1980. P. 179.

the patient is conscious, any fruit juice, sugar, honey, or candy may be given, with recovery occurring within minutes. If the patient is unconscious, intravenous glucose must be given. The patient must always be aware of the relationship between diet, insulin dosage, and activity level. To avoid the possibility of insulin shock, some form of sugar or hard candy should always be carried by the individual.

DIABETIC COMA

Diabetic coma is caused by actions opposite to those that lead to insulin shock. It occurs when extra food is eaten for which the insulin dosage did not provide, or when the insulin dosage was inadequate or omitted entirely. Infection or trauma in the diabetic can lead to diabetic acidosis and coma. Sometimes undetected diabetes can first manifest as diabetic coma. The symptoms are similar to insulin shock; the diagnosis is difficult to make unless the events prior to the onset of symptoms are known. The individual feels weak, nauseated, and may have a headache, abdominal pains, and skin that is flushed, dry, and hot. Rapid breathing and drowsiness follow, progressing to coma and, eventually, death. The urine is positive for glucose and acetone; the blood glucose level is always greater than 250 mg per 100 ml. Diabetic coma is a medical emergency and requires treatment by a physician in a hospital. The therapy includes large doses of regular insulin with smaller doses every hour until the blood glucose level is reduced to below 200 mg per 100 ml. Fluids and alkali therapy are given to correct the dehydration and severe acidosis.

These two acute complications are compared in Table 39-6.

FACTORS AFFECTING THERAPY

The treatment of juvenile-onset diabetes is a challenge that demands multidisciplinary attention. Support of both the patient and family is needed if therapy is to be effective. Often precipitated by an infectious and/or acute illness, juvenile diabetes is frequently difficult to control. Intercurrent infections may quickly and unexpectedly throw the young diabetic into an acidotic state. Insulin injections often contribute to the emotional response of both patients and their parents to

TABLE 39-6. Differential diagnosis of diabetic coma and hypoglycemic reactions

Features	Diabetic coma	Hypoglycemic reactions	
		Regular insulin	Modified insulin or oral agents
Onset	Slow (days)	Sudden (minutes)	Gradual (hours)
Causes	Ignorance Neglect of therapy Intercurrent disease or infection	Overdosage Omission or delay of meals Excessive exercise before meals	

Symptoms	Thirst, headache, nausea,
	  vomiting, abdominal
	  pain, dim vision,
	  dyspnea, constipation
		"Inward nervousness"
		Hunger, sweating
		
		Weakness
		Diplopia
		Blurred vision
		Paresthesia
		Psychopathic behavior
		Stupor and convulsions
			Fatigue, headache, nausea,
			  sweating (sometimes absent)

Signs	Florid face, air hunger
	  (Kussmaul's respiration)
	Finally, respiratory
	  paralysis
	Dehydration (dry skin)
	Rapid pulse
	Soft eyeballs
	Normal or absent reflexes
	Acetone breath
		Pallor
		Shallow respiration
		Sweating
		Normal pulse
		
		Eyeballs normal
		Babinski's reflex often present
			Skin may be dry

Source: *Diabetes Mellitus*. Indianapolis: Eli Lilly, 1980. P. 168.

the disease. Emotional factors may also influence the course of juvenile diabetes, particularly during adolescence when the restrictions imposed by the disease may be viewed as just another pressure from which to rebel [4]. Three changing factors, each operating independently but exerting a cumulative effect on both disease and therapy, contribute to the difficulties in the management of juvenile diabetes. Blood sugar levels are very labile in these children; hypoglycemia and hyperglycemia become real dangers. Physical activity is erratic in all children, but in diabetics it can quickly raise or lower insulin needs [5]. Nutritional requirements are constantly changing, influenced by growth spurts and hormonal changes.

Although the maturity-onset diabetic may present a less severe form of the disease, there are problems unique to this age group also. They may be overweight and sedentary, two factors that aggravate the diabetes. With weight loss and exercise, many of these diabetics can be advanced from insulin to oral agents to diet alone. Loneliness may be a problem in this older age group and meals may take on more importance than just nutrition or pleasure. In the elderly, eyesight may be failing, making written instructions and insulin injections difficult. The inclusion of family members and/or the public health nurse to help interpret and reinforce the diet and drug therapy for the diabetic can n difference between success and failure.

Dietary Recommendations

The nutritional needs of the diabetic are essentially the same as for the non-diabetic. A nutritionally complete diet of a variety of foods is best; special supplements and diet foods are not necessary. The amount, distribution, and timing of food intake are important, however, for both diabetics on insulin and those taking oral hypoglycemic agents. Since diet therapy will be a lifelong component of most diabetics' lives, it should remain as flexible as possible. In those diabetics requiring insulin, the insulin regimen should be adapted to the individual's basic eating habits whenever possible for maximum freedom of choice and optimal control [6].

EXCHANGE LISTS

To simplify meal planning for the diabetic, foods are grouped into six *exchange lists* (see the chapter appendix on pp. 674–679). Each item within an exchange list has the same amount of protein, fat, carbohydrate, and calories in the portion specified as any other item in that list. For example, one fruit exchange equals 10 gm of carbohydrate and 40 calories. Two small apricots are equal to one fruit exchange, as is one small orange. In a meal pattern that includes one fruit exchange as an afternoon snack, either one small orange or two small apricots could be eaten, or any other item in the fruit exchange list in the quantities specified.

Any food that is added in meal preparation must be calculated using the exchange lists. This includes homemade recipes (such as beef stew, tuna casserole, franks and beans) and foods eaten in restaurants (e.g., combination hamburgers, fried chicken dinners, submarine sandwiches, pizzas). This may seem difficult to do, but with more public awareness of nutrition in recent years it actually is quite simple. More and more products have nutrition labeling, which states the serving size, amount of protein, fat, carbohydrate, calories, vitamins, and minerals per serving (see Chap. 20). More canned fruits are being offered either packed in their own juices or in water. Many of the fast-food restaurant chains, because of consumer demand, have made available a breakdown of their products in terms of exchange lists [7, 8]. With practice and careful planning, the diabetic diet can be varied and delicious and will hardly seem like a diet at all.

RECENT REVISIONS

In 1950, the concept of exchange lists was first introduced and did much to simplify the planning and application of the diabetic diet. Recently, the exchange lists have been revised by the American Diabetes Association, the American Dietetic Association, and the National Institute of Health in view of newer knowledge of good nutrition. These revisions include the use of nonfat milk as the basic milk exchange; starchy vegetables now appear under the bread exchange list;

lean meat is the basic meat exchange, with medium-fat meat and high-fat meat forming two new categories; and the distinction between saturated and polyunsaturated fat in the fat exchange list. These changes reflect the new awareness of the role of fat and sodium in the etiology of chronic diseases.

Diet Prescription

The factors to consider when planning the diet prescription [9] include the individual's height and weight; caloric needs; division of calories into protein, fat, and carbohydrate; and division of nutrients into meals and snacks. From Fig. 39-2, determine the individual's weight and height and caloric needs. Next, the caloric allowance is divided into 20 percent for protein, 45 to 70 percent for carbohydrate, and 30 to 55 percent for fat. Meals usually contain between $\frac{2}{10}$ to $\frac{4}{10}$ of the carbohydrate and calories; snacks usually contain $\frac{1}{10}$ of the carbohydrate and calories. For those individuals on oral agents or diet alone, food is usually divided into three meals per day. For those diabetics taking insulin, the diet is divided into three meals and two snacks per day.

FIG. 39-2. Calculation of weight and height and caloric needs. (From *The Effective Application of Exchange Lists for Meal Planning.* Chicago: American Diabetes Association and American Dietetic Association, 1977. P. 19.)

I. Weight and height

Build	Women	Men	Children
Medium	Allow 100 lb for first 5 ft of height plus 5 lb for each additional in.	Allow 106 lb for first 5 ft, plus 6 lb for each additional in.	Chart growth pattern on graph every 3–6 months (Wetzel, Iowa, or Stuart)
Small	Subtract 10%	Subtract 10%	
Large	Add 10%	Add 10%	

II. Caloric needs (see appropriate chapters in Section VI for specific caloric requirements throughout the life cycle).
  A. For adults
    1. Basal calories equals desirable weight (lb) × 10.
    2. Add activity calories
      a. Sedentary equals desirable weight (lb) × 3.
      b. Moderate equals desirable weight (lb) × 5.
      c. Strenuous equals desirable weight (lb) × 10.
    3. Add calories for indicated weight gain, growth (pregnant women), or lactation.
    4. Subtract calories for indicated weight loss.
  B. For children
    1. Children vary markedly in their caloric needs depending on rate of growth and level of activity.
    2. Estimate caloric requirement from Recommended Daily Dietary Allowances.
    3. Adjust caloric intake as needed to maintain normal rate of growth.

The following examples illustrate how to calculate the number of grams each of protein, fat, and carbohydrate in a diet prescription (rounded off to nearest 5).

	Juvenile diabetic (2255 cal)	Maturity-onset diabetic (3000 cal)	Maturity-onset diabetic (1200 cal)
PROTEIN			
20% of calories ÷ 4 calories	$20\% \times 2255 = 451$ $\dfrac{451}{4} = 115$ gm	$20\% \times 3000 = 600$ $\dfrac{600}{4} = 150$ gm	$20\% \times 1200 = 240$ $\dfrac{240}{4} = 60$ gm
CARBOHYDRATE			
45% of calories ÷ 4 calories	$45\% \times 2255 = 1015$ $\dfrac{1015}{4} = 255$ gm	$45\% \times 3000 = 1350$ $\dfrac{1350}{4} = 340$ gm	$45\% \times 1200 = 540$ $\dfrac{540}{4} = 135$ gm
FAT			
35% of calories ÷ 9 calories/gram	$35\% \times 225 = 79$ $\dfrac{79}{9} = 9$ gm	$35\% \times 3000 = 1050$ $\dfrac{1050}{9} = 115$ gm	$35\% \times 1200 = 420$ $\dfrac{420}{9} = 45$ gm

Once the calories have been divided into the appropriate percentages of protein, carbohydrate, and fat, the next step is to translate these figures into exchanges. In insulin-dependent diabetics, it is particularly important to plan a carbohydrate-containing bedtime snack if they are using intermediate or long-acting insulin.

The 1200-calorie diabetic reducing diet would translate into the following daily food plan.

	MENU	EXCHANGE
Breakfast	1 soft-boiled egg	1 meat (med. fat)
	1 slice toast	1 bread
	4 oz orange juice	1 fruit
Midmorning	8 oz whole milk	1 milk plus 2 fat
Lunch	2 oz tuna fish	2 meat
	9 saltine crackers	1½ bread
	Lettuce and tomato	
	Iced tea	
Midafternoon	2 graham cracker squares	1 bread
	Fresh sliced apple	1 fruit
Dinner	3 oz broiled hamburger	3 meat
	¾ cup white rice	1½ bread
	Steamed broccoli	1 vegetable
	Coffee	
Bedtime	8 oz whole milk	1 milk plus 2 fat
	2 graham cracker squares	1 bread

It is very important for the daily meal plan to be practical and accepted by the patient. Consideration of life-style, cultural foods and habits, economics, and food preferences should be included when devising the diet. Since adherence to the dietary regimen is vital to good metabolic control, the patient should be included in its planning for best acceptance.

Case Studies

1. Betsey is a 10-year-old juvenile diabetic who is going on a camping trip with her Girl Scout troop. Besides her insulin, what other things might be useful to bring along for the treatment of her diabetes, and why? She has volunteered her mother to bring dessert to a cookout one evening after a hike: Which of the following would be best and why: fruit compote, cherry pie, or chocolate layer cake?

2. Mr. Jones, a 42-year-old man known to have diabetes mellitus, is brought into the emergency room unconscious. He is accompanied by his wife. What questions would you want to ask his wife and what laboratory tests would you want to perform to make the differential diagnosis of insulin shock versus diabetic coma?

3. A newly diagnosed maturity-onset diabetic complains that she will not be able to use any of her recipes anymore. How would you translate the following recipe into exchange lists?

STUFFED PEPPERS
3 large green peppers
½ lb ground beef
1 cup tomato juice
1 slice stale bread, in pieces
1 tsp salt
¼ tsp pepper
1 tbsp chopped onion

References

1. World Health Organization. *W.H.O. Expert Committee on Diabetes Mellitus.* Geneva: W.H.O., 1980. P. 7.
2. Human insulin. *Med. Lett. Drugs Ther.* 25:63, 1983.
3. From the NIH. Insulin and human growth hormone: Triumphs in genetic engineering. *J.A.M.A.* 245:1724, 1981.
4. Guthrie, D. W., and Guthrie, R. A. Diabetes in adolescence. *Am. J. Nurs.* 75:1740, 1975.
5. Koivisto, V. A., and Felig, P. Effects of leg exercise on insulin absorption in diabetic patients. *N. Engl. J. Med.* 298:79, 1978.
6. Nuttall, F. Q. Dietary recommendations for individuals with diabetes mellitus, 1979: Summary of report from the Food and Nutrition Committee of the American Diabetes Association. *Am. J. Clin. Nutr.* 33:1311, 1980.
7. Diabetic food exchange list for McDonald's restaurants. McDonald's System, Inc., 1977.
8. Midgley, W. On the fast food trail: How to handle eating on the go. *Diabetes Forecast* 32:20, 1979.

9. American Diabetes Association and American Dietetics Association. A guide for professionals: The effective application of "exchange lists for meal planning." 1977.
10. *Exchange Lists for Meal Planning*. American Diabetes Association and American Dietetic Association, 1976.

Suggested Readings

The American Diabetes Association/The American Dietetic Association Family Cookbook. Englewood Cliffs, N.J.: Prentice-Hall, 1980. P. 391.

Arbogast, K. K. *Exchange Lists and Diet Patterns.* New York: Van Nostrand Reinhold, 1980. P. 340.

Bohannon, N. V., Karam, J. H., and Forsham, P. H. Endocrine responses to sugar ingestion in man. *J. Am. Diet. Assoc.* 76:555, 1980.

Cook, K. A. Diabetics can be vegetarians. *Nurs. 79* October. Pp. 70–73.

Finsand, M. J. *The Complete Diabetic Cookbook.* New York: Sterling, 1980. P. 192.

Giordano, B. P., and Edwards, L. L. Meeting the needs of the parents of children with diabetes: A babysitter's course. *Diabetes Educ.* 6:26, 1980.

Gorsuch, A. N., et al. Evidence for a long prediabetic period in type I (insulin-dependent) diabetes mellitus. *Lancet* 2:1363, 1981.

Greene, G. Behavior modification for adult onset diabetes. *Diabetes Educ.* 7:11, 1981.

Guidelines for the nutritional management of diabetes mellitus: 1980. A special report from the Canadian Diabetes Association. *J. Can. Diet. Assoc.* 42:110, 1981.

Helsel, J., and Lansing, E. *The ABC's of Diabetic Cooking and Dining.* New York: Dell, 1979. P. 96.

High-fibre diets and diabetes (editorial). *Lancet* 1:423, 1981.

How diabetics can dine out gourmet style. *Institutions* 87:186, 1980.

Jackson, R. L., et al. Growth and maturation of children with insulin-dependent diabetes mellitus. *Diabetes Care* 1:96, 1978.

Jenkins, D. J. A., et al. Diabetic Diets: High carbohydrate combined with high fiber. *Am. J. Clin. Nutr.* 33:1729, 1980.

Manhire, A., et al. Unrefined carbohydrate and dietary fibre in treatment of diabetes mellitus. *J. Hum. Nutr.* 35:99, 1981.

McCarthy, J. A. Diabetic nephropathy. *Am. J. Nurs.* 81:2030, 1981.

McDonald, J. Alcohol and diabetes. *Diabetes Care* 5:629, 1980.

Nuttall, F. Q., and Brunzell, J. D. Special report: Principles of nutrition and dietary recommendations for individuals with diabetes mellitus: 1979. *Diabetes* 28:1028, 1979.

Sims, D. F. (ed.). *Diabetes: Reach for Health and Freedom.* St. Louis: Mosby, 1980. P. 128.

So, B., Chew, D., and Bright-See, E. Dietetic counseling of Chinese diabetic patients. *J. Can. Diet. Assoc.* 39:46, 1978.

Teller, J. Vegetarian meal planning for the diabetic. *Diabetes Educ.* 5:13, 1979.

Appendix

DRUGS MENTIONED IN CHAPTER 39:
DESCRIPTION OF THE ORAL HYPOGLYCEMIC SULFONYLUREA COMPOUNDS

Acetohexamide (Dymelor). This intermediate-acting compound is related to tolbutamide, but is longer acting. Onset: 3–4 hours; Peak: 3 hours; Duration: 12–14 hours.

Chlorpropamide (Diabinese). This agent is also related to tolbutamide, but is the longest-acting sulfonylurea compound. Onset: 1 hour; Peak: 3–6 hours; Duration: 72 hours.

Tolazamide (Tolinase).   Also related to tolbutamide, but this agent is five times more potent. Onset: 4–6 hours; Peak: 4–8 hours; Duration: 10 hours.

Tolbutamide (Orinase).   This short-acting antidiabetic agent lowers the blood sugar by stimulating the pancreas to produce and secrete insulin. Onset: 30 min.; Peak: 3–5 hours; Duration: 6–12 hours.

Depending on the agent used, it is important to space the carbohydrate intake to match the onset and peak actions of the medications. Especially for the intermediate and long-acting oral hypoglycemic agents, a bedtime snack should always be included.

LIST 1: MILK EXCHANGES

One exchange of milk contains 12 gm carbohydrate, 8 gm protein, a trace of fat, and 80 cal.

NONFAT FORTIFIED MILK	SERVING SIZE
Skim or nonfat milk	1 cup
Powdered (nonfat dry)	⅓ cup
Canned, evaporated skim milk	½ cup
Buttermilk made from skim milk	1 cup
Yogurt made from skim milk (plain, unflavored)	1 cup
LOW-FAT FORTIFIED MILK	
1% fat fortified milk (omit ½ fat exchange)	1 cup
2% fat fortified milk (omit 1 fat exchange)	1 cup
Yogurt made from 2% fortified milk (omit 1 fat exchange)	1 cup
WHOLE MILK (OMIT 2 FAT EXCHANGES)	
Whole milk	1 cup
Canned, evaporated whole milk	½ cup
Buttermilk made from whole milk	1 cup
Yogurt made from whole milk (plain, unflavored)	1 cup

LIST 2: VEGETABLE EXCHANGES

One exchange is ½ cup and contains about 5 gm carbohydrate, 2 gm protein, and 25 cal.

Asparagus	Greens (continued)
Bean sprouts	Mustard
Beets	Spinach
Broccoli	Turnip
Brussels sprouts	Mushrooms
Cabbage	Okra
Carrots	Onions
Cauliflower	Rhubarb
Celery	Rutabaga
Eggplant	Sauerkraut
Green pepper	String beans, green or yellow
Greens	Summer squash
Beet	Tomatoes
Chards	Tomato juice
Collards	Turnips
Dandelion	Vegetable juice cocktail
Kale	Zucchini

The following raw vegetables may be used as desired

Chicory	Lettuce
Chinese cabbage	Parsley
Cucumbers	Pickles, dill
Endive	Radishes
Escarole	Watercress

Starchy vegetables are found in the Bread Exchange List.

LIST 3: FRUIT EXCHANGES   One exchange contains 10 gm carbohydrate and 40 cal.

Apple	1 small
Apple juice	⅓ cup
Applesauce (unsweetened)	½ cup
Apricots, fresh	2 medium
Apricots, dried	4 halves
Banana	½ small
Berries	
Blackberries	½ cup
Blueberries	½ cup
Raspberries	½ cup
Strawberries	¾ cup
Cherries	10 large
Cider	⅓ cup
Dates	2
Figs, fresh	1
Figs, dried	1
Grapefruit	½
Grapefruit juice	½ cup
Grapes	12
Grape juice	¼ cup
Mango	½ small
Melon	
Cantaloupe	¼ small
Honeydew	⅛ medium
Watermelon	1 cup
Nectarine	1 small
Orange	1 small
Orange juice	½ cup
Papaya	¾ cup
Peach	1 medium
Pear	1 small
Persimmon, native	1 medium
Pineapple	½ cup
Pineapple juice	⅓ cup
Plums	2 medium
Prunes	2 medium
Prune juice	¼ cup
Raisins	2 tbsp
Tangerine	1 medium

LIST 4: BREAD EXCHANGES   One exchange contains 15 gm carbohydrate, 2 gm protein, and 70 cal.

BREAD	SERVING SIZE
White (including French and Italian)	1 slice
Whole wheat	1 slice
Rye or pumpernickel	1 slice
Raisin	1 slice
Bagel, small	½
English muffin, small	½
Plain roll, bread	1
Frankfurter roll	½
Hamburger bun	½
Dried bread crumbs	1 tbsp
Tortilla, 6 in.	1

CEREAL	
Bran flakes	½ cup
Other ready-to-eat unsweetened cereal	¾ cup
Puffed cereal (unfrosted)	1 cup
Cereal (cooked)	½ cup
Grits (cooked)	½ cup
Rice or barley (cooked)	½ cup
Pasta (cooked)	½ cup
Spaghetti, noodles, macaroni	
Popcorn (popped, no fat added, large kernel)	3 cups
Cornmeal (dry)	2 tbsp
Flour	2½ tbsp
Wheat germ	¼ cup

CRACKERS	
Arrowroot	3
Graham, 2½ in. square	2
Matzo, 4 in. × 6 in.	½
Oyster	20
Pretzels, 3⅛ in. × ⅛ in.	25
Rye wafers, 2 in. × 3½ in.	3
Saltines	6
Soda, 2½-in. square	4

DRIED BEANS, PEAS, AND LENTILS	
Beans, peas, and lentils (dried and cooked)	½ cup
Baked beans (canned, no pork)	¼ cup

STARCHY VEGETABLES	
Corn	⅓ cup
Corn on cob	1 small
Lima beans	½ cup
Parsnips	⅔ cup
Peas, green	½ cup
Potato, white	1 small
Potato, mashed	½ cup
Pumpkin	¾ cup
Winter squash, acorn or butternut	½ cup
Yam or sweet potato	¼ cup

PREPARED FOODS	SERVING SIZE
Biscuit, 2 in. diagonal (omit 1 fat exchange)	1
Corn bread, 2 in. × 2 in. × 1 in. (omit 1 fat exchange)	1
Corn muffin, 2 in. diagonal (omit 1 fat exchange)	1
Crackers, round butter type (omit 1 fat exchange)	5
Muffin, plain small (omit 1 fat exchange)	1
Potatoes, french fried, length 2–3½ in. (omit 1 fat exchange)	8
Potato or corn chips (omit 2 fat exchanges)	15
Pancake, 5 in. × ½ in. (omit 1 fat exchange)	1
Waffle, 5 in. × ½ in. (omit 1 fat exchange)	1

LIST 5: MEAT EXCHANGES

LEAN MEAT EXCHANGES

One exchange of lean meat (1 oz) contains 7 gm protein, 3 gm fat, and 55 cal.

Beef	Baby beef (very lean), chipped beef, chuck, flank steak, tenderloin, plate ribs, plate skirt steak, round (bottom, top), all cuts rump, spare ribs, tripe	1 oz
Lamb	Leg, rib, sirloin, loin (roast and chops), shank, shoulder	1 oz
Pork	Leg (whole rump, center shank), ham, smoked (center slices)	1 oz
Veal	Leg, loin, rib, shank, shoulder, cutlets	1 oz
Poultry	Meat (without skin) of chicken, turkey, cornish hen, guinea hen, pheasant	1 oz
Fish	Any fresh or frozen fish	1 oz
	Canned salmon, tuna, mackerel, crab and lobster	¼ cup
	Clams, oysters, scallops, shrimp	5 or 1 oz
	Sardines, drained	3
Cheeses containing less than 5% butterfat		1 oz
Cottage cheese, dry and 2% butterfat		¼ cup
Dried beans and peas (omit 1 bread exchange)		½ cup

MEDIUM-FAT MEAT EXCHANGES

One exchange of medium-fat meat (1 oz) contains 7 gm protein, 5 gm fat, and 75 cal.

Beef	Ground (15% fat), corned beef (canned), rib eye, round (ground commercial)	1 oz
Pork	Loin (all cuts tenderloin), shoulder arm (picnic), shoulder blade, Boston butt, Canadian bacon, boiled ham	1 oz
Liver, heart, kidney, and sweetbreads (these are high in cholesterol)		1 oz
Cottage cheese, creamed		¼ cup

Cheese	Mozzarella, ricotta, farmer's cheese, neufchatel, parmesan	1 oz/3 tbsp
Egg (high in cholesterol)		1
Peanut butter (omit 2 additional fat exchanges)		2 tbsp

HIGH-FAT MEAT EXCHANGES
One exchange (1 oz) contains 7 gm protein, 8 gm fat, and 100 cal.

Beef	Brisket, corned beef (brisket), ground beef (more than 20% fat), hamburger (commercial), chuck (ground commercial), roasts (rib), steaks (club and rib)	1 oz
Lamb	Breast	1 oz
Pork	Spare ribs, loin (back ribs), pork (ground), country style ham, deviled ham	1 oz
Veal	Breast	1 oz
Poultry	Capon, duck (domestic), goose	1 oz
Cheese	Cheddar types	1 oz
Cold cuts		4½ in. × ⅛ in. slice
Frankfurter		1 small

LIST 6: FAT EXCHANGES
One exchange contains 5 gm fat and 45 cal.

POLYUNSATURATED FATS	SERVING SIZE
Margarine, soft, tub, or stick[a]	1 tsp
Avocado (4 in. in diameter)[b]	⅛
Oil, corn, cottonseed, safflower, soy, or sunflower	1 tsp
Oil, olive[b]	1 tsp
Oil, peanut[b]	1 tsp
Olives[b]	5 small
Almonds[b]	10 whole
Pecans[b]	2 large whole
Peanuts[b]	
Spanish	20 whole
Virginia	10 whole
Walnuts	6 small
Nuts, other[b]	6 small
SATURATED FATS	
Margarine, regular stick	1 tsp
Butter	1 tsp
Bacon fat	1 tsp
Bacon, crisp	1 strip
Cream, heavy	2 tbsp
Cream, light	2 tbsp
Cream, sour	2 tbsp
Cream cheese	1 tbsp

SATURATED FATS (continued)	SERVING SIZE
French dressing[c]	1 tbsp
Italian dressing[c]	1 tbsp
Lard	1 tsp
Mayonnaise[c]	1 tsp
Salad dressing, mayonnaise type[c]	2 tsp
Salt pork	¾-in. cube

[a] Made with corn, cottonseed, safflower, soy, or sunflower oil only.
[b] Fat content is primarily monounsaturated.
[c] If made with corn, cottonseed, safflower, soy, or sunflower oil, can be used on fat-modified diet.

Chapter 40

CARDIOVASCULAR DISEASES

Nearly 40 percent of all persons living in the United States will eventually die of cardiovascular disease [1]. In 1979, the percent of total deaths from diseases of the heart and cerebrovascular diseases totaled 49.3 percent [2]. Also known as coronary artery disease, arteriosclerosis, or "hardening of the arteries," this disease is characterized by degenerative changes in the arteries caused by the deposition of lipids, carbohydrates, calcium, fibrous tissue, blood, and blood products. These changes result in a thickening of the lining of the artery wall, loss of elasticity, and progressive narrowing of the blood vessels supplying vital organs. Changes in the arteries may be generalized, or may be more localized to certain areas or organs, such as the heart, brain, kidneys, lungs, or extremities. Atherosclerosis, a common type of arteriosclerosis, affects the lining of the aorta, cerebral, and coronary blood vessels. When the damaged, narrowed vessel finally occludes completely, it blocks the passage of blood (and the nutrients and oxygen blood carries) and causes necrosis and death of the deprived tissue. Cerebrovascular accident, or stroke, is caused by the occlusion of an artery in the brain. When the blockage occurs in the coronary arteries in the heart, it results in *myocardial infarction*, death of the heart muscle, claiming more than half a million lives in the United States each year. A summary of heart facts is given in Table 40-1.

This chapter will present the pathogenesis of cardiovascular disease and the preventive and therapeutic measures used to treat it. Special emphasis is on the role of cholesterol and the current diet therapy used to lower plasma levels.

Chapters to review: Chapters 5, 11, 21.

Pathogenesis of Cardiovascular Disease

The process of arteriosclerosis is a slow one, beginning in early life and taking decades to develop [3]. Vessels become clogged by a material called *plaque*, a mixture of cells, scar tissue, and fat, which narrows the vessel's lumen. Symptoms appear when the tissues supplied by the diseased vessels do not receive enough oxygen or nutrients.

The wall of a healthy blood vessel is lined by endothelial cells, which produce *prostacyclin*, a type of prostaglandin that prevents circulating blood platelets from adhering and clumping to the vessel walls. This substance arises from the underlying smooth muscle layer; ironically, most of the arteriosclerotic plaques also arise from the smooth muscle. When the lining of endothelial cells is disrupted, such as by high blood pressure or by the toxic effects of circulating materials, such as high cholesterol levels, the production of prostacyclin is interrupted, allowing circulating platelets to adhere to the exposed underlying wall. The clumps of platelets may also trigger proliferation of cells from the smooth muscle layer. The fat present in the plaque is derived primarily from the fat in the large lipoprotein molecules circulating in the blood, particularly the low-density lipoprotein cholesterol fraction (see Table 40-2). The fat enters the developing plaque in proportion to its concentration in the blood or in increased amounts, if

TABLE 40-1. Selected heart facts

Cardiovascular disease cost (American Heart Association estimate)
 $26.7 billion in 1977.

Prevalence
 29,270,000 Americans have some form of heart and blood vessel disease.
  Hypertension: 23,660,000 (one in six adults)
  Coronary heart disease: 4,050,000
  Rheumatic heart disease: 1,770,000
  Stroke: 1,810,000

Cardiovascular disease mortality
 1,035,273 deaths in 1974 (54% of all deaths)
 1,036,900 deaths in 1977
  One-fourth of all persons killed by cardiovascular disease are under age 65.

Atherosclerosis
 Contributed to many of the 872,278 heart attack and stroke deaths in 1974.

Heart attack
 Caused 664,854 deaths in 1974.
  4,050,000 alive today have history of heart attack and/or angina pectoris.
  350,000 a year die of heart attack before they reach the hospital; average victim
   waits three hours before deciding to seek help.
  Over 1,000,000 Americans will have a heart attack this year; about 650,000 of
   them will die.

Stroke
 Killed 207,424 in 1974; afflicts 1,810,000.

Hypertension
 23,660,000 adults have it, but more than 7,000,000 do not know it.
  Of those who do know they have it, many are untreated or inadequately controlled.
  Only a minority have it under adequate control.
  For 90 percent of those with high blood pressure, science does not know the
   cause, but it is easily detected and usually controllable.

Major risk factors
 Blood pressure
  A person with systolic pressure over 150 has more than *twice* the risk of heart
   attack and nearly *four* times the risk of stroke of a person with a systolic pres-
   sure under 120.
 Cholesterol
  A person with blood cholesterol of 250 or more has about *three* times the risk of
   heart attack and stroke of a person with cholesterol level below 194.
 Cigarette smoking
  A person who smokes more than one pack a day has nearly *twice* the risk of heart
   attack and nearly *five* times the risk of stroke of a nonsmoker.

Source: American Heart Association. *Heart Facts*, Dallas, Texas, 1976.

the epithelial lining is disturbed. The high-density lipoprotein cholesterol component of the blood may actually help carry away fat from the developing plaque. Fat eventually becomes trapped by scar tissue in the plaque; calcium is also deposited and distorts the structure of the vessel wall.

RISK FACTORS   Although there is still considerable controversy over the influence of plasma levels of various lipoproteins and the development of cardiovascular disease, a

TABLE 40-2. The principal lipoproteins

	Size (nm)	Composition (%)				Origin
		Protein	Cholesterol	Triglyceride	Phospholipid	
Chylomicrons	75–100	2	5	90	3	Intestine
Very-low-density lipoprotein (VLDL)	30–80	10	12	60	18	Liver and small intestine
Intermediate-density lipoprotein (IDL)	25–40	10	30	40	20	VLDL
Low-density lipoprotein (LDL)	20	25	50	10	15	VLDL
High-density lipoprotein (HDL)	7.5–10	50	20	5	25	Liver

Source: W. F. Ganong, *Review of Medical Physiology*. Los Altos, Calif.: Lange, 1979. P. 230.

number of factors in recent years, including cholesterol-lowering regimens, have led to a decline in the cardiovascular death rate by more than 20 percent since 1968 [3]. These factors include improved in-hospital care; new, sophisticated measures by community-based units; better emergency medical services personnel; and improved surgical techniques. These factors are contributing to improved outcomes today, but it is probably changes in risk factors that have led to the decline in mortality from acute heart disease in the past 10 to 15 years [3].

The major risk factors, as given in Table 40-1, include cigarette smoking, elevated serum cholesterol, and hypertension (high blood pressure). Other factors, such as age, male sex, diabetes mellitus, personality profile, and heredity, also play a major role in determining an individual's risk of developing cardiovascular disease. The following section elaborates on these and other risk factors that contribute to the etiology of this complex disease.

HYPERTENSION

Hypertension, one of the most common chronic diseases affecting 24 million Americans, is one of the three major risk factors contributing to high and premature mortality from heart disease and stroke. The excessive use of salt in the American diet has been implicated as the main etiologic factor in the development of hypertension, although genetic and familial factors may also be involved [4]. It has been suggested that a low salt intake initiated early and continued throughout life may protect, to some degree, the 20 percent of children who are at risk of developing hypertension in adulthood [5]. This increased awareness of salt intake during childhood has led to the reduction or elimination of added sodium to infant and baby food by the major manufacturers.

COFFEE AND CIGARETTE SMOKING

Reports from a variety of studies on the role of coffee in the development of cardiovascular disease have been conflicting. In four recent studies, no association was shown between coffee drinking and heart disease [6–9], while retrospective studies on survivors of myocardial infarctions found a positive correlation [10, 11]. Caffeine has been shown to cause an increase in blood pressure [12] and, when combined with cigarette smoking, an increase in low-density lipoproteins (LDL) and a decrease in high-density lipoprotein (HDL) cholesterol [13]. It is not known whether the influence of coffee on the development of cardiovascular disease is due to associated factors related to the habit (such as stress or cigarette smoking) or to the coffee drinking itself.

EXERCISE

Obesity and a sedentary life-style have long been associated with the development of cardiovascular disease. The opposite has also been demonstrated; exercise and the maintenance of ideal weight can effectively lower the serum cholesterol level and minimize the development of atherosclerotic heart disease [14, 15]. Exercise has been shown to decrease triglyceride-rich prebetalipoproteins and cholesterol-rich betalipoproteins and increase cholesterol-rich alphalipoproteins (HDL, high-density lipoproteins) [16]. Exercise, therefore, can produce a change in the cholesterol-carrying character of the lipoproteins.

GENETICS

Genetic factors also influence an individual's susceptibility to cardiovascular disease. The dietary factors that contribute to increases in the serum level of cholesterol and triglycerides are potentiated in the genetically predisposed individual. A genetic influence should be suspected when the serum cholesterol level exceeds 350 mg per 100 ml.

Familial hypercholesterolemia occurs in the general population in a frequency of about 0.2 to 0.5 percent. It is inherited as an autosomal dominant disorder, affecting approximately 50 percent of the children of an affected parent carrying the gene. The presence of the disease is, of course, a predictor of early cardiovascular disease.

Familial hypertriglyceridemia is also an autosomal dominant trait and is often associated with obesity, diabetes, insulin resistance, and hyperinsulinemia. The basic defect causing this disease remains unclear.

Familial combined hyperlipidemia, also due to an autosomal dominant gene, causes an elevation of both cholesterol and triglycerides. The main treatment is the dietary restriction of both triglycerides and cholesterol.

Type I and type III hyperlipidemia are very rare conditions associated with the premature development of cardiovascular disease.

Genetic lipoproteinemias are diagnosed using the phenotype system, which may utilize lipoprotein electrophoresis or ultracentrifugation techniques. In addition, cholesterol and triglyceride determinations must also be made.

ORAL CONTRACEPTIVES

It has been found recently that oral contraceptives have the additional side effect of increasing the risk of venous thromboembolic disease, myocardial infarction, thrombotic stroke, and hemorrhagic stroke [17–19]. The use of oral contraceptives have been found to potentiate the associated risk of other factors also present, such as cigarette smoking or hypertension [20, 21]. These drugs cause such side effects by increasing the size of the intravenous clot formed in response to injury or other stimuli that lead to the thrombin formation [19]. This effect is due primarily to the estrogen component of oral contraceptives. It has been found that this increased risk continues even after the discontinuation of the long-term use of oral contraceptives [22].

ROLE OF DIET

FATS

Although the exact mechanism is yet unknown, it has been shown that the replacement of saturated fat in the diet with sources supplying polyunsaturated fatty acids is effective in lowering the serum cholesterol level [23–25]. There is still controversy over whether the total fat content of the diet should be lowered or just the ratio of polyunsaturated-saturated fatty acids altered to as much as 1.5:1.0 [26]. In areas of the world where the incidence of cardiovascular disease is low, the average diet is also low in total fat content. It seems logical to both decrease the total fat content of the diet and increase the percentage of polyunsaturated fats in this lowered intake, although this would be difficult to implement due to traditional high-fat and saturated-fat dietary patterns.

The risk for developing cardiovascular disease is increased with serum cholesterol levels above 200 mg/100 ml. Levels of high-density lipoproteins (HDL), which normally carry 20 percent of the total plasma cholesterol, have been correlated to be inversely proportional to risk—the higher the HDL levels, the lower the risk [27].

Other studies have shown that the lipid composition of the diet, particularly the high intake of animal fats and other saturated fats, affects the serum cholesterol concentration and the risk of coronary death [28].

Levels of low-density lipoproteins (LDL), which carry about two-thirds of the cholesterol in the blood but less protein, are directly proportional to increased risk [29].

CARBOHYDRATES

Carbohydrates have also been implicated in the development of cardiovascular disease. One study concluded that men with myocardial infarction or peripheral artery disease had consumed twice as much sugar as did controls [30]. Other studies have also shown this relationship, as well as correlating sugar intake with that of saturated fat [31]. A negative association has been observed between the average concentration of serum cholesterol and the average intake of complex carbohydrates (cereals and starchy vegetables). The average per capita consumption of sucrose in the United States is in excess of 110 lb per year, providing approximately 20 to 24 percent of the average daily caloric intake. It has been suggested that sucrose might increase the serum concentration of lipids by increasing blood pressure [32]. Experimentally induced hypertension causes an elevation in the serum levels of essential fatty acids, which decreases the ability of the liver to form triglycerides.

VITAMIN C, ALCOHOL, AND FIBER

Various components of the diet, other than fats, have recently been implicated in increasing the risk of developing cardiovascular disease. In the aged, vitamin C therapy resulted in decreased LDL-cholesterol and total cholesterol levels while increasing the HDL-cholesterol component [33]. Alcohol consumption, in moderation, is positively correlated with increased levels of HDL-cholesterol (high levels of which protect against cardiovascular disease) [34].

Increases in the type and amount of fiber in the diet have recently been shown to be effective in lowering various components of the plasma lipoproteins. The addition of citrus pectin, oat bran, or a combination of cereal brans caused a reduction in the serum total cholesterol [35–37]. The oat and combined cereal brans also produced a decrease in the LDL-cholesterol and triglyceride levels, without affecting the HDL-cholesterol levels [36, 37]. The use of dietary fiber may prove to be a palatable and inexpensive adjunct in the diet therapy of the hyperlipoproteinemias.

ZINC AND COPPER

A deficiency of copper can contribute to elevated serum cholesterol levels. An excess of zinc can cause a relative deficiency of copper by suppressing intestinal absorption. Copper deficiency causes an increase in plasma LDL levels and a decrease in HDL. Zinc supplementation may, therefore, not only induce the signs of copper deficiency, but also adversely affect cholesterol metabolism and lead to arterial vascular damage [38, 39].

Diet Therapy

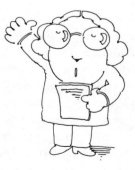

Hyperlipoproteinemia is an elevation of one or more of the lipoprotein components in the blood. This elevation may be caused by other diseases known to affect lipid metabolism, such as hypothyroidism, insulin-dependent diabetes, nephrotic syndrome, or obstructive liver disease. In this type of hyperlipoproteinemia, also known as "secondary," therapy is directed toward the underlying disorder. Diet therapy [40] is used to treat "primary" hyperlipoproteinemia, that is, an elevation not caused by another known disease process.

To determine the type (and, therefore, the specific therapy) of hyperlipoproteinemia, both cholesterol and triglyceride concentrations should be made. In addition, a chylomicron test may be helpful. Tables 40-3 and 40-4 outline the use of these laboratory values in determining the hyperlipoproteinemia type. To evaluate the effectiveness of the prescribed therapeutic diet, cholesterol and triglyceride measurements should be made every other week for about 6 weeks. A reduction of 15 percent or greater in these lipoprotein components suggests that the diet is successful and should be continued. The following is a discussion of

TABLE 40-3. Laboratory values in diagnosing hyperlipoproteinemia: concentrations of cholesterol, triglyceride, or low-density lipoproteins, which, if exceeded, clearly indicate hyperlipidemia

Age	Cholesterol (mg/100 ml)	LDL (mg/100 ml)	Triglyceride
1–19	230	170	150
20–29	240	170	200
30–39	270	190	200
40–49	310	190	200
50 +	330	210	200

Source: *The Dietary Management of Hyperlipoproteinemia.* DHEW Pub. No. (NIH) 78-110. Pp. vi and ix.

TABLE 40-4. Laboratory values in diagnosing hyperlipoproteinemia: type of hyperlipoproteinemia as suggested by cholesterol (C) and triglyceride (TG) levels

C high; TG normal	Type IIa
C high; TG 150–400	Type IIb, III, or IV
C high; TG 400–1000	Type III, IV, or V
C high; TG > 1000	Type I or V
C normal; TG high	Type IV (I or V)

Source: *The Dietary Management of Hyperlipoproteinemia.* DHEW Pub. No. (NIH) 78-110. Pp. vi and ix.

the types of hyperlipoproteinemias and each specific diet therapy. A summary of the diet therapy is given in Table 40-5.

TYPE I

This type of hyperlipoproteinemia, in which the cholesterol level is normal to high and the triglycerides are elevated, is caused by the inability to clear chylomicrons (dietary fat) from the blood. LDL and VLDL levels are normal. This is a rare, familial disease usually found in the young and may show accompanying symptoms, such as abdominal pain associated with fat digestion, enlarged spleen and liver, lipemia retinalis, and eruptive xanthomas. The etiology of this disorder is thought to be a genetic deficiency of lipoprotein lipase, responsible for clearing chylomicrons from the blood. There is no increase in atherosclerosis with this type of hyperlipoproteinemia.

The diet therapy for type I is aimed at reducing the level of dietary fat. MCT oil (triglycerides of medium chain length) is useful since it is absorbed directly into the portal vein and does not require chylomicron formation for transport. It may be used as an ingredient in pie crusts, cookies, salad dressings, or in broiling or frying. The total dietary fat intake should be limited to 25 to 35 gm per day. The polyunsaturated to saturated ratio is not important; cholesterol, protein, and carbohydrate intake is not restricted. Fat intake is usually divided as 5 oz of meat per day (total of 15 gm of fat) and 10 gm of fat from other low-fat foods. A sample of this diet regimen is given in Fig. 40-1.

688

TABLE 40-5. Summary of diets for types I–V hyperlipoproteinemia

	Type I	Type IIa	Types IIb and III	Type IV	Type V
Diet prescription	Low-fat, 25–35 gm	Low-cholesterol, polyunsaturated fat increased	Low-cholesterol; approximately 20% cal protein, 40% cal fat, and 40% cal carbohydrate	Controlled carbohydrate, 45% of cal; moderately restricted cholesterol	Restricted fat, 30% of cal; controlled carbohydrate, 50% of cal; moderately restricted in cholesterol
Calories	Not restricted	Not restricted	Achieve and maintain "ideal" weight; reduction diet if necessary	Achieve and maintain "ideal" weight; reduction diet if necessary	Achieve and maintain "ideal" weight; reduction diet if necessary
Protein	Total protein intake is not limited	Total protein intake is not limited	High-protein	Not limited other than control of patient's weight	High-protein
Fat	Restricted to 25–35 gm; kind of fat not important	Saturated fat intake limited; polyunsaturated fat intake increased	Controlled to 40% of cal; polyunsaturated fats recommended	Not limited other than control of patient's weight; polyunsaturated fats recommended	Restricted to 30% of cal; polyunsaturated fats recommended
Cholesterol	Not restricted	As low as possible; meat is the only source in the diet	Less than 300 mg; meat is the only source in the diet	Moderately restricted—300–500 mg	Moderately restricted—300–500 mg
Carbohydrate	Not limited	Not limited	Controlled; restrict concentrated sweets	Controlled; restrict concentrated sweets	Controlled; restrict concentrated sweets
Alcohol	Not recommended	May be used with discretion	Limited to 2 servings (substituted for carbohydrate)	Limited to 2 servings (substituted for carbohydrate)	Not recommended

Source: *The Dietary Management of Hyperlipoproteinemia.* DHEW Pub. No. (NIH) 78-110. U.S. Dept. of Health, Education, and Welfare, Public Health Service, and National Institutes of Health, 1978.

TYPE IIa

Type IIa hyperlipoproteinemia is a common form found at all ages and is characterized by elevated cholesterol levels (in the range of 300 to 600 mg per 100 ml) and normal triglyceride levels. VLDL levels are normal and LDL levels are elevated. It is often transmitted as an autosomal dominant trait. If the disease is genetically transmitted, it can often be detected before 1 year of age. Vascular disease often becomes evident early in life; xanthomas on the extensor tendons of the hands, the Achilles tendons, and the elbows may also appear early.

The diet therapy in type IIa is aimed at reducing the intake of cholesterol to less than 300 mg per day, decreasing the intake of saturated fats, and increasing the intake of polyunsaturated fats (see Tables 40-6 and 40-7). This is most easily accomplished by removing all eggs and most dairy products from the diet and supplementing with polyunsaturated fats. The aim is to achieve a high dietary polyunsaturated to saturated fatty acid ratio

$$\frac{\text{Linoleic acid}}{\text{Saturated fatty acids}} = \text{P/S ratio (1.5:1 or better)}$$

FIG. 40-1. Sample diets for hyperlipoproteinemia.

	BREAKFAST	LUNCH	DINNER	BETWEEN MEAL SNACK
Type I	Juice, skim milk, cereal, toast, jelly, sugar, coffee or tea	Fruit, skim milk; 2 oz poultry, fish, or lean meat; potato, bread, vegetable, jelly, sugar, allowed dessert	Skim milk; 3 oz poultry, fish, or lean meat; potato, bread, vegetable, jelly, sugar, allowed dessert	Skim milk, fruit or allowed dessert, bread with jelly or jam
Type IIa or IIb	Juice, skim milk, cereal, toast, allowed fat, jelly, sugar	Cooked poultry, fish, or lean meat; potato, bread, vegetable, allowed fat, allowed dessert, skim milk	Cooked poultry, fish, or lean meat; bread, vegetable, allowed fat	Skim milk, fruit or allowed dessert, bread, allowed fat
Type IIb or III	Juice, skim milk, cereal or toast, allowed fat	Poultry, fish, or lean, trimmed meat; potato, bread, vegetable, allowed fat, fruit	Poultry, fish, or lean, trimmed meat; potato, bread, vegetable, allowed fat, fruit, skim milk	
Type IV	Juice, skim milk, cereal or toast, allowed fat	Poultry, fish, or lean, trimmed meat; potato, bread, vegetable, allowed fat, fruit	Poultry, fish, or lean, trimmed meat; potato, bread, vegetable, allowed fat, fruit, skim milk	
Type V	Juice, skim milk, cereal or toast, allowed fat	Poultry, fish, or lean, trimmed meat; potato, bread, vegetable, allowed fat, fruit, skim milk	Poultry, fish, or lean, trimmed meat; potato, bread, vegetable, allowed fat, fruit, skim milk	Skim milk, bread or cereal

TABLE 40-6. Cholesterol in foods: amount of cholesterol present per 100 grams (3½ oz)

Food	Cholesterol (mg/100 gm)	Food	Cholesterol (mg/100 gm)
Egg yolk, dried	2950	Veal	90
Brains, raw	2000	Cheese (25–30% fat)	85
Egg yolk, fresh	1500	Milk, dried, whole	85
Egg yolk, frozen	1280	Beef, raw	70
Egg, whole	550	Fish, steak	70
Kidney, raw	375	Fish, fillet	70
Caviar or fish roe	300	Lamb, raw	70
Liver, raw	300	Pork	70
Butter	250	Cheese spread	65
Sweetbreads (thymus)	250	Margarine	65
Oysters	200	Mutton	65
Lobster	200	Chicken, flesh only, raw	60
Heart, raw	150	Ice cream	45
Crab meat	125	Cottage cheese, creamed	15
Shrimp	125	Milk, fluid, whole	11
Cheese, cream	125	Milk, fluid, skim	3
Cheese, cheddar	100	Egg white	0
Lard and animal fat	95		

Source: C. F. Church and H. N. Church, *Food Values of Portions Commonly Used* (12th ed.). Philadelphia: Lippincott, 1975. P. 186.

TABLE 40-7. Foods useful in low-cholesterol diets

Fruits: all are low in cholesterol

Vegetables: if prepared and served without butter, cream, lard, or suet. Vegetable-oil margarine, vegetable oils, and mayonnaise may be used for flavoring

Breads and cereals

Skim or nonfat milk, buttermilk, and cottage cheese to replace whole milk and cheese

Lean meat and lean fish

Marmalade, jelly, jam, syrup, and sugar may be used in place of butter and other fats, unless calories are restricted

Source: C. F. Church and H. N. Church, *Food Values of Portions Commonly Used* (12th ed.). Philadelphia: Lippincott, 1975. P. 186.

The carbohydrate and protein intake are not limited and alcohol may be used with discretion. A sample diet is given in Fig. 40-1.

TYPE IIb

This second division of type II hyperlipoproteinemia differs from type IIa by both the cholesterol and triglycerides being elevated. Both LDL and VLDL levels are elevated. Depending on the individual patient, either the diet for type IIa or, for a greater reduction in lipoproteins, the diet for type III may be used.

TYPE III

This fourth type is a relatively uncommon form. Type III hyperlipoproteinemia is usually familial and is transmitted as a recessive trait. Both cholesterol and triglyceride levels are elevated. A unique symptom is orange yellow streaking of the palmar creases. Signs of vascular disease often manifest in males before the age of 35 and in females 10 to 15 years later.

The diet therapy of type III involves an initial reduction to ideal body weight. The diet is low in cholesterol, with 40 percent of the calories each from fat and carbohydrate. Protein accounts for the remaining 20 percent, making it a high-protein diet. Alcohol may be substituted for carbohydrates in limited amounts. A sample diet is given in Fig. 40-1.

TYPE IV

Endogenous hyperlipemia is a very common pattern often seen after the second decade of life and associated with diabetes and premature atherosclerosis. Type IV is characterized by increases in both cholesterol and triglyceride fractions. VLDL levels are increased and LDL levels are either normal or increased. Almost half of all patients with type IV also have abnormal glucose tolerance tests and elevated levels of uric acid.

The initial diet therapy is geared at achieving ideal body weight. On the maintenance diet, carbohydrate makes up about 45 percent of the total calories; protein and fat are not restricted, but polyunsaturated fats are substituted for saturated fats and cholesterol is moderately restricted. Alcohol may be substituted for carbohydrate in limited amounts. A sample menu is given in Fig. 40-1.

TYPE V

This pattern may be familial or secondary to such acute metabolic disorders as nephrosis, alcoholism, diabetic acidosis, or pancreatitis. Both the cholesterol and triglyceride levels are elevated, as is the level of chylomicrons. VLDL levels are increased; LDL may be slightly increased. When this pattern is familial, symptoms may appear after age 20 and may resemble those of type I (enlarged liver and spleen, abdominal pain, and pancreatitis). An abnormal glucose tolerance test and elevated levels of uric acid are also often associated with type V hyperlipoproteinemia.

As with types III and IV, the initial goal of the diet therapy is the achievement of ideal body weight; this alone may bring the concentration of plasma lipids into normal range. Fat is both restricted and modified to 25 to 30 percent of the total calories, with polyunsaturated substituted for saturated and cholesterol moderately restricted. Carbohydrate accounts for 48 to 53 percent of the total calories and protein the remaining 21 to 24 percent (a high protein allowance). Alcohol is not recommended, as it may exacerbate the plasma triglyceride concentrations and abdominal pain. A sample diet is given in Fig. 40-1.

Conclusions and Recommendations

This chapter has presented the evidence for dietary modification in the treatment of cardiovascular disease. The application of these principles would also be good preventive medicine for most Americans, even those without overt symptoms of vascular disease. As recommended in other chapters, including Chap. 21, most Americans would live longer, healthier lives if their diets included less saturated and more polyunsaturated fats, less salt, and less refined sugar. The achievement and maintenance of ideal body weight is also a major preventive and therapeutic measure in this and many other diseases.

References

1. Department of Health, Education and Welfare. *The Surgeon General's Report on Health Promotion and Disease Prevention.* Washington, D.C.: U.S. Govt. Printing Office, 1979.
2. National Center for Vital Statistics. *Annual Summary for the United States, 1979.* Atlanta: Centers for Disease Control, 1979.
3. Wolinsky, H. Taking heart. *The Sciences* 21:6, 1981.
4. Dahl, L. K. Salt and hypertension. *Am. J. Clin. Nutr.* 25:231, 1972.
5. American Academy of Pediatrics, Committee on Nutrition. Salt intake and eating patterns of infants and children in relation to blood pressure. *Pediatrics* 53:115, 1974.
6. Dawber, T. R., Kannel, W. B., and Gordon, T. Coffee and cardiovascular disease: Observations from the Framingham study. *N. Engl. J. Med.* 291:871, 1975.
7. Klatsky, A. L., Friedman, G. D., and Siegelaub, A. B. Coffee drinking prior to acute myocardial infarction: Results from the Kaiser-Permanente epidemiological study of myocardial infarction. *J.A.M.A.* 226:540, 1973.
8. Yano, K., Rhoads, G. G., and Kagan, A. Coffee, alcohol and risk of coronary heart disease among Japanese men living in Hawaii. *N. Engl. J. Med.* 297:405, 1977.
9. Heyden, S., et al. Coffee consumption and mortality. *Arch. Intern. Med.* 138:1472, 1978.
10. Boston Collaborative Drug Surveillance Program. Coffee drinking and acute myocardial infarction. *Lancet* 2:1278, 1972.
11. Rosenberg, L., et al. Coffee drinking and myocardial infarction in young women. *Am. J. Epidemiol.* 111:675, 1980.
12. Robertson, D., et al. Effects of caffeine on plasma renin activity, catecholamines, and blood pressure. *N. Engl. J. Med.* 298:181, 1978.
13. Heyden, S., et al. The combined effect of smoking and coffee drinking on LDL and HDL cholesterol. *Circulation* 60:22, 1979.
14. Kramsch, D. M., et al. Reduction of coronary atherosclerosis by moderate conditioning exercise in monkeys on an atherogenic diet. *N. Engl. J. Med.* 305:1483, 1981.
15. Hartung, G. H., et al. Relation of diet to high-density lipoprotein cholesterol in middle-aged marathon runners, joggers, and inactive men. *N. Engl. J. Med.* 302:357, 1980.
16. Balart, L., et al. Serum lipids, dietary intakes, and physical exercise in medical students. *J. Am. Diet. Assoc.* 64:42, 1974.
17. Vessey, M. P. Female hormones and vascular disease: Epidemiological overview. *Br. J. Fam. Plan.* 6 [Suppl.]:1, 1980.
18. Royal College of General Practitioners' Oral Contraception Study. Further analysis of mortality in oral contraceptive users. *Lancet* 1:541, 1981.
19. Stadel, B. V. Oral contraceptives and cardiovascular disease. *N. Engl. J. Med.* 305:612, 1981.
20. Shapiro, S., et al. Oral contraceptive use in relation to myocardial infarction. *Lancet* 1:743, 1979.

21. Rosenberg, L., et al. Oral contraceptive use in relation to nonfatal myocardial infarction. *Am. J. Epidemiol.* 111:59, 1980.

22. Slone, D., et al. Risk of myocardial infarction in relation to current and discontinued use of oral contraceptives. *N. Engl. J. Med.* 305:420, 1981.

23. Bartz, W. M. The pathogenesis of hypercholesterolemia. *Ann. Intern. Med.* 80:738, 1974.

24. Shaper, A. G. Diet in the epidemiology of coronary heart disease. *Proc. Nutr. Soc.* 31:297, 1972.

25. Vegroesen, A. J. Dietary fat and cardiovascular disease: Possible modes of action of linoleic acid. *Proc. Nutr. Soc.* 31:323, 1972.

26. Krehl, W. A. The Nutritional Epidemiology of Cardiovascular Disease. In N. H. Moss and J. Mayer (eds.), *Food and Nutrition in Health and Disease.* New York: New York Academy of Sciences, 1977.

27. Blood lipids and coronary heart disease. *Nutr. Rev.* 36:239, 1978.

28. Shekelle, R. B., et al. Diet, serum cholesterol, and death from coronary heart disease. *N. Engl. J. Med.* 304:65, 1981.

29. More data show lipoproteins as cardiac risk factors. *J.A.M.A.* 239:1119, 1978.

30. Yudkin, J. Sucrose and cardiovascular disease. *Proc. Nutr. Soc.* 31:331, 1972.

31. Keys, A. Coronary heart disease in seven countries. *Circulation* 41 [Suppl. 1]:1, 1970.

32. Ahrens, R. A. Sucrose, hypertension and heart disease: A historical perspective. *Am. J. Clin. Nutr.* 27:402, 1974.

33. Horsey, J., Livesley, B., and Dickerson, J. W. T. Ischaemic heart disease and aged patients: Effect of ascorbic acid on lipoproteins. *J. Hum. Nutr.* 35:53, 1981.

34. Willett, W., et al. Alcohol consumption and high-density lipoprotein cholesterol in marathon runners. *N. Engl. J. Med.* 303:1159, 1980.

35. Stasse-Wolthuis, M., et al. Influence of dietary fiber from vegetables and fruits, bran or citrus pectin on serum lipids, fecal lipids, and colonic function. *Am. J. Clin. Nutr.* 33:1745, 1980.

36. Kirby, R. W., et al. Oat-bran intake selectively lowers serum low-density lipoprotein cholesterol concentrations of hypercholesterolemic men. *Am. J. Clin. Nutr.* 34:824, 1981.

37. Munoz, J. M., et al. Effects of some cereal brans and textured vegetable protein on plasma lipids. *Am. J. Clin. Nutr.* 32:580, 1979.

38. Klevay, L. M. Coronary heart disease: The zinc/copper hypothesis. *Am. J. Clin. Nutr.* 28:764, 1975.

39. Sandstead, H. H. Zinc, copper, and cholesterol. *J.A.M.A.* 245:1528, 1981.

40. Department of Health, Education, and Welfare. *The Dietary Management of Hyperlipoproteinemia* DHEW Pub., No. (NIH) 78-110, 1978.

Suggested Readings

American Health Foundation (ed.). *Plasma Lipids: Optimal Levels for Health.* New York: Academic, 1980. P. 187.

Anderson, J. T., Grande, F., and Keys, A. Cholesterol-lowering diets. *J. Am. Diet. Assoc.* 62:133, 1973.

Ellison, R. C., Newburger, J. W., and Gross, D. M. Pediatric aspects of essential hypertension. *J. Am. Diet. Assoc.* 80:21, 1982.

Ethanol and angina pectoris. *Nutr. Rev.* 34:300, 1976.

Farrand, M. E., and Mojonnier, L. Nutrition in the Multiple Risk Factor Intervention Trial (MRFIT). *J. Am. Diet. Assoc.* 76:347, 1980.

Feldman, E. B. (ed.). *Nutrition and Cardiovascular Disease.* New York: Appleton-Century-Crofts, 1976. P. 326.

Ferguson, J. M., Taylor, C. B., and Ullman, P.   *A Change for Heart: Your Family and the Food You Eat.* Palo Alto, Calif.: Bull Publishing, 1978. P. 192.

Flink, E. B., Brick, J. E., and Shane, S. R.   Alterations of long-chain free fatty acid and magnesium concentrations in acute myocardial infarction. *Arch. Intern. Med.* 141:441, 1981.

Friedman, M.   Type A behavior: A progress report. *The Sciences* 20:10, 1980.

Frohlich, E. D.   Physiological observations in essential hypertension. *J. Am. Diet. Assoc.* 80:18, 1982.

Glueck, C. J., Mattson, F., and Bierman, E. L.   Diet and coronary heart disease: Another view. *N. Engl. J. Med.* 298:1471, 1978.

Gupta, R. C., Bhagat, J. K., and Sharma, S. K.   Serum magnesium in ischaemic heart disease. *J. Indian Med. Assoc.* 75:55, 1980.

Gustafsson, I.-B., et al.   Effects of lipid-lowering diets on patients with hyperlipoproteinemia. *J. Am. Diet. Assoc.* 80:426, 1982.

Hausman, P.   *Jack Sprat's Legacy: The Science and Politics of Fat and Cholesterol.* New York: Marek, 1981.

Hill, M.   Helping the hypertensive patient control sodium intake. *Am. J. Nurs.* 79:906, 1979.

Hlatky, M. A., and Hulley, S. B.   Plasma cholesterol: Can it be too low? *Arch. Intern. Med.* 141:1132, 1981.

Kesteloot, H., and Geboers, J.   Calcium and blood pressure. *Lancet* 1:813, 1982.

Kinsella, J. E.   Dietary fat and prostaglandins: Possible beneficial relationships between food processing and public health. *Food Technol.* 35:89, 1981.

Levine, R. S., et al.   Cardiovascular risk factors among children of men with premature myocardial infarction. *Public Health Rep.* 96:58, 1981.

Lewis, B., et al.   Towards an improved lipid-lowering diet: Additive effects of changes in nutrient intake. *Lancet* 2:1310, 1981.

MacGregor, G. A., et al.   Double-blind randomized crossover trial of moderate sodium restriction in essential hypertension. *Lancet* 1:351, 1982.

Mann, G. V.   Diet-heart: End of an era. *N. Engl. J. Med.* 297:644, 1977.

Marier, J. R.   Water hardness and disease. *J.A.M.A.* 245:1315, 1981.

Morrison, J. A., et al.   Lipid and lipoprotein distributions in black adults. *J.A.M.A.* 245:939, 1981.

Moser, M.   Sodium restriction: Diuretics and potassium loss. *Arch. Intern. Med.* 141:983, 1981.

Norum, K. R.   Some present concepts concerning diet and prevention of coronary heart disease. *Nutr. Rev.* 36:194, 1978.

Olendzki, M. C., Toplin, H. G., and Buckley, E. L.   Evaluating nutrition intervention in atherosclerosis: Some theoretical and practical considerations. *J. Am. Diet. Assoc.* 79:9, 1981.

Oster, K. A.   Diet, cholesterol, and heart disease. *N. Engl. J. Med.* 304:1168, 1981.

Oster, K. A.   Atherosclerosis: Conjecture, data, and facts. *Nutr. Today* 16:28, 1981.

Ram, C. V. S., Garrett, B. N., and Kaplan, N. M.   Moderate sodium restriction and various diuretics in the treatment of hypertension. *Arch. Intern. Med.* 141:1015, 1981.

Richmond, F.   A political perspective on the diet/heart controversy. *J. Nutr. Educ.* 12:186, 1980.

Rossouw, J. E., et al.   The effect of skim milk, yoghurt, and full cream milk on human serum lipids. *Am. J. Clin. Nutr.* 34:351, 1981.

Sirtori, C., Ricci, G., and Gorini, S. (eds.).   *Diet and Atherosclerosis* (vol. 60). *Advances in Experimental Medicine and Biology.* New York: Plenum Press, 1975. P. 255.

Stone, N. J. *Fat Chance.* Chicago: Year Book, 1980. P. 88.

Tall, A. R., and Small, D. M. Plasma high-density lipoproteins. *N. Engl. J. Med.* 299:1232, 1978.

Taming the no. 1 killer. *Time Magazine* June 1, 1981.

Wilber, J. A. The role of diet in the treatment of high blood pressure. *J. Am. Diet. Assoc.* 80:25, 1982.

Chapter 41

THE ANEMIAS

Anemia is a condition in which there is a decrease in the oxygen-carrying capacity of the blood caused by a deficiency of red blood cells and/or hemoglobin. It should be considered a symptom of an underlying disorder and not a disease in itself. Slight anemia may not have any adverse effects on health, except to increase an individual's susceptibility to infection and decrease tolerance to strenuous exercise or work. It does, however, place the individual at increased risk for serious consequences if he or she suffers blood loss from other disease, an injury, or from childbirth. There are three main causes of anemia: (1) loss of blood (*hemorrhage*); (2) excessive destruction of red blood cells (*erythrocytes*) (*hemolysis*); and (3) impaired or reduced production of erythrocytes and hemoglobin (*dyshemopoiesis*). The nutritional anemias are of this third type. Iron-deficiency anemia is the most prevalent nutritional deficiency in the world today.

Chapters to review: Chapters 3, 7, 8, 9, 11.

Red Blood Cell Formation (Erythropoiesis)

Erythrocytes, red blood cells, have a life span of about 120 days. A normal level of erythrocytes and hemoglobin is maintained by the bone marrow as a dynamic balance between their formation and destruction and removal. About 40 percent of the bone marrow in the sternum, ribs, vertebrae, skull, and proximal ends of the femur and humerus are involved in blood production (*hematopoiesis*); fat cells occupy the remaining portion of the bone marrow. During times of increased demand for blood production, hematopoiesis is seen in marrow not normally engaged in blood production and can even occur in sites outside the marrow, including the liver and spleen. All cellular components of blood are thought to arise in bone marrow from undifferentiated cells, termed *stem cells*. Some stem cells differentiate and mature in the marrow, slowly acquiring more hemoglobin and eventually losing their nuclei before being released into the circulation as mature erythrocytes. Other cellular or formed elements of the blood include the platelets, responsible for blood clotting, and leukocytes, the white blood cells. Erythrocytes, platelets, and leukocytes are suspended in plasma, a transparent liquid that makes up about 55 percent of the blood's volume.

Mature red blood cells and their nucleated precursors are located in normal adult bone marrow. The hormone, *erythropoietin*, which is secreted by the kidneys, acts on the marrow precursors to maintain sufficient numbers of circulating red blood cells with adequate hemoglobin content to preserve normal tissue oxygen. The level of oxygen in the tissues directly influences the production of erythropoietin, not the number of red blood cells or hemoglobin concentration. The lack of oxygen (hypoxia) triggers production of erythropoietin. Hypoxia causes the kidney to release a *renal erythropoietic factor* (*REF*), which, in turn, converts an inactive form of erythropoietin in the blood to an active form. The active erythropoietin acts on the bone marrow, stimulating stem cells to differentiate and early erythrocytes (erythroblasts) to multiply and mature. The release

FIG. 41-1. Erythropoietin mechanism. (From E. E. Selkurt [ed.], *Basic Physiology for the Health Sciences* [2nd ed.]. Boston: Little, Brown, 1982.)

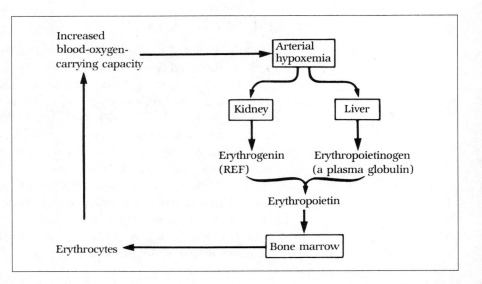

of increased numbers of oxygen-carrying cells (erythrocytes) into the blood alleviates the hypoxia and thereby turns off the production of erythropoietin (see Fig. 41-1). Other sources of erythropoietin or REF probably do exist, since red blood cell formation does continue after removal of the kidneys.

During the breakdown of erythrocytes, most of the components are effectively conserved and recycled. Some components cannot be effectively conserved or must be supplied de novo from dietary sources, such as the essential amino acids. A variety of nutrients are needed in the production of erythrocytes. The most important include iron, folic acid, and vitamin B_{12}; others also needed include pyridoxine, ascorbic acid, vitamin E, copper, and protein. Nutritional anemias result from the impaired or reduced production of erythrocytes and hemoglobin. The bone marrow activity is limited by a deficiency of one or more erythropoietic components due to its lack in the diet, increased loss (i.e., iron deficiency due to chronic blood loss), or malabsorption. Folic acid and vitamin B_{12} are essential in the synthesis and maturation of erythrocytes. When these vitamins are not present in sufficient amounts, the normal development of erythrocytes is impaired, with fewer and more immature erythrocytes resulting. Iron is an essential component of the hemoglobin molecule. When there is an insufficient supply of iron, there is a limit on the amount of new hemoglobin that can be synthesized. The end result will be normal erythrocytes, but each will contain a lowered complement of hemoglobin. Diet alone is rarely responsible for the development of anemia, although it may not be able to supply sufficient essential nutrients to meet increased needs caused by chronic blood loss (hemorrhoids, bleeding peptic ulcers), genetic disorders (sickle cell anemia), or abnormally high requirements (pregnancy, growth during childhood).

TABLE 41-1. Etiologic classification of types of anemia

Nutrient deficiency	Resultant deficiency
Iron	Microcytic and hypochromic
Folic acid *or* vitamin B_{12}	Macrocytic and normochromic (also termed *megaloblastic*)
Iron *and* folic acid *and* vitamin B_{12}	Macrocytic and hypochromic (also termed *dimorphic*)

Source: R. A. Rifkind, et al., *Fundamentals of Hematology.* Chicago: Year Book, 1976.

LABORATORY
EVALUATION

When an insufficient amount of iron is available during erythropoiesis, the red blood cells produced are small (*microcytic*) and pale (*hypochromic*). When there is only a lack of folic acid or vitamin B_{12}, the resulting erythrocytes are larger than normal (*macrocytic*), but contain a full complement of hemoglobin (*normochromic*). This type of anemia is termed *megaloblastic*, after the immature precursor of the erythrocytes, the megaloblast. When iron and vitamins B_{12} and folic acid are lacking, the resulting macrocytic hypochromic anemia is termed *dimorphic*. These anemias are summarized in Table 41-1.

Several measurements of blood components can be made to distinguish the type and severity of anemia present. A decrease in the hemoglobin concentration may be a sign of iron deficiency, but it is not conclusive. The *hematocrit*, or packed cell volume (PCV), is determined by centrifuging a sample of blood and then reading the height of the column of packed red cells (see Fig. 41-2). This value may be used to differentiate between iron and folate deficiency, or may be used with the hemoglobin value as a ratio (hemoglobin/PCV), giving the *mean corpuscular hemoglobin concentration* (MCHC). An MCHC value below 30 indicates a lack of hemoglobin and hypochromic anemia. The *red blood cell* (RBC) *count* is another useful measurement and indicates the number of red blood cells per cubic millimeter. The *mean corpuscular volume* (MCV) is given as the ratio of the packed cell volume/red blood cell count (PCV/RBC). A value greater than 95 indicates that the erythrocytes are larger than normal, suggesting a deficiency of either folate or vitamin B_{12}. Another useful measurement is the *reticulocyte count*. Reticulocytes are the last phase of the immature erythrocyte and are normally present in the blood as less than 1 percent of the total number of erythrocytes. They are present in greater numbers when the bone marrow is unusually active, such as during response to specific anemia therapy. A comparison of laboratory findings in normal and deficiency states is summarized in Table 41-2.

CLINICAL SYMPTOMS

Regardless of the cause or type of anemia, the symptoms are similar, reflecting a decrease in the transport of oxygen to the tissues. The clinical symptoms of

FIG. 41-2. Hematocrit tubes before and after centrifugation.

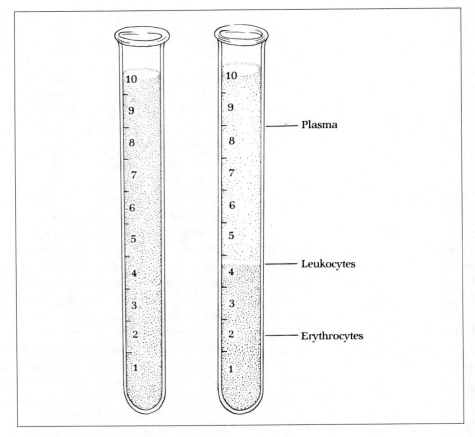

anemia are easy fatigability, pallor, and shortness of breath on exertion. Their severity is related to the degree of anemia and how rapidly it has developed. With iron-deficiency anemia, the skin, nails, and mucous membranes are pale, reflecting the reduction in circulating hemoglobin. Cardiac signs include tachycardia (rapid heartbeat), murmurs, and slight enlargement of the heart with eventual failure if the anemia becomes severe. Concurrent signs of nutritional deficiencies may also be present, such as *angular stomatitis*, *koilonychia*, and *glossitis*. Angular stomatitis is an inflammation of the oral mucosa or soft tissues of the mouth. Koilonychia are changes in the nails; they may become brittle, ridged, and concave or spoon shaped (Fig. 41-3). Glossitis is an inflammation of the tongue with atrophy of the papillae. Most of these symptoms are reversible with treatment of the anemia.

Iron Deficiency

Iron is an essential trace element that is vital to life. Its main role in human physiology is in the exchange of gases at the cellular level. Iron-containing compounds are involved in a wide variety of chemical reactions in the body;

TABLE 41-2. Laboratory findings in normal and deficiency states

Measurement	Normal range in women	Deficiency	
		Iron	Folate
Basic measurements			
Hemoglobin (Hgb), gm/dl	12–16	7	7
Packed cell volume (PCV), percent	36–47	28	22
Red blood cell count (RBC) × 10^6/cu mm	3.9–4.6	3.7	2.0
Derived values			
Mean corpuscular hemoglobin concentration (MCHC), percent	30–36	25	32
Mean corpuscular volume (MCV), μm	75–95	78	110

among the most important are *hemoglobin* and *myoglobin*, iron-protein complexes that combine reversibly with oxygen; the *cytochrome enzymes*, iron-protein complexes involved in electron transport; and *transferrin*, *ferritin*, and *hemosiderin*, iron-protein complexes that act as transport or storage forms of iron (see Chap. 6).

Nearly 70 percent of all iron in the body is found in the form of hemoglobin. Because iron is a vital component of hemoglobin, a deficiency of this element is reflected in a lowered level of hemoglobin, with anemia eventually resulting. A fall in the hemoglobin level represents a late manifestation of the iron-deficient state. Initially, iron stores become depleted, then iron-deficient erythropoiesis develops, and, finally, iron-deficiency anemia results.

ASSESSING IRON STATUS

Iron deficiency has been found to be the most common nutritional disorder [1] and the most important cause of anemia in the world [2, 3]. It has been estimated to affect 10 to 20 percent of the world's population [4]. Because hemoglobin levels alone are unreliable as a screening method for detecting iron deficiency, other guidelines must additionally be used. Simple iron deficiency causes a fall in the level of serum iron and a rise in iron-binding capacity. A ratio of these two parameters is termed the *transferrin saturation*. Because it fluctuates diurnally (varies according to hour of day or night) and falls with mild

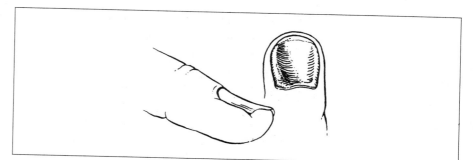

FIG. 41-3. Koilonychia, or spoon nails, may occur in iron-deficiency anemia. The nails become brittle, ridged, and concave. (From J. D. Judge, G. D. Zuidema, and F. T. Fitzgerald, *Clinical Diagnosis*. Boston: Little, Brown, 1982.)

FIG. 41-4. The quaternary structure of hemoglobin. The hemoglobin molecule is made up of four polypeptide chains. Two identical chains are called α-chains, and the other two identical chains are called β-chains. Each chain encloses a heme molecule. (From G. H. Schmid, *The Chemical Basis of Life: General, Organic, and Biological Chemistry for the Health Sciences.* Boston: Little, Brown, 1982.)

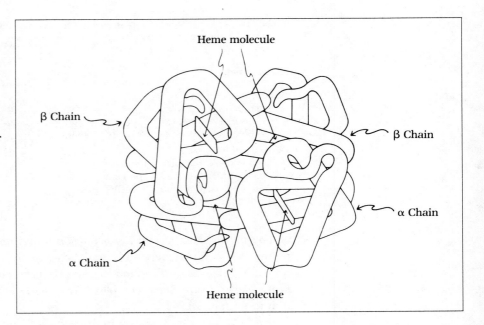

infection, this ratio has a limited use. The *free erythrocyte protoporphyrin* (*FEP*) has also been used to detect iron deficiency. Protoporphyrin is the complex that combines with iron to form hemoglobin (see Fig. 41-4). With a lack of sufficient iron, there is an increase of free erythrocyte protoporphyrin in the blood. FEP is a more reliable index than the transferrin saturation, but it may not be sensitive enough to detect milder degrees of iron deficiency. The most sensitive indicator used thus far is the *serum ferritin* level [5]. It falls with iron deficiency and rises with chronic infection, particularly inflammation and liver disease.

No one indicator can monitor the entire spectrum of iron status, from deficiency to overload. When only one parameter of iron-deficiency is used, few cases are detected. Two parameters give a better prediction of anemia and all three plus a clinical screening for chronic infective or inflammatory states would provide the most accurate results [6, 7]. A summary of the parameters of iron status in relationship to body iron stores is given in Table 41-3.

GROUPS AT SPECIAL RISK

Iron balance in the body is dependent on several factors: (1) iron requirements for hemoglobin production; (2) iron losses from physiologic and pathologic processes; and (3) the amount of iron absorbed from the intestine. The requirements for hemoglobin synthesis are greatest when there is rapid expansion of tissue and red cell mass, that is, during infancy, childhood, and pregnancy.

Infancy

Iron needs are great during infancy because of rapid growth and the expansion of the blood volume. Normal full-term infants (those born after 40 weeks of

TABLE 41-3. Parameters of iron status in relationship to body iron stores

Test	Normal	Iron depletion	Iron-deficient erythropoiesis	Iron-deficient anemia
Serum ferritin	60	<12	<12	<12
Transferrin saturation	35	35	<16	<16
Free erythrocyte protoporphyrin	30	30	>100	>100
Hemoglobin	>12	>12	>12	<12

Source: J. D. Cook and C. A. Finch, Assessing iron status of a population. *American Journal of Clinical Nutrition* 32:2115, 1979.

gestation) have a complement of iron stored during the last 4 weeks of gestation. This stored iron is mobilized during the rapid growth period of the first year. Premature infants (those born before 38 weeks of gestation) have less iron stored and may require supplemental iron from birth. The iron present in breast milk is extremely well absorbed, far better than the iron in fortified cow's milk formula or fortified commercial infant formula. It has been suggested that infants who are exclusively breast-fed may not require routine administration of supplemental iron [8], whereas normal term infants on other formulas should receive 1 mg/kg/day starting at about the third month of life. Low-birth-weight (under 2500 gm) or premature infants should receive 2 mg/kg/day from birth to maintain optimal hemoglobin levels [9].

Iron deficiency remains to be the most common cause of anemia among infants and children. The risk for developing iron deficiency is greatest after the first 2 months of life for small preterm infants and after 4 to 6 months in term infants. Iron supplementation should start no later than 2 and 4 months, respectively; iron-fortified cereal or iron-containing drops are good sources [10]. The American Academy of Pediatrics recommends screening for iron-deficiency anemia (hemoglobin < 11 gm/100 ml or hematocrit < 33%) between 9 and 12 months of age in term infants and between 6 and 9 months in premature or low-birth-weight infants [11].

Pregnancy

During pregnancy, demands are made on iron stores due to the needs of the growing fetus and placenta, the expanding maternal blood volume and red cell mass, plus blood losses at delivery. These requirements are superimposed on the nonpregnant baseline needs. Although the increased demands are in part offset by amenorrhea (the cessation of menses) and increased iron absorption, it is doubtful that needs can be met by dietary sources alone. During pregnancy, iron needs average about 3.5 mg per day, with a range of 2 to 4 mg. Iron requirements may reach 4 mg per day during the latter half of pregnancy. Total demands during pregnancy with a single fetus average 1000 to 1100 mg.

Both the fetus and placenta effectively parasitize folic acid and iron from the mother, even if she is grossly deficient [12]. Iron is transferred to the fetus against a concentration gradient; the placenta and fetus receive about one-sixth the total iron passing through the maternal plasma each day. The iron drain is greatest after the twentieth week of pregnancy. Maternal excretion accounts for about 200 mg, about 300 mg is transferred to the fetus, placenta, and its contained blood, and about 500 mg is utilized to increase the maternal blood volume [13]. The mode of delivery also influences iron balance. Vaginal delivery is associated with a loss of at least 500 ml of blood, or over 200 mg of iron; cesarean section is associated with at least a 1000 ml blood loss, or more than 400 mg of iron [13]. A portion of these needs can be met by iron stores, but in females these stores tend to be low or nonexistent. Without supplementation, the pregnant woman consuming an excellent diet will still finish pregnancy with an iron store deficit; if nutrition was less than excellent, frank iron deficiency anemia will develop.

When imposed on the physiologic stress of pregnancy, severe anemia has been reported to increase maternal morbidity and mortality, as well as cause a greater risk to the fetus [14, 15]. Pregnant women who are anemic are less able to withstand serious hemorrhage and have a greater incidence of premature deliveries, and the anemia may also have an adverse effect on birth weight [16].

Elderly

This age group is often considered to be particularly susceptible to iron deficiency. Some of the etiologic factors cited include poor diet, gastrointestinal blood loss, and reduced iron absorption. Studies have shown that when iron deficiency is found in the aged, it should be considered pathologic and not due to an age-related impairment of iron absorption from foods [17].

OTHER CAUSES OF IRON-DEFICIENCY ANEMIA

Iron-deficiency anemia can also occur due to acute or chronic hemorrhage (blood loss), or to malabsorption of iron. During an acute hemorrhage, fluid from surrounding tissues is drawn into the blood, causing a drop in the hemoglobin and red cell count. The rapid loss of 2 to 3 liters of blood is usually fatal, but can be sustained if spread over a period of hours. The treatment of a large acute hemorrhage requires blood transfusion.

Chronic hemorrhage results from the repeated loss of small amounts of blood. The most common causes include menorrhagia (heavy menstrual bleeding) and bleeding from the gastrointestinal tract (peptic ulcers, hemorrhoids, chronic aspirin consumption). The drop in hemoglobin is usually slow and progressive. Once diagnosed, either by the laboratory findings of hypochromic anemia or, if gastrointestinal, by the presence of occult (hidden) blood in the feces, the treatment includes therapy of the primary cause plus medicinal and dietary iron. Iron-deficiency anemia due to malabsorption most often occurs after gastrointestinal surgery and may take months or years to develop. The symptoms develop slowly and may go unrecognized because of the long-time interval since surgery.

TREATMENT OF IRON-DEFICIENCY

Prevention is the best treatment of iron-deficiency anemia in high-risk age groups. Preventive treatment includes supplementation of infants and the introduction of fortified or enriched foods at appropriate ages and supplementation of pregnant women from at least 20 weeks gestation until delivery. In uncomplicated adult cases, the preferred treatment, once iron-deficiency anemia is present, is with inexpensive, soluble iron salts such as ferrous sulfate, ferrous gluconate, or ferrous fumarate. The usual dose is 200 mg per day, expressed as elemental iron and taken after meals. Injections (parenteral administration) of iron compounds are indicated when there is intestinal malabsorption; gastrointestinal disease; when oral supplementation is irritating or ineffective; or when patient compliance is poor. The diet should be planned to maximize the iron intake and other factors aiding absorption (i.e., vitamin C and animal protein) and minimize inhibiting factors (i.e., binding agents such as tea, phytates, and phosphates). Food sources of iron and a discussion of factors influencing absorption are given in Chapter 6.

Anemias Due to Folate or Vitamin B_{12} Deficiency

This group of anemias is caused by a deficiency of folate or vitamin B_{12}, both of which are vital in the synthesis of proteins and nucleic acids and are, therefore, vital in the formation of new erythrocytes. Since vitamin C functions in the conversion of folic acid to its biologically active form, tetrahydrofolic acid, a deficiency of vitamin C would have a similar effect as a lack of folic acid. A deficiency of either folate or vitamin B_{12}, or both, interferes with the normal development and maturation of erythrocytes, resulting in anemia characterized by large, immature erythrocytes carrying a normal complement of hemoglobin (megaloblastic, normochromic anemia).

In Europe and North America these anemias are most often seen during pregnancy or as a result of malabsorption. In Asia, India, and Africa, the cause is more often malnutrition. As a group, these anemias are fairly rare compared to the overwhelming world-wide incidence of iron-deficiency anemia.

MEGALOBLASTIC ANEMIAS

FOLATE DEFICIENCY

This type of anemia occurs most frequently among populations consuming diets poor in animal protein and fresh, green vegetables and in association with protein-calorie malnutrition. It is more common among children and women than among men and is also associated with pregnancy. Megaloblastic anemia due to folate deficiency can also develop as a result of malabsorption of folic acid (due to surgical resection of the small intestine, tropical sprue, or idiopathic steatorrhea), when dietary intake is insufficient to meet demands, or when folic acid is destroyed by chronic drug therapy (i.e., anticonvulsants, oral contraceptives).

Glossitis and paresthesia are often present, as is the laboratory finding of megaloblastic (macrocytic) anemia. The plasma folate level is usually less than 3 ng per ml and the red cell folate is less than 100 ng per ml [18]. Treatment is usually 5 to 10 mg of folic acid per day, and iron may be needed as well. Food sources of folate should be utilized (see Chap. 7), as well as follow-up blood counts to detect relapses.

VITAMIN B_{12} DEFICIENCY

Vitamin B_{12} is found only in foods of animal origin and, therefore, individuals excluding meat, dairy products, and eggs risk developing this deficiency. The liver stores this vitamin; several years of a deficient diet are needed to deplete its large reserve. Strict vegetarians, or Vegans, may demonstrate a reduced plasma vitamin B_{12} level and a soreness of the mouth and tongue. Since vitamin B_{12} deficiency caused by diet alone is rare, other factors should be ruled out, such as gastric and intestinal function and impaired absorption by drug therapy. Parenteral administration of this vitamin may be required.

PERNICIOUS ANEMIA

Pernicious anemia is a type of megaloblastic anemia caused by a failure of gastric secretion of *intrinsic factor*. A failure to absorb vitamin B_{12} is due to lack of production of intrinsic factor by the gastric mucosa. Intrinsic factor is essential for the intestinal absorption of this vitamin. In some cases antibodies have been detected against the gastric mucosa, which is responsible for destruction of the mechanism producing intrinsic factor.

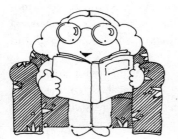

Pathophysiologic changes caused by pernicious anemia include extension of the active bone marrow into the shafts of the long bones; increased blood destruction; and deposition of iron in the liver, spleen, bone marrow, and kidneys. The gastric mucosa becomes thin and atrophic (from the Greek, *atrophia*, lack of nourishment) and there is a complete absence of hydrochloric acid (achlorhydria). In advanced stages, pernicious anemia can lead to degenerative changes of the posterior (dorsal) and lateral tracts of the spinal cord.

Pernicious anemia is more common among women than men; it occurs most frequently between 45 and 65 years of age. Weight loss and pale mucous membranes and skin are common symptoms. The tongue becomes painful, red and raw in appearance, and occasionally develops ulcers. In its late stages, the tongue becomes smooth and the mucous membranes atrophic (see Fig. 41-5). Another clinical feature includes paresthesia of the fingers and toes—numbness, tingling, and a "pins and needles" feeling.

The diagnosis of pernicious anemia is made by a low-plasma vitamin B_{12} level (<160 ng/L) and a normal plasma folate level. The Schilling test is also used; a positive test occurs when an oral dose of vitamn B_{12} labeled with radioactive cobalt shows decreased absorption and when absorption returns to normal when intrinsic factor is given simultaneously. After the diagnosis is confirmed, the treatment is cyanocobalamin (vitamin B_{12}), 1000 μg intramuscularly, for the

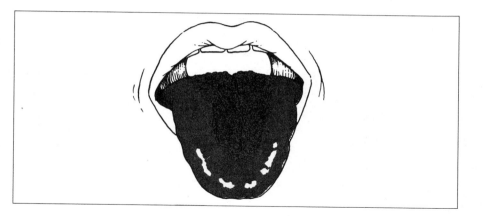

FIG. 41-5. Glossitis in pernicious anemia. In extreme cases, the tongue becomes pale and smooth, with the glossal papillae inflamed. (From J. D. Judge, G. D. Zuidema, and F. T. Fitzgerald, *Clinical Diagnosis.* Boston: Little, Brown, 1982.)

first week, then 250 μg weekly until the blood count is normal [18]. When the response is very rapid, iron stores may become depleted and concurrent iron therapy may also be required. Maintenance therapy includes cyanocobalamin, 1000 μg intramuscularly, every 4 to 6 weeks and regular blood counts every 6 months to avoid spinal degeneration. Folic acid is never given because it can mask the spinal degenerative changes.

Other Causes of Anemia

Although rare in Europe and North America, anemia due to malaria and hookworm infection are common in other parts of the world. A malarial attack, particularly when due to *Plasmodium falciparum*, is accompanied by hemolysis (the breakdown of erythrocytes), with anemia resulting. Hookworm infections effect anemia by the chronic blood loss at the site of attachment of the worm to the intestinal wall, plus the ingestion of blood by each worm daily. Improved sanitary conditions and hygiene, health education, and better housing and social environments can decrease the incidence of these illnesses and their resultant suffering.

A number of anemias are not due to a primary nutritional deficiency, but do have dietary implications. Such diseases as uremia, cancer, hepatic cirrhosis, and infection can all result in anemia due to hemorrhage, hormonal imbalance, increased hemolysis, or poor dietary intake. Genetic anemias resulting in abnormal hemoglobin may cause the individual erythrocytes to be fragile, with hemolysis leading to anemia. Sickle cell anemia is caused by the replacement of normal hemoglobin A by the abnormal hemoglobin S, resulting in a distortion of the red cell, hemolysis, and anemia. Thalassemia results when hemoglobin A is replaced by fetal hemoglobin (hemoglobin F), also resulting in accelerated hemolysis.

Case Studies

1. Nanette is the youngest of five children, ranging in age from 16 to 1½. Her mother is pregnant again. Nanette's father is a farmer and raises mostly rice,

the family's main food. What type of anemia do you think this family is most at risk for developing? Who do you think will develop it first? Why?

2. Mrs. Greene is 80 years old and lives alone in an urban housing project. Since both the telephone and utilities have increased their monthly bills while her social security check has remained the same, she has decided to cut down expenses by eating less expensive foods. Her diet consists mainly of tea, pastries, white bread, butter, and jam. What type of anemia would she most likely develop? Describe the symptoms and explain their development.

3. Joey is 9 months old and has been receiving a diet of whole milk and mashed fruit since birth. At his checkup this month by the pediatrician, what would you expect the laboratory evaluation of his blood to reveal? Would you change his diet and how?

4. Mrs. Smith, a 50-year-old woman, comes to the doctor's office complaining of weight loss, sore tongue, and "tingling" of the fingers and toes. What three laboratory tests would you want to order? A diagnosis of pernicious anemia is confirmed; can it be treated by diet? Explain.

References

1. Control of nutritional anaemia with special reference to iron deficiency. *WHO Tech. Rep. Ser.* No. 580. Geneva, 1975.
2. Finch, C. A. Iron deficiency anemia. *Am. J. Clin. Nutr.* 22:512, 1969.
3. Beaton, G. H. Epidemiology of Iron Deficiency. In A. Jacobs and M. Worwood (eds.), *Iron in Bio-Chemistry and Medicine.* New York: Academic, 1974. Pp. 477–528.
4. Cook, J. D., and Finch, C. A. Assessing iron status of a population. *Am. J. Clin. Nutr.* 32:2115, 1979.
5. Cook, J. D., et al. Serum ferritin as a measure of iron stores in normal subjects. *Am. J. Clin. Nutr.* 27:681, 1974.
6. Cook, J. D., Finch, C. A., and Smith, N. J. Evaluation of the iron status of a population. *Blood* 48:449, 1976.
7. Population screening for iron deficiency. *Nutr. Rev.* 35:271, 1977.
8. Diet and iron absorption in the first year of life. *Nutr. Rev.* 37:195, 1979.
9. National Research Council. *Recommended Dietary Allowances* (9th ed.). Washington, D.C.: National Academy of Sciences, 1980. P. 138.
10. Committee on Nutrition. Iron supplementation for infants. *Pediatrics* 58:765, 1976.
11. Committee on Standards of Child Health Care. *Standards of Child Health Care* (2nd ed.). Evanston, Ill.: American Academy of Pediatrics, 1972. P. 10.
12. Kitay, D. Z., and Harbort, R. A. Iron and folic acid deficiency in pregnancy. *Clin. Perinatol.* 2:255, 1975.
13. Scott, D. E., and Pritchard, J. A. Anemia in pregnancy. *Clin. Perinatol.* 1:491, 1974.
14. Gatenby, P. B. B., and Lillie, E. W. Clinical analysis of 100 cases of severe megaloblastic anaemia of pregnancy. *Br. Med. J.* 2:1111, 1960.
15. Llewellyn-Jones, D. Severe anaemia in pregnancy. *Aust. N.Z. J. Obstet. Gynaecol.* 5:191, 1965.
16. Luke, B. *Maternal Nutrition.* Boston: Little, Brown, 1979. Pp. 59–73.

17. Iron absorption and utilization in the elderly. *Nutr. Rev.* 37:222, 1979.

18. Davidson, S., et al. *Human Nutrition and Dietetics* (6th ed.). Edinburgh: Churchill Livingstone, 1975. Pp. 502–515.

Suggested Readings

Chopra, J. G., and Kevany, J.   International approach to nutritional anemias. *Am. J. Public Health* 61:250, 1971.

Cook, J. D., et al.   Serum ferritin as a measure of iron stores in normal subjects. *Am. J. Clin. Nutr.* 27:681, 1974.

Doswell, W. M.   Sickle cell disease: How it influences preoperative and postoperative care. *Nurs. '74* June. Pp. 19–22.

Elwood, P. C.   Anaemia. *Lancet* 2:1364, 1974.

Graiteer, P. L., Goldsby, J. B., and Nichaman, M. Z.   Hemoglobins and hematocrits: Are they equally sensitive in detecting anemias? *Am. J. Clin. Nutr.* 34:61, 1981.

Olszon, E., et al.   Food iron absorption in iron deficiency. *Am. J. Clin. Nutr.* 31:106, 1978.

Rosa, R. M., et al.   A study of induced hyponatremia in the prevention and treatment of sickle-cell crisis. *N. Engl. J. Med.* 303:1138, 1980.

Scott, D. E.   *Iron and Folic Acid Nutrition in Pregnancy.* Columbus, Ohio: Ross Laboratories, 1978.

Sjölin, S.   Anemia in adolescence. *Nutr. Rev.* 39:96, 1981.

Strauss, R. G.   Iron deficiency, infections, and immune function: A reassessment. *Am. J. Clin. Nutr.* 31:660, 1978.

Toy, L., Williams, T. E., and Young, E. A.   Nutritional status of patients with hemophilia. *J. Am. Diet. Assoc.* 78:47, 1981.

Voors, A. W., et al.   Hemoglobin levels and dietary iron in pubescent children in a biracial community. *Public Health Rep.* 96:45, 1981.

Chapter 42

RENAL DISEASE

The outlook for patients with progressive renal disease was somewhat bleak until the past 50 years or so. As the kidneys began to fail, patients would die a long and agonizing death, literally poisoned by the accumulation of their own toxic wastes. Since it was known that the kidneys normally rid the body of the excess by-products of the diet, it has long been reasoned that dietary restrictions might be able to modify the symptoms of uremia (the toxic accumulation of waste products) and prolong life. As early as 1844, a protein-restricted diet was tried but with little success. With the discoveries in biochemistry and nutrition during the early part of the twentieth century, diet therapy in renal disease proved to be more effective. The concepts of differing biologic value of various dietary proteins and the "all or none" nature of protein synthesis and essential amino acids made later attempts at protein restriction more fruitful. With the development of efficient hemodialysis and safe transplantation, the outlook for the patient with renal disease is much brighter today than it was even 10 years ago.

This chapter will present renal function, dysfunction, and the role of diet therapy in all phases of renal disease.

Chapters to review: Chapters 3, 6, 8, 10, 34.

Renal Function

The kidneys have the immense task of regulating the volume and composition of body fluids. Together with the lungs, which control the concentrations of oxygen and carbon dioxide, these two sets of organs maintain the body's internal environment. The kidneys accomplish their functions through three main pathways—*excretory, endocrine,* and *regulatory.*

EXCRETORY

The excretory functions of the kidney are clearly its most important. The kidney excretes a wide variety of metabolic waste products and precisely regulates the amount of body water and the concentration of sodium, potassium, chloride, bicarbonate, phosphorus, calcium, and many other minerals and organic molecules. The kidneys maintain the normal body pH by selectively excreting acid or base. Acid is excreted in the form of inorganic acid, usually sulfate, phosphate, ammonium, as well as hydrogen ions and organic acids. The kidneys control the excretion of the end products of protein metabolism, particularly urea, uric acid, creatinine, sulfates, and organic acids. This excretion and regulation of body fluids is carried out by filtration through the glomerulus. Compounds of molecular weight of 5000 or less are completely filtered by the glomerulus. The *glomerular filtration rate* (GFR) is used as an indicator of renal function (see Fig. 42-1).

The *creatinine clearance* (normal values = 95–105 ml/min) is often used as a measure of the GFR since this metabolite is filtered at the glomerulus but is neither secreted nor absorbed by the tubule. The creatinine clearance is also used as an indicator of the amount of dietary protein that should be prescribed in treating renal disease. By the time the GFR has dropped to 1.5 ml per min

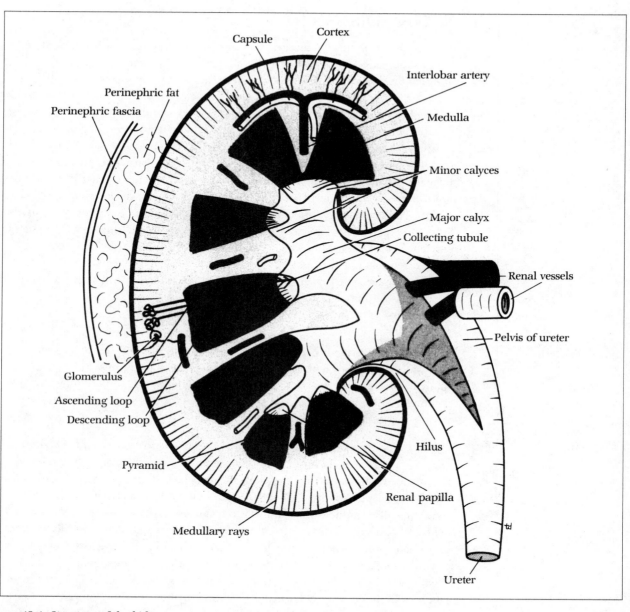

FIG. 42-1. Structure of the kidney and its functional unit, the uriniferous tubule.

A. Longitudinal section through the kidney. (From R. Snell, *Clinical Anatomy for Medical Students* [2nd ed.]. Boston: Little, Brown, 1981.)

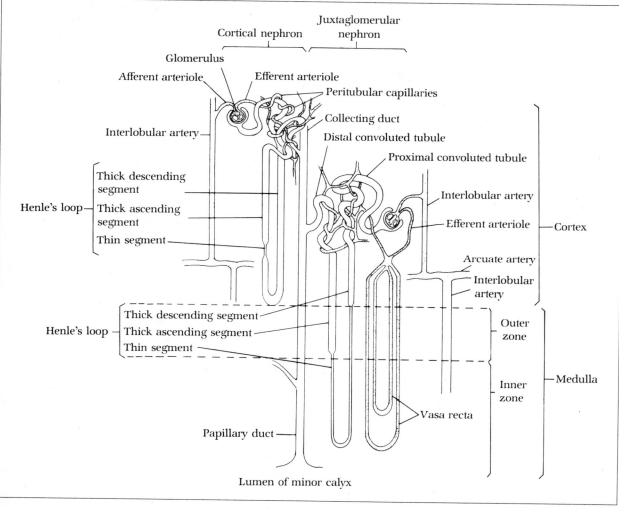

B. Uriniferous tubule with attendant blood supply. The uriniferous tubule has two distinct functional regions—the *nephron,* which is concerned with production of urine, and the *collecting tubule,* which is concerned with the hypertonic concentration of urine. (From M. Borysenko, et al., *Functional Histology* [2nd ed.]. Boston: Little, Brown, 1984.)

(creatinine clearance to 5 ml/min), the patient is severely uremic from the accumulation of metabolic toxins and electrolyte disturbances, and must have dialysis and/or transplantation for life to continue. By way of an extensive circulatory system, the kidney receives and processes about 25 percent of the entire cardiac output every minute. For this reason, the kidneys are particularly susceptible to destruction by vascular disease. The kidneys can function until as little as 10 percent of its nephrons, the functional units, remain and then the loss or impairment of homeostatic ability causes metabolic alterations affecting every system, tissue, and organ of the body. When the GFR falls to about one-tenth that found in health (10–12 ml/min in disease, 120 ml/min in health), clinical symptoms of renal disease appear.

ENDOCRINE

The endocrine functions of the kidney affect every organ and system of the body. The hormones produced by the kidney have diverse metabolic effects. *Renin* is one such hormone, produced by the juxtaglomerular apparatus of the kidney, as well as by the uterus and brain. Through its action on angiotensin, renin indirectly affects blood pressure by causing vasoconstriction. This hormone is the major regulator of aldosterone secretion; it also helps to regulate intrarenal blood flow, glomerular filtration rate, and sodium excretion. *Prostaglandins* are another group of hormones produced by the kidney. They inhibit sodium and water reabsorption, lower blood pressure, and alter intrarenal blood flow.

The kidney also has an essential role in *vitamin D* metabolism. It is in the kidney that the inactive form of vitamin D is hydroxylated for the second, and final, time to produce the active form. The first hydroxylation occurs in the liver, producing 25-hydroxycholecalciferol; in the kidney this compound is converted to 1,25-dihydroxycholecalciferol (or 1,25-dihydroxyvitamin D). The activated form of vitamin D then acts on the intestine where it enhances calcium and phosphorus absorption; in the bone, where it affects the deposit and mobilization of calcium and phosphorus; and in the kidney, where it enhances calcium reabsorption (see Chap. 5 for more detail). In renal disease, the second hydroxylation of the inactive form of vitamin D does not occur, causing impaired intestinal calcium absorption and leading to the development of *uremic osteodystrophy*, defective bone formation.

Another endocrine function of the kidney is its secretion of the glycoprotein, *erythropoietin*. This substance regulates erythropoiesis (red blood cell production) by the bone marrow and balances the hematocrit. The anemia that develops with kidney disease is most often due to the decreased production of erythropoietin.

REGULATORY

The kidney's regulatory and metabolic functions include the maintenance of electrolyte balance in the body by the excretion and selective reabsorption of sodium, potassium, chloride, and other ions; the maintenance of water balance; and the maintenance of acid-base equilibrium through selective excretion of excess acid. The kidney also has the ability to degrade such hormones as insulin, glucagon, gastrin, and parathyroid hormone. During periods of starvation or prolonged fasting, the kidney also becomes a producer of glucose (see Chap. 35).

Renal Dysfunction

Renal disease may be classified as *acute, chronic, congenital,* or *acquired,* depending on the etiology. The cause of renal failure may involve the kidney primarily or secondarily, resulting in temporary or permanent impairment of renal function. Various causes of renal failure have been grouped as *prerenal,* factors that decrease renal blood flow and thereby cause damage; *renal,* factors primarily causing damage directly to the kidney; and *postrenal,* those causes acting on the urinary system distal to the kidneys (ureters, bladder, urethra). These causes and classifications have been summarized in Tables 42-1 and 42-2.

TABLE 42-1. Causes of renal failure

Acute	Chronic	Primary	Secondary
Acute tubular necrosis	Polycystic kidney disease	Glomerulonephritis	Hypertensive nephropathy
Acute glomerulonephritis	Chronic glomerulonephritis	Pyelonephritis	Diabetes nephropathy
Acute urinary obstruction	Chronic urinary obstruction	Polycystic kidneys	Lupus nephritis
Occlusion of renal artery or vein	Severe hypertension	Hypernephroma	Gouty nephropathy
Acute pyelonephritis	Diabetes		
Bilateral cortical necrosis	Gout		
	Chronic pyelonephritis		

Source: D. J. Brundage, *Nursing Management of Renal Problems* (2nd ed.). St. Louis: Mosby, 1980. P. 17.

TABLE 42-2. Classification of causes of renal failure

Prerenal	Renal	Postrenal
Dehydration	Glomerulonephritis	Urinary tract infection
Hemorrhage	Pyelonephritis	Urinary tract obstruction
Shock	Polycystic kidneys	Urinary stones
Burns	Hypertensive nephropathy	
	Diabetic nephropathy	
	Nephrotoxic substances	
	Blood transfusion reactions	
	Wilms' tumor	
	Hypernephroma	
	Horseshoe kidney	
	Pregnancy-related disease	

Source: D. J. Brundage, *Nursing Management of Renal Problems* (2nd ed.). St. Louis: Mosby, 1980. P. 17.

Glomerulonephritis and pyelonephritis are among the most common causes of renal failure. The interrelationships between pathophysiology and clinical manifestations in renal disease are described further in Fig. 42-4.

ACUTE RENAL FAILURE

Acute renal failure is the sudden loss of renal function in an individual without a previous history of renal disease. It may be temporary or permanent, depending on the causative factors. It is more likely to be temporary if the disease causes acute necrosis of the tubules and if the decreased urine output (*oliguria*) only lasts less than 12 to 14 days. Damage is more likely to be permanent if the cortex of the kidney is involved and if the oliguria persists for longer than 2 weeks. The complete absence of urine (*anuria*) or severe oliguria suggests obstruction of both kidneys and is probably irreversible. The major causes of acute renal failure are given in Fig. 42-2.

Both food and fluid are restricted during the first 24 to 48 hours after the onset of symptoms. Fluid intake is given according to the volume of urine output and

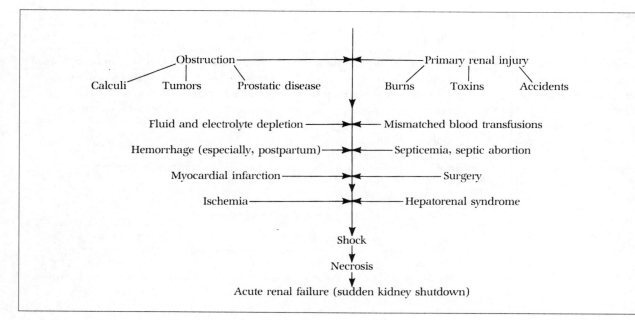

insensible losses. The caloric intake is increased as soon as possible, to prevent tissue breakdown and resultant hyperkalemia and to prevent increases in blood levels of nitrogenous substances. Calories should be supplied mainly as carbohydrates since carbohydrates do not require the kidneys for elimination of their end products of metabolism. Sodium is restricted when edema and hypertension are present. Proteins are allowed according to the blood urea nitrogen level. As the level falls, more dietary protein is allowed; as it rises, protein is restricted.

CHRONIC RENAL FAILURE

Chronic renal failure follows a more progressive course, although the onset may be either sudden or slow and insidious. Among the most common causes of chronic renal disease are those that are congenital (present at birth), secondary to systemic disease (such as essential hypertension and diabetes mellitus) or infection, or by obstruction in the lower urinary tract (such as prostatic enlargement or stricture of the urethra). *Glomerulonephritis*, characterized by diffuse inflammatory changes in the glomerulus, is one of the most common forms of renal disease and can be either acute or chronic. In its acute form, it usually follows a beta hemolytic group A streptococcal infection, mostly affecting individuals between the ages of 3 and 21. The symptoms of edema, hypertension, hematuria (presence of blood in the urine), and oliguria usually subside with bed rest; appropriate antibiotics; and sodium, protein, and fluid restriction. The young patient usually recovers without any residual problems. Chronic glomerulonephritis may progress from the acute form or occur independently. The highest incidence of the chronic form is among males under age 45. This form is characterized by the progressive destruction of the glomeruli and tubules of the kidney. Before progressing to end-stage renal disease and renal failure (requiring dialysis or transplantation for life to continue), chronic glomerulonephritis progresses to a stage termed the *nephrotic syndrome*, characterized by the loss of large amounts of protein in the urine. During the early stages of either acute or chronic glomerulonephritis, the diet therapy is the same. Fluids, sodium, potassium, and protein are all given in amounts reflected by clinical symptoms and laboratory values (see the diet therapy section, which follows). Carbohydrates are given liberally to spare tissue breakdown and for energy.

END-STAGE RENAL DISEASE   As discussed earlier, the kidney has a tremendous amount of functional reserve; only when a small portion of healthy nephrons remain does the accumulation of toxic wastes exceed the excretory ability. End-stage renal disease (ESRD) represents either the end of a long series of acute renal illnesses or the final stage of progressive chronic renal disease. In either case the results are similar; the work of the kidneys must be replaced by renal transplantation, by artificial kidneys (hemodialysis), or other means (peritoneal dialysis).

RENAL TRANSPLANTATION

Renal transplantation was first used successfully in this country in 1954 in Boston, performed between identical twins. Other transplantations that followed were not as successful due to tissue incompatibilities. During the past 30 years, much has been learned about tissue rejection, immunologic response to foreign tissues, and immunosuppressive drugs. In addition, improved surgical techniques, such as vascular suturing, have advanced renal transplantation from an experimental procedure to an accepted therapeutic practice. When successful, it is less expensive than hemodialysis and frees up a dialysis machine for another patient.

One of the greatest rewards of a successful renal transplant is the return to a normal, unrestricted diet. After the usual postsurgical bland diet, the patient progresses to solid foods and an essentially nonrestricted diet. During the immediate posttransplant period, however, the patient is placed on immunosuppressive therapy whose temporary side effects may need to be treated with appropriate diet therapy. Some of these side effects may include nausea and vomiting, intestinal ulceration, and diarrhea.

DIALYSIS
Hemodialysis

Hemodialysis, also called an "artificial kidney," is a machine that permits the filtering of water and solutes to or from the blood. The patient's blood is passed through a *dialyzer*, where wastes, excess electrolytes, and water cross the semipermeable membrane into the dialysate solution (see Fig. 42-1). The cleansed blood is then filtered for bubbles and returned to the patient. The entire procedure takes about 4 to 6 hours and must be repeated about three times per week.

Hemodialysis was first used in 1913, but only became a practical therapeutic regimen when cellophane (for the semipermeable membrane) and heparin (for anticoagulation) were discovered. During the past 20 years, several new types of hemodialysis machines have been developed and improved, as well as the perfection of surgical techniques that connect an artery and vein in the forearm to allow access to the circulation. Many patients feel well enough on hemodialysis to return to work, full-time or part-time, and as many as 80 percent of all patients are still alive after 5 years of treatment. In addition, dietary restrictions can be liberalized (see section on diet therapy).

Special problems arise when the hemodialysis patient is a child, particularly concerning the nutritional management (see the diet therapy section, which follows). The protein, sodium, and potassium allowed are adjusted to the etiology of the renal failure, residual renal function, weight, age, urinary output, medications, and other treatments [2]. The high carbohydrate allowance may lead to dental caries; protein requirements are constantly fluctuating due to rapid periods of growth. The problems and challenges are many, particularly with this age group; for this reason, pediatric renal nutrition has evolved into a distinct subspecialty of dietetics.

One of the biggest problems with hemodialysis is its cost. About 62,000 patients were on hemodialysis in 1981, costing over $1 billion annually [1]. By the end of the 1980s, these figures could rise to at least 90,000 patients, costing between $4 and $5 billion annually. In 1973, the Social Security Act was amended to give Medicare benefits to anyone suffering from kidney failure, regardless of age. Medicare pays for 80 percent of hospitalization and treatment and 100 percent of transplantation costs. Hospital-based hemodialysis is estimated to cost about $25,000 per year; home hemodialysis, about $18,000 per year. Various methods are being developed to help keep down the cost of this treatment, including the design of simpler and more effective dialysis equipment and the encouragement of more home treatments through education and special training programs.

Peritoneal Dialysis

This method of dialysis utilizes the body's own semipermeable membrane, the peritoneum, which surrounds most of the internal organs (see Fig. 42-3). The dialysate solution is instilled into the peritoneal cavity where, by osmosis and diffusion, metabolic wastes, electrolytes, and water pass into the solution. In adults, about 2 liters of dialysate are usually used and are kept within the abdominal cavity for 20 to 40 minutes [3]. The solution is then removed by gravity drainage. For acute conditions, the procedure is usually continuous for 36 to 72 hours; chronic, intermittent dialysis usually lasts 10 to 12 hours, three to five times per week [4].

Peritoneal dialysis is an accepted, safe alternative to hemodialysis and is used in the treatment of acute or chronic renal failure. Although it is a safe and simple procedure, this type of dialysis is expensive, time-consuming, and uncomfort-

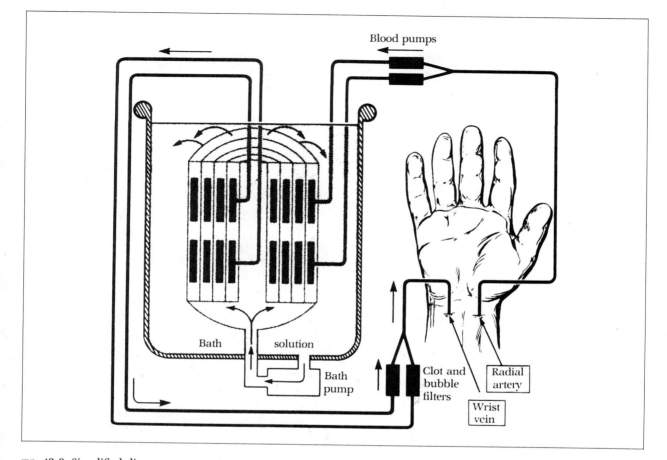

Blood pumps

Bath   solution

Bath
pump

Clot and
bubble
filters

Radial
artery

Wrist
vein

FIG. 42-3. Simplified diagram
of a twin-coil apparatus for
hemodialysis (an artificial kidney). (From E. Selkurt, *Basic
Physiology for the Health Sciences* [2nd ed.]. Boston: Little,
Brown, 1982.)

able. Improvements are being developed, including indwelling catheters, home
training programs, and automatic cycling machines.

The interrelationships between pathophysiology and clinical manifestations in
renal disease are given in Fig. 42-4.

Diet Therapy in Renal Disease
OBJECTIVES AND GOALS

Since renal disease is a constantly changing process, the prescribed diet therapy
must be adaptable to these changes to be truly therapeutic [5]. During the
predialysis phase of end-stage renal disease, the basic objectives of diet therapy
include decreasing the work load of the diseased kidney(s) by lowering the
amounts of metabolic waste products that must be excreted (urea, uric acid,
creatinine, electrolytes); replacing vital substances excreted in the urine due to
impaired renal function (e.g., protein, sodium); and supplying enough vital
nutrients to maintain body functions without placing additional stress on the
kidneys for their excretion (e.g., protein to maintain muscle mass, potassium to
maintain cardiac function).

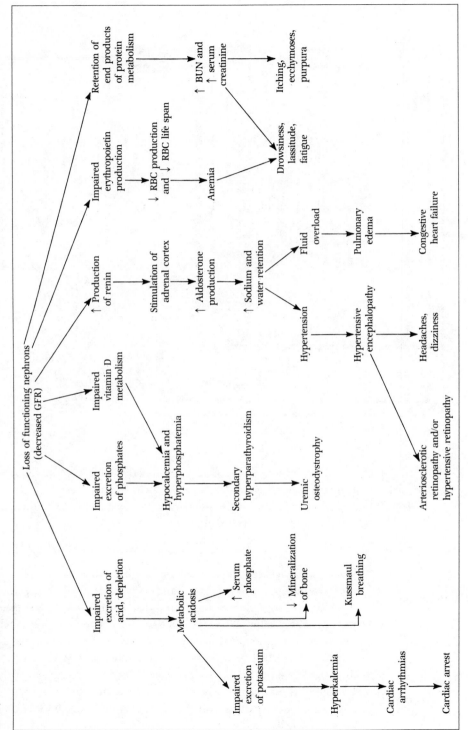

FIG. 42-4. Interrelationships between pathophysiology and clinical manifestations in renal disease. (From B. Luke, *Case Studies in Therapeutic Nutrition.* Boston: Little, Brown, 1977.)

Chronic hemodialysis (or more recently, home peritoneal dialysis) poses another type of picture. The clinical and biochemical status of the dialysis patient is related to several factors—the duration and frequency of dialysis, residual renal function, and adherence to prescribed diet and drug regimens.

The nephrotic syndrome differs from end-stage renal disease and dialysis in that there is neither nitrogen retention nor hypertension. Just as uremia is a stage of renal disease, regardless of etiology, so is nephrotic syndrome. Symptoms include albuminuria, hypoalbuminemia, hypercholesterolemia, and massive edema. The edema is due to two factors. (1) The constant loss of serum albumins into the urine causes a decrease in the colloidal osmotic pressure of the blood, with consequent edema. (2) The inability of the kidney to excrete sodium results in sodium retention and edema, compounding the effects of the hypoalbuminemia. Clinical edema becomes evident when the serum albumin level falls below 2 gm/100 ml. The basic dietary objectives in the treatment of nephrotic syndrome are to supply dietary protein in amounts equal to that lost in the urine and to correct the low plasma protein levels, and to restrict dietary sodium intake to prevent retention and further edema.

PROTEIN RESTRICTION

In end-stage renal disease, because of the impaired excretion of the end products of protein metabolism (urea, uric acid, creatinine, sulfates, and organic acids) with a potentially toxic accumulation of these wastes, the *quality* and *amount* of dietary protein allowed is restricted. At the same time carbohydrates and fats, which do not require the kidney for excretion of their metabolic waste products, are given liberally to avoid the breakdown of tissue proteins for energy production. The decision to implement protein restriction is based on clinical symptoms (i.e., anorexia, nausea) and certain biochemical limits, such as a creatinine clearance of less than 25 ml per minute and/or a blood urea nitrogen greater than 100 mg/100 ml. Daily protein intake is often adjusted to the level of the creatinine clearance.

The protein used is of the highest biologic value, following the principles established by two Italian physicians, Giordano and Giovanetti (the G-G diet) in the 1960s [6, 7]. If the minimum amount of protein (as low as 6.10 gm of protein per day) containing all the essential amino acids is supplied, the patient utilizes the waste nitrogen in his blood for the synthesis of nonessential amino acids needed by the body. Urea accumulation is counteracted by the body's recycling of nitrogenous wastes in the blood. Nitrogen equilibrium is maintained with a minimal amount of protein and without loss of muscle mass (tissue nitrogen) if adequate calories are supplied by dietary fats and carbohydrates. The foods prescribed most often on the G-G diet are milk and eggs; meat, fish, and poultry are used sparingly because, although they contain all the essential amino acids, they also include many nonessential amino acids, which place an additional burden on the kidneys for the disposal of their nitrogenous waste products. Grains and legumes are not used because not only are they incomplete proteins, but they are also high in potassium and their inclusion would further aggravate already elevated levels. Other foods containing protein of low biologic value are also restricted because they only contribute to the urea overload. With strict adherence to the diet, there is a reduction in the blood urea nitrogen (BUN) and concurrent improvement of clinical symptoms. A diet with such severe protein restriction is deficient in many vitamins and minerals and, therefore, these are often prescribed.

During chronic hemodialysis, the dietary protein allowance is 1.2 gm per kg body weight [8]. This amount maintains nitrogen equilibrium and replaces the amino acids lost in the dialysate during treatment. Foods are also chosen from those having the highest biologic value, although milk is given sparingly because it contributes fluid and has high levels of sodium, potassium, and phosphate. It has recently been shown that morbidity (illness) is increased in hemodialysis patients that have a high blood urea nitrogen; morbidity can be decreased by more efficient removal of urea and the intake of adequate protein and other nutrients [9].

The nephrotic syndrome presents a completely different type of problem from end-stage renal disease without dialysis—that of excessive protein loss. The amount of protein prescribed for patients with the nephrotic syndrome should both correct the low plasma protein levels plus replace the amount equal to that lost in the urine. The amount prescribed is usually based on 1 gm protein/kg body weight/day, plus the amount lost in the urine.

PHOSPHATE RESTRICTION

Impaired excretion of phosphates together with impaired vitamin D metabolism leads to hyperphosphatemia and hypocalcemia in the patient with end-stage renal disease. If this is allowed to continue, secondary hyperparathyroidism develops, with uremic osteodystrophy resulting. The therapy to counteract these blood abnormalities is twofold. First, dietary sources of phosphates are restricted. This is easy to accomplish since most phosphates are found in dietary proteins, which have already been restricted to minimal amounts. Second, an aluminum hydroxide gel (Amphojel) may be prescribed. This preparation binds phosphates in the gastrointestinal tract so they are excreted, unabsorbed, in the feces. In addition, this gel has a low sodium content (0.8 mEq/L), so it will not interfere with the dietary regimen of sodium restriction.

Dietary phosphates are restricted in the hemodialysis patient also. The clinical and biochemical status of the hemodialysis patient is related to several factors, including prescribed drug and dietary regimens. Some patients do not adhere to drug regimens, such as the regular use of Amphojel, and their clinical and biochemical health reflects this (elevated levels of phosphate and uric acid in the serum causing joint pains, uremic osteodystrophy). Using Amphojel in cooking (e.g., medicated cookies) [10] may make it more palatable and acceptable to the patient while still accomplishing its therapeutic action. The Ca $\times$ P product (serum calcium value times the serum phosphorus value) is a useful clinical indicator [11]. Precipitation of calcium phosphate crystals into soft tissue, vasculature, and joints (uremic osteodystrophy) occurs when this number exceeds 40, and it may reach as high as 75 to 80. A high Ca × P product indicates the need for better control of serum values through diet and/or drug therapy.

CALORIC INTAKE

Liberal intake of carbohydrates and fats should be encouraged in the patient with renal disease. These nutrients have a protein-sparing action, that is, they spare protein to build and repair tissue while supplying the calories needed for energy production. Since they do not require the kidney for the metabolism of their waste products (carbon dioxide and water) and do not add to the urea load, they can be used freely in the diets of patients with kidney disease. If calories provided are insufficient, tissue catabolism will result with liberation of nitrogenous wastes into the bloodstream; this will further aggravate the uremia. It is difficult to get the severely ill uremic patient to consume carbohydrates and fats if nausea and vomiting are a problem, but every effort should be made to make the diet as palatable as possible.

The inclusion of ample amounts of carbohydrates and fats is also important with the hemodialysis patient to avoid the breakdown of tissue proteins for energy production. Sugar and whipped cream can be added to fruits, and butter and sauces to vegetables. Although the protein allowance is increased during hemodialysis, low-protein, low-electrolyte breads can be used, supplying little nutritional value but adding variety and serving as carriers for jellies, jams, honey, and preserves. The use of special deglutenized wheat starch in baking broadens the variety of food available to the hemodialysis patient. Also available are low-protein, low-electrolyte pastas (for use with butter or cream sauces) and cereals (topped with butter, brown sugar, cream).

FLUID RESTRICTION AND ELECTROLYTE BALANCE

Before all residual function of the kidneys is lost, the fluid intake must be regulated to their remaining fluid excretory ability. When the glomerular filtration rate (GFR) is reduced, the fluid intake must be decreased. In addition, insensible losses of water via the lungs, skin, and feces, as well as in vomitus and/or diarrhea (if present) must be included in calculating the correct amount of fluid to prescribe. The concurrent disease processes and the actions of prescribed medications must also be considered. Renal hypertension is related to an increased production of renin, which in turn results in sodium and water retention from increased aldosterone production and is also one of the side effects of the antihypertensive drug, methyldopa (Aldomet). Dietary sodium is restricted to prevent further retention and consequent edema. Decreased cardiac function combined with fluid overload can lead to acute pulmonary edema or congestive heart failure. Diuretic therapy combined with sodium restriction counteracts this possibility. Supplemental potassium is given to replace that lost by the action of the diuretic and to avoid the complication of hypokalemia.

On maintenance hemodialysis many patients lose all residual function soon after starting, making the fluid restriction component of the diet paramount. Some patients, including those with the diagnosis of polycystic kidney disease (a congenital malformation of the kidneys), may still excrete fluids and this must be considered in calculating the fluid allowance. In patients with no residual function, indiscretions can quickly lead to fluid overload, pulmonary edema, and congestive heart failure. Even close adherence to the prescribed 500 ml, plus an amount equal to the urine output usually results in mild fluid retention and a weight gain of a pound or more per day between treatments. Dietary sodium is also restricted to help control fluid retention and avoid hypertension. Although the protein allowance has been liberalized, vegetables of low biologic value (corn, peas, beans) are still excluded because of their high sodium content. Commercial salt substitutes are not recommended because they contain potassium chloride. Hyperkalemia is a potential danger for the hemodialysis patient because it could lead to sudden death by cardiac arrest. Since potassium is found in so many foods (meats, fruits, vegetables), the patient should receive careful instruction regarding choice of foods, size of portions, and methods of preparation. The potassium content of some foods can be reduced by *leaching;* by soaking raw potatoes before cooking, the potassium content can be reduced by as much as 75 percent [12]. Canned fruits and vegetables lose some of their potassium in the canning process. Some vitamins (such as ascorbic and folic acids) are lost during hemodialysis and may be given as a supplement.

The nephrotic syndrome patient is usually placed on a fairly strict sodium restriction (i.e., 800 mg/day for a 100-gm protein diet). With sodium so severely restricted, fluids can be given ad libitum.

Case Studies

1. Mrs. Jameson is a 42-year-old schoolteacher on maintenance hemodialysis. During today's visit to her doctor she complains of weakness and pains in her knees and fingers. What laboratory tests would you want to order, and what values would you expect to find?

   On further questioning, Mrs. Jameson admits that she does not regularly take the prescribed Amphojel. Why is this medication important in renal disease and what other ways could you suggest she take it?

2. Mary Jane is a 12-year-old sixth grader who has polycystic kidney disease (a congenital disorder). She is on a 40-gm protein, 1000-mg sodium diet, with a high carbohydrate and fat allowance. She has volunteered to bring one of the desserts for her Girl Scout Halloween party. Which of the following would be best and why—pound cake, mint candy, chocolate layer cake, marshmallows, sugar wafers, peanut brittle, lemon meringue pie.

3. Mrs. Abernathy is a 60-year-old grandmother with end-stage renal disease. She has consistently had decreased levels of calcium (hypocalcemia) and elevated levels of phosphate (hyperphosphatemia). She now has a bowing of

her legs, which resembles rickets. Explain the pathophysiology of these developments and how they relate to altered vitamin D metabolism.

References

1. Jones, B. The high cost of kidney care. *The New York Times*. April 26, 1981.
2. Hetrick, A., Frauman, A. C., and Gilman, C. M. Nutrition in renal disease: When the patient is a child. *Am. J. Nurs.* 79:2152, 1979.
3. Valtin, H. *Renal Dysfunction.* Boston: Little, Brown, 1979. P. 244.
4. Brundage, D. J. *Nursing Management of Renal Problems* (2nd ed.). St. Louis: Mosby, 1980. P. 128.
5. Luke, B. *Case Studies in Therapeutic Nutrition.* Boston: Little, Brown, 1977. Pp. 3–22.
6. Giordano, C. Use of exogenous and endogenous urea for protein synthesis in normal and uremic patients. *J. Lab. Clin. Med.* 62:231, 1963.
7. Giovanetti, S., and Maggiore, Q. A low-nitrogen diet with proteins of high biological value for severe chronic uremia. *Lancet* 1:1000, 1964.
8. Kluthe, R., et al. Protein requirements in maintenance hemodialysis. *Am. J. Clin. Nutr.* 31:1812, 1978.
9. Lowrie, E. G., Laird, N. M., and Parker, T. F. Effect of the hemodialysis prescription on patients' morbidity. *N. Engl. J. Med.* 305:1176, 1981.
10. Cost, J. S. *Dietary Management of Renal Disease: A Controlled Protein, Sodium, and Potassium Cookbook.* New York: C. B. Slack, 1975. Pp. 29–38.
11. Hampers, C. *Long-term Dialysis.* New York: Grune & Stratton, 1973. Chap. 10.
12. Louis, C. J., and Dolan, E. M. Removal of potassium in potatoes by leaching. *J. Am. Diet. Assoc.* 57:42, 1970.

Suggested Readings

Alexander, R. S. *Case Studies in Medical Physiology.* Boston: Little, Brown, 1977. Pp. 91–106.

Blumenkrantz, M. J., et al. Nutritional management of the adult patient undergoing peritoneal dialysis. *J. Am. Diet. Assoc.* 73:251, 1978.

Bock, G. H., et al. Hemodialysis in the premature infant. *Am. J. Dis. Child.* 135:178, 1981.

Bodnar, D. M. Rationale for nutritional requirements for patients on continuous ambulatory peritoneal dialysis. *J. Am. Diet. Assoc.* 80:247, 1982.

Brundage, D. J. *Nursing Management of Renal Problems.* St. Louis: Mosby, 1980.

Burton, B. T. Nutritional implications of renal disease. *J. Am. Diet. Assoc.* 70:479, 1977.

Cadwallader, A. Dietary therapy for the individual on hemodialysis. *Behav. Med. Update* 3:12, 1981.

Chambers, J. K. Assessing the dialysis patient at home. *Am. J. Nurs.* 81:750, 1981.

Corea, A. L. Current trends in diet and drug therapy for the dialysis patient. *Nurs. Clin. North Am.* 10:469, 1975.

de St. Jeor, S. T., et al. *Low Protein Diets for the Treatment of Chronic Renal Failure.* Salt Lake City: University of Utah Press, 1970.

Decreased taste acuity in chronic renal patients. *Nutr. Rev.* 39:207, 1981.

Farrington, K., et al. Vitamin A toxicity and hypercalcemia in chronic renal failure. *Br. Med. J.* 282:1999, 1981.

Fat-soluble vitamin nutrition in patients with chronic renal disease. *Nutr. Rev.* 39:212, 1981.

Fürst, P., et al. Principles of essential amino acid therapy in uremia. *Am. J. Clin. Nutr.* 31:1744, 1978.

Giordano, C. The role of diet in renal disease. *Hosp. Pract.* November, 1977. Pp. 113–119.

Hodges, R. E. (ed.). *Nutrition: Metabolic and Clinical Applications.* New York: Plenum Press, 1979. Pp. 409–457.

Kopple, J. D. Nutritional therapy in kidney failure. *Nutr. Rev.* 39:193, 1981.

Luke, B. *Case Studies in Therapeutic Nutrition.* Boston: Little, Brown, 1977. Pp. 3–22.

Luke, B. Nutrition in renal disease: The adult on dialysis. *Am. J. Nurs.* 79:2155, 1979.

Panel report on nutritional support of patients with liver, renal, and cardiopulmonary disease. *Am. J. Clin. Nutr.* 34:1235, 1981.

Pickering, L., and Robbins, D. Fluid, electrolyte, and acid-base balance in the renal patient. *Nurs. Clin. North Am.* 15:577, 1980.

Riemold, E. W. Chronic progressive renal failure. *Am. J. Dis. Child.* 135:1039, 1981.

Spitzer, M. E., Dickinson, B. B., and Rogers, P. W. *A Renal Failure Diet Manual Utilizing the Food Exchange System.* Springfield, Ill.: Thomas, 1976.

Valtin, H. *Renal Dysfunction: Mechanisms Involved in Fluid and Solute Imbalance.* Boston: Little, Brown, 1979.

Valtin, H. *Renal Function: Mechanisms Preserving Fluid and Solute Balance in Health* (3rd ed.). Boston: Little, Brown, 1983.

Winters, R. *Principles of Pediatric Fluid Therapy* (2nd ed.). Boston: Little, Brown, 1982.

Chapter 43

MENTAL AND PHYSICAL HANDICAPS

Many studies have shown that the nutritional status and the dietary intake of physically or mentally handicapped individuals are frequently inadequate. The cause most often is the physical disability. Although many of the factors that may lead to physical or mental disabilities have been reduced or eradicated during the past 25 to 30 years, the problem still remains. Depending on the criteria used, the proportion of children estimated to have special needs is about 20 percent of the whole child population [1]. Other factors or illnesses that may become manifest in adulthood or affect the elderly population add up to a large segment of the world's population with some degree of disability. A disability becomes a handicap when it puts the individual at a disadvantage in his or her particular environmental circumstances. For a child this is particularly important, since the disability may adversely affect the child's development and capacity to learn and adjust to life. The home environment and the mastery of feeding skills are two factors that will help lay the foundation toward a healthier and more productive future. When a handicap disables an adult, the attainment of independence in the activities of daily living is the key to successful rehabilitation; the mastery of self-feeding skills is central to that goal.

Chapters to review: Chapters 11, 23, 24, 28.

Causes of Feeding Disabilities
CEREBROVASCULAR DISEASE

As discussed in Chap. 41, the accumulation of lipids, fibrin, calcium, and other materials forming plaques in arteries and vessels can lead to vascular occlusion and tissue death, secondary to arteriosclerosis. When vessels in the brain are involved, the result is termed a *cerebrovascular accident*, cerebral thrombosis, or stroke. Brain damage may also be caused by *cerebral embolism*, which occurs when a blood clot from another area of the body becomes dislodged and blocks a vessel in the brain. Both cerebral thrombosis and cerebral embolism cause tissue death of the area supplied by the occluded vessel. Immediately after the occlusion, the symptoms of cerebral dysfunction are observed; these symptoms are headache, nausea and vomiting, convulsions, and coma. Specific symptoms are related to the site of the injury. *Hemiplegia*, paralysis of one side of the body, is common. Other symptoms may include *aphasia*, the impaired ability to relay thoughts and ideas into words and sentences, and *apraxia*, the inability to perform purposeful movements. Recovery frequently occurs, particularly if the treatment during the initial, acute phase was comprehensive. Some of the paralysis may subside after 2 to 3 weeks, but at least 6 months should lapse before improvement is considered maximal. Some residual neurologic damage usually remains, contributing to poor dietary intake. Specific nutritional problems associated with cerebral thrombosis or embolism include muscle wasting due to inactivity; possible tissue breakdown (decubitus ulcers); and secondary to prolonged bed rest, decalcification of bones; and difficulty with self-feeding during the convalescence period.

CEREBRAL PALSY

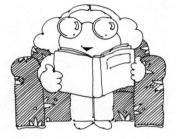

Cerebral palsy may be caused by developmental defect or cerebral degeneration in utero; it may also be due to birth trauma, infection, jaundice, asphyxia, or an unknown cause. In severe cases, the symptoms are present at birth and include irritability, vomiting, and difficulty in nursing. These children are particularly susceptible to infections and may die early in infancy. Milder forms of the disease may not be suspected until the child does not progress normally, such as failing to sit up by 6 months of age or not walking or talking by 1 year. *Athetoid movements* (from the Greek, *athetos*, meaning "out of place") are involuntary motions characterized by recurrent, slow, continual change of position of the hands, feet, fingers, toes, and other parts of the body. This symptom of cerebral palsy does not usually appear until age 2 or 3. Convulsions may also be present.

This disorder is classified into three types: (1) *spastic* (the cortex of the brain is affected most severely); (2) *ataxic* (the cerebellum is predominantly involved); and (3) *athetoid* (the basal ganglia are affected). Most cases are a mixture of types. *Spastic weakness* (from the Greek, *spastikos*, meaning "to draw in") is the most common clinical manifestation and is caused by increased stretch reflexes and irritability of the muscles. When an attempt is made to move an arm or leg in a certain direction, the action may be blocked by the inadvertent contraction of antagonistic muscles. Because of this, movement is generally limited in patients with spastic cerebral palsy. In the athetoid type, involuntary motor activity is the predominant feature, increasing caloric requirements to almost twice that of normal. Other problems that may complicate the diet therapy of children with cerebral palsy include poor control of throat and tongue muscles, inability to chew and swallow correctly, poor appetite, dental problems, and inability to feed.

MUSCULAR DYSTROPHY

The *muscular dystrophies* are inherited diseases characterized by progressive weakness due to the degeneration of muscle fibers. The metabolic defect has not yet been identified. The pathologic changes include degeneration of skeletal and cardiac muscle and increases in connective tissue and fat deposition. Classification is made according to individual clinical manifestations and genetic patterns. Differential diagnosis is usually made by muscle biopsy. There are two major varieties and a number of other minor categories. In the *Duchenne*, or *pseudohypertrophic*, form, only boys are affected; the gene is recessive and sex-linked. Symptoms appear when the child attempts to walk, due to weakness of the muscles of the pelvic girdle. The weakness progresses throughout childhood, until by adolescence the individual is usually confined to a wheelchair. In the other major form, *Landouzy-Déjerine*, or *fascioscapulohumeral*, both sexes are equally affected, but symptoms do not usually start until adolescence. Weakness of the muscles of the shoulder girdle is more prominent than leg weakness and, unlike the Duchenne form, the facial muscles are usually affected. The progression of the Landouzy-Déjerine form is much slower, but the clinical manifestations are variable from patient to patient. Eating handicaps are much more severe in this second form since, in addition to affecting the muscles of the trunk, it involves movement of the arms at the shoulders and the muscles of the face.

MULTIPLE SCLEROSIS

Characterized by patches of demyelination of the brain and spinal cord, *multiple sclerosis* is a slowly progressive disease marked by remissions and exacerbations. The cause is not known, although it has been attributed to viral or toxic factors. The onset of symptoms occurs between the ages of 20 and 40 in the majority of cases. Vague symptoms, such as minor visual disturbances, difficulties with bladder control and walking, and transient weakness of an extremity, may occur months or years before the disease is diagnosed. The most frequent presenting symptom is a tingling or burning sensation (*paresthesias*) involving the face or extremities, a weakness or heaviness of the limbs, or visual disturbances. Mental changes, such as apathy, lack of judgment, or inattention, indicate involvement of the pathways of emotional control. *Scanning speech*, slow enunciation with the tendency to hesitate at the beginning of a word or syllable, is common. Transient paralysis of the eye muscles and atrophy of the optic nerve are among some of the visual changes. Muscular weakness and spasticity result in a stumbling gait; tremor is common and is intensified with purposeful motion. Most patients live several decades after the disease has been diagnosed. The course of multiple sclerosis is variable; remissions may last 10 years or longer. Nutritional problems during periods of exacerbation include difficulty in activities of daily living, such as food preparation and eating.

PARKINSON'S DISEASE

Parkinson's disease is a disorder of the central nervous system, characterized by slowness and little purposeful movement, weakness, tremor, and muscular rigidity. The cause is unknown in the majority of cases but in some, it is the sequelae of encephalitis or poisoning with carbon monoxide. This disease usually occurs in middle-aged and elderly individuals.

The symptoms of Parkinson's disease are so striking as to be considered diagnostic. In extreme cases, the individual has a wide-eyed, unblinking expression. The muscles of the face are almost immobile; often the mouth is held partially open, with saliva drooling from the corners. The patient walks in short, shuffling steps with the arms held stiffly at the sides and the trunk bent slightly forward. All voluntary movements are slowed, particularly those involving the small muscles (i.e., the fingers). There is muscular rigidity throughout the body; when an attempt is made by another individual to passively move an extremity, the response is a series of jerks (*cogwheel rigidity*). An involuntary tremor, frequently involving the fingers, gives a characteristic "*pill-rolling*" movement. It is most severe at rest and may disappear temporarily with voluntary movement. Fatigue or emotional excitement intensifies the tremor; it may be inhibited by conscious effort for short periods and is not seen during sleep. Joint changes secondary to rigidity are common, as is impairment of speech. The nutritional problems created by this disease are varied, from poor control of eating utensils to the inability to prepare meals. Since mental capabilities remain unchanged with this disease, the patient with Parkinson's may feel extremely frustrated with his inability to successfully accomplish even simple tasks of daily living.

MYASTHENIA GRAVIS

Myasthenia gravis is another muscular disorder of unknown etiology. It occurs most often during early adult life, but may strike in children or the elderly of either sex. It is characterized by fluctuating muscle weakness, which frequently improves with the administration of cholinergic drugs. Symptoms fluctuate from one day to the next and are often worse at the end of the day. Some of the more common symptoms include limb weakness, impairment of speech (*dysarthria*), and difficulty in swallowing (*dysphagia*). Although some cases are rapidly fatal, due to respiratory failure or aspiration, many individuals go into remission and their lives are little affected. The dysphagia and limb weakness cause difficulties in meal preparation and self-feeding.

RHEUMATOID ARTHRITIS

Rheumatoid arthritis, a chronic systemic disease of unknown etiology, is characterized by overgrowth of connective tissue at various locations in the body. The symptoms include pain, swelling, and tenderness of the joints of the fingers, wrists, knees, and feet (see Fig. 43-1). There are juvenile and adult forms of the disease; the former has a more favorable prognosis. During an exacerbation, the affected joints are warm, reddened, and may contain fluid. The severity of symptoms is related to the level of activity; they are most severe after the individual has been inactive and lessen after activity has been resumed. Pain in the affected joint causes secondary "splinting" of adjacent muscle groups, often resulting in flexion deformities. Severe muscle weakness is also seen, due to pain and the active rheumatoid process within the muscle. Spontaneous remissions are frequent. Treatment is essentially symptomatic at this time. Since this disease mostly affects the joints of the fingers and wrists, as well as the feet, the individual may experience difficulty in meal preparation and eating due to poor or weak grasp and difficulty in flexion at the wrists.

MENTAL RETARDATION

Severe mental retardation may result from any number of causes or it may be due to unknown factors. Lack of oxygen at birth (*birth asphyxia*), birth trauma, prenatal malnutrition, or toxic exposure are all possible etiologic factors. Chromosomal abnormalities, such as *Down's syndrome*, often result in severe mental retardation and delayed physical development. Many of the congenital metabolic disorders, such as *phenylketonuria,* result in mental retardation when left untreated or when therapy is initiated too late (see Chap. 45). The nutritional problems of this group of children are twofold; in addition to difficulties in self-feeding, the diseases themselves may pose special nutritional demands. Conditions that contribute to feeding disabilities are summarized in Table 43-1.

FIG. 43-1.
A. Rheumatoid arthritis.
B. Osteoarthritis. These conditions weaken muscle control of the hand and fingers, making simple tasks, such as grasping a glass or picking up food from a plate, impossible. (From R. D. Judge, G. D. Zuidema, and F. T. Fitzgerald, *Clinical Diagnosis.* Boston: Little, Brown, 1982.)

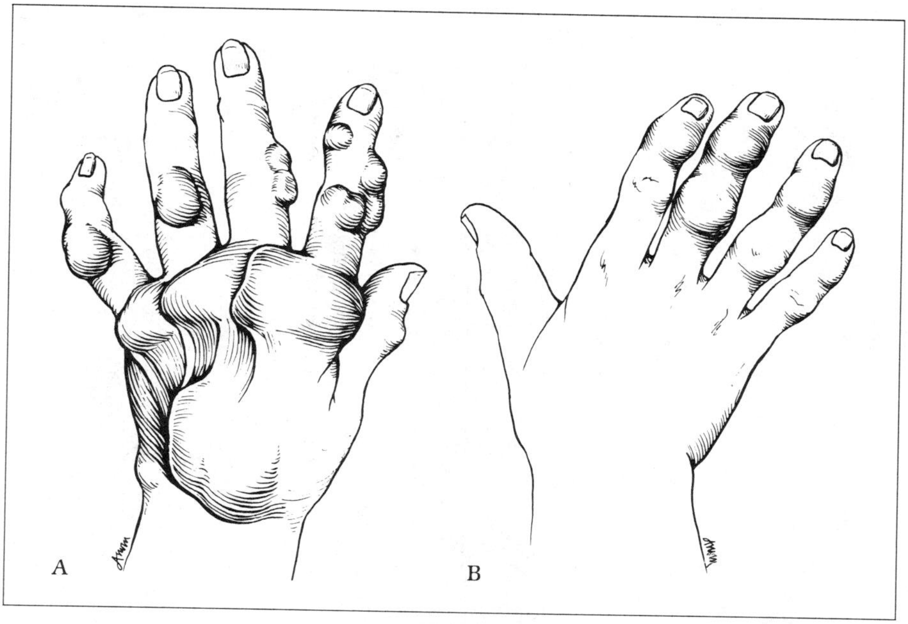

CONGENITAL AND
TRAUMATIC PHYSICAL
PROBLEMS

Congenital physical anomalies, such as cleft lip and cleft palate, present another area of great nutritional challenge. Before surgery is done to correct these deformities, these infants must use special adaptive nipples to ensure adequate oral intake. *Traumatic physical disabilities*, such as spinal cord injuries, also present challenges for nutrition and self-feeding.

Developmental Stages of Eating
ROOTING REFLEX

Nature has endowed the human infant with a variety of reflexes to ensure his ability to eat, and therefore survive, at birth. If any of these reflexes are malfunctioning, eating disorders will result. Abnormal oral-motor patterns are summarized in Table 43-2. Fully developed and present at birth, the *rooting reflex* is elicited by lightly touching either of the newborn's cheeks. The infant responds by turning his head toward the direction of the stimulus (usually a nipple), opening his mouth, extending his tongue, and bringing up one hand to his mouth. This reflex is very strong at birth and normally disappears completely by the third month of life. If the rooting reflex continues after 7 months of age, it may indicate damage of the central nervous system, particularly the cortical area of the brain. When the reflex continues beyond its normal period, as is sometimes seen in children with cerebral palsy, it can interfere with the eating process and the development of a normal sucking pattern.

SUCKLING REFLEX

Suckling is another reflex present at birth. It can be elicited by stimulating the area of the mouth, such as the lips or cheeks. Suckling is a continuous process

TABLE 43-1. Handicapping conditions and feeding disabilities

Handicapping condition	Feeding disabilities				
	Inability to suck, close lips	Inability to bite, chew, swallow	Poor grasp	Poor hand-mouth coordination	Poor trunk and upper extremities control
Cerebrovascular accident (stroke)					
With facial paralysis	+	+			
With hemiplegia on dominant side	+	+	+	+	+
Cerebral palsy					
Athetoid type	+	+	+/−	+	++
Ataxic type			+/−	++	++
Spastic type				+/−	
Traumatic spinal cord injury					
Paraplegia					
Quadriplegia			+	+	+
Muscular dystrophy					
Duchenne's	++	+	++	++	++
Fascioscapulohumeral	+	+	+	+	++
Multiple sclerosis	+		+	+	++
Parkinson's disease	+	+	+	+	++
Myasthenia gravis			+	+	
Rheumatoid arthritis			+	+	+/−
Severe and profound mental retardation	+	+	+	+	+

Key: + = moderate; + + = severe; +/− = variable.
Source: L. Anderson, et al., *Nutrition in Nursing.* Philadelphia: Lippincott, 1972. P. 289.

TABLE 43-2. Abnormal oral-motor patterns

Pattern	Definition	Problems	Normal counterpart
Jaw thrusting	A strong, downward extension of the lower jaw	May occur when food is presented or while food is in the mouth; the child may have difficulty closing the mouth to take in food	Normal, full opening of the jaw
Tongue thrust	A strong extension and protraction of the tongue before or during feeding; the tongue appears thick and bunched; the force and emphasis in suckling are greater during the "out" phase rather than the "in" phase (the opposite is true in the normal child)	Difficulty inserting nipple or spoon; ejection of food during feeding; problems in cup drinking	Sucking and an easy extension-retraction swallowing pattern; tongue is protruded at the time of swallowing
Tonic bite reflex	Strong closure of the jaw following stimulation of teeth or gums	Difficulty reclosing and opening the mouth after the reflex occurs; trouble releasing food after biting down; biting down when something touches the face, tongue, or lips	Phasic bite reflex
Lip retraction	A firm drawing back of the lips, which forms a tight line over the mouth	Inability to use the lips in sucking and swallowing	Thought to be the inactivity of the lips seen in babies under the age of 6 months
Tongue retraction	Drawing the tongue into the pharyngeal space	Difficulty managing food in the mouth; sometimes, serious difficulty in breathing; may prevent insertion of a nipple	Tip of tongue is normally even with the gums, and close to the lower lip; the tongue pulls back slightly from this position as the spoon enters the mouth and during swallowing
Nasal regurgitation	Loss of food or liquid through the nose during sucking and swallowing, because of abnormalities of the soft palate or poor coordination of sucking and swallowing	Difficulty retaining food	Loss of food through the nose during vomiting or spitting up

Note: The abnormal patterns do not occur in the normal infant. Each, however, has a normal counterpart.
Source: *Dietary Modifications in Disease: Mental and Physical Disabilities*, Columbus, Ohio: Ross Laboratories, 1979. P. 14.

involving closure of the lips to seal out air, the maintenance of the nipple against the hard palate by the tip of the tongue, and a pumping movement of the back of the tongue, which rhythmically pulls the liquid from the nipple to the back of the mouth and directly into the throat. Nasal breathing is continuous throughout the suckling process, without any interruptions. Liquid does not accumulate in the mouth. This reflex is normally observed until about the fifth month of life.

Problems that interfere with normal suckling include failure of the lips to seal out air, lack of coordination of the tongue in maintaining the nipple against the hard palate, or weakness of the tongue muscles resulting in ineffective pumping action needed to pull the liquid from the nipple. If difficulties are encountered, the infant should be placed in a flexed position, with the knees, hips, and neck relaxed and bent slightly. Better coordination and relationship between body parts will result.

SUCKING REFLEX

Sucking is a further development of the suckling reflex. It begins when the muscles of eating have developed sufficient strength and coordination to adapt to a change in the texture of food, such as when strained fruits and cereals are introduced. The creation of a vacuum seal by the lips in the front of the mouth and the soft palate closing the nasal passageway, combined with a pumping action of the tongue, result in negative pressure within the mouth. Sucking is similar to suckling, except that sucking is not a continuous process. Food is accumulated in the mouth; when there is a sufficient amount, there is a pause in the breathing cycle to permit swallowing. When food is propelled to the back of the pharynx, the *swallowing reflex* is triggered. The second, involuntary, stage of swallowing involves the simultaneous sealing of the nasal and windpipe passages. Breathing begins again as the food passes down the esophagus. This last phase is characterized by peristaltic action of the muscles of the esophagus and the relaxation of the cardiac sphincter leading to the stomach.

Structural problems, such as cleft palate or lip (before surgery), may interfere with the establishment of an effective seal to form a vacuum. Other diseases that may also cause an inability to close the lips or suck include muscular dystrophy (particularly the fascioscapulohumeral form), multiple sclerosis, Parkinson's disease, stroke, and cerebral palsy. Adaptive equipment and special instructional therapy [2] can help overcome these difficulties.

BITE REFLEX

A fourth reflex present at birth is *biting movements*, also termed the *phasic bite reflex*. It involves the rhythmic opening and closing of the jaws with oral stimulation, and it gradually disappears by 5 or 6 months of age. The biting reflex precedes chewing, which normally occurs between age 7 and 10 months, simultaneously with the eruption of teeth. The biting reflex is normal during the first 6 months of life, but can cause problems if it persists in older children. Such problems include interference with chewing, dental hygiene treatments, and speech therapy [3]. Solid foods may increase the frequency of the reflex; a pureed diet may provide a temporary solution. This type of diet, however, limits the normal development of muscles required for chewing solid foods. With successful teaching, the pureed diet should be replaced with chopped or solid foods as soon as the bite reflex is controlled.

SPOON FEEDING

Spoon feeding requires additional muscular strength and coordination. The suckling reflex may be triggered by the sight of food and the movement of the tongue may make initial attempts ineffectual. The new texture of solid or strained food may cause the infant to cough or gag at first. Between 4 and 6 months of age, the infant can better control the tongue to be motionless in anticipation of food and can effectively scrape food off the spoon with his lips. The tongue forms a central depression to help carry the food back to the pharynx.

CHEWING MOVEMENTS

By the seventh month of age, chewing movements begin to develop. These movements are not a reflex action like the preceding stages, but are a learned skill. Chewing allows the diet to be advanced from liquids and semisolid foods to solid foods and greater variety. If these skills are not mastered, the child's eating habits remain at the infant stage of development.

Before teeth have erupted, chewing is actually a combination of the phasic bite reflex and sucking. Food is mashed against the hard palate and mixed with saliva, without much lateral movement within the mouth. By 6 or 7 months of age, the tongue begins rolling laterally to the teeth and eventually becomes adept at transferring food. The motion of the jaws becomes more lateral and rotary than vertical. The infant learns to use his lips more effectively, including keeping them closed while chewing.

If any of the stages preceding chewing are missing, effective chewing will fail to develop. Dental or neuromuscular problems will also interfere with chewing. Inadequate chewing causes maldigestion due to inadequate mechanical breakdown of food and surface exposure to digestive enzymes. Intensive physical and occupational therapy may help overcome some of these problems.

GAG REFLEX

The *gag reflex*, also present at birth, fades at about the seventh or eighth month of life in coordination with the development of normal chewing movements. It never completely disappears throughout life, remaining as a safety valve to prevent food from being inhaled into the lungs (*aspiration*).

When this reflex is hyperactive, as often seen in brain-injured children and adults, it interferes with the eating process. When it is hypoactive, as seen in children with Down's syndrome or after tube feedings, it can be potentially dangerous to the individual. Special instructional methods may help overcome this problem [2].

DRINKING

Drinking involves much more muscular control and coordination. Before 12 months of age, the movement of the lips, tongue, and jaws may still be uncoordinated, resulting in ineffectual drinking. As the jaw is stabilized by biting the edge of the cup and lip function improves, the child of 15 to 18 months loses less fluid when eating. By 2 years of age, the child can effectively hold a cup between his lips, moves the tongue upward rather than protruding it, and has attained jaw stabilization.

Any physical disabilities with the lips, tongue, jaw stability, or swallowing reflex will result in difficulties in drinking. Programs to strengthen, control, and coordinate the muscles involved will aid in mastering this skill.

Special Nutritional Problems
WEIGHT CONTROL

Perhaps the two most common nutritional problems observed among individuals with mental or physical handicaps are underweight and overweight. Children with cerebral palsy and Down's syndrome are often overweight, probably due to a combination of an imbalanced diet and a low level of physical activity. The child with athetoid type cerebral palsy may be underweight due to excessive activity. Obesity can be a deterrent in physical therapy for individuals with muscle weakness. The opposite is also true; underweight only potentiates inactivity in those with muscular problems. Optimal weight for height and age can only be achieved and maintained by overcoming feeding disabilities, provision of a balanced diet, and a program of regular, individualized activity.

DENTAL HYGIENE

Problems with the teeth and gums may be congenital or acquired. Poor dental development is a consequence of several diseases, including Down's syndrome. Poor occlusion and frequent dental caries are frequently caused by excessive intake of concentrated sweets and may interfere with normal eating patterns. A hyperactive gag reflex, often present in children with cerebral palsy, may preclude adequate oral hygiene.

SPECIAL DIETS

Patients who have lost voluntary control of bowel and bladder function, such as the quadriplegic and paraplegic, must regulate fluid and roughage intake as part of control training. Other diseases, such as cerebrovascular accident, may require dietary fat or sodium modification. Drug therapy for specific diseases may cause increased requirements of various nutrients or malabsorption of others. The fluid and fiber content of the diet is important with physical disabilities to prevent the complication of constipation. All of these factors, in addition to the feeding limitation imposed by the disease process, must be taken into consideration when planning diets for the mentally or physically disabled.

ADAPTIVE EQUIPMENT

When muscle control of the hands or fingers is affected, as in rheumatoid arthritis, myasthenia gravis, and Parkinson's disease, a variety of adaptive equipment can help make self-feeding easier (see Fig. 43-2). Plastic or heavy paper dishes may be easier to control than china or breakable dishes; if tremors or spasticity is a problem, adhesive tape or suction cups can aid in anchoring. Glasses and cups should only be filled to about one-fourth capacity to prevent spilling, and a *glass holder* may be helpful (see Fig. 43-2). For those individuals having difficulty grasping small objects, the handles of eating utensils can be

FIG. 43-2. Some types of adaptive equipment to aid in self-feeding.
A. Glass holder.
B. Rocker knife.
C. Food guard.

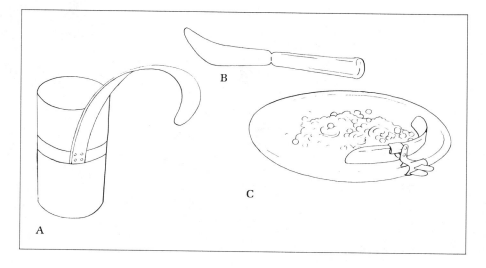

built up with cloth or foam rubber. Silverware with extra large handles is also available. A *band of elastic* or fabric made to fit snugly around the hand can be useful in holding a fork, spoon, or toothbrush. For patients who have lost motion ability at the wrist, a spoon bent at a 90 degree angle permits food to be brought to the mouth without bending at the wrist. The hemiplegic patient often has difficulty cutting meats; a *rocker knife* and *food guard* may help make this patient independent in self-feeding. A rocker knife (see Fig. 43-2) does not require the use of a fork to hold the meat or other food while it is being cut. The food is cut by pressing down on the blade and rocking it until it cuts through. A food guard (see Fig. 43-2) creates a barrier to help in filling a fork or spoon and to prevent food spillage. Spill-proof drinking cups with lids and weighted bases may also be helpful. For children with sucking and swallowing difficulties, a variety of special nipples and straw attachments are available.

References

1. Mitchell, R. G.   Antecedents of handicap. *Lancet* 1:86, 1981.
2. Gallender, D.   *Eating Handicaps: Illustrated Techniques for Feeding Disorders.* Springfield, Ill.: Thomas, 1979.
3. Gallender, C. W., and Gallender, D.   *Dietary Problems and Diets for the Handicapped.* Springfield, Ill.: Thomas, 1979. Pp. 46–47.

Chapter 44

NEOPLASTIC DISEASES

Cancer is the broad term used to cover all malignant neoplastic diseases. In its various forms, cancer affects both sexes and all age groups. In 1982, over 430,000 deaths in the United States were caused by cancer, ranking it second only to cardiovascular disease as the leading cause of death in the United States [1]. Figure 44-1 gives the incidence of cancer and deaths by site and sex.

Cancer is being diagnosed earlier and treated more aggressively and effectively than ever before. As a consequence, therapy often results in chronic or intermittent side effects, which may produce physiologic and nutritional problems that persist for many years or even the patient's lifetime. The maintenance of good nutritional status is central in achieving an optimal quality of life; both immediate and long-term diet therapy for the cancer patient are aimed toward this goal.

This chapter will explore the effects of cancer and cancer therapies on nutritional status, as well as methods of diet therapy for this disease. In addition, the current knowledge linking various dietary factors to the development of cancer will be presented.

Chapters to review: Chapters 10, 11, 35, 36, 37.

Effects of Cancer

One of the most direct effects of cancer on nutritional status is by the partial or complete obstruction of some portion of the gastrointestinal tract. Until surgical intervention is done to relieve the obstruction, hyperalimentation or tube feedings to a site distal to the blockage is necessary to maintain intake. Tumor growth within or leading to or from any of the gastrointestinal organs will impair their function and cause secondary maldigestion and malabsorption. Tumors of the pancreas and bile duct interfere with the digestion and absorption of fats and fat-soluble vitamins. Fat malabsorption soon leads to increased excretion of calcium and magnesium. Protein and vitamin B_{12} absorption may also be impaired if the pancreas is involved.

Fluid and electrolyte imbalances are often seen in cancer patients. Anemia and hypoalbuminemia may also be present. The latter is the result of a decreased capacity of the liver to produce albumin, losses of albumin from the body in excess of synthetic capacity, and the dilution of albumin by ascites and edema [2]. Electrolytes may be lost through tumor drainage or by diarrhea. Vitamin levels may be depressed secondary to poor intake or abnormal losses by the kidney or gastrointestinal tract. The immune response is frequently depressed in cancer patients, further complicated by the deleterious effect of malnutrition and cancer therapy on the defense systems against infection. Improved nutritional status usually results in improved immune responses. Diet therapy is paramount before, during, and after treatment to aid in host resistance, healing, and rapid convalescence. Some of the effects of neoplastic diseases on nutritional status are given in Table 44-1.

Weight loss is another common systemic effect of cancer. In part, it is the result

FIG. 44-1.
A. 1982 estimated cancer incidence by site and sex.
B. 1982 estimated cancer deaths by site and sex. (From E. Silverberg, Cancer statistics, 1982. *CA* 32:15, 1982. Courtesy of the American Cancer Society.)

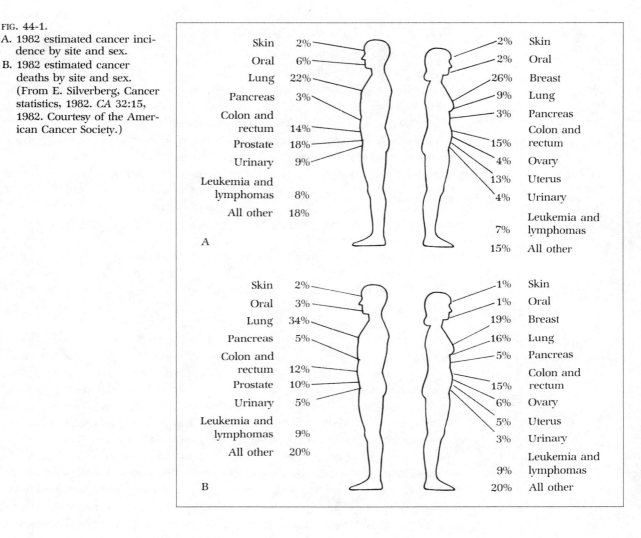

of anorexia and cancer cachexia. In patients with cancers of the gastrointestinal tract, the resultant malabsorption and maldigestion can easily lead to weight loss. In patients with tumors outside the gastrointestinal tract, this relationship is not as clear. The metabolic rate is greater in cancer patients than in other patients, and when this factor is combined with lower intakes associated with inactivity imposed by the disease, weight loss may result [3].

A number of metabolic changes also occur due to the effects of cancer. Defects in protein synthesis, altered glucose metabolism, delayed and prolonged insulin secretion, and increased growth hormone concentrations have been reported [4, 5]. Alternations in metabolism are seen in these patients, interfering with the normal utilization of protein, fats, and carbohydrates [6]. Iron metabolism is also affected, altering hemoglobin synthesis and iron-containing enzymes [6].

TABLE 44-1. Some effects of neoplastic diseases on nutritional status

I. Cachexia (weakness, extreme weight loss, and tissue wasting) secondary to anorexia

II. Malnutrition associated with impaired food intake secondary to obstruction

III. Malabsorption associated with
   A. Deficiency of pancreatic enzymes or bile salts
   B. Infiltration of small bowel by neoplasms, such as lymphoma or carcinoma
   C. Fistulous bypass of small bowel
   D. Gastric hypersecretion inhibiting pancreatic enzymes (in Zollinger-Ellison syndrome)
   E. Blind loop secondary to partial upper small bowel obstruction

IV. Protein-losing enteropathy (e.g., in gastric carcinoma, lymphoma, or with lymphatic obstruction)

V. Electrolyte and fluid-balance disturbances associated with
   A. Persistent vomiting in obstruction
   B. Vomiting secondary to increased intracranial pressure from tumors
   C. Small-bowel fluid losses from fistulas
   D. Diarrhea associated with hormone-secreting tumors (e.g., carcinoid, medullary thyroid carcinoma) and villous adenoma of the colon
   E. Inappropriate antidiuretic hormone secretion associated with certain tumors
   F. Hyperadrenalism secondary to excessive corticotropin or corticosteroid production by tumors

Source: M. E. Shils, Nutrition and Neoplasia. In R. S. Goodhart and M. E. Shils (eds.), *Modern Nutrition in Health and Disease* (5th ed.). Philadelphia: Lea & Febiger, 1973.

LOCALIZED EFFECTS

The cancerous tumor preferentially utilizes the body's protein stores and essential nutrients at the expense of normal healthy tissue. Negative nitrogen balance for the healthy tissue results, but the tumor is actually in positive balance.

SYSTEMIC EFFECTS

A common, almost characteristic, systemic effect of cancer is the development of *anorexia* (loss of appetite), resulting in progressive wasting of tissues. Often first noted even before a malignancy is detected or when a tumor is relatively small, the anorexia is not related to any intestinal obstruction, endocrine disorder, or alteration in intestinal absorption. This effect has been attributed to abnormalities of taste and smell, alterations in hypothalamic control of food intake, and unknown factors related to the cancer [7–9]. Regardless of its cause, anorexia, or *cancer cachexia* as it is sometimes called, perpetuates a vicious cycle of malnutrition in these patients.

Another symptom frequently associated with anorexia in cancer patients is an *altered sense of taste*. Lowered serum zinc or copper levels have been implicated in alterations in taste and smell sensations [10]. Altered sensitivity to sweet, sour, and bitter have also been reported [11]. Studies have also shown that most high-protein foods, cereal products, and sweet foods are generally less palatable to cancer patients with food aversions [12]. Altered taste may result from antineoplastic drug use or from radiation therapy, and often is reversible after the end of the cycle of therapy. Individual likes and dislikes, as well as cravings and aversions produced by the malignant state, should be incorporated into meal planning to make the diet therapy of these patients both enjoyable and therapeutic.

Effects of Treatment
RADIATION

Radiotherapy acts against cancer by altering the chemical bonds necessary for the synthesis and reproduction of DNA. At the time of mitosis (cell division), the irradiated cell dies. Those tissues in the body with the most rapid turnover (those that are the most mitotically active) are therefore the most susceptible to radiotherapy. The bone marrow and gastrointestinal mucosa have the highest turnover rate.

HEAD AND NECK

The head and neck are particularly sensitive to radiotherapy. A predictable radiation reaction occurs, directly related to the type of radiation, dosage, size of the field, and volume of tissue being treated. The most common symptoms include sore, painful throat; dry mouth; altered sense of taste; and loss of appetite. There may also be ulceration of the oral tissues and bleeding. The symptom that probably has the greatest effect on the patient is the altered sense of taste, also termed *mouth blindness.* This effect has been described as unequal alterations in taste sensitivity, with bitter and acid tastes being most susceptible, and salty and sweet tastes being less affected. Mouth blindness, which can result in profound nutritional and psychological effects, disappears in most patients within 1 year after cessation of radiotherapy [13]. The mechanism of taste alteration may be due to radiation-induced damage of the microvilli of the taste cells or their surfaces [14].

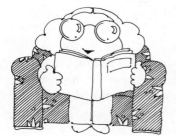

The salivary glands are also very sensitive to radiotherapy, resulting in decreased salivation and a change in quality to a viscous, acidic mixture. The combined reactions of altered quantity and quality of saliva, irritation of the mucosa, and altered composition of the oral bacterial flora all lead to increased caries formation [13]. The teeth, both developing and mature, are affected by radiotherapy. In developing teeth, radiation causes direct cellular damage; in mature teeth, there is a denaturing of the organic components and a change in the mitotic stage of development. As a result, patients undergoing radiotherapy may experience an increased sensitivity of their teeth to sweets, hot, and cold.

High-dose radiation therapy to the head and neck is often associated with significant weight loss, for one or more of the reasons previously cited. The therapeutic management is usually supportive, aimed at relieving symptoms and preventing further complications. Good oral hygiene, including the use of mouthwashes with a dilute hydrogen peroxide solution, may help prevent infection. Prophylactic dental care should be initiated before beginning the course of radiation therapy. Daily fluoride treatments should be continued after therapy and as a follow-up at home. The teeth should be kept as clean as possible by frequent brushing and use of dental floss. The dry mouth due to decreased salivary secretions (xerostomia) may be helped by the use of sugarless gum or candy drops. Alcohol and tobacco should be limited or avoided to prevent further irritation of inflamed tissues. If an oral infection does occur, cultures should be taken and appropriate antibiotics administered promptly. The consistency of food may have to be adjusted to facilitate swallowing during acute phases of inflammation.

THORAX

When portions of the thorax are irradiated, including the lungs, chest, esophagus, and mediastinum, the most common side effect influencing dietary intake is esophageal irritation. Dysphagia, or difficulty swallowing, is the usual symptom of this side effect, occurring after 2 or 3 weeks of therapy and subsiding about 2 weeks after cessation of treatment. More serious effects on esophageal structure may also occur, including ulceration or perforation. To prevent these complications, the esophagus may be shielded during radiotherapy. Topical relief may be achieved through the use of viscous xylocaine or chloroseptic (topical anesthetics) prior to eating. The consistency of the diet should be adjusted to the degree of dysphagia; tube feedings may be necessary.

ABDOMEN AND PELVIS

As mentioned earlier, the gastric mucosa is extremely sensitive to radiation, second only to bone marrow. Some of the symptoms, including ulcer formation, nausea and vomiting, and diarrhea, may persist throughout the course of therapy. A delayed reaction to radiation therapy is *radiation-induced enteritis*, which may present as chronic diarrhea or as complete or partial bowel obstruction. The pathophysiologic changes behind radiation-induced enteritis include decreased enzyme activity, altered absorption, vascular abnormalities, and decreased transit time. Alternations in the normal gastrointestinal flora, resulting in bacterial overgrowth, may add to the postradiation problems.

The therapy for radiation-induced gastrointestinal injury is aimed at minimizing symptoms and preventing further complications. The use of antiemetics, tranquilizers, and antidiarrheal drugs may be useful. Prompt correction of fluid and electrolyte imbalances and signs of infection is imperative. Surgery may be necessary to treat ulcerations if medical treatment fails. Recently, a low-residue, low-fat, gluten- and lactose-free diet has been shown to be effective in patients with radiation enteritis [15]. Hyperalimentation may also be useful in these patients.

SURGERY

This method of treatment, whether used alone or in combination with radiation and/or chemotherapy, often results in altered function of the area involved, and may often lead to the psychological problems of altered body image.

Surgery in the head and neck area can cause a variety of problems. Difficulties in chewing and swallowing are almost universal. Surgical removal of part of the tongue makes eating difficult and less enjoyable, due to poor control and fewer numbers of taste buds. The speech may be garbled and foods limited to liquids.

Some patients may be dependent on tube feedings for the rest of their lives; these feedings should be warm or at room temperature, and administered slowly to prevent diarrhea. Surgery on the esophagus causes its own set of problems. When both vagus nerves must be sacrificed with surgery at the lower end of the esophagus, bacterial overgrowth of the upper small bowel, diarrhea, and steatorrhea may result, as well as gastric atony and hypoacidity. The use of MCT (medium-chain triglyceride) oil and small, frequent feedings may be helpful.

Gastric surgery causes a myriad of problems, as discussed in Chap. 38. The patient may experience the "dumping syndrome," further aggravating poor dietary intake. Malabsorption and chronic deficiencies of iron, calcium, and fat-soluble vitamins may develop due to changes in gastric acidity and a lack of intrinsic factor. Vitamin B_{12} should be given intramuscularly, and special anti-dumping diets, supplemental calcium, iron, fat-soluble vitamins, and pancreatic enzymes may be helpful.

Surgical removal of part of the small bowel causes problems with absorption and fluid and electrolyte balance. The prognosis is in a large part dependent on the capacity of the remaining bowel to hypertrophy and compensate. Adequate nutrition must be maintained during this period, and can be accomplished by hyperalimentation. Surgery of the terminal ileum results in poor absorption of vitamin B_{12} and bile salts. Intramuscular vitamin B_{12} is necessary, and the use of a low-fat diet and MCT oil may reduce the steatorrhea. Surgery of the large bowel often results in fluid and electrolyte imbalances, particularly magnesium. This element may be given intramuscularly to prevent magnesium depletion.

Surgical removal of part of the pancreas (pancreatectomy) leads to the development of diabetes mellitus and fat and protein malabsorption. The diet therapy must include the principles of both cancer and diabetes mellitus to be effective.

CHEMOTHERAPY

The drugs used to treat cancer are among the most potent and destructive available. Adequate nutrition before, during, and after treatment helps ensure maximal therapeutic action. As shown in Table 44-2, chemotherapeutic drugs often cause nausea, vomiting, and anorexia, as well as tissue irritation, malabsorption, and diarrhea. Certain drugs, such as the antifolate agents, selectively bind folic acid, producing megaloblastic anemia. Others may cause iron deficiency through blood loss. Because many of these drugs are given on a continuous, cyclic basis, adequate nutrition may have to be maintained with hyperalimentation.

A summary of some of the consequences of cancer treatment predisposing to nutrition problems is given in Table 44-3.

Methods of Diet Therapy

As previously discussed, nutritional problems are almost inevitable with the diagnosis of cancer. Pretreatment, intratreatment, and posttreatment diet therapy is essential for maximal effectiveness of all modes of therapy. Because both treatment and disease may interfere with traditional methods of diet therapy

TABLE 44-2. Alimentary tract effects of cancer chemotherapeutic agents

Effect	Adriamycin	Asparaginase	BCNU	Bleomycin	Busulfan	Cyclophosphamide	Cytarabine	Dactinomycin	Daunorubicin	CDDP (Cisplatin)	Hydroxyurea	Methotrexate	Mithramycin	Procarbazine	Vinblastine	Vincristine
Anorexia	x	x	x			x		x		x		x	x	x		
Nausea	x	x	x	x	x	x	x	x	x	x	x	x	x	x	x	
Diarrhea								x				x		x		
Mucositis	x			x				x	x	x		x	x			
Abdominal pain												x				
Intestinal ulceration																
Vomiting	x	x	x			x	x	x	x	x	x		x			

Source: M. E. Shils, Nutrition and Neoplasia. In R. S. Goodhart and M. E. Shils (eds.), *Modern Nutrition in Health and Disease* (6th ed.). Philadelphia: Lea & Febiger, 1980.

used with other diseases (i.e., radical surgery and/or high-dose radiation), other methods must be utilized. Because many of these patients are more seriously ill for prolonged periods of time, closer monitoring of nutritional status, such as daily electrolyte determinations, nitrogen intake and output, and renal function, is vital.

Enteral feeding (feeding via gastrointestinal route), may be accomplished by the use of a small-bore pediatric feeding tube inserted through various routes—nasogastric, pharyngostomy, esophagostomy, gastrostomy, or jejunostomy [16]. The feeding may be given as a bolus or as a continuous infusion. The latter is preferred if the patient is in poor nutritional state before therapy. *Elemental diets*, also called a chemically defined diet, may be considered for those patients with decreased digestive capacity. Due to the high osmolarity of these solutions, however, and the possible complications of diarrhea and abdominal distress, these feedings should be initiated at quarter strength or less. Lactose-free preparations, such as Ensure or Isocal, are best tolerated. The advantages of enteral feeding include their relative low cost, ability to be administered both at home and in the hospital, and utilization of the normal mechanisms for nutrient absorption. The disadvantages include the possibility of nasopharyngeal and mucosal irritation, pulmonary aspiration, fluid overload, and abdominal cramping.

Parenteral feeding (feeding by vein) is indicated when the patient cannot tolerate enteral feeding or when adequate amounts or concentrations of nutrients cannot be achieved. Chapter 35 discussed this method in detail. In cancer patients, this mode of diet therapy has proven to be particularly useful. Its use has been reported to correct the taste abnormality so common among cancer patients

TABLE 44-3. Consequences of cancer treatment predisposing to nutrition problems

I. Radiation treatment
   A. Radiation of oropharyngeal area—destruction of sense of taste and impaired intake
   B. Radiation of abdomen and pelvis—bowel damage (acute and chronic), with diarrhea, malabsorption, stenosis, and obstruction
II. Surgical treatment
   A. Radical resection of oropharyngeal area—dependency on tube feeding
   B. Esophagectomy and esophageal reconstruction
      1. Gastric stasis secondary to vagotomy
      2. Malabsorption
      3. Fistula development or stenosis with long-term dependency on tube feeding
   C. Gastrectomy
      1. Dumping syndrome
      2. Malabsorption
      3. Hypoglycemia
   D. Intestinal resection
      1. Jejunum—decreased efficiency of absorption of many nutrients
      2. Ileum
         a. Vitamin B_{12} deficiency
         b. Bile salt losses
      3. Massive bowel resection
         a. Malabsorption
         b. Malnutrition
      4. Ileostomy and colostomy—complications of salt and water balance
   E. Blind loop syndrome
   F. Pancreatectomy
      1. Malabsorption
      2. Diabetes mellitus
   G. Ureterosigmoidostomy
      1. Hyperchloremic acidosis
      2. Potassium depletion
III. Chemotherapy treatment
   A. Corticosteroids and other hormones—fluid and electrolyte problems
   B. Antimetabolites and other agents
      1. Gastrointestinal damage
      2. Anemias

Source: Adapted from M. E. Shils, Nutrition and Neoplasia. In R. S. Goodhart and M. E. Shils (eds.), *Modern Nutrition in Health and Disease* (6th ed.). Philadelphia: Lea & Febiger, 1980.

[17]. Chemotherapy is better tolerated and can be given in increased amounts [18]. Immunologic function has also been shown to improve in cancer patients given hyperalimentation, suggesting that depressed functioning is probably related to malnutrition [19]. Hyperalimentation has been shown to reverse nutritional and metabolic defects caused by cancer [20]. This method of feeding does carry risks and possible complications, including the possibility of fluid and electrolyte imbalances, complications in placement, and sepsis.

Theoretical Dietary Causes of Cancer

The incidence of most cancers varies from one country to another. For example, the incidence of stomach cancer is much higher in Japan than in the United

States, and the incidence of colon cancer is greater in the United States than in Africa. These variations suggest environmental or genetic factors as causative agents. In studies done on migrant populations, the group will take on the incidence rate of the new country [21]. It appears then that environmental factors may predominate, and since environmental factors can be changed, perhaps the incidence of cancer can be reduced or even eliminated.

Several mechanisms have been suggested by which foods might influence the development of cancer [22]. One theory suggests that ingested food might contain carcinogens, as intentional or unintentional additives, or as natural toxic substances. Foods may also contain substances that of themselves are not carcinogenic but may be converted during digestion, processing, or cellular metabolism. The components of the diet, including type and amount of protein, fat, carbohydrate, and fiber may also influence the development of cancer by altering the gastrointestinal environment (see Chap. 25).

The Delaney Clause of the 1958 amendment to the Pure Food, Drug, and Cosmetic Act prohibits the use of any compound for which there is evidence of carcinogenicity. Many additives were in common usage when the Delaney Clause was passed, and were placed on the GRAS (generally-recognized-as-safe) list. With more testing, even some of these additives that were "grandfathered" in have since been proven carcinogenic and taken off the market (see Chap. 19). The use of an acceptable artificial sweetener has posed a special problem. Cyclamates have already been banned, and an acceptable substitute is yet to be found. The current trend seems to be toward accepting the risk that saccharin might slightly increase the incidence of cancer, rather than giving up its use all together [23]. This thinking may lead to a modification of the Delaney Clause, from banning all additives with any carcinogenic potential to developing a risk-to-benefit policy.

Unintentional additives are more difficult to control or even identify. Substances that fall into this category include heavy metals from processing or air or water pollution, pesticides, radioactive compounds, residues from packaging, and the like. Through epidemiologic studies, perhaps more will be learned about the cause and effect of these substances.

Various components of the diet have been implicated as etiologic factors in the development of cancer. Research has produced conflicting evidence, perhaps influenced by the differences in the populations studied—urban versus rural, sedentary versus physically active. Other factors may also potentiate or negate the effects of diet, such as air and water pollution; presence of elements in the water supply and soil; other foods in the diet; and genetics. One of the first individuals to suggest a diet and cancer link was Dr. D. P. Burkitt, with his observations on the relationship between the high-fiber diet of Africans and their low incidence of colon cancer [24]. Other investigators have not always agreed with his hypothesis. The consumption of animal protein has also been linked to cancer, suggesting that intestinal bacteria, permeability of the intestinal mucosa, and bile salts may interact with the components of a high–animal protein diet. Nitrites and nitrates, often used in processing meats, have long been implicated in the development of cancer [25]. High-fat diets and, recently, severe constipation have both been linked to the development of breast cancer [26, 27]. Coffee has been implicated in pancreatic cancer [28].

It is most likely a combination of factors, including increased susceptibility of certain individuals, specific agents, and unique conditions, which lead to the development of cancer, rather than a single cause.

Conclusions

This chapter has illustrated the central role nutrition has in the therapy of and convalescence from cancer. Optimal nutrition can make other therapies more effective, boost immunologic response, and aid in healing. Perhaps more than in any other disease, nutrition before, during, and after cancer treatment is vital for maximal therapeutic response.

References

1. Silverberg, E.   Cancer statistics, 1982. *CA* 32:15, 1982.
2. Shils, M. E.   How to nourish the cancer patient. *Nutr. Today* May/June 1981. Pp. 4–15.
3. Lundholm, K., et al.   Skeletal muscle metabolism in patients with malignant tumor. *Eur. J. Cancer* 12:465, 1976.
4. Schein, P. S., et al.   Cachexia of malignancy: Potential role of insulin in nutritional management. *Cancer* 43 [Suppl.]:2070, 1979.
5. Carter, A. C., et al.   Metabolic parameters in women with metastatic breast cancer. *J. Clin. Endocrinol. Metab.* 40:260, 1975.
6. Munro, H. N.   Tumor-host competition for nutrients in the cancer patient. *J. Am. Diet. Assoc.* 71:380, 1977.
7. DeWys, W. D., and Walters, K.   Abnormalities of taste sensation in cancer patients. *Cancer* 36:1888, 1975.
8. Morrison, S. D.   Control of food intakes in cancer cachexia: A challenge and a tool. *Physiol. Behav.* 17:705, 1976.
9. Brennan, M. F.   Uncomplicated starvation versus cancer cachexia. *Cancer Res.* 37:2359, 1977.
10. Henkin, R.   Newer Aspects of Copper and Zinc Metabolism. In W. Mertz and W. E. Cornatzer (eds.), *Newer Trace Elements in Nutrition.* New York: Dekker, 1971. Chap. 12.
11. Williams, L. R., and Cohen, M. H.   Altered taste thresholds in lung cancer. *Am. J. Clin. Nutr.* 31:122, 1978.
12. Vickers, Z. M., Nielsen, S. S., and Theologides, A.   Food preferences of patients with cancer. *J. Am. Diet. Assoc.* 79:441, 1981.
13. Donaldson, S. S.   Nutritional consequences of radiotherapy. *Cancer Res.* 37:2407, 1977.
14. Conger, A.   Loss and recovery of taste acuity in patients irradiated to the oral cavity. *Radiat. Res.* 53:338, 1973.
15. Donaldson, S. S., et al.   Radiation enteritis in children: A retrospective review, clinicopathologic correlation, and dietary management. *Cancer* 35:1167, 1975.
16. DeWys, W. D., and Kubota, T. T.   Enteral and parenteral nutrition in the care of the cancer patient. *J.A.M.A.* 246:1725, 1981.

17. Russ, J. E., and DeWys, W. D.   Correction of taste abnormality of malignancy with intravenous hyperalimentation. *Arch. Intern. Med.* 138:799, 1978.
18. Copeland, E. M., et al.   Intravenous hyperalimentation as an adjunct to cancer chemotherapy. *Am. J. Surg.* 129:167, 1975.
19. Copeland, E. M., MacFadyen, B. V., and Dudrick, S. J.   Effect of intravenous hyperalimentation on established delayed hypersensitivity in the cancer patient. *Ann. Surg.* 84:60, 1976.
20. Brennan, M. F.   Total parenteral nutrition in the cancer patient. *N. Engl. J. Med.* 305:375, 1981.
21. Gori, G. B.   Diet and cancer. *J. Am. Diet. Assoc.* 71:375, 1977.
22. Oace, S. M.   Diet and cancer. *J. Nutr. Educ.* 10:106, 1978.
23. Cohen, B. L.   Relative risks of saccharin and calorie ingestion. *Science* 199:983, 1978.
24. Burkitt, D. P.   Epidemiology of cancer of the colon and rectum. *Cancer* 28:3, 1971.
25. Gunby, P.   Nitrosoureas suspected in stomach cancer. *J.A.M.A.* 245:1714, 1981.
26. Dickerson, J. W. T.   Nutrition and breast cancer. *J. Hum. Nutr.* 33:17, 1979.
27. Petrakis, N. L., and King, E. B.   Cytological abnormalities in nipple aspirates of breast fluid from women with severe constipation. *Lancet* 2:1203, 1981.
28. MacMahon, B., et al.   Coffee and cancer of the pancreas. *N. Engl. J. Med.* 304:630, 1981.

Suggested Readings

Bloch, A. S.   Practical hints for feeding the cancer patient. *Nutr. Today* 16:23, 1981.
Chernoff, R.   Nutrition and the cancer patient. *J. Can. Diet. Assoc.* 40:139, 1979.
Costa, G., and Donaldson, S. S.   Current concepts in cancer: Effects of cancer and cancer treatment on the nutrition of the host. *N. Engl. J. Med.* 300:1471, 1979.
Daly, K. M.   Oral cancer: Everyday concerns. *Am. J. Nurs.* 79:1415, 1979.
Donaldson, S. S., et al.   A study of the nutritional status of pediatric cancer patients. *Am. J. Dis. Child.* 135:1107, 1981.
Fishman, J., and Anrod, B.   *Something's Got to Taste Good: The Cancer Patient's Cookbook.* Kansas City, Mo.: Andrews & McMeel, 1981. P. 221.
Gori, G. G.   The cancer and other connections . . . if any. *Nutr. Today* 16:14, 1981.
Hankin, J. H., and Rawlings, V.   Diet and breast cancer: A review. *Am. J. Clin. Nutr.* 31:2005, 1978.
Hegedus, S., and Pelham, M.   Dietetics in a cancer hospital. *J. Am. Diet. Assoc.* 67:235, 1975.
Hoover, R., and Hartge, P.   Non-nutritive sweeteners and bladder cancer. *Am. J. Pub. Health* 72:382, 1982.
Larsen, G. L.   Rehabilitation for the patient with head and neck cancer. *Am. J. Nurs.* 82:119, 1982.
Panel report on nutritional support of patients with cancer.   *Am. J. Clin. Nutr.* 34:1199, 1981.
Rose, J. C.   Nutritional problems in radiotherapy patients. *Am. J. Nurs.* 78:1194, 1978.
Rosenbaum, E. H., et al.   *Nutrition for the Cancer Patient.* Palo Alto, Calif.: Bull Publishing, 1980. P. 112.
Rosenberg, L., et al.   Breast cancer and alcoholic beverage consumption. *Lancet* 1:267, 1982.
Segaloff, A.   Managing endocrine and metabolic problems in the patient with advanced cancer. *J.A.M.A.* 245:177, 1981.
Soukop, M., and Calman, K. C.   Nutritional support in patients with malignant disease. *J. Hum. Nutr.* 33:179, 1979.

Symposium: Nutrition in the causation of cancer. *Cancer Res.* 35 [Part 2]:3237, 1975.

A taste aversion can develop during cancer chemotherapy. *Nutr. Rev.* 37:40, 1979.

Walker, A. M., et al. An independent analysis of the National Cancer Institute Study on non-nutritive sweeteners and bladder cancer. *Am. J. Pub. Health* 72:376, 1982.

Welch, D. Nutritional consequences of carcinogenesis and radiation therapy. *J. Am. Diet. Assoc.* 78:467, 1981.

Wollard, J. J. (ed.). *Nutritional Management of the Cancer Patient.* New York: Raven Press, 1979. P. 204.

Chapter 45

CONGENITAL METABOLIC DISORDERS

The term *inborn errors of metabolism* was first used by Garrod at the turn of the century to describe a group of genetically transmitted biochemical disorders [6]. Many of these diseases have dramatic pathologic and clinical manifestations that are the direct result of the biochemical disorder. In studying various inborn errors, many normal biochemical pathways have been elucidated, as well as the structure and function of a variety of enzymes and other key molecules.

Most of the inborn errors of metabolism are characterized by a decrease in or an absence of a specific enzyme or enzymes. This may be caused by deficient enzyme synthesis or the production of an abnormal enzyme with no functional abilities. There may only be partial loss of enzyme activity, or an abnormal binding of excessive amounts of cofactors. The incidence of most of these diseases is very low, as shown in Table 45-1, partially due to the technical limitations of screening for enzymes or amino acids in the blood, urine, or spinal fluid. As techniques are developed and improved, there may be an increase in the number and variety of inborn errors that are detected.

This chapter will present the more common inborn errors of metabolism, or congenital metabolic disorders. Many rare disorders will not be discussed due to limitations of space; the suggested readings at the end of the chapter elaborate on all of the inborn errors in greater detail. The underlying cause or defect will be discussed as well as the clinical and pathologic results, and therapy, when known.

Chapters to review: Chapters 3, 4, 5, 11, 34, 39, 40.

Disorders of Protein and Amino Acid Metabolism

The genetic diseases of protein and amino acid metabolism produce a wide variety of clinical manifestations. Some interfere with the normal development of the central nervous system, and lead to mental retardation, while others cause no abnormality in intellect. The majority of inborn errors are present at birth and may produce severe illness and even death at a very early age. For this reason, early detection and treatment are especially important. Phenylketonuria is the most common inborn error of protein metabolism; all others are comparatively rare. A summary of all known inborn errors of amino acid metabolism is given in Table 45-2.

PHENYLALANINE

Phenylketonuria (PKU), a disease inherited as an autosomal recessive trait affecting between 1 in 10,000 and 1 in 25,000 births, was first described by Følling in 1934 [1]. This disorder is caused by the decreased or absent functional capacity of the enzyme *phenylalanine hydroxylase*, which converts phenylalanine (an essential amino acid) to tyrosine (a nonessential amino acid precursor of melanin, thyroxine, and epinephrine). As a result, unmetabolized phenylalanine and alternate products of phenylalanine metabolism build up in the blood. These alternate products are *phenylpyruvic acid* (the deamination product of phenylalanine), *phenyllactic acid* (the reduction product of phenylpyruvic acid), and

TABLE 45-1. Incidence of selected inborn errors of metabolism

Inborn error	Estimated incidence	Total reported
Phenylketonuria	1:10,000–25,000	
Alkaptonuria	2–5:1,000,000	600+
Histidinemia	1:10,000–24,000	
Cystinuria	1:7000–20,000	
Maple syrup urine disease	5–10:1,000,000	50+
Hartnup disease	1:26,000	
Homocystinuria	1:160,000–270,000	
Diabetes mellitus	1:2500	
Galactosemia	1:60,000–75,000	
Galactokinase deficiency	1:40,000–50,000	
Essential fructosuria	1:130,000	
Tangier disease		17
Tay-Sachs disease (Ashkenazi Jews)	1:60	

phenylacetic acid (the product of the decarboxylation and oxidation of phenylpyruvic acid). Phenylacetate is conjugated in the liver with glutamine and excreted in the urine as phenylacetylglutamine; the presence of the keto acid, phenylpyruvate, in the urine gives the disease its name. Phenylpyruvate can be detected in the urine by adding a few drops of ferric chloride ($FeCl_3$); a green color indicates a positive test. The level of phenylpyruvate in the urine is indicative, but not diagnostic, of PKU. The disease is detected, most often by the third or fourth day after birth, by the Guthrie test, which measures the level of unmetabolized phenylalanine in the blood [2]. Infants with phenylalanine levels over 30 mg per dl are diagnosed as having "classic" PKU; with levels between 15 and 30 mg per dl, they are grouped as having variant, atypical PKU, or hyperphenylalaninemia. Recently, more sensitive determination of phenylalanine hydroxylase activity by liver biopsy has been used. When there is a complete absence of phenylalanine hydroxylase activity (as seen in classic PKU), strict lifetime control of dietary phenylalanine intake may help prevent any development of intellectual deficit (the most common clinical consequence of PKU). Individuals with any residual enzyme function (variant PKU, or hyperphenylalaninemia) may benefit from strict treatment early in life and should then be able to tolerate a more liberalized or normal diet later in life without harm.

One of the most serious consequences of untreated PKU is the retardation of normal mental development. The exact mechanism of the central nervous system damage is yet unknown. It may be due to high blood levels of unmetabolized phenylalanine or its alternate derivatives, or to the inhibition of tyrosine metabolism. Mental retardation can be prevented by instituting a diet during the first 3 months of life that strictly limits the amount of phenylalanine allowed. It has been strongly advised to take whatever steps necessary to reduce phenylalanine levels below 15 mg per dl to avoid excess phenylalanine exposure in these

TABLE 45-2. Inborn errors of amino acid metabolism

Disorder	Enzyme defect	Manifestations
Phenylketonuria	Phenylalanine hydroxylase	Blond hair, blue eyes, eczema, $FeCl_3$, mental retardation
Tyrosinosis (Medes), Tyrosinosis	p-Hydroxyphenylpyruvic acid oxidase	Urinary reducing substance Hepatic cirrhosis, renal Fanconi syndrome
Alkaptonuria	Homogentisic acid oxidase	Dark urine, reducing substance, ochronosis, arthritis
Albinism	Tyrosinase (melanocyte granules)	Lack of pigment (local or universal), skin, hair, and eyes
Histidinemia	Histidase	Speech retardation, $FeCl_3$, may have mental retardation
Isovalericacidemia	Isovaleryl CoA dehydrogenase	Mental retardation, odor, convulsions, coma, death*
Maple syrup urine disease	Branched-chain keto-acid decarboxylase	Urinary odor, coma, flaccidity, opisthotonos
Hypervalinemia	Valine transaminase	Mental retardation, death*
Propionic-acidemia	Propionyl CoA carboxylase	Recurrent vomiting and ketosis, thrombocytopenia, neutropenia, osteoporosis, mental retardation, death*
α-Methyl-β-hydroxybutyric-aciduria	α-Methylaceto-acetyl CoA thiolase	Intermittent acidosis, ketosis, hyperglycinemia syndrome, mental retardation
β-Methylcrotonyl glycinuria	β-Methylcrotonyl CoA carboxylase	Failure to thrive, dermatitis, ketosis, acidosis, death*
Methylmalonic-acidemia	Methylmalonyl CoA isomerase	As in propionic-acidemia
Nonketotic hyperglycinemia	Glycine cleavage enzyme	Convulsions, cerebral palsy, mental retardation, death*
Oxalosis	Glyoxylate carboligase	Renal calculi, renal failure
Hyperprolinemia	Proline oxidase, Δ'-pyrroline-5-carboxylic acid dehydrogenase	Nephropathy, deafness, mental retardation
Hydroxyprolinemia	Hydroxyproline oxidase	Small kidneys, hematuria, mental retardation
Pyroglutamicacidemia	Glutathione synthetase	Chronic acidosis, ataxia, mental retardation
Argininosuccinicaciduria	Argininosuccinase	Trichorrhexis nodosa, seizures, mental retardation
Citrullinemia	Argininosuccinate synthetase	Mental retardation, death*
Hyperammonemia	Carbamylphosphate synthetase, ornithine transcarbamylase	Episodic coma, mental retardation
Hyperlysinemia	Lysine α-ketoglutarate reductase	Convulsions, hypotonia, growth retardation
Cystathioninuria	Cystathionase	Mental retardation; may be normal
Homocystinuria	Cystathionine synthase	Ectopia lentis, thromboembolism, failure to thrive, mental retardation
Sacrosinemia	Hepatic sarcosine dehydrogenase	Mental retardation, vomiting, failure to thrive

Note: In each instance, it is recognized that there may be heterogeneity in which multiple forms of a defective enzyme may lead to different phenotypic manifestations. For instance, in the decarboxylation of the branched-chain keto acids, a complete deficiency leads to classic maple syrup urine disease; a different level of defect leads to a milder disease, known as branched-chain ketoaciduria. In this table, only one form has been listed.

*The disorders designated as causing death are those in which a rapid fulminating course often complicates early infancy.

Source: W. L. Nyhan, Disorders of Amino Acid Metabolism. In A. M. Rudolph (ed.), Pediatrics (16th ed.). New York: Appleton-Century-Crofts, 1977. P. 674.

children during the early critical period of brain development, the first 2 postnatal years [3]. Once mental retardation has occurred, the outlook for improvement is poor; dietary treatment may have some beneficial effect on behavioral disturbances and seizure activity only.

The first low phenylalanine diet for PKU was used in 1953 [4]. An adequate diet very low in phenylalanine causes a rapid disappearance of all abnormal biochemical features. Various preparations are available commercially as balanced, low-phenylalanine mixtures, such as Lofenalac by Mead Johnson Laboratories (see Table 45-3). The dietary regimen should be adapted to the needs of each child, based on specific biochemical tests and the progress of his or her physical and mental growth. The goals of diet therapy include the absence of phenylpyruvic acid in the urine, normal phenylalanine blood levels (between 1 and 2 mg/dl as compared to 15 to 63 mg/dl if untreated), and normal physical and mental growth. Overzealous restriction of dietary phenylalanine has been shown to cause anemia, growth retardation, malnutrition, cutaneous changes, hypoglycemia, and even death. For this reason, all therapy, particularly dietary, should be under the supervision of experienced health professionals. With variant PKU, the diet can be liberalized or even changed to a normal, nonrestricted diet usually by the time the child is 6 years old. By this time, high levels of phenylalanine are no longer injurious to the developed brain.

Maternal PKU can be particularly harmful to the developing fetus, causing intrauterine growth retardation, mental retardation, cardiac malformations, and microcephaly (retarded head growth) [5]. The outcome is related to the mother's blood levels of phenylalanine as well as other factors. For women in their childbearing years with PKU, strict control is important in preventing mental and physical retardation of their unborn children.

TYROSINE

Several defects of tyrosine metabolism have been reported. Although rare, their study has provided important information regarding normal pathways of tyrosine metabolism. In *tyrosinosis*, large quantities of tyrosine are excreted in the urine, due to the absence of either of the liver enzymes, *p*-hydroxyphenylpyruvate hydroxylase, or tyrosine transaminase. *Tyrosinemia* may be caused by delayed maturation of tyrosine-metabolizing enzymes in the premature infant; it may accompany scurvy or liver disease. In tyrosinemia, plasma levels of tyrosine are elevated. The defect is probably enzymatic, although the exact mechanism is not known. The symptoms of tyrosinemia include enlargement of liver and spleen, cirrhosis of the liver, abnormalities of tyrosine and methionine metabolism, defects in renal tubular reabsorption, rickets, elevated serum levels of protein and phosphate, and the excretion of amino acids in the urine. Most of these patients die from liver failure or tumors, usually in early childhood. Dietary restriction of tyrosine and its precursor, phenylalanine, may slow degenerative liver changes and improve renal function in some patients.

Alkaptonuria, the third inherited metabolic disorder of tyrosine metabolism, has been noted in the medical literature as early as the sixteenth century. This

TABLE 45-3. The composition of Lofenalac

Nutrients	Value per 100 gm Lofenalac powder
Proximate analysis	
Calories	450.00
Total nitrogen (equivalent to approximately 15 gm protein)	2.40
Fat (gm)	18.00
Carbohydrate (gm)	57.00
Minerals	
Calcium (gm)	0.65
Phosphorus (gm)	0.50
Iron (gm)	0.01
Sodium (gm)	0.30
Potassium (gm)	0.80
Chlorine (mg)	0.50
Magnesium (gm)	0.087
Copper (gm)	0.0003
Zinc (gm)	0.002
Phenylalanine (mg)	60–100
Vitamins	
A (U.S.P. units)	1080.00
D (U.S.P. units)	288.00
Ascorbic acid (mg)	36.00
Thiamin hydrochloride (mg)	0.33
Riboflavin (mg)	1.30
Niacinamide (mg)	2.88
Pyridoxine hydrochloride (mg)	0.36
Calcium pantothenate (mg)	2.30
Folic acid (mg)	0.036
Biotin (mg)	0.022
E (mg)	3.60
Choline chloride (mg)	108.00
B_{12} (mg)	3.23
Amino acids[a]	
L-Tyrosine (gm)	0.82[b]
L-Tryptophan (gm)	0.20[b]
L-Methionine (gm)	0.51
L-Arginine (gm)	0.34
L-Histidine (gm)	0.27
L-Lysine (gm)	1.58
L-Leucine (gm)	1.45
L-Isoleucine (gm)	0.78
L-Threonine (gm)	0.81
L-Valine (gm)	1.19

[a] Average values from analysis of nine batches by the Amino Acid Analyzer.
[b] Values from six batches assayed microbiologically.

disease also formed the basis of Garrod's theories concerning the inheritable metabolic disorders—that genetic factors specify chemical reactions and human biochemical individuality [6]. The absence of the enzyme, *homogentisate oxidase,* results in the excretion of homogentisic acid in the urine. The urine is oxidized to a brownish-black pigment when exposed to air. During infancy, alkaptonuria may be suspected by finding such stains on a wet diaper. Ferric chloride ($FeCl_3$) will cause the homogentisic acid–containing urine to turn a characteristic deep blue. Although this disease is present at birth, it is usually asymptomatic until the third decade, when a generalized pigmentation of connective tissue (*ochronosis*) by a black polymer of homogentisic acid occurs. Degeneration of the pigment-containing cartilage often leads to the development of severe osteoarthritis. At the present time, the treatment is nonspecific, although some restriction of dietary protein may reduce homogentisic acid formation.

HISTIDINE

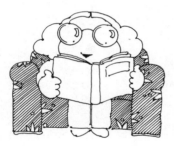

Histidinemia, first described in 1961, is an inherited disorder of histidine metabolism [7]. It occurs in $1:10,000–17,000$ births and is caused by inadequate or absent liver *histidase* activity. Under normal conditions, histidine is converted by histidase to urocanic acid, which is then further metabolized to formiminoglutamic acid and, ultimately, to glutamic acid. The lack of histidase activity causes elevated levels of unmetabolized histidine in the blood and urine, as well as increased urinary excretion of alternative histidine derivatives; these derivatives are imidazole pyruvic acid, imidazole acetic acid, and imidazole lactic acid. The urine gives a positive ferric chloride ($FeCl_3$) test, and because of this, histidinemia is sometimes misdiagnosed as phenylketonuria, which also gives a positive test. In addition, the ferric chloride test is not always conclusive, since this metabolic pathway is not fully developed in the newborn period. The definitive diagnosis of histidinemia is made by the direct assay of histidase in the skin [8].

The clinical manifestations of histidinemia include behavior disturbances, scholastic failure, speech impairment, and some degree of mental retardation. During childhood, there may be a propensity to infections, short stature, and seizures. Current therapy includes the dietary restrictions of histidine, an amino acid that is essential for infants and young children, but not for adults.

As a result of normal changes in renal function during pregnancy, elevated levels of histidine and other amino acids are found in the urine. This is a normal occurrence during pregnancy and is not due to any metabolic defect.

GLYCINE

At least four different congenital disorders of metabolism result in elevated levels of glycine in the body fluids. These include *propionic-acidemia*, *methylmalonic-aciduria* (both termed *ketotic hyperglycinemia syndrome*), *nonketotic glycinemia*, and *isovaleric-acidemia*. All four of these disorders present clinically as overwhelming illness in early infancy.

Propionic-acidemia is caused by a deficiency of *propionyl-CoA carboxylase,* which catalyzes the formation of methyl-malonyl CoA from propionyl CoA. It is characterized by high serum levels of propionate, and plasma glycine concentrations as great as 10 times normal. Such symptoms as acidosis, ketonuria, and vomiting occur as early as 18 hours after birth. Osteoporosis and mental retardation may develop later. The therapy includes correction of the acidosis and a diet restricted in isoleucine, valine, threonine, and methionine, since they are all metabolized through this same propionyl CoA to methylmalonyl CoA pathway.

Several different forms of methylmalonic-acidemia have been defined, with clinical manifestations similar to propionic acidemia. Ketoacidosis may occur very early in the newborn period, and may lead to coma and death if untreated. Seizures, mental retardation, chronic infections, and growth retardation are common later symptoms. High plasma and urinary levels of methylmalonic acid are found in this disorder, due to a defect in *methylmalonyl CoA mutase*, the enzyme that catalyzes the methylmalonyl CoA to succinyl CoA. *Vitamin B_{12} is a* coenzyme for this reaction. Some patients respond well to large doses of vitamin B_{12}, others do not. Patients in this second group may be treated successfully with diets restricted in threonine, leucine, isoleucine, valine, and methionine.

BRANCHED-CHAIN AMINO ACIDS

There are four known genetically produced defects in the metabolism of the branched-chain amino acids, leucine, valine, and isoleucine. Hypervalinemia, intermittent branched-chain ketonuria, and isovaleric acidemia have been reported in only one, three, and four cases, respectively. Because they are so rare, they will not be discussed here. The fourth known defect, *maple syrup urine disease*, has been reported in over 50 cases, and has an estimated incidence of about five to ten per 1 million births. This disease is due to the absence or reduced activity of *alpha keto acid decarboxylase*, which catalyzes the oxidative decarboxylation of all three branched-chain amino acids. As a result, leucine, isoleucine, and valine are present in high concentrations in the blood and urine; the keto acid analogues are also found in the urine.

These infants appear well at first, but characteristic symptoms appear by the end of the first postnatal week. In addition to the biochemical abnormalities, these infants become difficult to feed, have irregular respirations, become lethargic, and develop convulsions. The skin, urine, and hair have a characteristic odor, similar to maple syrup or caramel. If untreated, the disease progresses rapidly to death in 2 to 4 weeks. It is imperative that diagnosis be made quickly so that treatment may be initiated as soon as possible. The therapy includes removing all dietary sources of valine, leucine, and isoleucine from the diet until the plasma levels of these essential amino acids return to normal. These amino acids are then replaced in the diet in amounts only to meet, not to exceed, physiologic requirements. There is no evidence that the dietary restrictions for these amino acids could ever be eased. When therapy is initiated during the first postnatal week, the outlook is good.

SULFUR-CONTAINING
AMINO ACIDS

Three inborn errors of metabolism are known involving cystine and methionine, the sulfur-containing amino acids. *Cystinuria* (also termed *cystine-lysinuria*) is caused by a defect in the renal reabsorptive mechanisms of cystine, lysine, arginine, and ornithine. As a result, the excretion of these amino acids in the urine is greatly increased. There may also be a defect in the intestinal transport of these amino acids. The major complication of this disease is the precipitation of cystine crystals in the kidney tubules, forming cystine calculi. *Cystinosis* (also known as *cystine storage disease*) differs from cystinuria in that cystine crystals are deposited in tissues and organs throughout the body, as well as in the kidney tubules. Death may come at an early age due to acute renal failure. *Homocystinuria* is the second most common inherited disorder of amino acid metabolism, second to phenylketonuria. This disorder is due to a defect of *cystathionine* synthase, resulting in free homocystine and elevated levels of its precursor, methionine. The presence of homocystine in the blood causes increased adhesiveness of platelets. The major complications of homocystinuria are caused by occlusion of coronary, renal, or cerebral arteries or veins. Death may also result from this increased clotting tendency. Some patients with homocystinuria respond to large doses of pyridoxine (vitamin B_6) (100 to 500 mg/day) [9]. In those patients who do not respond, a diet restricted in methionine and supplemented with cystine may be beneficial.

AMINO ACID TRANSPORT

Hartnup disease, named for the first family described with this disorder, involves the abnormal transport of certain amino acids in the intestines and renal tubules. The urine has a characteristic pattern of amino acid excretion. The clinical manifestations of this disorder, which include the development of pellagra, photosensitivity, psychiatric abnormalities, and sometimes mental retardation, do not appear until age 6 or 8. The urinary excretion of tryptophan, histidine, phenylalanine, tyrosine, leucine, isoleucine, valine, alanine, glutamine, asparagine, threonine, and serine are 5 to 10 times normal. The symptoms of this genetic disorder are completely reversible with nicotinamide and a high-protein diet.

**Disorders of
Pyrimidine Metabolism**

Hyperuricemia, also known as gout, has been known since antiquity. This genetically transmitted disorder may be primary, due to the overproduction or diminished renal clearance of uric acid; or secondary, in association with catabolic states such as leukemia, or with chronic renal insufficiency. This disease is mostly seen in adult males, occurring in women only after menopause. *Lesch-Nyhan syndrome*, a type of hyperuricemia seen in children, has only been recognized since 1964. Both types exhibit symptoms of acute arthritis, blood in the urine (hematuria), and urinary obstruction. In addition, children with Lesch-Nyhan syndrome also show signs of mental retardation, cerebral palsy, and self-destructive biting behavior. Prenatal diagnosis of this disease is possible; it is an X-linked recessive trait. Diet therapy has been shown to have little value in these disorders. Colchicine is the drug used for acute gouty arthritis; Allopurinal is used for hyperuricemia.

Disorders of Carbohydrate Metabolism

Diabetes mellitus is a chronic disorder that initially involves abnormalities of carbohydrate metabolism, and later involves abnormalities of the vascular system. It is thought that this fairly common disorder, with an estimated incidence of 1:2500, may be due to a genetic abnormality, but other theories are still being considered. This disease is discussed at length in Chap. 39.

Several inborn errors of metabolism result in abnormal carbohydrate metabolism and the symptom of *mellituria*, the presence of sugar in the urine. This symptom may also appear under normal conditions, as seen in the newborn or premature infant and during pregnancy; or it may be temporary, accompanying impaired liver function, sepsis, or gastrointestinal diseases.

Galactosemia is caused by the genetic lack of the enzyme, galactose-1-phosphate uridyl transferase. Clinical symptoms appear soon after the initiation of milk feedings, since the principal dietary source of galactose is the disaccharide lactose in milk. Lactose is hydrolyzed in the intestines into its component monosaccharides, galactose and glucose. In addition to the inability to effectively utilize galactose for energy, other alternative derivatives result, including the reduction of free galactose to the sugar alcohol galactitol, which leads to the development of cataracts. This unfortunate complication may begin as early as a few days after birth. The initial symptoms of galactosemia include enlargement of the liver (hepatomegaly), jaundice, vomiting, diarrhea, and lethargy. Death may result from infection or liver failure. Retardation in physical and mental growth may result if the child survives. The diagnosis of galactosemia is made by measuring the level of the affected enzyme in the red blood cells. The treatment includes the elimination of galactose or lactose from the diet to avoid the accumulation of derivatives in the tissue. Milk substitutes such as soybean formulas, casein hydrolysates, and meat-based preparations may be used. Careful avoidance of all galactose-containing and lactose-containing foods is vital. At the present time, this restriction is for life. With treatment, the complications such as adverse effects on physical and mental development are absent to mild. The cataracts may improve, but some residual damage is common.

Pentosuria and *fructosuria* are two rare genetic disorders. In pentosuria, small amounts of arabinose, xylose, and ribose can be detected in the urine. In fructosuria, the sugar fructose is found in the urine. These rare diseases do not require treatment.

The *glycogen storage diseases* are a group of hereditary disorders that involve the aberrant synthesis and degradation of glycogen in the body. Thirteen different types have been described, indicating differences in clinical manifestations and tissue distribution of the defective enzyme (see Table 45-4). With the exception of type IX, all of these disorders appear to be autosomal recessive traits; type IX is sex-linked. Types O, I, III, IV, VI, IX, XI, and XII primarily affect the liver;

TABLE 45–4. Types of glycogen storage disease

Type	Enzymatic defect	Defect demonstrated in			
		Red blood cells	White blood cells	Liver	Muscle
O	UDPG—glycogen transferase			Yes	Yes
IG	Glucose-6-phosphatase	No	No	Yes	Yes
IIa	Lysosomal α-1,4 glucosidase	No	Inconstant	Yes	Yes
IIb	Lysosomal α-1,4 glucosidase	No	Inconstant	Yes	Yes
III	Amylo-1,6-glucosidase and/or oligo-1,4→1,4 glucantransferase	Yes	Yes	Yes	Yes
IV	Amylo-1,4→1,6-transglucosylase	Yes	Yes	Yes	Yes
V	Myophosphorylase	No	No	No	No
VI	Hepatic phosphorylase	No	Yes	Yes	No
VII	Phosphofructokinase	Yes	Yes	No	Yes
VIII	Phosphohexosisomerase				Yes
IX	Phosphorylase kinase	No		Yes	No
X	Phosphorylase kinase				Yes
XI	Phosphoglucomutase			Yes	
XII	Cyclic-AMP-dependent kinase			Yes	

Source: J. B. Sidbury, Glycogenoses. In A. M. Rudolph (ed.), *Pediatrics*. New York: Appleton-Century-Crofts, 1977. P. 729.

TABLE 45-5. Symptoms and treatments of glycogen storage disease

Type	Symptoms	Treatment
I (also known as von Gierke's disease)	Massive hepatomegaly Failure to thrive Severe hypoglycemia Hyperuricemia ↑ Plasma lipids	Surgical Continuous infusion of glucose
II	Massive cardiomegaly Hypotonia	Symptomatic
III	Massive hepatomegaly Hypoglycemia Muscle wasting and weakness	High-protein diet
IV	Progressive hepatic cirrhosis Hypotonia	Symptomatic
V (also known as McArdle's disease)	Painful cramps with strenuous exercise Myoglobinuria after strenuous exercise	Symptomatic
VI	Massive hepatomegaly Hypoglycemia Growth retardation	High-protein and high-carbohydrate diet
VII	Identical to type V	Symptomatic
VIII	Similar to type V	
IX	Similar to types I, III, and VI	High-protein diet
X	Similar to type V	

types II, V, VII, VIII, and X affect the muscles. Because failure to maintain a normal blood glucose is a common feature, the principal diet therapy is frequent, high-carbohydrate meals. A summary of symptoms and treatments is given in Table 45-5.

Disorders of Lipid and Lipoprotein Metabolism

The *familial hyperlipoproteinemias* are among the most common groups of inherited disorders. They comprise six genetically distinct diseases causing an elevation in the plasma cholesterol or triglyceride level. Chapter 4 presents these disorders in detail.

Another group of inherited diseases of lipid metabolism involves lowered levels of lipoproteins. *Abetalipoproteinemia* is caused by absent transport mechanisms of triglyceride from the intestine and liver, resulting in the lack of VLDL, LDL, and chylomicrons from the plasma. The clinical manifestations include fat malabsorption and retinitis pigmentosa (a degeneration of the retina of the eye, leading to eventual blindness). Treatment with vitamin E may prevent some of the consequences. *Familial hypobetalipoproteinemia* is transmitted as an autosomal dominant trait. This disease is characterized by lowered levels of LDL, VLDL, triglycerides, and fat-soluble vitamins. The clinical symptoms are similar to those of abetalipoproteinemia, but much milder. *Tangier disease*, another genetic disorder of lipid metabolism, involves the presence of abnormal plasma proteins and widespread lipid storage. This disease is characterized by enlarged orange tonsils, enlarged liver and spleen, and infiltration of the cornea of the eye. The treatment for abetalipoproteinemia and Tangier disease includes a low-fat diet, supplemented with linoleic acid, and vitamins A, E, and K. The treatment for familial hypobetalipoproteinemia is primarily symptomatic.

Another group of inherited disorders of lipid metabolism having the common clinical symptoms of retarded mental development, and enlarged liver and spleen are known as the *sphingolipidoses*. All of these may be diagnosed prenatally. The most common of these disorders is *Tay-Sachs disease*, with an incidence of 1 in 60 persons of Ashkenazi Jewish ancestry. It is caused by the absence of *N*-acetylgalactosaminidase in affected tissues. The hallmark of this disease is severe and progressive mental retardation, accompanied by an enlargement of the head. The mental deterioration usually begins at about age 6 months. By the end of the second year, patients become blind and die soon after. Therapy using enzyme replacement is still in experimental stages. *Gaucher's disease* is another disorder of this group, characterized by the excessive accumulation of the glycolipid, glucocerebroside, in various organs and tissues. Clinical symptoms include enlarged liver and spleen as well as osteoporotic erosion of the long bones, spine, and hip joints. This disease has been divided into three types, by infant, childhood, and adult variations. Replacement enzyme therapy using glucocerebrosidase has shown promising results. *Niemann-Pick disease* is characterized by abnormal accumulation of excessive quantities of sphingomyelin in various organs and tissues. The liver and spleen are enlarged and the pulmonary and central nervous system are also involved. The disease is caused by the absence of the enzyme, sphingomyelinase. No effective therapy has yet been devised. The last of these disorders is *Fabry's disease*, caused by the abnormal accumulation of the glycolipid, ceramidetrihexoside, in the tissues. Clinical symptoms include hard reddish-purple lesions around the umbilicus, severe and progressive renal failure, cardiac dysfunction, cataracts, and gastrointestinal disorders. Female carriers of this gene may have only mild symptoms or none at all. Replacement enzyme therapy is still experimental, but results are encouraging.

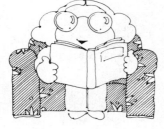

Cystic Fibrosis

This genetically transmitted disease is one of the most common long-term illnesses among infants and children, and most often malnutrition is a primary manifestation. Cystic fibrosis occurs in nearly 1 out of every 2000 live births and affects the mucus and sweat glands of the body. An abnormally thick mucus is secreted by the mucous glands, most frequently obstructing air passages in the lungs and the narrow ducts of the pancreas. Because of these obstructions severe respiratory infections are common, as is malabsorption due to the lack of pancreatic enzymes in the gastrointestinal tract. These children also produce sweat that is abnormally high in sodium chloride; this can lead to sodium depletion and collapse under strenuous conditions.

Between 80 and 90 percent of all cystic fibrosis patients suffer from pancreatic insufficiency, resulting in intestinal malabsorption and poor nutrient utilization. Although all three pancreatic enzymes (amylase, protease, and lipase) are usually missing or present in insufficient quantities, the decrease in lipase activity results in the worst clinical effects. The resulting steatorrhea causes malabsorption of fat-soluble vitamins, essential fatty acids, bile salts, and some minerals. The basic objectives in the diet therapy of cystic fibrosis are as follows:

1. To provide adequate protein for growth and development, and optimal resistance to infection
2. To provide adequate calories to spare dietary protein for tissue building and repair
3. To minimize electrolyte loss by controlling steatorrhea and vomiting, with restriction of dietary fats
4. To maintain electrolyte balance with replacement therapy as needed

Since most cystic fibrosis patients are young, the need for ample dietary protein for normal tissue repair and growth cannot be overemphasized. Adequate calories must be provided by dietary fats and carbohydrates to spare dietary protein for growth. Chronic infection and malabsorption of as much as 50 percent of dietary intake, compounded by an acute febrile period, can put the cystic fibrosis patient into a catabolic state of negative nitrogen balance. Between acute episodes, the level of dietary protein should be about 6 to 8 gm/kg body weight/day. Acute episodes require a higher allowance. The high-protein foods of choice in fulfilling the diet prescription are those that provide maximum protein, vitamins, and minerals, while keeping dietary fats to a moderate to minimal level. Broiled, stewed, or roasted meats, fish, and fowl are best. Skim milk is recommended, although whole milk may be used as tolerated. Such foods as hot dogs, luncheon meats, sausages, bacon, and oil-packed tuna may cause gastrointestinal upsets because of their high content of fat and spice; these foods should be avoided if possible. Eggs may be used freely in baking, cooking, and in main dishes. Cholesterol levels in these patients may be low, and eggs contribute not only protein, minerals, and vitamins to the diet, but also this essential nutrient. Adequate dietary protein is also needed for optimal action of supplemental pancreatic enzymes. If there is insufficient dietary protein to combine with free hydrochloric acid, trypsin is destroyed by peptic digestion.

Malabsorption of dietary fats is one of the hallmarks of cystic fibrosis, with resultant steatorrhea, osteoporosis, and lowered serum levels of fat-soluble vitamins. Vitamin K levels may be low secondary to fat malabsorption, decreased bile availability, and decreased synthesis by normal bacterial flora that are destroyed by antibiotic therapy. The level of dietary fat tolerated must be individualized for each patient. Restriction to about 50 percent of normal often results in improved symptoms. MCT oil has been used successfully with these patients.

Probana, a special infant formula, is used with infants diagnosed with cystic fibrosis.

Because as much as 50 percent of all calories may be malabsorbed, the caloric allowance for these patients should be increased by at least 50 to 75 percent. The liberal use of monosaccharides (glucose, fructose, sucrose) helps to meet this increased need; monosaccharides are found in fruits, honey, and corn syrup.

Excessive loss of electrolytes is also characteristic of this disease. Sodium-rich and potassium-rich foods should be used liberally in the diet.

As a genetic disease, the clinical signs of cystic fibrosis are present at birth, and resemble those of celiac disease. With a continuous program of antibiotics, pancreatic enzymes, physical therapy, and nutritional support, many more of these children are now able to reach adulthood and lead nearly normal lives.

Conclusions

The inherited diseases demonstrate how powerful the genetic influence is on health and well-being. Since nutrition and biochemistry are both relatively new sciences, so is the study of the inborn errors of metabolism. As more is learned about metabolic pathways, genetics, and enzyme replacement therapy, treatment for these diseases will improve. Now and in the future, diet therapy plays an important role in the therapeutic regimen of these disorders, offering hope and a better quality of life to the patients and their families.

References

1. Følling, A.   Uber Ausscheidung von Phenylbrenztraubensaure in den Harn als Stoffwechselanomalie in Verbindung mit Imbezillitat. *Z. Physiol. Chem.* 227:169, 1934.
2. Guthrie, R., and Susi, A.   A simple phenylalanine method for detecting phenylketonuria in large populations of newborn infants. *Pediatrics* 32:338, 1963.
3. Gütler, F., and Wamberg, E.   On indications for treatment of the hyperphenylalaninemic neonate. *Acta Paediatr. Scand.* 66:339, 1977.
4. Bickel, H., Gerrard, J., and Hickmanns, E. M.   Influence of phenylalanine intake on phenylketonuria. *Lancet* 2:812, 1953.
5. Lenke, R. R., and Levy, H. L.   Maternal phenylketonuria and hyperphenylalaninemia: An international survey of the outcome of untreated and treated pregnancies. *N. Engl. J. Med.* 303:1202, 1980.
6. Garrod, A. E.   The incidence of alkaptonuria: A study in chemical individuality. *Lancet* 2:1616, 1902.
7. Ghadimi, H., et al.   An inborn error of histidine metabolism mimicking phenylketonuria. Abstract from the meeting of the European Society for Pediatric Research, Atlantic City, N.J., 1961.
8. Ito, F., Aoki, K., and Eto, Y.   Histidinemia: Biochemical parameters for diagnosis. *Am. J. Dis. Child.* 135:227, 1981.
9. Rudolph, A. M. (ed.).   *Pediatrics* (16th ed.). New York: Appleton-Century-Crofts, 1977, p. 684.

Suggested Readings

Acosta, P. B., and Elsas, L. J.   *Dietary Management of Inherited Metabolic Disease.* Atlanta: ACELMU Publishers, 1976. P. 83.

Acosta, P. B., et al. Nutrition in pregnancy of women with hyperphenylalaninemia. *J. Am. Diet. Assoc.* 80:443, 1982.

Berry, H. K. The diagnosis of phenylketonuria. *Am. J. Dis. Child.* 135:211, 1981.

Catching up on an inborn error. *FDA Consumer* 14:19, 1980.

Chase, H. P., Long, M. A., and Lavin, M. H. Cystic fibrosis and malnutrition. *J. Pediatr.* 95:337, 1979.

Fällström, S.-P., Lindblad, B., and Steen, J. On the renal tubular damage in hereditary tyrosinemia and on the formation of succinylacetoacetate and succinylacetone. *Acta Paediatr. Scand.* 70:315, 1981.

Francis, D. E. M. *Diets for Sick Children* (3rd ed.). Oxford, England: Blackwell, 1976. P. 434.

Ghadimi, H. K. Histidinemia: Biochemistry and behavior. *Am. J. Dis. Child.* 135:210, 1981.

Goodman, S. I., et al. The treatment of maple syrup urine disease. *J. Pediatr.* 75:485, 1969.

Hansen, R. G. Hereditary galactosemia. *J.A.M.A.* 208:2077, 1969.

Heffernan, J. F., and Trahms, C. M. A model preschool for patients with phenylketonuria. *J. Am. Diet. Assoc.* 79:306, 1981.

Hubbard, V. S., and Mangrum, P. J. Energy intake and nutrition counseling in cystic fibrosis. *J. Am. Diet. Assoc.* 80:127, 1982.

Kline, J. J., et al. Arginine deficiency syndrome. *Am. J. Dis. Child.* 135:437, 1981.

Larter, N. Cystic fibrosis. *Am. J. Nurs.* 81:525, 1981.

Lloyd, J. K. Dietary problems associated with the care of chronically sick children. *J. Hum. Nutr.* 33:135, 1979.

Moynahan, E. J. Acrodermatitis enteropathica: A lethal inherited human zinc-deficiency disorder. *Lancet* 2:399, 1974.

Nyhan, W. L. (ed.). *Heritable Disorders of Amino Acid Metabolism: Patterns of Clinical Expression and Genetic Variation.* New York: Wiley, 1974.

Queen, P. M., Fernhoff, P. M., and Acosta, P. B. Protein and essential amino acid requirements in a child with propionic acidemia. *J. Am. Diet. Assoc.* 79:562, 1981.

Reyzer, N. Diagnosis: PKU. *Am. J. Nurs.* 79:1895, 1978.

Schvett, V. (ed.). *Low Protein Cookery for Phenylketonuria.* Madison, Wis.: University of Wisconsin Press, 1977.

Scriver, C. R., and Clow, C. L. Phenylketonuria: Epitome of human biochemical genetics. *N. Engl. J. Med.* 303:1336, 1980.

Solomons, N. W., et al. Some biochemical indices of nutrition in treated cystic fibrosis patients. *Am. J. Clin. Nutr.* 34:462, 1981.

Sorscher, E. J., and Breslow, J. L. Cystic fibrosis: A disorder of calcium-stimulated secretion and transepithelial sodium transport? *Lancet* 1:368, 1982.

Stanbury, J. B., Wyngaarden, J. B., and Fredrickson, D. S. (eds.). *The Metabolic Basis of Inherited Disease* (4th ed.). New York: McGraw-Hill, 1978.

von Wendt, L., et al. Prenatal brain damage in nonketotic hyperglycinemia. *Am. J. Dis. Child.* 135:1072, 1981.

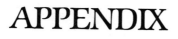

APPENDIX

ANSWERS TO CASE STUDIES

Chapter 35

1. a. BEE = 655 + (9.6 × W) + (1.8 × H) − (4.7 × A) (for women)
   = 655 + (9.6 × 50) + (1.8 × 157.5) − (4.7 × 24)
   = 1305.7 calories/day before surgery
   b. Increased by 20 percent after surgery = (.20)(1305.7) = 261.1
   1305.7 + 261.1 = 1566.8 calories/day after surgery

2. a. Essential fatty acid deficiency.
   b. Children have greater demands for normal growth and development in addition to the requirements imposed by the disease process.

3. a. BEE = 66 + (13.7 × W) + (5 × H) − (6.8 × A) (for men)
   = 66 + (13.7 × 90.9) + (5 × 183) − (6.8 × 30)
   = 2022.3 calories/day before the accident
   b. Increased by 100 percent after the accident = 4044.6 calories/day
   c. Protein requirements = 2 gm/kg/day
   = (2)(90.9) = 181.8 gm/day
   d. 182 gm protein × 4 calories/gm = 728 calories from protein
   4045 calories − 728 calories = 3317 calories remaining
   1658 calories from carbohydrate, at 4 calories/gm, = 414.5 gm of carbohydrate
   1658 calories from fat, at 9 calories/gm, = 184.2 gm of fat.

4. a. Initial BEE = 900 calories/day
   Increased 30 percent = (.30)(900) = 270; 270 + 900 = 1170 calories/day
   b. Fever of 6° above normal; 7 to 8 percent increase in BEE/degree = (6)(7) = 42 percent to (6)(8) = 48 percent increase
   Total BEE = (1170)(.42) = 491.4 + 1170 = 1661.4 to (1170)(.48) = 561.6 + 1170 = 1731.6 calories/day

Chapter 36

1. Both arms = 9% × 2 = 18%. Ideal caloric intake = (25 × 59) + (40 × .18) = 1482.2
   3.2 gm/kg/day × 59 = 188.8 gm of protein/day
2. Dairy products would be excellent choices since they provide both protein of high biologic value and ample calcium, which is usually low in the elderly and is lost from the skeleton during bed rest. Ice cream and creamed soups would be good for additional calories so protein can be spared for tissue repair.
3. Low serum potassium may be one consequence and is manifested by muscle weakness, irritability, paralysis, and rapid heartbeat (tachycardia). The loss of fluids and proteins can also result in dehydration and lethargy.

Chapter 38

1. a. High-fat foods—deep-fried chicken, potato salad, and ice cream.
   b. She should follow a low-fat, low-calorie, high-protein, and high-carbohydrate diet.
   c. The blockage of bile passage into the duodenum may have caused some fat malabsorption, and, therefore, lower levels of vitamin K and an increased tendency toward prolonged bleeding times.

2. Parietal cells in the stomach are the site of the production of intrinsic factor, the glycoprotein that binds vitamin B_{12} and is required for its absorption by the ileum. When intrinsic factor is not produced, vitamin B_{12} is not absorbed. As a result, the bone marrow cannot produce mature red blood cells and releases the large immature precursors (macrocytes) into the bloodstream instead.

3. a. Rice cereal.
   b. Cornstarch puddings, homemade ice cream, fresh fruits.
   c. Cakes, biscuits, and breads made with wheat, rye, oats, or barley flour or any foods containing those grains.

Chapter 39

1. Betsey, in addition to telling her troop leader about her diabetes, should always carry some hard candy to help prevent insulin shock. The increased exercise of a hiking trip may cause insulin requirements to decrease, making her normal dose too high and causing hypoglycemia. Betsey's mother should bring fruit compote. It is the least concentrated carbohydrate food of the three choices.

2. a. What were the events prior to the onset of symptoms?
   b. Has he been taking his insulin? Following his diet?
   c. Has he been sick (fever, vomiting, infection)?
   Laboratory tests: blood glucose level, urinalysis.

3.
	EXCHANGES
3 large green peppers	3 vegetable
½ lb ground beef	8 meat
1 cup tomato juice	2 vegetable
1 slice stale bread	1 bread
1 tsp salt	—
¼ tsp pepper	—
½ cup chopped onion	1 vegetable

Chapter 41

1. a. Megaloblastic anemia.
   b. Those individuals experiencing rapid growth and, therefore, an expanding red cell mass.
   c. Nanette, because of her age, and her pregnant mother.

2. a. Both iron-deficiency and megaloblastic anemias.
   b. Her diet is deficient in iron, folic acid, and vitamin B_{12}; it also contains a binding agent (tea). Her symptoms would include fatigue, pallor, lethargy, glossitis, and paresthesia.

3. a. Iron-deficiency anemia.
   b. Yes, I would change his diet by adding iron-fortified formula until age 12 months and introducing iron-enriched cereal.

4. a. Plasma vitamin B_{12}, plasma folate, and a Schilling test.
   b. Pernicious anemia cannot be treated by diet because it is due to a defect in absorption; therapy is by intramuscular injections of cyanocobalamin.

Chapter 42

1. a. The laboratory tests that should be ordered include serum phosphate; hemoglobin, hematocrit, and complete blood count; blood urea nitrogen (BUN). Both the phosphate and urea nitrogen may be elevated; the hemoglobin and hematocrit are probably decreased. The elevated phosphate level would explain the joint pain (uremic osteodystrophy). The weakness is most likely due to anemia (decreased erythrocyte production and decreased red blood cell life span) and the elevated urea nitrogen levels.

b. Amphojel binds phosphates in the gastrointestinal tract and counteracts the development of uremic osteodystrophy. It may be used in special recipes, such as medicated cookies, to make it more acceptable.

2. Pound cake, chocolate layer cake, peanut brittle, and lemon meringue pie are too high in protein or electrolytes. Better choices (high in carbohydrates, low in protein and sodium) would be mint candy, marshmallows, or sugar wafers.

3. The second, and final, hydroxylation of the inactive form of vitamin D, which should occur in the kidney, does not take place with renal disease. As a result, a type of vitamin D deficiency develops, including decreased absorption of calcium from the intestines, impaired calcium and phosphorus balance in the blood, and altered bone formation. The elevated levels of phosphate and decreased serum calcium causes secondary hyperparathyroidism and resultant uremic osteodystrophy.

GLOSSARY

acetoacetic acid   A ketone acid normally produced in small amounts as a product of fat metabolism; produced in excessive amounts when carbohydrate oxidation is inadequate.

acetone, or dimethylketone   Formed by the decarboxylation of acetoacetic acid; normally present in minute quantities, but accumulates when fatty acid degradation is excessive or incomplete.

acetyl CoA   Formed from the oxidation decarboxylation of pyruvic acid, it is an important part of the Krebs cycle (TCA cycle), is a precursor in the biosynthesis of fatty acids and sterols, and it gives rise to acetoacetic acid. Also called *active acetate.*

achlorhydria   The absence of hydrochloric acid in the stomach.

acid   A substance that donates protons (H ions); a strong acid dissociates completely into H^+ and its other components; a weak acid does so only slightly.

acidosis   A pathophysiologic condition characterized by a fall in the pH of body fluids or a decrease in the body's alkali reserve. May be caused by several states that produce excesses in various acids, including diabetes mellitus (ketone bodies), renal insufficiency (phosphoric, sulfuric, and hydrochloric acids), respiratory disease (carbonic acid), and prolonged strenuous exercise (lactic acid).

acquired obesity   Fatness due to familial eating habits.

acrolein, or acrylic aldehyde   Formed in the decomposition of glycerol; a liquid of characteristic pungent odor.

actin (Latin *actus,* motion)   One of the protein constituents of the muscle fibril; together with myosin, responsible for the contractile muscle mechanism.

actinomysin   The muscle mechanism of contraction and relaxation, composed of actin and myosin.

active site   That part of an enzyme to which the substrate or cofactor is linked in normal enzymatic activity.

active transport   The movement of substances against a concentration gradient, a process requiring energy.

adenosine phosphates   Sources of high-energy phosphate for cellular activity and muscular movement. *ADP* (adenosine diphosphate) is composed of two molecules of phosphate and one molecule each of adenine and D-ribose. *ATP* (adenosine triphosphate) is composed of three phosphate molecules and one molecule each of adenine and D-ribose.

adipocytes   The major cell structures found in fatty connective tissue.

adipose tissue   A type of connective tissue that serves as a depot for fat storage, an insulator against heat loss, and a padding for support and protection of internal organs.

adolescence (Latin *adolescere,* to grow up)   The period from puberty to maturity.

adult bovine   Beef greater than 12 months of age; classified by maturity classes A to E.

aerobic metabolism (Greek *aeros,* air)   Metabolism requiring oxygen, particularly oxidation of fatty acids.

agar   A polysaccharide obtained from seaweed; undigestible by humans; used in foods and as a culture medium.

aging   The holding of meat for 48 hours after slaughter to increase its tenderness.

air cell   A pocket of air formed between the shell and the shell membranes of an egg as it cools and its contents contract.

aleurone   The outer row of thick-walled cells of the endosperm that is removed with bran during the milling process; contains oil and nongluten protein.

alginates   Another polysaccharide obtained from seaweed; used as a thickener and stabilizer in food products.

alpha helix   The spatial configuration of the polypeptide chains of proteins, held together by hydrogen bonds between carboxyl and amino groups of different amino acids; resembling a hollow cylinder with radiating side groups.

amenorrhea   The absence of menstruation; termed *secondary* when due to exogenous factors (i.e., weight reduction, athletic training).

amino sugars   A sugar in which a hydroxyl group has been replaced with an amino group ($-NH_2$); e.g., glucosamine, galactosamine.

aminopeptidase   An enzyme found in the intestinal mucosa that catalyzes the hydrolysis of polypeptides with a free amino group, producing a free amino acid and a smaller peptide.

amphipatic   The characteristic of a compound containing hydrophobic and hydrophilic chemical groups, making it miscible in both water and hydrocarbon (lipid solvents).

amylase   The enzyme that catalyzes the hydrolysis of starch to sugar.

amylopectin   The branched-chain glucose component of starch, consisting of alpha-1,6 branched linkages and alpha-1,4 linked glucose units.

amyloplasts   A storage granule containing food in the form of starch, found in the cytoplasm of a plant cell.

amylose   The straight chain glucose component of starch, consisting of alpha-1,4 linked glucose units.

anabolism   The conversion of nutritive material into complex living matter; constructive metabolism.

anadromous   Fish that are born in fresh water, swim to the sea for their adult life, and return to their birthplace to spawn.

anaerobic metabolism   Metabolism in the absence of oxygen, particularly the oxidation of carbohydrates.

angular stomatitis   Inflammation of soft tissues (oral mucosa) of the mouth, particularly the corners of the lips; often seen with riboflavin deficiency and with anemias.

anions   Electrolytes that carry negative charges and can accept electrons.

anorexia Loss of the desire to eat.

anorexia nervosa (Greek *orexis*, appetite) Lack of appetite and aversion to food resulting in self-induced starvation; usually caused by an unresolved emotional conflict.

anthocyanin A group of color pigments (glycosides) that give rise to red, pink, purple, and blue in plants and flowers.

anthoxanthins A group of three structurally related color pigments— flavones, flavonols, and flavonones. Their color ranges from pale yellow to almost colorless, and is found in fruits and vegetables.

antibodies Immunoglobulins that react with and destroy specific antigens.

antioxidant A substance that delays or prevents the process of oxidation; some commonly used antioxidants include vitamin C (ascorbic acid), vitamin E (tocopherol), lecithin, butylated hydroxyanisole (BHA), and butylated hydroxytoluene (BHT).

apoferritin (Greek *apo*, derived from, related to) A protein in the intestinal mucosa capable of binding and storing iron as ferritin.

appetite (Latin *appetere*, to desire, seek) The desire to eat.

appetite center The lateral hypothalamus of the brain, which controls the desire to eat.

arachidonic acid An essential fatty acid, consisting of 20 carbon atoms and four double bonds; a constituent of lecithin, cephalin, and the lipids of the brain, liver, and other organs; a precursor of the prostaglandins.

Argentaffin cells Specialized cells present in the stomach and intestines. They produce 5-hydroxytryptamine, which stimulates the motility of the gastrointestinal tract.

astacin Red pigment found in lobster and salmon.

ATP (adenosine triphosphate) An intermediate compound in the production of energy for muscular work.

autocatalytic The acceleration of a chemical reaction by one or more products of the same reaction.

avidin A protein found in raw egg white that binds the vitamin biotin making it biologically unavailable; denatured by heat and other agents.

axial ratio The proportion of length to width in the three-dimensional shape of a protein molecule.

baby beef Beef that is 8 to 12 months of age.

beriberi The disease resulting from a deficiency of thiamin and characterized by a combination of neurologic, cardiac, and cerebral manifestations.

berries A classification of fruits in which the seeds are contained in the mass, and the layers of the pericarp are succulent and pulpy.

beta-hydroxybutyric acid Formed by the reduction of acetoacetic acid in fat metabolism; excessive production results during inadequate carbohydrate oxidation.

bile A substance secreted by the liver and utilized in the duodenum in the emulsification, digestion, and absorption of dietary fats.

biliary achalasia Failure of the sphincter of Oddi to release.

biliary dyskinesia Spasm of the sphincter of Oddi.

bilirubin The main pigment of bile, normally present in stool, and formed by the reduction of biliverdin.

biliverdin A bile pigment formed from hemoglobin or reduced in the liver to bilirubin.

biologic value (BV) The relative nutritional value of an individual protein compared to a standard protein, usually hen's egg, with a BV of 100.

blastoderm The germination portion of the fertilized egg.

blastodisk The germination portion of the unfertilized egg.

bran The outer layer of the grain, containing mostly cellulose, and some protein and minerals.

bromeline A proteolytic enzyme found in fresh, raw pineapple, used as a meat tenderizer.

brown-fat Metabolically active adipose tissue capable of uncoupling oxidation and phosphorylation in order to warm itself; found in hibernating animals.

brush border Special surface in the small intestine, composed of microvilli for absorption of metabolites that result from the digestive process.

bulbs A group of vegetables in which the food reserve is stored in specialized stems (e.g., garlic and onions).

bulgur Wheat that has been cooked, dried, and the bran partially removed; the kernels are then cut fine, medium, or coarse or left whole.

butterfat The lipid content of milk and milk products.

buttermilk The milk remaining after churning butter.

calf Beef that is 3 to 8 months of age.

candling The process of viewing an egg before a light source in a darkened room to evaluate yolk centering and movement; clarity, firmness, and defects of the white; integrity of the shell and its normality; and the depth and regularity of the air cell.

carbohydrases The enzymes that hydrolyze complex carbohydrates and polysaccharides into simple sugars.

carboxypeptidase An exopeptidase, synthesized by the pancreas, which catalyzes the hydrolysis of polypeptides with a terminal carboxyl group, to form smaller peptide units and amino acids with a free carboxyl group.

cardiac beriberi A deficiency of thiamin with predominantly cardiac decompensation.

cardiac sphincter A circular ring of muscle located at the base of the esophagus at the entrance to the stomach.

caries (Latin *caries*, decay) The destruction of teeth; molecular death of dental tissue.

carotenoids Several pigments with slightly different chemical structures, all precursors of vitamin A. Their intense red color is due to the conjugated (alternating) double bonds.

casein (Latin *caseus*, cheese) The principal protein of milk, precipitated as calcium caseinate by the enzyme, rennin, leaving the residual clear fluid, whey.

catabolism The breaking down of complex compounds by the body with the release of energy; destructive metabolism.

cations Electrolytes that carry positive charges and can donate electrons.

cellulose The polysaccharide-supporting structure of plant tissues; it yields glucose on complete hydrolysis; on partial hydrolysis, it yields *cellobiose*.

cementum Bony tissue covering the root of a tooth.

cereal grain Grasses that are grown for their edible seeds.

chalazae (Greek for hailstone, hard lump) Spiral cords formed from the shell membranes attaching at the shell, serving to both cushion and suspend the yolk and embryo of the egg, while still allowing them to revolve.

chief cells A specialized type of cell present in the gastric mucosa of the ileum where pepsinogen, the inactive precursor of pepsin, is formed and secreted.

chlorophyll The color pigment found in green plants, responsible for photosynthesis.

chloroplasts The plant cell structure that contains chlorophyll and the enzymes for photosynthesis.

cholecalciferol Vitamin D_3, the main form of vitamin D found in animals; it develops in skin when exposed to ultraviolet light.

cholecystokinin The hormone that causes contractions of the gallbladder and the release of concentrated bile into the duodenum.

cholesterol An unsaturated monohydric alcohol of the class of sterols; the chief sterol in the body found in all tissues; a constituent of animal fat, bile, gallstones, nervous tissue; important in metabolism and can be activated to form vitamin D.

chromoplasts Specialized structures containing the red, yellow, and orange color pigments.

churning The process of aggregating the fat globules of milk to form butter.

chylomicrons The largest of the blood lipids, composed of triacylglycerol and smaller amounts of cholesterol, phospholipid, and protein; synthesized in the intestine and which serve to transport triacylglycerol to sites of utilization; omegalipoproteins.

chyme The liquefied acid food mass.

chymotrypsin An intestinal proteolytic enzyme formed from chymotrypsinogen by the action of trypsin. This endopeptidase preferentially hydrolyzes peptide linkages of the aromatic amino acids tyrosine, phenylalanine, and tryptophan.

cirrhosis (Greek *kirrhos*, orange-colored) Accumulation of fat in the liver, destroying the normal hepatic architecture and function.

cis From the Latin, meaning "on this side"; a prefix used to designate geometric isomers with a double bond between carbon atoms, indicating that a given atom or radical is located on the same side of the carbon axis.

clabbered milk The curdling of milk into curds and whey by heat, acid, or the enzyme, rennin.

coagulation   The change from a liquid to a more solid state, as accompanying denaturation in heating egg proteins. In proteins, denaturation followed by precipitation out of solution; the irreversible process of changing from a liquid to a solid.

coenzyme   A nonprotein organic molecule, which may be a vitamin, whose presence is necessary for the activity of many enzymes; a prosthetic group of an enzyme.

cofactor   An overall term for the nonprotein fraction of an enzyme, a prosthetic group, firmly attached to the protein portion of the enzyme, coenzyme, easily dissociated.

collagen   The insoluble protein of connective tissue, skin, bones, cartilage, and tendons; resistant to digestive enzymes, but hydrolyzed to gelatin by boiling.

collenchyma   A type of ground cell with thick, fibrous walls important in the support of growing plants and photosynthesis.

complete protein   A protein food containing all essential amino acids.

compound lipid   A lipid compound plus a nonlipid substance.

conalbumin   An egg white protein characterized by its ability to bind divalent and trivalent metallic ions, such as iron; inhibits the growth of microorganisms.

condensation   A chemical reaction involving a combination between two molecules or parts of the same molecule.

cones   The light receptors in the retina of the eye for vision in bright light, and for color.

conformation   The relative development of the muscular and skeletal systems, used as a factor in grading muscle meats.

congenital lactose intolerance   Absence of the enzyme lactase at birth, resulting in permanent lactose intolerance.

conjugated protein   A protein combined with a nonprotein substance.

converted rice   Processing rough rice prior to milling by parboiling; permeation of nutrients in the bran into the endosperm.

cover fat   The exterior layer of fat that helps muscle or lean tissue retain moisture and protects it from the action of microorganisms. Also known as the *separable fat*.

cretinism   A condition caused by a deficiency of thyroid hormone before birth, and characterized by small stature, a large protruding tongue, dry skin, hoarse cry, poor muscle tone, and mental retardation.

crude fiber   The residue remaining after a food sample has been treated in the laboratory with a solvent, hot acid, and hot alkali.

cutin   A hydrophobic fatty acid polymer found on the dermal surface of some plants, which helps limit moisture loss.

dark-cutting beef   Beef from an animal that has been stressed to deplete muscle glycogen immediately before slaughter; less lactic acid is formed, and a higher final pH results. Meat of this type is dark in color and sticky in texture.

deaminate The removal of an alpha amino group from an amino acid; occurs chiefly in the liver.

decarboxylate The removal of a carboxyl group from a molecule, usually amino acids.

dehydration The condition resulting from excessive body fluid loss.

denaturation An alteration in the structure of a protein, resulting in a change in chemical, physical, and biologic properties; may be brought about by heating, freezing, irradiation, pressure, or treatment with organic solvents.

dental plaque Transparent film on the surface of tooth enamel composed of bacteria and polysaccharides.

dentin The calcified tissue forming the major portion of the tooth; it is covered by enamel above the gums and by cementum below the gums.

dermis The outer layer of cells on plants that provides mechanical protection; it may be epidermis, or the softer, mature peridermis.

developmental obesity Fatness due to the cumulative result of positive energy balance. Also termed *simple obesity*.

dextrins Formed during digestion or dry heat (e.g., toasting), this polymer of glucose is intermediate in structure between starch and maltose.

dietary fiber The sum of all components of food (mostly polysaccharides and lignin) that are not digested by the gastrointestinal tract.

diffusion The movement of substances to equalize concentrations on both sides of a membrane; a process not requiring energy.

digestion The process by which foods are broken down, both mechanically and chemically, into smaller molecules for absorption via the gastrointestinal tract.

dimorphic Existing as two distinct structural forms, such as anemia caused by iron and folate deficiency, causing macrocytic, hypochromic anemia.

dipeptidase An exopeptidase that hydrolyzes dipeptides into free amino acids.

disaccharides A sugar formed by the glycosidic linkage of two monosaccharides, with the elimination of a molecule of water.

disulfide bonds The bond formed as the result of the union of two parallel peptide chains by a sulfur-sulfur linking of two cysteine groups.

drupes From the Greek *dryppa*, meaning alive, it is a type of fruit with a single seed surrounded by a fleshy pericarp (e.g., plums and peaches).

dry beriberi A deficiency of thiamin, with predominantly neuromuscular symptoms.

durum semolina Middlings of durum wheat, ground to a certain size.

durum wheat A unique type of wheat with a high-protein content and extreme hardness.

dynamic equilibrium The continuous synthesis and degradation of body constituents even at constant composition.

dyshemopoiesis (Greek *dys*, impaired) Abnormal formation of red blood cells.

elastin   The protein base of yellow elastic tissue found in lung matrix, blood vessel walls, and ligaments; insoluble in water, but hydrolyzed by the enzyme elastase.

elderly gravida   A pregnant woman 35 years of age or older; at special risk for developing complications because of her age.

electrolyte   Any substance that dissociates into its component ions when dissolved in a fluid.

emulsification   The process of breaking up particles of an immiscible liquid into smaller ones, so that they remain suspended in another liquid. Emulsifying agents, such as bile salts and lecithin, break up lipids, facilitating its digestion.

emulsion (Latin *emulgere*, to milk out)   One liquid suspended within another liquid; achieved by lowering the surface tension or breaking up the particles of an immiscible liquid into smaller ones so they remain suspended in solution.

enamel   The calcified substance that covers the crown of the tooth.

endomysium (Greek *endon*, inside + *mys*, muscle)   The connective tissue surrounding the fibers of a muscle bundle, or fasciculus.

endopeptidase   A class of proteolytic enzymes that preferentially split peptide bonds in the middle of a protein; pepsin, trypsin, chymotrypsin.

endosperm   The inner portion of the grain kernel, composed of starch granules embedded in a matrix of protein.

enrichment   The addition of vitamins and minerals to a cereal product to the level present prior to milling.

enterokinase   An intestinal enzyme that converts the zymogen, trypsinogen, to the active enzyme trypsin.

enzymes   Proteins, produced by a lining organism, capable of catalyzing certain chemical reactions that occur in the cell.

epimysium (Greek *epi*, on, upon)   The sheath of connective tissue surrounding a muscle.

ergocalciferol   Vitamin D_2, the chief vitamin D precursor found in plants.

erythroblast (Greek *erythros*, red)   An early, nucleated precursor of the erythrocyte.

erythrocyte   The mature, oxygen-carrying cell of vertebrate blood that contains hemoglobin, which is responsible for blood's red color.

erythropoiesis   The process by which mature erythrocytes are formed.

erythropoietin   A hormone produced by the kidney and possibly other sites in the body that stimulates the production of erythrocytes by the bone marrow.

essential amino acids   An amino acid that cannot be synthesized by the body, or not at a sufficient rate commensurate with normal growth.

essential fatty acids   Polyunsaturated fatty acids necessary for growth, reproduction, healthy skin, and proper utilization of fats; linoleic acid cannot be synthesized by the body, and serves as precursor of arachidonic and linolenic acids; all three are considered essential fatty acids.

ethylene gas   Used to artificially ripen fruits and vegetables harvested early.

evaporated milk   Milk with 60 percent of its original water content removed.

exopeptidase   A class of proteolytic enzymes that preferentially hydrolyzes peptide bonds to free an amino group or a carboxyl group at the end of a protein; aminopeptidase, carboxypeptidase.

external signals   Factors such as social customs, conscious or unconscious emotional drives, habits, and environment that override the physiologic mechanisms of appetite and hunger.

farina   A cereal made from wheat middlings.

fasciculus   A bundle of fibers separated by connective tissue.

fatty acids   Acids derived from the saturated series of open-chain hydrocarbons; classified by the number of carbon atoms and the number of double bonds between them.

favism   A disease occurring in persons with glucose 6-phosphate dehydrogenase deficiency of erythrocytes when fava beans are eaten; manifests as an acute hemolytic anemia.

fecundability   The monthly probability of conception.

fecundity   The ability to reproduce.

fermentation   The oxidation of carbohydrate under anaerobic or partially anaerobic conditions; also termed glycolysis.

ferritin   A protein-iron complex found in tissues; a storage form of iron similar to hemosiderin; a water-soluble iron-protein complex.

fertility   The capacity to conceive or induce conception.

fibrils   Linear bundles of cellulose molecules, forming a crystalline arrangement.

fibrous proteins   Insoluble animal proteins very resistant to digestion by proteolytic enzymes; e.g., silk, wool, skin, hair, nails, hooves, quills, connective tissue, and bone.

finfish   Fish with bony skeletons.

finish   The appearance of fat and its distribution within meat; one of the factors evaluated in determining meat quality and grade.

fluoridation   The addition of fluoride to water (1–2 ppm) to reduce the incidence of dental caries.

fluorosis   The mottling of dental enamel as the result of excessive intake of fluorine, usually greater than 2.5 ppm or 2.5 mg per day.

fortification   The addition of vitamins and minerals to a cereal product to a level greater than that present prior to milling.

fructosan   A polysaccharide yielding only fructose on hydrolysis (e.g., inulin).

fructose   The hexose monosaccharide found in fruits and honey, and obtained on hydrolysis of sucrose to glucose and fructose.

galactose   The hexose monosaccharide linked with glucose in the disaccharide, lactose (milk sugar); seldom found free in nature.

gallstones   The crystal precipitates of excess amounts of cholesterol.

gastric lipase   Another enzyme produced by the chief cells of the stomach, which hydrolyzes triacylglycerols to short-chain and medium-chain fatty acids.

gastrin A hormone, produced by the gastric glands in the stomach, which induces secretion of gastric juices.

gelatin The product of the hydrolysis of collagen from cartilage, bone, tendon, and skin; considered an incomplete protein and of poor biologic value because it lacks tryptophan and is low in cystine and tyrosine.

gelatinization The changes that occur when starch is heated in water.

gelation The solidification of a *sol,* a colloidal system with water or liquid as the dispersing medium.

geriatrics (Greek *geras,* old age; *iatrikos,* of physician) Pertaining to the process of aging; the branch of medical science concerned with aging and its diseases.

germ layer Contains the embryo of the grain kernel; this layer is the richest in fat, and is high in protein, sugar, and minerals.

gerontology (Greek *gerontos,* old man) The study of the phenomena and problems of aging.

gestation (Latin *gestare,* to carry or bear) Pregnancy.

gingivitis Inflammation of the gums, making them more prone to bacterial infection.

gliadin A component of the protein gluten, found in wheat, oats, rye, and barley; lacking in lysine.

globular proteins Complex proteins characterized by the presence of peptide chains that are folded or coiled into compact three-dimensional structures; enzymes, oxygen-carrying proteins, and protein hormones.

glossitis An inflammation of the tongue; may be due to a deficiency of one or more of the B-complex vitamins.

gluconeogenesis The formation of glucose from noncarbohydrate sources such as glucogenic amino acids and glycerol.

glucose The hexose monosaccharide naturally occurring in plant tissues, the major sugar in the blood, and the preferred energy source.

gluten The protein component of some cereal grains that gives flour an elastic quality; composed of gliadin and glutenin.

glutenin A component of gluten, with more disulfide bonding than gliadin.

glycogen A branched-chain polysaccharide composed of glucose units; the chief form of carbohydrate storage in animals, particularly in the liver and muscles.

glycogenesis The formation of glycogen.

glycogenolysis The breakdown of glycogen.

glycolysis The anaerobic breakdown of glucose or glycogen.

glycosuria The presence of sugar in the urine.

goblet cells Specialized cells that produce acid glycoproteins to protect and lubricate the lining of the intestines.

goiter Enlargement of the thyroid gland.

goitrogens   Foods that interfere with the use of thyroxine, including peanuts, rutabagas, cabbage, cauliflower, and brussels sprouts.

grana   The specialized pigment containing granules found in chloroplasts and chromoplasts.

green shrimp   Fresh shrimp.

grits   A cereal product made by grinding corn to a coarse consistency.

groats   Oat grain with the hull removed.

hard wheat   A type of wheat, high in protein, with greater resistance of the endosperm to grinding (due to increased hydrogen bonding).

hardening   The process of saturating the unsaturated bonds of a lipid, making it more solid, crystalline; hydrogenation.

HDL (high-density lipoprotein)   Also termed an alphalipoprotein; composed of cholesterol, phospholipid, and triacylglycerol; transports phospholipids in the plasma bound to protein.

heat stroke   A syndrome caused by excessive heat exposure and dehydration and characterized by high fever, lack of perspiration, convulsions, and eventually death.

hematocrit (Greek *haimatos*, pertaining to blood + *krit*, from *krinein*, to separate)   The volume percentage of erythrocytes in blood.

hematopoiesis   The formation of blood; hemopoiesis.

heme iron   The iron found in hemoglobin; present exclusively in animal tissues.

hemochromatosis (Greek, *haima*, pertaining to blood)   A chronic disease of impaired iron balance, characterized by excessive deposits of iron in the body, resulting in enlarged and scarred liver, graying pigmentation of the skin, diabetes mellitus, and eventual heart failure.

hemoglobin   The oxygen-carrying pigment of erythrocytes.

hemolysis   The excessive destruction of erythrocytes.

hemorrhage   The acute loss of blood; bleeding.

hemosiderin   A protein-iron complex found mainly in the liver, spleen, and bone marrow; a storage form of iron; unlike ferritin, hemosiderin is insoluble and granular.

hepatocrinin   The hormone that stimulates the secretion of bile from the liver.

hexose   A six-carbon sugar, with the empirical formula, $C_6H_{12}O_6$.

hominy   A type of grits made from white corn.

homogenation   The dispersion and uniform suspension of two or more immiscible substances, such as water and lipid in milk; emulsification of the lipid in milk.

hunger   The physiologic longing for food.

hydrogen bonding   The link formed due to the attraction of hydrogen to oxygen within a polypeptide chain of protein; responsible for the secondary structure of proteins.

hydrogenation   The process by which molecular hydrogen is added to the double bonds of unsaturated fatty acids; hardening.

hydrolysis   The breaking of bonds with the addition of water.

hydrophilic   The characteristic ability to hold or attract water.

hyperkalemia   An elevated serum potassium level.

hypertension   Elevated blood pressure.

hyperthermia   An increase in body temperature above normal.

hypochromic   A lack of color, as occurs when there is an incomplete complement of hemoglobin in the erythrocytes.

hypochromic anemia   A type of anemia caused by a deficiency of iron and characterized by pale erythrocytes due to a reduced hemoglobin content.

hypogeusia   Impaired sense of taste.

hypokalemia   A decreased serum potassium level.

hyposmia   Impaired sense of smell.

hypothalamus   The region of the brain controlling appetite and satiety.

hypoxia   Lack of oxygen.

infancy   The first year of life after birth.

intercellular spaces   The spaces between plant cells that allow the exchange of gas between the internal and external environments.

internal signals   The physiologic response of appetite and satiety to blood levels of nutrients.

intrinsic factor   A substance normally present in gastric fluid that facilitates the absorption of vitamin B_{12} in foods.

iodine number   The number of grams of iodine taken up by 100 gm of fat; a reflection of the degree of saturation of the fatty acids of a particular lipid.

iodopsin   The photosensitive pigment in cones (also know as *visual violet*).

ionic bonds   The link between positively and negatively charged residues that come into juxtaposition.

isoelectric point   The pH of a solution at which a dipolar ion, such as an amino acid, carries both negative and positive charges, and bears a net charge of zero.

juvenile gravida   A pregnant woman 18 years of age or younger; at nutritional risk because her own growth is not yet finished.

keratins   The insoluble protein of hair, hooves, nails, and feathers; resistant to digestive enzymes; contains a large amount of sulfur.

keratomalacia   Changes in the eye resulting from vitamin A deficiency, including clouding, thinning, and eventual perforation of the cornea.

ketone bodies   Acetoacetic acid, betahydroxybutyric acid, and acetone.

ketosis   A condition characterized by the accumulation of ketone bodies in the blood and urine leading to acidosis; caused by a disturbance in carbohydrate metabolism and incomplete fatty acid oxidation.

koilonychia (Greek *koilos*, hollow or concave)   A deformity of the nails characterized as spoon-shaped; associated with iron-deficiency anemia.

lactalbumin   One of the milk proteins, resembling serum albumin; easier to digest than casein and accounting for one-half of the total protein in human milk; it has advantages in infant feeding.

lactase The enzyme normally present in the brush border of the small intestine, responsible for hydrolyzing lactose into glucose and galactose.

lactation amenorrhea The absence of menstruation caused by the hormones involved with breast-feeding.

lactoglobulin One of the milk proteins, found only in milk, and containing a high proportion of the amino acid, cysteine; this protein is usually the offending agent in incidences of cow's milk allergy.

lactose The disaccharide that occurs naturally only in the milk of mammals; glucose and galactose.

lamb An animal of the ovine species less than 14 months of age.

lathyrism A disease caused by the consumption of large quantities of certain types of sweet peas (vetches), characterized by spastic paralysis of the legs, tremors, paresthesias, bone deformities, and ruptured blood vessels.

LDL (low-density lipoprotein) The lipoprotein complex that transports cholesterol in the plasma. Also termed a betalipoprotein.

leaching The extracting, or washing, of soluble materials from a substance.

lecithin, or phosphatidylcholine A phospholipid, containing glycerol, fatty acids, phosphoric acid, and choline; widely distributed, especially in nerve cells.

leucoplast A specialized body within a plant cell whose function is to produce and store food.

libido Sexual desire.

lignin A noncarbohydrate substance, resistant to chemical breakdown; found in wood and certain vegetables.

limiting amino acid The amino acid present in the least amount, limiting protein synthesis.

linoleic acid An essential fatty acid of 18 carbon atoms and two double bonds; occurs in the glycerides of linseed oil, as well as soybean, cottonseed, safflower, and fish oils.

linolenic acid An essential fatty acid that can be synthesized from linoleic acid; composed of 18 carbon atoms and three double bonds, and found mainly in the glycerides of linseed oil.

lipases Fat-splitting enzymes that catalyze the hydrolysis of fats into fatty acids and glycerol; found in pancreatic juice, blood plasma, stomach, and certain plants.

lipemia An increased level of lipid in the blood.

lipid A member of the group of organic compounds insoluble in water and soluble in fat solvents; of nutritional importance are the essential fatty acids, triacylglycerols, lecithin, carotene; and the steroids, including cholesterol, bile acids, adrenocortical hormones, and sex hormones.

lipoproteins A group of compounds of conjugated proteins consisting of a lipid and a protein; most important are the alphalipoproteins (HDL), betalipoproteins (LDL), and omegalipoproteins (chylomicrons).

lumen The channel within a tubular organ, such as in an artery or intestine.

lyse To unbind, loosen, disintegrate; dissolution.

lysozyme An enzyme present in egg white with the ability to hydrolyze certain bacterial cell walls.

macrocytic Abnormally large, immature erythrocytes; when present in large quantities in the peripheral blood, they are characteristic of folic acid or vitamin B_{12} deficiency.

maillard reaction Nonenzymatic browning; the reaction between proteins and amino acids forming brown pigments; occurs on heating or prolonged storage.

maltose The disaccharide composed of two molecules of glucose, formed as an intermediate product of starch hydrolysis; not found free in nature.

mannose The hexose monosaccharide found in some legumes; does not occur free in nature.

marbling The pattern of distribution of fat throughout the muscle.

masa harina Corn that has been soaked in an alkaline solution, rinsed, drained, dried, and ground into meal.

maternal impressions The belief that the unborn child will be marked by the unfulfilled maternal desire for a particular food.

MCT (medium-chain triglyceride) Consists of a carbon chain of 8 to 10 atoms in length; may be absorbed in the absence of bile salts directly into the circulation; used in diet therapy of fat malabsorption and steatorrhea.

menarche The age at which menstruation begins.

menopause The age at which menstruation ceases.

metabolic alkalosis or acidosis An imbalance of acid-base in the body resulting from alterations in the renal regulation of acid and base.

metmyoglobin The oxidized form of myoglobin, occurring when cut meat is exposed to air.

micelle A unit of structure composed of an oriented arrangement of molecules; a submicroscopic structural unit of protoplasm.

middlings Chunks of endosperm free of bran and germ; they become flour when pulverized.

milk-alkali syndrome A possible complication of prolonged, excessive intake of milk and soluble alkali; elevated serum calcium, alkalosis, and renal insufficiency.

milk lamb A lamb less than 3 months of age.

milk tetany A condition seen in infants given undiluted cow's milk, resulting in excessive blood levels of phosphate, causing tetany.

milliequivalents The atomic weight of a substance divided by its valence.

monosaccharides Simple sugars; a single sugar unit that cannot be hydrolyzed further; classified by the number of carbon atoms in its structure.

monounsaturation (monoethenoid) Having one double bond within the structure of a fatty acid.

morbidly obese An individual 100 pounds or more overweight for his or her height and sex.

mutton Lamb over 2 years of age.

myoglobin A form of hemoglobin occurring in the muscle fibers, which holds oxygen in the muscles.

myosin Part of the contractile muscle mechanism, acting in concert with actin, as actinomyosin; after death, its coagulation leads to rigor mortis.

myristic acid A saturated fatty acid of 14 carbons, found in butter, coconut oil, and nutmeg.

NAD Nicotinamide adenine dinucleotide.

NADP Nicotinamide adenine dinucleotide phosphate.

native protein A protein in its original state that has not been altered in composition or properties.

nephron The functional unit of the kidney.

net protein utilization (NPU) The proportion of nitrogen intake retained in the body.

neutral fats Triacylglycerol, diacylglycerol, and monacylglycerol.

nitrogen balance The measurement of the nitrogen equilibrium in the body.

nonessential amino acids An amino acid that can be synthesized in the body with an adequate source of nitrogen.

nonheme iron The iron found in vegetables, grains, and all nonanimal products.

nonshivering thermogenesis The process by which brown fat (or like tissue) generates its own heat by dissipating energy into its own tissues; seen in hibernating animals and newborn infants.

normochromic Normal content of hemoglobin in the blood.

obese (Latin, *obesus*, from *ob*, over-, and *esum*, to eat) An individual 50 percent or more overweight for height and sex.

oil Simple lipids that are liquid at room temperature.

oleic acid A monounsaturated fatty acid of 18 carbons found widely in nature in both animal and plant fats and oils.

organic acids (volatile and nonvolatile) Include citric, malic, oxalic, succinic, and give the plant its unique flavor.

osmosis (Greek *osmos*, to thrust or push) The movement of a solvent through a membrane from a dilute to a more concentrated solution.

osmotic pressure The pressure that is created when two solutions of different concentrations of the same substance are separated by a membrane permeable to the solvent only.

osteomalacia A condition, also known as "adult rickets," resulting from a decrease in the amount of available calcium, causing faulty ossification.

osteoporosis Deossification of bone with resultant enlargement of marrow, decreased thickness of cortex, and structural weakness.

oven spring The rapid rise in volume during the first 10 to 12 minutes of baking.

overweight An individual 20 percent or more above ideal weight for height and sex.

oxidation The chemical reaction involving the removal of hydrogen, the addition of oxygen; the loss of electrons or an increase in valence.

oxymyoglobin The form of myoglobin found in living tissue in equilibrium with myoglobin; the oxygenated form of myoglobin.

palmitic acid A saturated fatty acid of 16 carbons found in both plant and animal fats.

palmitoleic acid A monounsaturated fatty acid of 16 carbons found predominantly in animal fats.

pancreatic amylase (also known as amylopsin) An enzyme produced by the pancreas, which hydrolyzes starch to dextrins and maltose.

papain A proteolytic enzyme found in fresh, raw papaya; used in tenderizing meats.

parenchyma A type of ground cell, with the specialized functions of photosynthesis, storage, and wound healing.

parietal cells The sole source of hydrochloric acid in the stomach.

passive transport Diffusion through a membrane without the use of energy, from a higher to a lower concentration.

pasteurization The heat treatment of milk to destroy all pathogenic organisms and most of the nonpathogenic organisms.

pectic substances Include pectic acid, pectin, and protopectin. They are acid derivatives of the sugar galactose, and are used as an emulsifying and thickening agent.

pellagra Deficiency disease caused by lack of niacin and characterized by dermatitis, diarrhea, and dementia.

pentosans (hemicellulose) A complex carbohydrate composed of five-carbon monosaccharides (pentoses); not digested by humans.

pentose A five-carbon monosaccharide; components of nucleic acids following hydrolysis of wood and straw; and as an intermediate metabolite in glucose metabolism.

pepsin The proteolytic enzyme formed from pepsinogen by hydrochloric acid in the stomach.

peptide bond A bond joining two amino acids coupled by the carboxyl group of one to the amino group of another, with the loss of water; the bonds in polypeptide chains of protein.

peptization The liquefaction of a gel to a sol; the breaking up of large molecules, with a resultant thinning out of the gel structure.

Peyer's patches Lymph nodes present beneath the intestinal mucosa of the ileum, which help protect against bacterial invasion.

pharyngeal lipase An enzyme found in the mouth that hydrolyzes triglycerides into free fatty acids and monoglycerides and diglycerides.

phloem A portion of the fibrovascular tissue system involved in the transport of food within plant structures.

phosphorylation The formation of an energy-rich phosphate bond; energy obtained from oxidation of protein, fats, or carbohydrates is trapped in these bonds, to be released as needed.

photophobia   Sensitivity to bright light, an early symptom of vitamin A deficiency.

phytates   A derivative of inositol found in certain plants and cereal husks; it forms insoluble compounds with certain minerals, particularly calcium, phosphorus, iron, and magnesium.

pica   The craving for nonfood substances or foods in excessive quantities, usually associated with pregnancy.

plasma   The fluid component of the blood.

plastids   Organized bodies within the cytoplasm involved in the production and storage of food, photosynthesis, and color.

polysaccharide   Carbohydrates containing 10 or more monosaccharide units; those of nutritional importance include starch, glycogen, and cellulose.

polyunsaturation (polyethenoid)   The state of having two or more double bonds within the structure of a fatty acid.

pomes   A type of fruit with an enlarged, fleshy pericarp surrounding the seeds (e.g., apples and pears).

porphyrin   A derivative of the substance porphin, containing four pyrrolelike units linked by C-H groups or methane bridges; porphyrins are found in hemoglobin (with iron in the center of the ring) and chlorophyll (with magnesium in the center of the ring).

presbycusis (Greek *presby*, old man; *akousis*, hearing)   The decrease in hearing acuity that occurs with advancing age.

presbyopia (Greek *presby* + *ops*, eye)   Decreased power of accommodation due to impaired elasticity of the crystalline lens of the eye.

primary low lactase activity   A decline in the amount and activity of lactose after early childhood, when the major skeletal growth spurt is completed.

primary structure   The specific sequence of amino acids linked by peptide bonds.

proteases   A class of enzymes that splits proteins.

proteolytic   The rupture of peptide bonds with the addition of water and fragmentation of the protein molecule.

protoporphyrin   One of the components of hemoglobin, requiring an atom of iron in the center of its structure.

P/S ratio   The proportion of polyunsaturated to saturated fatty acids in a fat or fat-containing food.

ptyalin   A starch-splitting enzyme in saliva that hydrolyzes starch into dextrins and maltose. Also known as *salivary amylase*.

quaternary structure   The spatial relationship among the separate chains, each with its own primary, secondary, and tertiary structures.

quick-cooking rice   Rice that has been cooked to gelatinize the starch, then dried; the porous structure of the processed rice allows rapid rehydration.

quick oats   Flakes made from particles of the whole grain.

rancidity   The chemical change in fats or oils resulting in a disagreeable taste, color, or odor; may be caused by hydrolysis or oxidation.

reactive (emotional) obesity   Overeating in response to tension, life situations, or an underlying emotional illness.

regular oats   Flaked whole groats.

rennin   The enzyme present in gastric juice responsible for the clotting of milk; *rennet* is an enzyme preparation of pepsin and rennin obtained from the stomach of a calf or lamb; it is used in the preparation of cheese.

reproductive biologic age   A woman's chronologic age minus her age of menarche.

residue   The distinctive side chain of amino acids.

respiratory alkalosis or acidosis   An imbalance of acid-base in the body resulting from alterations in the normal pulmonary excretion of carbon dioxide.

reticulocyte   The last developmental stage of the immature erythrocyte.

rhodopsin   The photosensitive pigment in rods (also known as *visual purple*).

rickets   Faulty calcification of bones due to inadequate vitamin D and/or poor absorption of calcium and phosphorus; characterized by stunted growth, bowing of the legs, enlargement of the wrists and ankles, and a hollow chest.

rigor mortis (Latin, stiffness of death)   The stiffening of muscle, especially skeletal, after death.

ripening   The process by which fruits and vegetables are brought to the peak of maturity.

rods   The light receptors in the retina of the eye for vision in dim light.

satiety center   The ventromedial hypothalamus of the brain, which controls the desire to stop eating.

saturation   The absence of any double bonds.

sclerenchyma   A type of ground cell that contains lignified walls.

scurvy   The disease resulting from a deficiency of vitamin C, and characterized by a weakening of collagenous structures and hemorrhaging.

secondary structure   The unique folding of the polypeptide chain, intrinsically related to its biologic activity.

semipermeable membrane   A membrane between two fluid compartments that is permeable to water, but not to some of the dissolved solutes.

senescence (Latin, *senescere*, to grow old)   The state of being elderly.

senile (Latin, *senilis*, aged)   Pertaining to, or characteristic of old age.

shellfish   Mollusks and crustaceans.

simple protein   Proteins composed entirely of amino acids or derivatives of amino acids.

skim milk   Whole milk with most of the fat removed.

soap   The salt of one or more fatty acids with an alkali or metal; may be insoluble or soluble.

soft wheat   A type of wheat, with lower protein content than hard wheat.

sorting   The separating of eggs by sizes and grades.

spores   Vegetative cells.

spring wheat   Wheat that is planted in the spring and harvested in the late summer; usually of the hard type.

standards of identity   All foods termed a particular name (e.g., catsup, mayonnaise, white bread) must contain mandatory ingredients, which do not have to appear on the label.

starch   The storage form of carbohydrates in plants; the polysaccharide composed of glucose units of amylose and amylopectin.

stearic acid   A long-chain saturated fatty acid of 18 carbons found in animal fats as the triacylglycerol, *stearin*.

steatorrhea   The presence of fat in the stool, caused by biliary insufficiency, pancreatic insufficiency, or by a failure of the active absorptive processes in the intestinal mucosa.

striae (Latin, furrow)   Stretch marks or streaks caused by the stretching and rupture of the elastic fibers in the skin.

succus entericus   The alkaline, enzyme-rich juice produced by the glands of Brunner and Lieberkuhn of the intestinal mucosa.

sucrose   The disaccharide of glucose and fructose; table sugar or granulated sugar.

tannins   An astringent compound, found in some plants, capable of precipitating collagen and producing dark-colored compounds with ferric (iron) salt.

tertiary structure   A protein's spatial conformation in three dimensions.

tetany (Greek *tetanos*, stretched)   Intermittent muscle cramps with pain caused by a reduction in the blood calcium level and resultant increased neuromuscular activity.

texture   The moisture content of plant tissue.

tomalley   The lobster's liver; the green sac that becomes apparent on cooking.

toxin   A poisonous substance produced by animal or plant cells; if bound to the cell, termed *endotoxin*; if readily separable, termed *exotoxin*.

trans   From the Latin, meaning "on the other side"; a prefix used to designate geometric isomers when a given atom or radical is on the opposite side of the carbon axis.

transamination   The transfer of an amino group from one compound to another, catalyzed by the enzyme, transaminase; the process by which the body is able to use urea and synthesize the nonessential amino acids.

transferrin (Latin *trans*, through, across + *ferrum*, iron)   A glycoprotein that transports iron in the blood to the spleen and liver for storage, to the bone marrow for hemoglobin synthesis, or to other tissues for their use; also called siderophilin or siderophyllin.

triacylglycerol (triglyceride)   A lipid in which the glycerol molecule has attached three fatty acids.

trypsin   The endopeptidase, formed from the actions of enterokinase on trypsinogen and secreted by the pancreas into the small intestine, which catalyzes the hydrolysis of peptide linkages containing the carboxyl group of lysine and arginine.

turgor   The pressure of fluid-filled vacuoles against the cell wall (crispness).

underweight   An individual 10 percent or more below his or her ideal weight for height and sex.

unsaturation   The presence of one or more double bonds.

veal   Beef less than 3 months of age.

vitamin   Organic substances present in foods in minute quantities that perform specific functions for normal metabolism; a dietary essential coenzyme necessary for the functioning of an enzyme system.

VLDL (very-low-density lipoprotein)   Also termed a *prebetalipoprotein;* transports triacylglycerols in the blood plasma.

waxes   Simple lipids; esters of fatty acids with certain alcohols; usually hard and brittle and become pliable upon warming.

Wernicke's syndrome   Thiamin deficiency frequently seen in alcoholics resulting in confusion; incoordination of muscle action, particularly in walking; paralysis of the oculomotor nerve; and other degenerative changes in the central nervous system.

wet beriberi   A deficiency of thiamin with predominantly neuromuscular symptoms and edema.

whey   The fluid remaining after the curd is removed from coagulated milk; contains no fat, little protein, but most of the original lactose present in the milk before processing.

whole milk   Fluid milk containing 3.5% butterfat.

winter wheat   Wheat that is planted in the fall and harvested in the early summer; may be of the hard or soft variety.

xerophthalmia (Greek *xeros*, dry + *ophthalmos*, eye)   A thickening and drying of the conjunctiva, often caused by vitamin A deficiency.

xylem   A portion of the fibrovascular tissue system involved in the transport of water within plant structures.

yearling   Lamb 1 to 2 years of age.

yogurt   A curdled, fermented milk product made by inoculation with *Streptococcus thermophilus, Bacterium bulgarius,* and *Plocamo bacterium yoghouri.*

zymogen   A proenzyme, or an inactive form or precursor of an enzyme, which on reaction with an appropriate agent, liberates the enzyme in active form.

INDEX

INDEX